# Resuscitation Greats

Edited by

## Peter J.F Baskett

BA MB BCh (Cantab)
MB BCh BAO (The Queen's University of Belfast)
FRCA FRCP FCEM.
Consultant Anaesthetist Emeritus, Frenchay Hospital and The Royal Infirmary, Bristol.

## Thomas F. Baskett

MB BCh BAO (The Queen's University of Belfast)
FRCS(C) FRCS(Ed) FRCOG FACOG DHMSA
Professor, Department of Obstetrics and Gynaecology,
Dalhousie University, Halifax,
Nova Scotia, Canada.

*Published by*: Clinical Press Ltd. Redland Green Farm, Redland, Bristol, BS6 7HF, UK.

*British Library Cataloguing in Publication Data*

A catalogue record for this book is available from the British Library

ISBN-13:     978-1-85457-049-9
EAN:   9781854570499

These articles were originally published in the journal *Resuscitation* and are reproduced with the kind permission of *Elsevier* and the authors

'Death may usurp on nature many hours,
And yet the fire of life kindle again
The o'pressed spirits.'

William Shakespeare
Pericles Act 3, scene 2 1609


'The suspension will more frequently last forever,
unless the power of life is restored to action
by some application of art.'

John Hunter
Philosophical Transactions 1776;66:413


'It is clear that when patients are in this condition, trembling upon the very
brink of destruction, there is but little time for you to think what ought to be
done, these are the moments in which it becomes your duty not to reflect, but to
act. Think now, therefore, before the moment of difficulty arrives. Be ready
with all the rules of practice, which those very dangerous cases require.'

James Blundell
The Principles and Practice of Obstetricy London: E.Cox. 1834 p336


'Hearts too good to die'

Claude Beck
JAMA 1947;135:985-6

# PREFACE

*"There is nothing new under the sun" (Anon)*

It has been said that the Irish never forget history, and the English never learn from it. In the case of resuscitation most of us are guilty of dismissing history and therefore not learning from it. It is salutory to find that electricity was considered beneficial in cardiorespiratory arrest by Charles Kite and Herholdt and Rafn in the 18th century but defibrillation and cardiac pacing were not introduced into clinical practice until 200 years later. In the same era Benjamin Pugh perfomed tracheal intubation for neonatal resuscitation and Dr Monro in Scotland used blind oral intubation with a curved silver cannula for resuscitating the apparently drowned. It was over a century later that tracheal intubation came into regular clinical practice, thanks in no small way to Sir Ivan Magill who anaesthetised patients undergoing facial plastic reconstructive surgery as an aftermath of injury in the trenches in the 1914-1918 war. Jean Henri Dunant drew up the humanitarian principles governing the Red Cross and treatment of the injured and the captured, but 150 years later there is still abuse of these worthy principles. As Douglas Chamberlain reminds us in his 2003 Fitzwilliam Lecture to the Royal College of Physicians, we were 'never quite there'.

In 1997 one of us (PJFB) took over the role of Editor-in-Chief of the journal *Resuscitation* which had become the Official Journal of the European Resuscitation Council under the Editorship of his predecessor, Douglas Chamberlain. PJFB decided to establish a series of articles featuring the 'Resuscitation Greats'. The aim was to tell the story of those who had made significant contributions to the art and science of resuscitation over the centuries since early biblical times. If possible, the story would feature the subjects' personality and quirks as well as their contribution to resuscitation. Articles were solicited by the Editor and some were submitted voluntarily. The qualification to be a featured subject was to be dead, nearly dead or well into retirement- although one or two have bent the rules!. Thus, the majority of those featured, perforce, have had no say in the matter!
The first article was published in 2000 and there has been one published almost every month since then. Brother Tom (TFB), an obstetrician and gynaecologist and medical historian has written more articles in the series than any one else. Together we decided to produce this book which is a compilation of all the articles in historical order, published between 2000 and 2007. Clearly there will be those we have missed, but it is intended that the series should continue in the journal and perhaps, in the fullness of time, a second edition may be published. Since the original publication in the journal Henning Ruben, Vladimir Negovsky, Peter Safar and Frank Pantridge have died.

The editors are grateful to Anne Lloyd, Publishing Editor of *Resuscitation* for arranging transfer of copyright from Elsevier to Clinical Press, the publishers of this book, to Paul and Lois Goddard of Clinical Press, to Jo Frankland at Elsevier, to all of the authors who gave their permission freely for republication of their article(s) in this book, to Yvette Baskett who did a lot of typing for two stubborn editors, and to Cathy Kelly who has been secretary to, and manager of, TFB for some years.

Peter J F Baskett                                    Thomas F Baskett
Stanton St Quintin, Wiltshire, UK          Halifax, Nova Scotia, Canada
 2007                                                      2007


**The editors are most grateful for the generous educational grants from Laerdal Medical and ZOLL Medical Corporation which have enabled publication of this book**

# FOREWORD

There are relatively few books or articles devoted to the history of cardiopulmonary resuscitation (CPR) and related fields of medicine, making this book a refreshing and welcome addition to the subject. The historical vignettes or chapters have been written by experts and through their eyes, we get unique insight into the lives and works of the historical figures that have shaped the field of resuscitation over the last several hundred years. The editors have collated the vignettes from articles published in the journal *Resuscitation* and have arranged them carefully in date order, thus clarifying the sequence of events that led to modern-day resuscitation. Anatomists, physiologists, anaesthetists, surgeons, physicians, engineers and industrialists - the Resuscitation Greats cover the full spectrum of the medical world plus the occasional emperor, emphasizing the multidisciplinary nature of CPR. This blend of known and unknown pioneers has shaped resuscitation or reanimation as we know it today. Between them, they have contributed to every facet of CPR: airway; ventilation; chest compressions; defibrillation; post resuscitation care; education; and the organisation of emergency medical services.

It is often said that those who work in resuscitation today stand on the shoulders of those who have come before us. This book emphasises the breadth of those shoulders - the people and the events that enable modern day educators and researchers of resuscitation to build on the work that has come before them.

The editors are to be congratulated for assembling these articles in a book that will both serve as a valuable reference and a source of enlightenment. From medieval to modern times, this is an amazing collection of discoveries, methods, heroes, and even the occasional individual considered at the time to be a villain, whose stories must be heard.

William H. Montgomery, MD   Honolulu, Hawaii, United States
Jerry Nolan, MD   Bath, United Kingdom
Petter A. Steen, MD   Oslo, Norway

# About the Editors:

The Baskett brothers were born in Belfast, and grew up in the small village of Hillsborough, County Down, Northern Ireland.

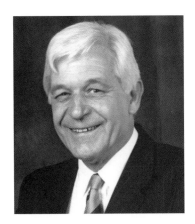

**Peter John Firth Baskett** was educated at Belfast Royal Academy and Campbell College, Belfast. He was awarded his rugby colours at Campbell, but little else. He studied the basics sciences of medicine at Queens College, Cambridge, got his rugby colours there and took up rowing on a part-time basis and managed to win an oar in the low grade echelons of rowing. This oar is 4 metres long and has dictated the dimensions of the staircase of his house ever since. He completed his clinical studies at The Queen's University of Belfast. After a period of training in physiology, emergency medicine, general practice and anaesthesia in Belfast and Bristol, he was appointed Consultant Anaesthetist at Frenchay Hospital and The Royal Infirmary, Bristol and Clinical Lecturer in the University of Bristol. He now holds the post of Consultant Emeritus.

He was President of the Association of Anaesthetists of Great Britain and Ireland and Founder Chairman of the European Resuscitation Council and has been Honorary Secretary, Chairman and President of a number of organisations in anaesthesia, emergency and disaster medicine, military medicine and resuscitation and has travelled widely. After his retirement from the National Health Service, he introduced the ALS course from the European Resuscitation Council into 22 countries.

He has now retired from clinical practice and is really a 'has been'. He spends his time being Editor-in-Chief of *Resuscitation* and pottering somewhat aimlessly in his home and garden in an old vicarage in a small village in Wiltshire with his family.

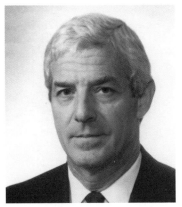

**Thomas Firth Baskett** was born during the Second World War and spent the first few weeks of his life in a cot under a heavy dining room table during the air raids on the Belfast shipyards. He was later evacuated to the country, making him an unwitting pioneer of future perinatal outreach programmes.

Educated at Belfast Royal Academy he gained his colours in rugby and athletics but no academic distinction. Under modern standards he would not have been accepted into medical school. Happily unaware of this he was admitted to medicine at the Queen's University of Belfast and qualified in 1964. He undertook six years of postgraduate training in Northern Ireland in obstetrics and gynaecology with some surgery and general practice.

Facing one of those cycles of over supply in his chosen specialty in the National Health Service he emigrated to Canada in 1970. He spent 10 years in Winnipeg and in 1980 moved to Dalhousie University in Halifax, Nova Scotia where he is currently a Professor of Obstetrics and Gynaecology. In 1997 he completed the Diploma in the History of Medicine from the Worshipful Society of Apothecaries of London and was awarded the Maccabean Prize and the Osler Medal. He is a former President of the Society of Obstetricians and Gynaecologists of Canada and has written widely on clinical obstetrics and the history of medicine.

# TABLE OF CONTENTS

# THE RESUSCITATION GREATS IN ALPHABETICAL ORDER

Ahnefeld, Fritz
Alexander, Czar
Apgar, Virginia

Ballasa, Janos
Beck, Claude
Bell, Alexander Graham
Bernard, Claude
Bible, Holy
Blundell, James
Brook, Morris

Caroline, Nancy
Cathcart, Lord
Chaemides, Leon
Chamberlain, Douglas
Cobb, Leonard
Cullen, William

Dunant, Jean -Henri

Elam, James
Eve, Frank

Fay, Thomas
Frey, Rudolf
Fitzpatrick Lecture
Galenius Claudius
Gray, Thomas Cecil
Guedel, Arthur
Gurvich,Naum

Hall, Marshall
Harvey, William
Hernholdt, John Daniel
Hillman, Harold
Holmberg, Stig
Hooke, Robert
Howard, Benjamin
Humane Societies
Hunter, John

Ibsen, Bjorn

Jackson Rees, Gordon
Jude, James

Kirschner, Martin
Kite, Charles
Knickerbocker, Guy
Koenig, Franz
Kouwenhoven, William
Kuhn, Franz

Laerdal, Asmund
Landsteiner, Karl
Larrey Baron Dominique Jean
Latta, Thomas
Lavoisier, Antoine Laurent de
Leale, Charles Augustus
Lind Bjorn
Lown, Bernard

Maass Friedrich
Mackintosh, Sir Robert
Mac William, John Alexander
Magill, Sir Ivan
Matas, Rudolph
Mayou, John
Mechanical devices for chest compression
Mundy, Baron Jaromir

Nagel, Eugene
Negovsky, Vladimir
Neilsen, Holger Louis

O 'Dwyer, Joseph
O'Shaughnessy, William

Pantridge, Frank
Paracelsus, Phillipus Aureolus
Paré, Ambroise
Pasha, Cemil Topuzla
Pask, Edgar

Percy, Baron Pierre Francois
Priestley, Joseph
Pugh, Benjamin

Rasn, Carl Gottlieb
Ringer, Sidney
Ruben, Henning

Safar, Peter I
Safar, Peter II
Schafer, Edward Sharpey
Scheele, Carl Wilhelm
Schiff, Moritz
Schultze, Bernard
Seldinger, Sven- Ivar
Sellick, Brian
Silvester, Henry
Snow, John

Trendelenberg, Friedrich

Vesalius, Andreas
Von Esmarch, Johan Friedrich August

Woods, Sir Robert

Zoll, Paul

# LIST OF AUTHORS AND THEIR AFFILIATIONS

**Pilar Acosta**
Universidad Autónoma de Tamaulipas, Tampico, México.
**Ana Graciela Alzaga**
Universidad Autónoma de Tamaulipas, Tampico, Mexico.
**David Baker**
Department of Anaesthesia, SAMU de Paris, Hôpital Necker, Enfants Malades, Paris, France.
**John Ballance**
Orchid Bank, Woolhope, Hereford, U K.
**Peter J.F. Baskett**
Stanton Court, Stanton St Quintin, Chippenham, Wiltshire, UK.
**Thomas F. Baskett**
Department of Obstetrics and Gynaecology, Dalhousie University, Halifax, Nova Scotia, Canada.
**Christian W. Bayer**
Klinik für Anaesthesiologie, Klinikum der Johannes Gutenberg Universität, Langenbeckstr, Mainz, Germany.
**Pervin Bozkurt**
Department of Anaesthesiology and Reanimation, Istanbul University Cerrahpasa Medical Faculty, Istanbul, Turkey.
**Pierre Carli**
Department of Anaesthesia, SAMU de Paris, Hôpital Necker, Enfants Malades, Paris, France.
**Jean-Bernard Cazalaà**
Department of Anaesthesia, SAMU de Paris, Hôpital Necker, Enfants Malades, Paris, France.
**Douglas Chamberlain**
Prehospital Research Unit, Lansdowne Hospital, Cardiff, UK.
**Stafford I. Cohen**
Harvard Medical School and Beth Israel Deaconess Medical Center, Boston, USA.
**Diana Coke**
Royal Humane Sociey, Brettenham House, Lancester Place, London, UK.
**Tim M Craft**
Consultant in Anaesthesia and Intensive Care, Royal United Hospital, Bath, UK.
**Jonathan E. Davis**
Department of Emergency Medicine, Stanford University Medical Center, Stanford, California, USA.
**Wolfgang Dick**
Klinik für Anaesthesiologie, Klinikum der Johannes Gutenberg Universität, Langenbeckstr, Mainz, Germany.
**Mickey S. Eisenberg**
Department of Medicine, University of Washington Medical Center, Emergency Medicine Service, Seattle, USA.
**Gary Enever**
Royal Victoria Infirmary, Newcastle upon Tyne, UK.
**Markus Figl**
Ludwig Boltzmann Institute for Experimental and Clinical Traumatology and Trauma Research Center of the Austrian Workers Compensation Board, Vienna, Austria.
**Fernando Eugênio dos Santos Cruz Filho**
Instituto Nacional de Cardiologia Laranjeiras, Ministry of Health of Brazil, Rio de Janeiro, Brazil.
**Judith M. Fisher**
336 Primrose Drive, Pleasant Hill, California 94523, USA.
**Robert E. Fromm Jr**
Sections of Cardiology, Pulmonary and Critical Care Section, Baylor College of Medicine, Department of Emergency Services, The Methodist Hospital, Houston, Texas, USA.
**Gillian R. Hamilton**
Dalhousie University, Halifax, Nova Scotia, Canada.
**Russell Harrison-Paul**
The University of Nottingham School of Nursing, Nottingham, UK.
**Johan Herlitz**
Sahlgrenska University Hospital, Division of Cardiology, Sweden.
**D. Karcher**
J Van Rijswijcklaan, Antwerp. Belgium.
**Mustafa Karatepe**
Department of History of Medicine and Deontology, Pamukkale University Medical Faculty, Denizil, Turkey.
**Mihaly Kis**
Department of Surgery, Dalhousie University, Halifax, Nova Scotia, Canada.

**Tore Laerdal**
Laerdal Medical, Stavanger, Norway.
**Yaroslav A Leschenko**
Department of Anaesthesiology and Intensive Care Medicine, Dnepropetrovsk State Medical Academy, Ukraine.
**A. Lowenthal**
J Van Rijswijcklaan, Antwerp, Belgium.
**Walter Mauritz**
Department of Anaesthesiology and Intensive Care Medicine, Lorenz Boehler Trauma Centre, Vienna, Austria.
**M.D.J. McKechnie**
Department of Accident and Emergency Medicine, The Royal Infirmary of Edinburgh, UK.
**Wendy Moore**
18 Glenshiel Road, London, UK.
(Author " The Knife Man: Blood, Body-Snatching and the Birth of Modern Surgery" Bantam Press)
**Fritz Nagele**
Department of Obstetrics and Gynaecology, University of Vienna, Austria.
**Ulf  Nyman**
Department of Radiology, University of Lund, Sweden.
**Linda E. Pelinka**
Department of Anaesthesiology and Intensive Care Medicine, Lorenz Boehler Trauma Centre, Vienna, Austria.
**Yolanda Perkins**
Autonomous University of Tamaulipas, Tampico, Tamaulipas, Mexico.
**Martin von Planta**
St. Johanns-Vorstadt, Basel, Switzerland.
**Linda Quan**
Emergency Services, Children's Hospital and Regional Medical Center, Seattle, Washington, USA.
**Colin Robertson**
Department of Accident and Emergency Medicine, The Royal Infirmary of Edinburgh, UK.
**Peter Safar**
University of Pittsburgh, Safar Center for Resuscitation Research, Pittsburgh, USA.
**Gloria A. Salazar**
Universidad Autónoma de Baja California, Tijuana, Mexico.
**David A.E. Shephard**
Department of Anaesthesia, Prince County Hospital, Summerside, PEI, Canada.
**Mario Sicuro**
Dirigente Mecico I livello, UAO Cardiologia, Ospedale Maggiore San Giovanni Battista, Turin, Italy.
**George Sternbach**
Department of Emergency Medicine, Stamford University Medical Centre, Stamford, CA 94305-5239
**Andreas Thierbach**
Klinik für Anaesthesiologie, Klinikum der Johannes Gutenberg Universität, Langenbeckstr, Mainz, Germany.
**Nina Tjomsland**
Byggstein 12. N-4042 Hafrsfjord, Norway.
**Erkan Tomatir**
Department of Anaesthesiology and Reanimation, Pamukkale University Medical Faculty, Denizli, Turkey.
**Alexander V Tsarov**
Department of Anaesthesiology and Intensive Care Medicine, Dnepropetrovsk State Medical Academy, Ukraine.
**Ludmila V. Ussenko**
Department of Anaesthesiology and Intensive Care Medicine, Dnepropetrovsk State Medical Academy, Ukraine.
**Federico Vallejo-Manzur**
Automomous University of Tamauipas, Tampico, Tamaulipas, Mexico.
**Joseph Varon**
Clinical Professor of Medicine, The University of Texas Health Science Center at Houston, Texas, USA.
**David J. Wilkinson**
The Boyle Department of Anaesthesia. St Bartholomew's Hospital, London, UK.
**Desmond Writer**
Formerly Professor, Department of Anaesthesia, Dalhousie University, Halifax, Nova Scotia, Canada.
**John Zorab**
Holmray Cottage, Park Street, Iron Acton, Bristol, UK.

# The Early Years

In the early years there was life and there was death, and to most people both of these states were ordained by the gods. Disease and death were visited upon individuals or groups by vengeful gods as punishment for errant human behaviour. Resuscitation was either forbidden or, if performed, was felt to be undertaken by God, with man merely the instrument through which God's will was imposed. The first article in this book outlines the references to resuscitation in biblical times and it should be noted that Elijah prayed to God before attempting to resuscitate the child: 'And the Lord hearkened unto the voice of Elijah, and the soul of the child came into him again, and he revived'.

Attempts at resuscitation must have gone on for millennia and Egyptian mythology records Isis resuscitating her husband Osiris by blowing into his mouth. It seems likely that attempts to revive apparently stillborn infants may be the oldest form of resuscitation and the mouth-to-mouth technique has probably been applied, to some extent instinctively, since antiquity by midwives caring for women during labour. Mouth-to-mouth respiration on the newborn was clearly described by the man-midwife **Benjamin Pugh** in 1754, detailing almost exactly the same technique recommended in modern resuscitation manuals. However, William Hunter (1718-1783), the influential Scottish obstetrician who taught in London, dismissed mouth-to-mouth resuscitation as the method 'practised by the vulgar to restore stillborn children'.

The classic period of Greek medicine (460-136 BC) produced the Hippocratic corpus that introduced the concept that disease was not incurred as the wrath of the Gods but pathological processes that had signs and symptoms. The chief function of the physician was diagnosis and prognosis and to support the natural healing forces of the body. **Galen** (130-200 AD) extended the work of Hippocrates, Aristotle and others to explore the anatomical basis of the body in health and disease. Unfortunately due to religious and legal restrictions his experiments were conducted mostly on animals, and much of his anatomical and physiological writings were flawed and limited by his extrapolation from the animal to the human. In 177 AD he used bellows to inflate the lungs of dead animals to study respiration but not to resuscitate. Some 16 centuries later bellows were to become the preferred method of ventilatory resuscitation, endorsed by the Royal Humane Society of London. Galen's principles held sway until the 16th century when the work of **Andreas Vesalius** and **William Harvey** emerged during the Renaissance and contributed to the enlightenment of the 17th century. Vesalius revolutionised anatomy with his dissection and experiments on the human body. In animal experiments he clearly described tracheotomy and ventilation via this route as the key to restoring both respiratory and circulatory function. **Robert Hooke** extended the observations of Vesalius and proved that it was the air itself forced into the lungs that was necessary for cardiac and respiratory function - rather than the mechanical action of ventilation. Some 70 years after the work of Vesalius, William Harvey established the circulation of the blood. He urged investigators to draw their conclusions 'not from the tenets of the philosophers, but from the fabric of nature...' Mind you, anatomical and physiological experimentation could still be a risky business in the 16th century. Miguel Servetus (1509-53), the Spanish physician and theologian, was burned at the stake by Calvin for describing the pulmonary circulation, along with other theological misdemeanours.

The history of discovery is full of 'near-misses'. Such was the case with **John Mayow** who showed that part of atmospheric air, 'the nitro-aerial spirit', was necessary to sustain life. This spirit was identical to that required to support combustion. For when an animal and a taper in flame were placed under the same glass dome the taper flame was extinguished at the same time as the animal developed cardio-respiratory arrest. John Mayow died at the age of 35 and it was to be 100 years more before the 'nitro-aerial spirit' was identified as life-giving oxygen by **Priestley, Scheele** and **Lavoisier**.

Robert Hooke was to become curator of the Royal Society in London which was founded in 1660. This group of gifted all round scientists included Robert Boyle, Isaac Newton, Thomas Willis, Richard Lower and Christopher Wren. In addition to the work described previously in this section these men laid down many of the scientific foundations for the medical discoveries in the next two centuries.

# The earliest records

## Judith M. Fisher

Myth — traditional story concerning the early history of a people or explaining a natural or social phenomenon and typically involving supernatural beings or events (OED).

Resuscitation attempts may be as old as man himself. The earliest medical records are in the papyri from ancient Egypt around 4000 years ago. Once the first written records were analysed, references to men driving out evil spirits to restore life, were frequent. This might have been by making loud noises or by beating the patient [1] but also by methods resembling resuscitative efforts, such as Isis restoring her husband Osiris by breathing into his mouth (Egyptian mythology). Even earlier, cave drawings (Palaeolithic drawings in the El Pindal caves in Spain), suggest that man may have sited the heart as the source of life [2].

Even before Elijah, references were made in both the Bible and Pentateuch to the breath of life [3]. In Genesis, in the second account of creation, God is said to have "...breathed into his nostrils the breath of life" when forming Adam (though not when forming the animals). We now get into the inevitable discussion of many early mythologies and their meaning. Was the Bible written as an explanation for life? Few people are such fundamentalists as to believe every word is fact. However, stories were recorded, often based on myths that had been handed down from generation to generation.

In the 11th and 12th centuries BC, the Hebrew midwife was known as a 'Shiphrah' derived from two separate words, the first She-Paru, meaning 'Israel multiplied' and the second Puah, a derivation of Mepiah, to revive [4]. Midwives would revive infants with their own respiration when the child was thought to be dead.

The basis of many myths are factual, although their content may be far fetched. The 'facts' behind many early scripts were based on what was known of life at the time, their traditions and practices. It is likely that the concept of 'Breath of Life' was based on current custom.

The most frequently quoted early example of resuscitation comes from later in the Hebrew's history, when their nomadic life had been exchanged for a more settled existence in towns and villages. In the first book of Kings [5], we read about the prophet Elijah, who laid himself upon the dying son of his land-lady, "..and his illness was so severe that there was no breath left in him". The story goes on to describe how Elijah first prayed then stretched himself along the sick child. "...and the soul of the child came into him again, and he revived". Although there is no mention of mouth-to-mouth contact, as in the next account, it is likely that both Elijah and Elisha used similar methods, since Elijah was Elisha's mentor and teacher. The second book of Kings [6] describes a more explicit resuscitation event in the life of the prophet Elisha (about the 8th Century BC). "And when Elisha came into the house, behold the child was dead, and laid upon his bed. He went in therefore, and shut the door upon the twain, and prayed unto the Lord. And he went up and lay upon the child, and put his mouth upon his mouth, and his eyes upon his eyes, and his hands upon his hands; and he stretched himself upon him; and the flesh of the child waxed warm. Then he returned, and walked in the house once to and fro; and went up, and stretched himself upon him; and the child sneezed seven times, and the child opened his eyes.".....

The Talmud, a compilation of post-biblical writings until around 500 AD, discusses the problem of "assisting in the breathing delivery" [7] and states "The new-born is held so it should not fall on the earth and one blows into his nostrils".

Not only was mouth-to-mouth resuscitation used but it seems that tracheotomy was well known in ancient times. McClelland [8] writes about the period of legend dating back to 2000 BC when the Egyptians were recorded as using reeds in the windpipe through a hole in the skin. He recalls Homer (356 BC) talking of cutting open the trachea to relieve choking persons and Alexander the Great is meant to have punctured the trachea of a soldier with the tip of his sword when he saw the man was choking from a bone lodged in his throat. Later in the 16th century he talks of Andreas Vesailius restoring animals to life by putting tubes into the trachea.

We may be celebrating 40 years of modern mouth-to-mouth resuscitation, but do not let us think that we are celebrating a new idea!

## References

[1] Varon J, Sternbach G. Cardio-pulmonary resuscitation: lessons from the past. J Emerg Med 1991;9:503–7.
[2] Lyons AS, Petrucelli RY. Medicine: An Illustrated History. New York: Abrams, 1978.
[3] Paraskos. Biblical Accounts of Resuscitation. J. Hist. Med. Allied Sci. 1992;47:310–321 (ISSN 0022-5045).
[4] Respiratory Resuscitation in Ancient Hebrew Sources. Rozen Z. Davidson J.T. 3.
[5] The Bible. 1 Kings Chapter 17:17.
[6] The Bible. 2 Kings Chapter vs 32–35.
[7] Babylonian Talmud, Shabbath 128b.
[8] McClelland RMA. Tracheostomy, it's management and alternatives. In: Proceedings of the RSM, vol. 65, 1972:401.

# Galen and the origins of artificial ventilation, the arteries and the pulse

George L. Sternbach    Joseph Varon    Robert E. Fromm Jr    Mario Sicuro
Peter J.F. Baskett

Most of the early discoveries made in the area of resuscitation relate to pulmonary physiology, with emphasis on ventilation [1]. Although some references to artificial ventilation can be traced to biblical times, it is in the works of the Greek physician Galen, following on from the theories of Hippocrates and Aristotle, that investigation in this area really begins. Galen introduced physicians to the anatomical concept of disease. This is centred on the doctrine that a detailed knowledge of the structure of the body is fundamental in understanding illness. His teachings were to remain authoritative for almost 15 centuries.

Claudius Galenius, commonly known as Galen, was born in Pergamon, in Asia Minor (now Western Turkey), in the year 130 during the reign of the Roman Emperor Hadrian [2]. The city of Pergamon, now named Bergama, was celebrated for its temple dedicated to Aesculapius, its school of medicine, and its ancient library [3]. Galen was a bright child and by the age of 14 had mastered the classic teachings in philosophy and mathematics [4]. He studied medicine in Pergamon, and, after his father's death, at the major medical learning centers of the ancient world, including Smyrna, Corinth and Alexandria.

When he arrived in Alexandria, human dissection, which had previously been practised, was no longer permitted. Deprived of the opportunity to study anatomy directly, Galen assumed that human organs were identical to those of animals. This error was to hinder the progress of human anatomy, and indeed physiology, for centuries.

Having completed his medical education, he returned to Pergamon, where he was charged with the treatment of wounded gladiators in the Great Circus. This allowed him some opportunity for enhancing his anatomical knowledge and surgical skills. In 161, he moved to Rome, where his reputation as a physician was to be made. There he lectured, wrote, experimented, and attended various Roman dignitaries, most notably the Emperor Marcus Aurelius. Although it is believed that Galen lived until the year 210, the exact year and place of his death are unknown.

He is described as a man of 'enormous industry, great sagacity, with a quick perception and boundless self-confidence' [5]. The latter quality gained him both followers and enemies. Galen was a prolific writer who was the author of more than 500 treatises. The body of his surviving works forms half of all the remaining ancient Greek medical writings. Eighty-three of his works are extant and acknowledged to be genuine [3]. He wrote on medical subjects, but also on ethics, philosophy, logic and grammar. Considering himself the natural heir to Hippocrates, he delighted in quoting the ancient Greek philosophers in his works [2].

In the field of cardiorespiratory physiology, his outstanding works related to the use of respiration, the blood in the arteries and the origin and description of the pulse. These topics are dealt with in his various treatises [6–9] and they have been translated by a number of scholars down the ages. A most comprehensive recent translation of Galen treatises, with argument and reasoning as to the precise meanings intended in the original works, is to be found in the work of Furley and Wilkie [11], and in the translation by May of Galen's work on the use of the parts of the body [12].

The physiology of respiration interested Galen greatly. He demonstrated that air entered mechanically into the expanded chest cavity on inspiration. Quiet respiration was performed mainly by the diaphragm, but forced breathing involved the intercostal muscles as well. He imagined, though, that air also entered the skull through the cribriform plate and passed out again by the same channel, carrying off humors from the brain into the nose [6,12]. This belief may have been handed down from the teachings of Hippocrates in his work, De Morso Sacro X, and reinforced by Galen as a result of his own observation that, in vivisected animals, the brain moves in time with respiration. Some of this cerebral air was thought to be combined with vital spirits in the anterior ventricles of the brain, and finally exuded from the fourth ventricle [2,6–8]. The lungs also served the important function of cooling the heart — "I have shown that respiration is useful to animals for the sake of the heart, which to some extent required the substance of the air and besides needs very greatly to be cooled because of its burning heat" [6,8,9,11–13].

Galen wrote on the trachea, termed the 'rough artery' due to its cartilaginous rings, "I shall now tell why nature joined to these vessels a third one which originates from the pharynx and is called the rough artery by some and bronchus by others" [12]. He recognized it as the vessel for both breathing and phonation. "Thanks to the rough arteries, the lung lacks nothing necessary for an instrument both of the voice and the respiration" [12]. The trachea served as a conduit for air, unlike the arteries and veins (the smooth arteries). "Now, are you not astonished when the rough artery alternately draws air into the lungs and gives it out, and when the nostrils and the whole mouth act similarly, nor do you think it strange or paradoxical that the air is dismissed through the very channel by which it was admitted just before" [7,14].

In Greek medical belief, there was an undefined spirit called *pneuma*. Having neither substance nor texture, it was drawn into the lungs by breathing. From the lungs, it entered the left side of the heart, and then the arteries. Galen believed that crude air began the transformation to *pneuma* after it had first undergone elaboration in the lungs [6,11,12]. The metamorphosis was completed when air mixed with blood in the heart. Proof that the arteries contain blood is generally agreed to be Galen's most important contribution to medical science. Until his investigations, blood was thought to be carried only by the veins which Aristotle believed were 'tubes of flesh' with pores which had been formed by the passage of blood. His predecessors, including

Aristotle and Erasistratus, believed that arteries served as the conduits only for *pneuma*.

Galen had observed, however, that blood had emerged after an artery was pierced and there was no sign of *pneuma* [6,11]. He argued the case that if *pneuma* was present in the arteries, there would have to be some sign of it. The reactionary supporters of the theories of Erasistratus, who believed that *pneuma* alone would be in the arteries in the normal state of the body, replied that all the *pneuma* would have emerged rapidly and silently at the initial time of puncture. But this argument was countered by Galen who pointed out that the animal continued to live (apparently without life-giving *pneuma*) after the artery continued to bleed [6,10].

In about the year 177, Galen used bellows to inflate dead animals' lungs [8,15]. He did this not in an effort to revive the animals, but to demonstrate the function of the pulmonary system. Following a description of the expansion and contraction of the trachea with insufflation, Galen wrote, "You can clearly see this for yourself, even after the animal is dead, if you blow air through the rough artery into the whole lung and then empty it out again by pressure" [6,12]. Similarly, with expansion of the lungs, "If, when the animal is already dead you blow air in through the larynx, you will, of course, fill the rough arteries and you will see the lung expanded to its greatest extent while the smooth arteries and the veins in the lung maintain their size unchanged" [6,12]. These investigations led at least one observer to declare that Galen "must have been very close indeed to discovering the usefulness of artificial ventilation" [15].

Galen was an avid experimenter, and stressed the pre-eminence of independent observation over dogma. Regarding the vena cava, for example, he wrote, "I think you will marvel the more if instead of relying entirely upon words, you are willing to dissect some animals and see this wondering thing for yourself" [6,12]. When undertaking, "the actual investigations of the parts of the lung", he indicated that, "of course it is perfectly clear to everyone that we ought to make such an investigation by dissecting animals" [6,12]. One scholar feels this represents "an excellent example of Galen's untroubled assumption that in order to discuss a structure in man, it is sufficient to have it dissected in animals" [12]. Though some criticism may be laid around his interpretation of results, there is no doubt he was a hands-on vivisector using dogs or pigs. He advocated that students should practice on cadavers first. He did not like to practice vivisection on apes because "the spectacle is hideous" [10].

Nevertheless Galen did make mistakes. In attempting to assess whether the brain was dependent on the heart, he occluded the common carotid arteries but ignored the vertebral arteries — although he knew of their existence and pathway [10]. This shortcoming was pointed out by Versalius some 1300 years later [16].

He also erroneously deduced from his experiments with arterial cannulation that the pulse was carried in the walls of the arteries rather than due to the pulsatile flow of blood. Harvey in his classical work, 'De Motu Cordis', pointed out this error of deduction [17].

Galen held a strong belief in a rational system ordering the universe. He wrote of "Nature, who does nothing without good reason" [6,12]. In this, he reflected the Aristotelian declaration that nature does nothing in vain. He believed in the concept of technology, which assumed that the structure of every part of the functioning body was preconceived and followed a purposeful plan. As such, he had a teleological explanation for much of what he observed. The main difficulty with Galen's anatomic concepts was that he often made the observed structure of the human body fit in his erroneous theories of physiology and the religious philosophy of the day.

As such, he made many mistakes concerning the structure of the internal organs. For example, although there is normally no direct connection between the right and left heart chambers, Galen described openings (he termed them 'pits' or 'pores') in the dividing septum to fit his theoretical system, in which blood had to pass from one side of the heart to the other. Because his theories require that *pneuma* somehow find its way into the veins, he pre-supposed that the interventricular pores allowed the spiritual essence to pass into that part of the bloodstream. "The pits to be seen in the heart, especially in the partition dividing it, were formed for the sake of the communication of which I have spoken" [6,12].

By virtue of his experimentation and writing, Galen laid down many of the principles of scientific investigation. His writings constituted an encyclopaedic knowledge of the medical art up to his time, with his own commentaries and additions. The effect was to add to and consolidate all existing medical knowledge. All his treatises were written with a great assurance that conveyed an impression of finality.

Though his anatomical studies were the best among ancient anatomists, because Galen's precepts and observations came to be held as sacrosanct, his influence ultimately became an obstacle to progress. For over a millennium after his death, no one challenged the medical doctrine of Galen's concepts. Medieval physicians saw in his works the authoritative answers to the challenging questions in medicine. Instead of rejecting his irrationalities and conjectures, they clung to them. When Andreas Vesalius (1514–1564), the great Flemish anatomist, demonstrated that Galen's description of the hip bone was wrong, he apologized for deviating from Galen's teaching by stating that man had changed shape over the intervening centuries by wearing tight trousers! [3].

Although Galen was subsequently held to account for such attitudes, recent observers have been charitable. One wrote that "the price we pay for our great men is that later generations make tyrants of them" [5]. Another of his translators lamented that the "appearance of an outstanding genius who far outstrips his predecessors and contemporaries is naturally followed by a longer or shorter period during which there is little or no progress" [12].

Galen's authority stood unchallenged until the 16th century. It was then that Paracelsus (1493–1541), the iconoclastic Swiss physician broke away completely from Greek classical medicine. He symbolically burned the works of Galen in the presence of his students at Basel. This was the most dramatic attack on the Galenic teachings, and was to gain Paracelsus much enmity.

Following his death, Galen's works were widely translated into Arabic. Ibn-an-Nafis, a 13th century Arab physician, seems to have been the first to reject Galen's contention that interventricular septum contained pores [5]. Vesalius [16] too, was finally to deny their presence. William Harvey's definitive proof in 1628 [17] that these pores did not exist became most damaging to the Galenic doctrine.

Although Galen did not conduct experiments in assisted ventilation as such, his anatomical studies and observations of respiratory physiology served as the basis for important subsequent investigations in ventilation. Ironically, both Paracelsus and Vesalius, who were to do much to discredit Galen's medical concepts, were pre-eminent among those who used experimental methods to perform assisted ventilations. Their use of bellows ventilation was, in turn, to stimulate John Hunter's subsequent work in 1771 [19]. The history of ventilatory support was to progress from that point [18,20].

## References

[1] Varon J, Sternbach GL. Cardiopulmonary resuscitation: lessons from the past. J Emerg Med 1991;9:503–7.

[2] Elliott JS. Outlines of Greek and Roman Medicine. London: John Bale, Sons & Danielsson Ltd, 1914.

[3] Gordon BL. Medicine Throughout Antiquity. Philadelphia, FA: Davis Company, 1949.

[4] Eisenberg MS. Life in the Balance. New York: Oxford University Press, 1997:38.

[5] Allbutt TC. Greek Medicine in Rome. London: Macmillan, 1921.

[6] Galenius C. De usu partum.

[7] Galenius C. De naturalibus facultibus.

[8] Galenius C. De usu respirationis.

[9] Galenius C. De placitis Hippocratis et Platonis.

[10] Galenius C. De usu pulsuum.

[11] Farley DJ, Wilkie JS. Galen on Respiration and the Arteries. Guildford, Surrey, UK: Princeton University Press, 1984.

[12] May MT. Galen on the Usefulness of the Parts of the Body (translated). Ithaca: Cornell University Press, 1968.

[13] Galenius C. De Instrumento Odoratus.

[14] Brock AJ. Galen on the Natural Faculties. New York: GP Putnam's Sons, 1916.

[15] Baker AB. Artificial respiration: the history of an idea. Med Hist 1971;15:336–46.

[16] Vesalius A. De corporis humanica fabrica VII. XIX, 1543.

[17] Harvey W. De motu cordis, 1628.

[18] Davis JE, Sternbach GL, Varon J, Fromm RE. Paracelsus and mechanical ventilation. Resuscitation 2000;47(1):3–6.

[19] Hunter J. Proposals for recovery of people apparently drowned, Phil Trans Roy Soc., 1776;66:412.

[20] Sternbach GL, Varon J, Fromm RE, Baskett PJF. The humane societies. Resuscitation 2000;45(2):71–5.

# Paracelsus and mechanical ventilation

Jonathan E. Davis    George L. Sternbach    Joseph Varon    Robert E. Froman Jr.

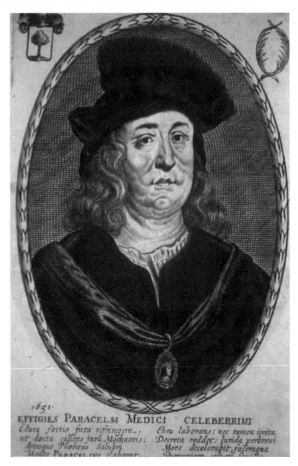

EFFIGIES PARACELSI MEDICI    CELEBERRIM
Clara fortis fata refringere.. Eheu laborans: nec tamen irrita
ut docta callens juri Machaonis: Decreta reddet: lurida perhorrui
Artesque Phoebeas Salubri    Mors decolorabit rabiemque
Morte Paracelsus elaborat.

The 16th century is generally agreed to mark the beginning of the modern era in medicine. Paracelsus, one of the most controversial of medical practitioners, lived during this period, the beginning of the Renaissance. Some attribute to him one of the breakthrough advances leading to what we now know as artificial respiration.

Born Phillipus Aureolus Theophrasus Bombastus von Hohenheim in 1493, in Einseideln, a small town near Zurich, Paracelsus was among the most erratic of Renaissance figures. The name Paracelsus is though to originate from the prefix *para*, meaning beyond, and the name Celsus, referring to Aulus Cornelius Celsus, a first century Roman medical writer [1]. Paracelsus is recognized as an important reformer of medicine and given praise as the father of biochemistry, pharmacology, toxicology and therapeutics. However, he was also known for quarreling with and antagonizing his peers and inconsistency in his teachings. Consequently, it has been said of him that "there are few medical men of whom so much of good and evil has been said" [2].

Paracelsus began his study of medicine under the tutelage of his father. At the age of 23, he is said by some to have earned his doctoral degree under Leonicenus at Ferrara [1,3]. Others question, as to what extent, he even experienced a conventional medical education. "Although it is thought that he studied in Ferrara and obtained a doctorate of medicine from that university", notes one scholar, "there is no convincing evidence to support this claim" [4]. As a physician, Paracelsus began to travel throughout Europe, practicing and acquiring a deeper knowledge of both traditional and folk medicine. Such travel was "according to the custom of the scholastics of those times, to visit the universities and hear the most celebrated professors" [2]. Paracelsus is criticized for his travels, for "instead of frequenting the schools, young Paracelsus sought the conversation of clever women, barbers, renovators, magicians, achymists (sic), though, in whose society, he boasted he had obtained valuable secrets" [2].

Paracelsus always maintained a conflicting relationship with traditional doctrines. For example, he chose to deliver his lectures in German rather than Latin, the accepted standard of the time. In order to capture sympathy for his scientific ideas, he sometimes included political viewpoints in his writings. In a tract on epilepsy, he exploited the prevalent anticlericism of the time to denounce the church and monastic orders for their extravagance and neglect of the poor [4].

He was appointed *Stadtartzt*, or town physician and Professor of Physic and Surgery of Basel in 1527. There he performed the dramatic gesture of publicly burning the works of Galen and Avicenna in the presence of his students. The teachings of Galen had remained the standard in medical thought and theory for 15 centuries. Specifically, Paracelsus rejected the ancient Greek humoral concept, to which Galen had adhered. This professed that illness was caused by insult to the delicate balance between the four bodily humors (phlegm, blood, yellow and black bile). In Galenic theory, treatment was aimed at the restoration of this balance, mainly via herbal-based remedies [5].

Paracelsus, on the contrary, proposed a chemical based theory of disease and its therapy. In Paracelsian theory, specific elements of the macrocosm (the universe) affect aspects of the microcosm (the body). Therapy was aimed at combating the macrocosmic element that affected the microcosm with an extensive pharmacopeia composed largely of various metals and minerals. In this way, Paracelsus discounted witchcraft, preferring the substitution of rational chemical therapeutics, including substances such as opium, arsenic, sulfates, lead, iron and various other metal salts. He refined the use of mercurials to combat the 16th century syphilis epidemic. Administering milder, chemically altered forms of mercury, he circumvented the often severe untoward effects produced by the more potent liquid mercury. Paracelsus is also credited with recognizing geographic variations of disease, associating cretinism with endemic goiter, distinguishing between mental defect and acquired mental illness, and appreciating the concept of occupational disease through his recognition of silicosis in miners.

Fundamental to Paracelsian thought was the condemnation of all teachings not based on experimentation. He believed, "Medicine can only be learned from that which the eyes can see and the fingers touch…Practice should not be based on speculative theory, theory should be derived from practice" [1]. Ironically, this precisely reflects advice put forward by Galen, though subsequently ignored by centuries of his followers. Galen urged his students to perform their own observations "instead of relying entirely upon words" [6]. In general, however, Paracelsus had little regard for the teachings of the ancients. "Of what avail is the rain that fell a thousand years ago?", he enquired rhetorically. "That which falls at present avails" [7].

As a consequence of his radical views and teachings, Paracelsus was forced to leave Basel in 1528, only one year after being appointed *Stadtartzt*. He did so under the threat of arrest by outraged colleagues. He spent the remainder of his life wandering through Europe, vacillating between bouts of drunkenness and periods of lucency, when he professed his radical views. In traveling from town to town, he viciously attacked the incompetence and profiteering of local physicians and apothecaries [8]. Consequently, he was soon forced to uproot yet again. Although the specifics of his death are apocryphal, Paracelsus apparently succumbed to a wound sustained in a tavern brawl in Salzburg in 1541 [3].

At the time of his death, few of his important works had been published, and Paracelsus was known primarily as the author of a dozen astrological tracts [4]. However, chiefly because his followers thought that he had achieved miraculous cures, his fame grew posthumously. Consequently, manuscripts that he had left behind in various towns during his travels were sought out and published, and a significant body of his writings survives [9].

Nonetheless, for centuries after his death, Paracelsus remained a controversial figure, vilified by many. In 1856, Renouard assessed Paracelsus as follows, "He made more noise in the world while he lived than many savans (sic) of superior merit, and, after his death, he obtained a celebrity which his writings are far from justifying" [2]. More recent opinion has been more favorable, as typified by the position of William Osler, who observed that, though Paracelsian doctrine had little immediate effect on the practice of medicine, "it made men think and Paracelsus stirred the pool as had not been done for fifteen centuries" [10].

Paracelsus refined earlier techniques of mouth-to-mouth ventilation that had been described in antiquity [11,12]. He did so by introducing a mechanical device to support respiration. By inserting the nozzle of a bellows into the nostrils of apneic patients, he attempted to inflate their lungs [11].

In about the year 177 AD, Galen had used bellows to inflate dead animals' lungs. He did so to study the functioning of the pulmonary system rather than in any effort to revive the animals [13]. Paracelsus, by contrast, is reported to have attempted the use of bellows in a resuscitation effort. He is said in 1530 to have inserted a fireside bellows into the nostril of an apneic patient to support ventilation [11]. In part because these bellows were partially occluded with cinders, the effort was unsuccessful.

More than two centuries later, this method was refined by John Hunter, who utilized a double-chambered bellows of his own design to ventilate experimental animals. His device induced both positive pressure ventilation and negative-pressure exhalation [14]. Bellows ventilation was codified by the Royal Humane Society of London in 1783 as the preferred method of ventilatory resuscitation. It was to remain the Society's recommended method for resuscitating drowning victims until 1837 [14].

If Paracelsus did, indeed, institute such therapy, his influence in resuscitation was seminal. Unfortunately, no reference to the bellows experiment can be found in his existing writings. In assessing this experiment, one author notes that "over the years, many discoveries have been credited to Paracelsus by his adherents, but in most instances it has not been easy to substantiate their claims" [7]. Although his efforts were met with limited success, an era of mechanically assisted ventilation was born.

# References

[1] Davis A. Paracelsus: a quintecentennial assessment. J R Soc Med 1993;86:653–6.
[2] Renouard PV. History of Medicine from the Origin to the Nineteenth Century. Cincinnati: Moore Wistach, Keys & Co, 1856:358–70.
[3] Garrison FH. History of Medicine, fourth ed. Philadelphia: W.B. Saunders, 1929.
[4] Webster C. Bare heads against red hats: a portrait of Paracelsus. Clio Medica 1998;48:54–75.
[5] Gerstner P. Paracelsus. J Lab Clin Med 1989;114:209–10.
[6] May MT. Galen on The Usefulness Of The Parts Of The Body. Ithaca: Cornell University Press, 1968.
[7] Gravenstein JS. Paracelsus and his contributions to anesthesia. Anesthesiology 1956;26:805–11.
[8] Feder G. Paradigm lost: a celebration of Paracelsus on his quincentenary. Lancet 1993;34:1396–7.
[9] Debus AG. The French Paracelsans. Cambridge: Cambridge University Press, 1991.
[10] Bliss M. William Osler: A Life in Medicine. Oxford: Oxford University Press, 1999.
[11] Price JL. The evolution of breathing machines. Med Hist 1962;6:67–72.
[12] Baker AB. Artificial respiration, the history of an idea. Med Hist 1971;15:336–51.
[13] Sternbach GL, Varon J, Fromm, RE. Galen and the origins of artificial ventilation. Resuscitation, in press.
[14] Sternbach GL, Varon J, Fromm RE, Baskett, PJF. The humane societies. Resuscitation, in press.

# Andreas Vesalius, the concept of an artificial airway

Federico Vallejo-Manzur    Yolanda Perkins    Joseph Varon    Peter Baskett

Andreas Vesalius (Fig. 1) was born in Brussels on December 31, 1514 into a family with a great tradition in the field of medicine [1,2]. His great grandfather, paternal grandfather and his father were all court physicians. His father worked for Charles V and Margaret of Austria [3]. Vesalius was born Andreas van Wesel which later was converted into a Latin equivalent, according to the custom of that time, to Andreas Vesalius [4]. As Vesalius' father was frequently away from home following the court of the emperor to different campaigns in Austria or Spain, his mother Isabel Crabbe became the greatest influence in his childhood. She encouraged him to read the extensive collection of ancient medical treatises [1,4,5]. Even as a child Vesalius had great fascination for anatomy. In the fields near his home he found dead animals on which he frequently did dissections [6].

Vesalius received his early education in Brussels at the school of the Brothers of the Common Life and at age 13 he entered the Castle College of the University of Louvain. During this period of time he studied Greek, Latin, Hebrew, rhetoric, philosophy mathematics and music and displayed a great interest in natural science, especially in anatomy, by dissecting mice, rats and dogs [1,5,7].

In the fall of 1533, after obtaining a master's degree in arts from the University of Louvain, he travelled to France to enrol in the medical school of the University of Paris, among the most distinguished and conservative in Europe [4]. Immediately after he entered the school, his interest in anatomy grew exponentially. He learned the subject from the most distinguished professors of his era: Jacobus Sylvius who was the first to teach anatomy with a cadaver and John Guinter who translated the most illustrious medical books from Greek into Latin. Their teaching was based on the medieval approach where unskilled barber-surgeons performed the dissections while the instructor sat above, reading from the writings of Galen whose teaching was held as divine and indisputable [2,5]. The young Vesalius began to be frustrated with this hands free method. Because of the lack of materials for dissection, the young adventurous student made expeditions to the Cimetiere des Innocents where he and his friends used to steal bones from graves [4]. On one occasion when he went to Montfaucon, the place where the bodies of executed criminals were deposited, he and his friends were attacked by fierce dogs but Vesalius was not afraid of risking his life in the pursuit of science. Soon he became an expert in the osseous system, and he was able to name and describe any part of the skeleton blindfolded [3].

The young Vesalius was firmly convinced that the best way of learning anatomy was by practising dissections in cadavers, substituting the place of ignorant barbers. 'Tangitis res vestries minibus, et his credit' (You touch with your own hands and trust in them) [8]. Very soon his talents were recognized by both professors and students; and at his third anatomy session, he was requested to take charge of the dissection [3]. The cadaver with which Vesalius made his debut, as he noted in De Fabrica, was a 'prostitute of fine figure in the prime of life who had been hanged'. The dissection was an astonishing success, and was followed by several more [4]. His fame started to grow day by day, and he became particularly expert in dissections of the extremities (Fig. 2) and the abdomen. These were the first steps in transforming the young anatomy student to be a reformer in the knowledge of anatomy [2]. His professor and friend John Guntier described Vesalius as 'a young man, by Hercules of great cine, learned in both languages (Greek and Latin), and very skilled in the dissection of bodies' [5].

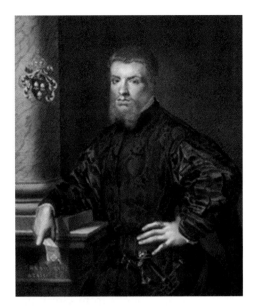

Fig. 1. Andreas Vesalius.

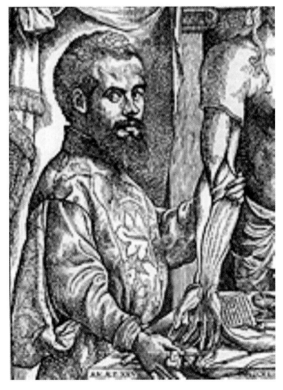

Fig. 2. Vesalius with an upper extremity dissection.

After several dissections, Vesalius started raising doubts about the Galenic theories, but he kept these feelings to himself because of the powerful Galenic influence around him [6].

Andreas Vesalius was close to obtaining his bachelor degree in medicine when the Emperor Charles V invaded France causing the start of the Franco-German War in 1536. This situation forced Vesalius to leave Paris [4,5].

In order to continue his studies, Vesalius returned to the University of Louvain [1]. One night in secret, he acquired a human skeleton from the gallows outside the walls of Louvain where criminals were executed and burned. The theft was done piecemeal and in the ensuing days he prepared and assembled the pieces into a complete skeleton. He was accompanied by his friend Reguier Gemme, who later became a famous mathematician. Grave robbing was punished severely in those times, so he convinced the authorities that he had brought the skeleton from Paris [3,4]. In 1536 Vesalius conduced the first public anatomical dissection to have been held in Louvain for 18 years. He performed the dissection himself and lectured at the same time [3]. He received his bachelor degree in medicine in the spring of 1537 [7]. Vesalius wrote his first book during this period; this book was named *A Paraphrase on the Ninth Book of Rhazes*. It dealt with illnesses from head to foot.

From Louvain, Vesalius went to Venice for a short period, where he practiced minor surgery and during this period of time, he met his compatriot Johannes Stephan van Calcar, an artist who was studying at Titans studio. After Venice he moved to Padua in order to receive his medical doctorate; he passed the set of three rigorous examinations with honours. Immediately he became Professor of Surgery and Anatomy at the University of Padua [1].

Based on his dissections and drawings and with the help of his friend van Calcar, Vesalius published *Tabulae Anatomicae Sex*, which consisted of the six charts that he used for his anatomy class. *Tabulae Anatomicae Sex* contained three charts of the arterial, venous and portal circulations drawn by Vesalius and three charts of the skeleton drawn by his friend, the artist van Calcar. This book became the first hand-drawn textbook for his students [6–8]. In the numerous public and academic dissections that Vesalius performed during his academic period it became clear to him that the anatomical teachings of Galen were wrong [8,9].

## 1. Contributions to airway management and resuscitation

There are no historical references to the exact date of the following events, but we believe they occurred during Vesalius's prolific academic period between his graduation from Padua and the publication of *De Fabrica*.

Vesalius described his technique for keeping an experimental animal alive to examine its thoracic contents. This description was published later in book VII of *De Humani Corporis Fabrica* [10] (Fig. 3).

'......But that life may in a manner of speaking be restored to the animal, an opening must be attempted in the trunk of the arteria aspera, into

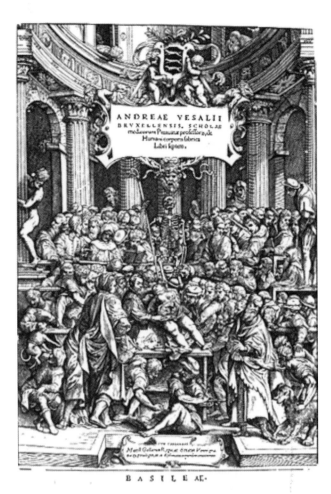

Fig. 3. Illustration of De Humanis Corporis Fabrica.

In 1543, after 4 years of meticulous preparation and elaboration he completed his masterpiece *De Humani Corporis Fabrica*. *De Fabrica* included seven books with 11 large plates and 300 illustrations [6]. Henry Sigerist, a renowned Swiss medical historian, has emphasized that *De Fabrica* marked a turning point in the history of medicine, or rather, it was the starting point of a new medical science [16]. This masterpiece gave Vesalius an important place in the Renaissance Culture [8]. The true identity of the artist who drew the illustrations of the book has been a matter of great controversy among historians, but it has been thought that Titus and his students were the artists that completed this work [5]. To seek the best publisher and printer of his time: Johannes Opornimus, Vesalius had to travel to Basel in Switzerland where *De Fabrica* was finally published [17]. That same year Vesalius published a compact version of *De Fabrica* for his students. This work was named *Epitome* [7].

*De Fabrica* was published in the same year that Copernicus published *De Revolutionibus Orbium Coelestium*, which showed that the sun, and not the earth, was the centre of the solar system. Versalius and Copernicus challenged the traditions of their respective sciences and both of them were severely attacked by traditionalist critics [8,18].

The reactions to *De Fabrica* were severe, especially from his master and old friend Sylvius, an ardent Galenist who said 'Let no one give heed to that very ignorant and arrogant man who, through his ignorance, ingratitude, impudence, and impiety denies everything his deranged or feeble vision cannot locate'. In 1546 in 'The Letter of China Root' Vesalius brilliantly defended his criticisms of Galen [5,19]. With the publication of *De Fabrica*, Vesalius corrected anatomical mistakes which had held sway for 13 centuries, and he started to put anatomical, physiological and surgical investigations down the right channel [6].

which a tube of reed or cane should be put; you will then blow into this, so that the lung may rise again and the animal take in the air....'

'...Indeed, with a slight breath in the case of this living animal the lung will swell to the full extent of the thoracic cavity, and the heart become strong and exhibits a wondrous variety of motions. So, with the lung inflated once and the second time, you examine the motion of the heart by sight and touch as much as you wish. And as I do this (the anatomical dissection) and take care that the lung is inflated at intervals, the motion of the heart and arteries does not stop...' [10].

In these paragraphs Andreas Vesalius described what appears to be one of the first attempts at a surgical airway performed with the purpose of preserving lung ventilation and circulatory function by artificial means as an experiment [11–15].

## 2. Other clinical discoveries

Although his clinical career was not extensive, Vesalius was among the first to note and describe an aneurysm and he is credited with reviving the ancient Hippocratic technique of draining an empyaema of the thorax. Vesalius also contributed greatly to the anatomical nomenclature. He linked the appendix to a worm (vermiformis), alveolus (a compartment in a honeycomb, to a tooth socket), choana (a funnel for the posterior nasal openings), incus (an anvil) and mitral valve (shaped like a bishop's mitre). As a student he discovered the spermatic vessels. He also described correctly the hip bone, revalidated the Hippocratic theory that the brain could be injured without a fracture of the skull, refuted the Galenic teaching that the jaw was composed of two bones, not one, and that the sternum has seven segments rather than the three that exist. He also raised doubts on the Galenic theory of the permeability of the interventricular septum. This helped his student Colombus to describe the pulmonary circulation and William Harvey to elucidate the circulation of the blood. What is claimed to be the oldest skeletal preparation in the world is believed to have been prepared by Vesalius [6,9,16,20].

During the reign of Phillip II, Vesalius gained notorious fame as a clinician because of two celebrity patients. The first was Henri II, King of France, who had received a severe head injury in a Royal jousting match. Vesalius was sent to Paris to assist another renowned physician, Ambrosie Paré, to evaluate the situation. As soon as Vesalius arrived in Paris he did a preliminary examination using a clean white cloth which he put in the King's mouth, asking the King to bite on it. He then jerked it out. Henri II threw his arms back and shouted in pain. This technique appears to be a method of eliciting the head flexion sign to demonstrate meningeal irritation. With this finding of reflex extension, Vesalius predicted that the King would die in the next few days. This happened 8 days after the consultation [20].

The second case happened around 1562 when the son of Phillip II, Don Carlos, had an accident while running downstairs headlong into a wall. After the accident Don Carlos developed persistent fever, and was treated by a famous Spanish physician without any favourable results. Vesalius thought that the Prince's trouble stemmed from pressure on the eyeball. It is possible that this may have arisen from sinusitis. He incised the patient's left orbit and drained the wound of pus. Later the right orbit was drained, and the fever resolved immediately [4].

## 3. Pilgrimage and death

During the next 2 years, Vesalius continued practising medicine at the court; he was often invited to practise dissection and to try to resolve clinical puzzles. His career was at its height. He was a wealthy, famous physician of the Spanish court, who had received many honours, he was the author of one of the masterpieces of the Renaissance, and was beloved by his patients and family, when tragedy struck [3].

One of the most remarkable stories of Vesalius dissections concerned that of a Spanish nobleman who had died. Vesalius requested permission from the nobleman's family to perform an autopsy to find the cause of death. The autopsy was performed in the presence of witnesses. When the heart was exposed the

witnesses saw the heart beating, and they concluded that the patient was still alive. The horrified family accused Vesalius of murder and took the case to the Inquisition. King Phillip II interceded to obtain a commutation of the sentence. There is no doubt that, without the King's help, the sentence would have been execution by burning at the stake. Instead in order to atone and save his life, Vesalius had to make a pilgrimage to Jerusalem to cleanse his sin [1].

In 1564, Vesalius embarked on this pilgrimage to Jerusalem. After travelling to Jerusalem, he learned that he could return to his former position in Padua because the position was open following the death of Fallopius. Vesalius apparently became very ill during the extended and stormy voyage in which food and water supplies were depleted. He died of an unknown cause on October 14, 1564 at the age of 50, shortly after reaching the island of Zante near Greece [5].

## References

[1] Simeone FA. Andreas Vesalius: anatomist, surgeon, Count Palatine, and Pilgrim. Am J Surg 1984;147:432–40.

[2] Sherzoi H. Andreas Vesalius (1514–1567). J Invest Surg 1999;12:131–2.

[3] Norwich I. Andreas Vesalius. A bio-bibliographic study. S Afr Med J 1967;41:431–40.

[4] Bendiner E. Andreas Vesalius: man of mystery in life and death. Hosp Prac 1986;21:199–234.

[5] Silverman ME. Andreas Vesalius and *De Humani Corporis Fabrica*. Clin Cardiol 1991;14:276–9.

[6] Menzoian JO. Lest we forget: the contributions of Andreas Vesalius and Ambroise Paré to my surgical practice. Am J Surg 1999;178:85–91.

[7] Van Helden A. Vesalius Andreas. Galileo Project, 1995. Accessed September 3, 2002. Available from: http://es.rice.edu/ES/humsoc/Galileo/Catalog/Files/vesalius.html.

[8] Lasky II. The martyrdom of doctor Andreas Vesalius. Clin Orthop 1990;259:304–11.

[9] Sternbach GL, Varon J, Fromm RE, Sicuro M, Baskett PJF. Galen and the origins of artificial ventilation, the arteries and the pulse. Resuscitation 2001;49:119–22.

[10] Vesalius A. De Corporis Humani Fabrica 1543 VII, XIX, p 658.

[11] Hermreck AS. The history of cardiopulmonary resuscitation. Am J Surg 1988;156:430–6.

[12] DeBard ML. The history of cardiopulmonary resuscitation. Ann Emerg Med 1980;9:273–5.

[13] Somerson SJ, Sicilia MR. Historical perspectives of the development and the use of mechanical ventilation. AANA J 1992;60:83–94.

[14] Chen K, Sternbach GL, Fromm RE, Varon J. Mechanical ventilation: past and present. J Emerg Med 1998;16:453–60.

[15] Varon J, Sternbach GL. Cardiopulmonary resuscitation: lessons from the past. J Emerg Med 1991;9:503–7.

[16] Rahilly RO. Commemorating the fabrica of Vesalius. Acta Anat 1993;148:228–30.

[17] Clark H. Foiling the pirates: the preparation and publication of Andreas Vaesalius's *De Humani Corporis Fabrica*. Library Q 1981;51:301–11.

[18] Cassirer EA. The place of Vesalius in the culture of the renaissance. Yale J Bio Med 1944;16:101–29.

[19] Kornell M. Illustrations from the wellcome library. Vesalius' method of articulating the skeleton and drawing in the collection of the wellcome library. Med His 2000;44:97–100.

[20] Norwich I. A consultation between Andreas Vesalius and Ambroise Paré at the death bed of Henri II, King of France, 15 July 1559. S Afr Med J 1991;80:245–7.

# Ambroise Paré and the arrest of haemorrhage

Thomas F. Baskett

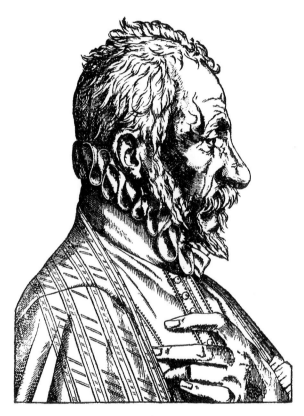

Ambroise Paré (1510–1590)

There can be few more basic aspects of resuscitation than the control and arrest of haemorrhage from wounds – either traumatic or surgical. Some 450 years ago the French surgeon, Ambroise Paré, applied ligatures to major bleeding vessels in battle wounds and limb amputations instead of the crude and cruel use of cautery. Paré started his career as a barber-surgeon with the French army in 1537 and for the first 15 years followed the standard teaching and used cautery with red hot irons heated in fire to staunch bleeding following amputation. He was repelled by the intense pain this caused the soldiers and also noted the serious secondary haemorrhage that often occurred when the scab sloughed away after the initial healing. He noted that the ancient physicians, Hippocrates and Celsus, had advocated the ligature of vessels in a variety of situations, including wounds [1], although this had not been applied to limb amputation – one of the commonest surgical procedures in the 16th century. Paré first used this method to control bleeding following an amputation he did in 1552. He did not publish the technique until 1564 in his *Dix Livres de la Chirurgie* and, indeed, it is mentioned almost casually in one of his texts [2]:

> A shot from a culverin passed through the tent of Monsieur de Rohan, which hit a gentleman's leg, which was of his trainee; which I was faine to finish the cutting off, which was done without applying hot irons......The camp being broken up, I returned to Paris with my gentleman whose leg I had cut off, I dressed him and God cured him; I sent him to his house merry with a wooden leg, and was content saying that he escaped good cheap, not to have been miserably burnt.

In the 16th century, one of the essential pieces of every military surgeon's equipment was the bullet forceps known as *Bec de Corbin* (Crow's Beak). As the name implied these forceps were fashioned with a shape rather like a crow's beak and used to explore wounds and to find and withdraw any bullets lodged therein [3]. Paré modified this instrument so that the tips of the forceps were suitable for grasping and closing the mouths of blood vessels allowing their ligation (Fig. 1). His instructions following amputation of the limb were as follows [2]:

> How to stanch the bleeding when the member is taken off: When you have cut off and taken away the member, let it bleed a little according to the strength of the patient, that so the rest of the part may afterwards be less obnoxious to inflammation and other symptoms: Then let the veins and arteries be bound up speedily and straightly as you can;

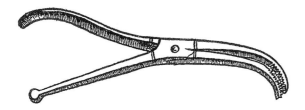

*The Crowes beake fit for to draw the vessells forth of the flesh wherein they lye hid, that so they may be tyed or bound fast.*

Fig. 1. Illustration of Paré's ligature forceps. From *The Apology and Treatise of Ambroise Paré* [2].

that so the course of the flowing blood may be stopped and wholly stayed. Which can be done by taking hold of the vessels with your Crowes beake. The ends of the vessels lying hid in the flesh, must be taken hold of and drawn with this instrument forth of the muscles whereinto they presently after the amputation withdrew themselves, as all parts are still used to withdrawn themselves toward their originals. In performance of this work, you need take no great care, if you together with the vessels comprehend some portion of the neighboring parts, as of the flesh, for hereof will ensue no harm; but the vessels will so be consolidated with the more ease, than if they being bloodless parts should grow together by themselves. To conclude, when you have drawn them forth, bind them with a strong double thread.

Predictably, Paré's technique of ligature application was criticized by those less dextrous than himself. However, as the knowledge of anatomy increased and the course and pressure points for major arteries became known, assistants could apply pressure to reduce or stop bleeding and facilitate application of the ligature. Paré comprehensively dismantled the arguments against ligature in his great work *The Apologie and Treatise of Ambroise Paré Containing the Voyages made into Divers Places* [2].

Ambroise Paré was born in Bourg-Hersent, on the outskirts of the city of Laval in the northern province of Maine, France. His father was a barber and his elder brother, Jean, was a master barber-surgeon in Vitré. Paré's early education was basic and he did not learn Latin or Greek – languages of the medical texts of that time. It is likely that he was an apprentice to a barber-surgeon, possibly his older brother, before moving to Paris in 1532. There he served a short apprenticeship with a barber-surgeon before becoming a resident surgeon in the Hôtel Dieu, the ancient monastic foundation which became the largest public hospital in Paris [4]. He worked in this position for three years and gained considerable experience, including midwifery in which he made the signal contribution of re-introducing internal podalic version into obstetrics [5]. Leaving the Hôtel Dieu in 1536 Paré soon embarked upon his career as a military surgeon which ultimately led to him serving as surgeon to four Kings of France. His first military campaign took him to Turin in 1537. At that time the standard treatment for gunshot wounds contaminated with gun powder, which was thought to be inherently infectious, was to irrigate and sterilise the wound with boiling oil. As a young surgeon in his first military campaign Paré followed this teaching, but when he ran out of oil he was forced to improvise as follows [2]:

Now at that time I was a fresh water soldier, I had not yet seen wounds made by gun-shot at the first dressing.... I was willing to know first, before I applied it how the other chirurgions did for the first dressing, which was to apply oil of elders, the hottest that was possible into the wounds; in so much that I took courage to do as they did. At last I ran out of oil, and was constrained instead thereof, to apply a digestive of yolks of eggs, oil of roses and turpentine. In the night I could not sleep in quiet, fearing some default in not cauterizing, that I should find those to whom I had not used the burning oil dead empoisoned; which made me rise very early to visit them, where beyond my expectation I found those to whom I had applied my digestive medicine, to feel little pain, and their wounds without inflammation or tumour, having rested reasonably well in the night: the others to whom was used the said burning oil, I found them feverish, with great pain and tumour about the edges of their wounds. I then resolved with myself never so cruelly, to burn poor men wounded with gunshot.

Thus, the young military surgeon in his first encounter with gun shot wounds, was forced by circumstances to improvise and to perform one of the first, albeit modified, randomized controlled trials. His combination of observation, logic, compassion and common sense led him to an improved and more humane method of treatment.

In 1541 Paré was able to leave the army with enough funds to sit the examination and be admitted to the community of barber-surgeons [6]. This was the lowest of the three medical hierarchies in France at that time. The faculty of physicians were university educated and 'did not work with their hands'. The second tier was the surgeons belonging to the College of St. Côme, who confined themselves to minor surgery. The lowest group, the barber-surgeons, while theoretically having the least education, performed most of the major surgery, including amputations [7]. As Paré's reputation grew he was elected, without fee or examination, to the College of St. Côme – a rare honour, indicative of his standing in the surgical community of Paris. Paré married and settled in the parish of St. André des Art on the left bank of the River Seine studying anatomy and practising as a barber-surgeon. However, his skill as a military surgeon frequently led to his recall by the army over the next 32 years.

He published a number of works on anatomy and surgery but it was his *Apologie and Treatise* published in 1585 which represented his collective experience and surgical teachings acquired over almost 50 years of both civilian and military surgery. Paré may have been the first to write of the condition known as 'phantom limb'-the pain experienced in the limb after amputation: *"Verily it is a thing wonderous strange and prodigious, and which will scarce be credited, unless by such as have seen with their eyes and heard with their ears the patients who have many months after the cutting away of the leg, grievously complained that they yet felt exceeding great pain of that leg so cut off"*. [2] He is also credited with discovering the principle of the tourniquet for amputation of the limb [1]: *"Let them be tied with a straight ligature a little above that place of the member which is to be cut off, with a strong and broad fillet like that which women usually bind up their hair withall"* [2].

Paré married in 1541 and had three children by his first wife with only one daughter surviving infancy. After the death of his first wife he remarried at the age of 63 and had six further children, only two daughters surviving. Of his several grandchildren none studied medicine or surgery.

Paré was a Huguenot but he outwardly conformed to Catholicism and remained uninvolved in religious controversy. In August 1572, during the St. Bartholomew's Day Massacre of French Huguenots in Paris, King Charles IX, who had unleashed the Catholic forces, protected Paré by hiding him in his rooms saying "it is not right for a man so useful to the world to perish in such a manner".

Paré died at the age of 80 on 20 December 1590 and was buried in the church of St. André des Arts [8]. On 29 July, 1840 a bronze statute of Ambroise Paré was unveiled in his home town, Laval. Appropriately for a surgeon who frequently credited his success to divine assistance the base of the statue carries one of Paré's most frequent quotations: 'Je le pansay, Dieu le guerit', (I dressed him, God healed him). One of his biographers, Geoffrey Keynes, summarized his career as follows: "He was in fact, by virtue of his personality and his independent mind, the emancipator of surgery from the dead hand of dogma" [2].

## References

[1] Majno G. The Healing Hand: Man and Wound in the Ancient World. Cambridge: Harvard University Press, 1975. p 362–3.

[2] Paré A. The Apologie and Treatise of Ambroise Paré Containing the Voyages Made into Divers Places. With Many of his Writings Upon Surgery. (Edited by Geoffrey Keynes) Chicago: The University of Chicago Press, 1952 pp 23–24, 34–35, 147, 150–1.

[3] Doolin W. The first hurdle: the arrest of haemorrhage. J Irish Med Soc 1956;38:92–8.

[4] Hamby WB. Ambroise Paré: Surgeon of the Renaissance. St. Louis: W.H. Green Inc, 1967.

[5] Baskett TF. On the Shoulders of Giants: Eponyms and Names in Obstetrics and Gynaecology. London: RCOG Press, 1996, p 172–3.

[6] Graham H. The Story of Surgery. New York: Doubleday, Doran & Co Inc, 1939. p140–7.

[7] Shampo MA. Ambroise Paré: Father of Modern Surgery. J Pelvic Surg 1998;4:186–8.

[8] Shah M. Premier Chirugien du Roi: the life of Ambroise Paré (1510–1590). J R Soc Med 1992;85:292–4.

# William Harvey

## M.D.J. McKechnie    C. Robertson

William Harvey (1578–1657) was Britain's great Renaissance man. He has a claim to be the outstanding figure and leader of biological advances in 17th century European medicine, and perhaps the greatest of the early experimental scientists. His demonstration of the circulation of the blood, built on the work of Vesalius and Fabricius and exposing a new physiology, is the finest achievement of Renaissance anatomy. The convulsive effect of his revolutionary work convinced subsequent investigators that medical science and its methodologies had to be reassessed, and new foundations built.

Harvey was born in Folkestone on 1st April 1578, the eldest of nine children. William's early schooling is assumed to have been local, but aged ten he entered the oldest school in England, the King's School in Canterbury where he received a humanist education, reading and writing Latin and gaining a working knowledge of Greek. In May 1593, aged 16, he entered Gonville and Caius College, Cambridge where he studied dialectics and physic, before passing onto medicine proper on receiving a medical scholarship. He graduated B.A. in 1597.

The epicentre of medical education at this time was Padua, and on his 22nd birthday, Harvey enrolled as a student of the leading anatomist of the day, Fabricius. There he learned and absorbed Aristotelian approaches to the study of nature, particularly with regard to comparative anatomy and embryology. From Fabricius, Harvey used dissection to discover how organs worked and became interested in the '*action, function and purpose*' of the parts. In particular, he learned about the valves of the veins from the man who in 1574 had believed himself their first discoverer, and who had begun to demonstrate them in the human subject four or five years later. The full significance of this, for the circulation of the blood, was left to Harvey later to prove.

On 25th April 1602, Harvey graduated M.D. with great distinction, first in the list of English students. His diploma, signed by Fabricius, is in the library of the Royal College of Physicians of London. It gave him leave '*To practise and teach arts and medicine in every land and seat of learning*'. The degree allowed Harvey to incorporate as M.D. at Cambridge, which he did before the year was out.

He settled in Ludgate and became a Candidate or Member of the College of Physicians, a prerequisite along with the doctorate, to practice as a physician in London. He had the serendipitous good fortune to marry, on 24 November 1604, Elizabeth Browne. Elizabeth's father, Dr Lancelot Browne, was Physician to the recently enthroned first monarch of a United Kingdom, King James VI of Scotland and I of England.

After returning to London, Harvey engaged in medical practice and in 1607 was elected a Fellow of the Royal College of Physicians, and in 1609 became physician to St. Bartholomew's Hospital. In 1615 he was appointed Lumleian Lecturer in Anatomy and Surgery to the Royal College, including conducting public dissections. In 1618 he became Physician Extraordinary to James VI of Scotland and I of England and, when Charles I succeeded the latter, he was made Physician in Ordinary.

In 1628 he published, at the Frankfurt book fair, his 72 page volume, *Exercitatio Anatomica de Motu Cordis et Sanguinis in Animalibus* (An Anatomical Essay Concerning the Movement of the Heart and the Blood in Animals), or as it came to be known, *De Motu Cordis.* With the touch paper thus lit, and a receptive and hungry audience throughout Europe, principally in Italy, and the incursion of observations that did not square with the teachings of Galen, the publication and dissemination of ideas within *De Motu Cordis* allowed the birth of modern investigation and experimentation, obeying Harvey's exhortations to see for oneself and '*not from the tenets of Philosophers but from the fabric of Nature.*'

*De Motu Cordis* was not only an exciting statement of a new belief, but also an expression of the way in which physiological truth could be determined, and in incorporating these two methods it has been described as the most important medical work ever written. Nevertheless, it was regarded by many as fanciful and raised doubts about his reliability as a sober clinician, with the result that his practice declined.

To understand the importance and significance of Harvey's hypothesis and demonstration, it is worth recalling the ancient classical model of the blood system still adhered to around 1600.

Ancient Greek and Galenic physiology believed there to be two types of blood, venous and arterial, with distinct pathways and functions relating to the three chief body centres: the liver, heart and brain. These were thought to be responsible for nutrition and growth, vitality, and sensation and reason, respectively. Nourishment and growth were secured by the venous blood originating in the liver, while vitality was conveyed to the body parts by the arterial blood originating in the heart. Arterial life-giving blood contained *spirituous air* or pneuma and blood, and, like venous blood was thought to spread to all parts of the body when needed. This blood did not return to the heart, but was used up in these areas of need. It can thus be seen that there was no question of the blood circulating around the body. Rather, with their separate origins and well-defined functions, the belief was that the venous and arterial bloods were expended. Galenists believed that the blood's movement through the arteries could be explained by an innate *'pulsative faculty'* within the arteries themselves, and that the heart did not pump blood out nor even drive blood through the arteries, but instead sucked blood in during diastole.

This theory had, however several major difficulties. How did the venous blood and air of arterial blood reach the left ventricle of the heart? If air was required for arterial blood, then how did it get there? How did venous blood pass from the right side of the heart to the left?

Galen stated that blood seeped through the interventricular septum, but was unable to explain the pulmonary circulation, there being, it was thought, only enough blood leaving the right side of the heart to sustain the lungs. The function of the pulmonary vein was to convey air from the lungs to the left side of the heart, the resultant mixture of pneuma and blood in the left ventricle being arterial. The 'sooty vapours' produced by this process were exhaled after travelling back whence they came, via the same pulmonary vein. That these anatomical doctrines held sway for so long in the absence of sound evidence says much for the systematic and comprehensible ways in which they were taught and presented.

In the *Fabrica* (1543), Vesalius noted that the vena cava did not arise from the liver and he questioned the permeability of the interventricular septum. Colombo, through vivisection, concluded that systole was the heart's active phase, and Servetus conceived the idea of the pulmonary circulation, which Cesalpino supported along with heart valve action, and the use of the term *circulatio*. In Padua in 1603, Fabricius published his famous description of the valves of the veins, with illustrations later famously copied by his student, Harvey.

Harvey's Paduan experiences set him at the forefront of learned medicine, where Galenic ideas were challenged by Fabricius' Aristotelianism. He had also begun to probe the circulatory system. He had gradually become convinced that the blood circulates, rather than ebbs and flows as previously. He concluded that the heart worked as a muscle with the ventricles contracting and expelling blood in systole rather than sucking it in during diastole. The arterial pulse was the shockwave of the beating heart and not the artery's own intrinsic pulsative faculty.

*De Motu Cordis* falls into two parts, first pointing out Galen's flaws, then turning to experiment to announce Harvey's discovery of the circulation of the blood.

In particular, the work demonstrates uniquely how scientific method could lead to correct interpretation. Harvey asked how air and sooty vapours could be kept apart in the pulmonary vein since, when opened, neither could be seen in that vein, but blood alone. Further, frog vivisections showed the action of the atria and ventricles and the reality of the pulmonary circulation of the blood, while the amount of blood forced out of the heart in an hour far exceeded its volume in the whole animal. Indeed, so much blood left the heart in a minute that it could not possibly be absorbed by the body and continually be replaced by blood made in the liver from chyle.

This quantitative evidence established the constant circulation of the blood; if not then the arteries and body would explode under the pressure.

"Since all things, both argument and ocular demonstration, show that the blood passes through the lungs and heart by the force of the ventricles, and is sent for distribution to all parts of the body, where it makes its way into the veins and porosities of the flesh, and then flows by the veins from the circumference on every side to the centre, from the lesser to the greater veins, and is by them finally discharged into the vena cava and right auricle of the heart, and this in such a quantity or in such a flux and reflux thither by the arteries, hither by the veins, as cannot possibly be supplied by the ingesta, and is much greater than can be required for mere purposes of nutrition; it is absolutely necessary to conclude that the blood in the animal body is impelled in a circle, and is in a state of ceaseless motion".

What could not be demonstrated was the display of the complete cycle of the circular movement of the blood. Harvey lacked accurate knowledge of the capillary connection between arteries and veins, though he spoke of them. Malpighi, professor of medicine in Pisa, and Leeuwenhoek later saw and described the capillaries with the early microscope. In *De Pulmonibus* in 1661, Malpighi described the fine texture of blood vessels, the missing link in Harvey's theory, and thus provided decisive confirmation of the circulation of the blood. Harvey however, in a simple experiment, had already shown that such a connection must exist.

By ligating a forearm extremely tightly so that no arterial blood could flow below the ligature down the arm, it was then loosened so that arterial blood flowed down the arm, but venous blood did not move back above the ligature. When tight, the veins in the arm below the ligature had appeared normal, but now became swollen, showing that blood had poured down the arteries and back up the arm within the veins. Therefore, there had to be as yet undiscovered routes at the extremities for blood to pass from arteries to veins. He also demonstrated that the valves in the veins always directed blood back to the heart. Having displayed the circulation and the one-way valve system, Harvey was then able to explain that his practical discovery had far reaching effects in altering conceptions of disease. In Chapter XVI of *De Motu Cordis* he states that there are certain problems connected with

"contagious poisoned wounds, the bites of serpents and rabid animals, lues venerea and the like. We sometimes see the whole system contaminated, though the part first infected remains sound. Whence it appears that the contagion impressed upon or deposited in a particular part, is by-and-by carried by the returning current of blood to the heart, and by that organ is sent to contaminate the whole body".

This is quite a clear modern picture of septicaemia, bacteraemia, toxaemia and focal infection.

In 1633 Harvey was commanded by King Charles I to accompany him to Scotland for his Scottish coronation in Edinburgh. It is conjectured, though there is no documentation to support the probability, that he would have been formally introduced to Dr John Makluire, a prominent Edinburgh physician, who during the King and Court's subsequent sojourn in Edinburgh in 1641, may have facilitated the medically celebrated occasion of the visit paid to the Court by the young Hugh Montgomery, eldest son and heir of Hugh,

2nd Viscount Montgomery of the Ards in Ireland. This was the visit during which the cavity in the chest wall of the young man, dating from a childhood injury, and exposing his beating heart both to view and to touch, was examined by Harvey and demonstrated to the King in person. Harvey, at the time of his second visit to Edinburgh in 1641, had already been collecting material for his second book, *De Generatione Animalium*. This incorporated an account of his historic examination of the exposed heart of the young Hugh Montgomery, described explicitly by Harvey as 'this wonderful experiment'. Harvey's account reads:

"A noble young gentleman, son and heir to the honorable the Vice-Count of Mountgomery in Ireland, when he was a child, had a strange mishap by an unexpected fall, causing a fracture in the ribs on the left side: the bruise was brought to a suppuration, whereby a great quantity of putrified matter was voided out, and this putrefaction gushed out for a long while together out of the wide wound. This person of honour, about the eighteenth or nineteenth year of his age, having been a traveller in Italy and France, arrived at last at London: having all this time a very wide gap open in his breast, so that you might see and touch his lungs (as it was believed)".

When I came near him, and saw him a sprightly youth, with a good complexion, and habit of body, I supposed, some body or other had framed an untruth. He discovered all to me, and opened the void part of his left side, taking off that small plate, which he wore to defend it against any blow or outward injury.

Where I presently beheld a vast hole in his breast, into which I could easily put my three forefingers, and my thumb; and at the first entrance I perceived a certain fleshy part sticking out, which was driven in and out by a reciprocal motion, whereupon I gently handled it in my hand.

Being now amazed at the novelty of the thing, I search it again and again, and having diligently enough enquired into all, it was evident, that that old and vast ulcer (for want of the help of a skilfull physician) was miraculously healed, and skinned over with a membrane on the inside, and guarded with flesh all about the brimmes or margent of it. By its pulse, and the difference or rhythm thereof, or the time which it kept, (and laying one hand upon his wrest, and the other upon his heart) and also by comparing and considering his respirations, I concluded it to be no part of the lungs, but the cone or substance of the heart.

Harvey was said to be a small, swarthy sharp-eyed man, rapid in utterance and short of temper. He constantly fingered the dagger he always wore, but was always ready to instruct any that were modest and respectful to him. He had numerous idiosyncrasies including; keeping sugar in his salt cellar, combing his hair while walking about the fields instead of indoors, and treating his own gout by immersing his legs in a bucket of cold water and afterwards roasting them in front of a fire. He was said to be addicted to the newly-arrived coffee.

In 1645 Harvey was elected to the honourable position of warden of Merton College at the University of Oxford, but because of the tumult of the Cromwellian Civil War, he held this position for only a year. The surrender of Oxford in 1645 marks the period of Harvey's severance from the Court and his gradual retirement from public life, occasioned in part by his being affected with gout, from which he suffered recurrent attacks. During this time he was preparing *De Generatione Animalium* (1651).

The College of Physicians was promised, by an anonymous donor, a library of books, a museum of numerous objects of curiosity, and a variety of surgical instruments. Before the building was completed the generous benefactor became known, and the College responded in 1652 by commissioning Harvey's statue. Still feeling indebted to him, the College chose Harvey as its President in 1654, but he declined because of his deteriorating health. His attacks of gout increased, and he died on 3 June 1657, of a cerebral haemorrhage. He was buried in the family vault at the Church of St. Andrew, Hempstead, Essex.

"... it (De Motu Cordis) marks the break of the modern spirit with the old traditions. No longer were men to rest content with careful observation and with accurate description; no longer were men to be content with finely spun theories and dreams, which serve as a common subterfuge of ignorance; but here for the first time a great physiological problem was approached from the experimental side by a man with a modern scientific mind, who could weigh evidence and not go beyond it, and who had the sense to let the conclusions emerge naturally but firmly from the observations". (Sir William Osler, 1849–1919).

## Acknowledgements

With grateful thanks to John Dallas, Rare Books Librarian at the Royal College of Physicians of Edinburgh.

## Further Reading

Harris CRS. The heart and the vascular system in ancient Greek medicine; from Alcmaeon to Galen. Oxford: Clarendon Press, 1973.

Franklin KJ. (Trans.) De Circulatione Sanguinis by William Harvey. Oxford: Blackwell, 1958.

Keynes G. The life of William Harvey. Oxford: Clarendon Press, 1966.

McHarg JF. In search of Dr. John MakLuire. Wellcome, University of Glasgow, 1997.

Porter R. The greatest benefit to mankind; a medical history of humanity from antiquity to the present. Fontana, 1999.

Ellis H. A History of Surgery. Greenwich Medical Media, 2001.

James DG. To the immortal memory of Dr. William Harvey (1578–1657). Hospital Update Plus, June 1992, pp. 70–71.

# Robert Hooke and the origins of artificial respiration

Thomas F. Baskett

That respiratory action was necessary for human life must have been evident in the pre-historic era. From the time of Vesalius, it was known that artificial inflation of the lungs was required to keep an experimental animal alive in order to examine its thoracic contents. In studying the anatomy and function of the heart and lungs, it was observed that thoracotomy led to collapse of the lungs and death of the animal within a short time. Vesalius found that by making an incision in the trachea and passing a tube of reed or cane through the opening the lungs could be reinflated: "But that life may in a manner of speaking be restored to the animal … you will then blow into this, so that the lung may rise again and the animal take in air. Indeed, with a slight breath in the case of this living animal the lung will swell to the full extent of the thoracic cavity, and the heart become strong and exhibit a wondrous variety of motions" [1].

Robert Hooke was among the most brilliant of a gifted group of British scientists in the latter part of the 17th century, which included Robert Boyle, Isaac Newton, Thomas Willis and Christopher Wren. He was curator of the Royal Society of London for 20 years and in this position he regularly produced scientific experiments to accommodate the wide variety of interests of the membership. In one such sequence of experiments, he turned his attention to the problems of artificial respiration, more than a century after the work of Vesalius. Hooke demonstrated this technique to the fellows of the Royal Society in October 1667. Using a pair of bellows attached to a pipe in the trachea of a dog he showed that as long as the lungs were inflated the motion of the heart was normal. Upon removing the bellows "the lungs would presently grow flaccid, and the heart begin to have convulsive motions: but upon renewing the motion of the bellows the heart recovered its former motion, and the convulsions ceased" [1]. At this time, it was felt that the mo-

tion of the lungs was necessary to promote the circulation of blood and that it was the movement of the lungs, rather than the presence of the air within them, that was essential for cardiac function.

On 24 October 1667, Hooke again demonstrated this experiment to fellows of the Royal Society but extended his study to demonstrate that it was the supply of air within the lungs rather than their motion that was essential [2]:

> I caused another pair of bellowes to be immediately joyn'd to the first, by a contrivance, I had prepar'd, and pricking all the outer-coat of the lungs with the slender point of a very sharp pen-knife, this second pair of Bellows was mov'd very quick, whereby the first pair was always kept full and always blowing into the lungs; by which means the lungs also were always kept very full, and without any motion; there being a continual blast of air forc'd into the lungs by the first pair of bellows, supplying it as fast, as it could find its way quite through the coat of the lungs by the small holes pricked in it, as was said before. This being continued for a pretty while, the dog, as I expected, lay still, as before, his eyes being all the time very quick, and his heart beating very regularly; but, upon ceasing this blast, and suffering the lungs to fall and lye still, the dog would immediately fall into dying convulsive fits; but be as soon reviv'd again by the renewing the fullness of his lungs with the constant blast of fresh air.

Thus, Hooke was the first to show that the motion of the heart and the movement of the lungs were independent of each other. In the final paragraph of his short communication to the Society, Hooke outlined the possibility of extra-corporeal respiration; "I shall shortly further try, whether the suffering the blood to circulate through a vessel, so as it may be openly exposed to the fresh air, will not suffice for the life of an animal; and make some other experiments, which, I hope, will thoroughly discover the genuine use of respiration; and afterwards consider of what benefit this may be to mankind" [2].

Hooke's previous experiments with combustion had shown that fresh air was essential for burning charcoal. Using bellows directed at a charcoal fire Hooke demonstrated that adding fresh air increased the fire, but if air was removed the fire ceased despite the vigorous use of bellows. He also showed that by adding "satiated" air, rather than fresh air, the fire would be extinguished. Thus, 100 years before the discovery of oxygen Hooke drew the analogy between fresh and satiated air in combustion and for respiration in animals:

> Somewhat like this is observable in the life of animals, who live no longer than they have a constant supply of fresh air to breath, and, as it were, blow the fire of life; for so soon as that supply is wanting, the fire goes out, and the animal dies, and all the other vital functions cease; as one may presently see if he puts a small animal as a bird, or the like, into a small glass and covers it close; for in a short time the air becomes satiated, and is no longer fit for respiration; but though the animal breath it as before, and pant and move his lungs as before; yet if the air be not fresh, the fire of life with extinguish [3]."

Here again, Hooke observed that movement of the lungs was not essential to life but rather the passage of fresh air into the lungs:

> Some learned philosophers and physicians have been of the opinion, that the use of breathing was for nothing else, but that by the motion of the lungs the blood might be kept circulating which past through them, or that the steams of the blood might be carried off, which it could not when it was full of steams; but by many trials of I have proved that neither of those are at all the cause of death of the creature, but only the want of fresh air. For whether the lungs move or not move, if fresh air be supplied the animal lives, if it be wanting, it dies [3].

Robert Hooke was born on 18 July 1635 at Freshwater, Isle of Wight where his father was rector of the parish. He was described as a sickly child and throughout his life suffered from headaches, vertigo and intestinal irritability. For the first 6 years of his life he was fed largely milk and fruit. He showed scholastic promise and his father steered him toward a career in the ministry, but young Robert was more interested in tinkering with machines and instruments, as well as showing an inherent talent for sketching and painting. He took a brass clock to pieces, studied its mechanism, and built a wooden replica that was still working 60 years later [4]. His father died when Robert was 13, following which he entered Westminister School and became fluent in Latin and Greek as well as displaying obvious ability in mechanics and mathematics. At the age of 18, he went to Christ Church, Oxford, as a chorister. In this capacity, he acted as a servant to one of the fellows and assisted Thomas Willis in his laboratory. Willis later studied the central nervous system and described the blood vessels at the base of the brain; 'The Circle of Willis'. Hooke's mechanical skill brought him to the attention of Robert Boyle who he assisted in the construction of Boyle's air pump and the later enunciation of Boyle's Law. At this stage of his life, Hooke had very limited financial means and he left Oxford without graduating. However, in 1663, he was awarded the MA from Oxford and in 1691 the degree, Doctor of Physics, in the Doctors's Commons [3,5].

The Royal Society of London was founded in 1660 and the exclusive group of members met regularly in Gresham College. In 1662, Robert Hooke was appointed curator, as the members needed someone to design and conduct experiments for their regular meetings and Hooke needed the annual stipend that the position carried. In this position, to some extent a servant to the gentleman members, Hooke's talent for mechanical innovation and the design and building of the equipment necessary to carry out experiments was invaluable. The range of subjects that took his attention included astronomy, geology, biology, optics, the nature of air, the laws of falling bodies, diving-bells and methods of telegraphy. He developed the universal joint and formulated Hooke's Law of the extension and compression of elastic bodies. Samuel Pepys was a member of the Royal Society who admired and acknowledged Hooke's ability in his diary [6].

In the medical realm, Hooke discussed the potential value of auscultation 150 years before Laennec's treatise on the stethoscope [3]:

> There may also be a possibility of discovering the internal motions of actions of bodies by the sound they make, who knows but that as in a watch we may hear the beating of the balance and the running of the wheels and the striking of the hammers, and the grating of the teeth and a multitude of other noises; who knows, I say, but that it may be possible to discover the motions of the internal parts of bodies, whether animal, vegetable or mineral by the sound they make, that one may discover the works performed in the several offices and shops of a man's body, and thereby discover what instrument or engine is out of order more ... and somewhat more of encouragement I have also from experience, that I have been able to hear very plainly the beating of a man's heart.

In his capacity as curator of the Royal Society, Hooke corresponded with Anton van Leeuwenhoek who frequently reported his findings with early microscopy to the Society [7]. This stimulated Hooke's own investigation with the microscope, one of which involved observations on urinary sediments. He noted, in response to the age-old problem of urinary calculi, that further study by "physicians or chemists" might lead to an alternative to the brutal pre-anaesthetic era of lithotomy by discovery of a substance that could "... dissolve stone without hurting the bladder" [3].

No known portrait of Hooke exists. Although his name is printed 'Hook' in the edition of the *Philosophical Transactions* carrying his classical observations, his signature in

(517)                    *Numb.* 28.

# PHILOSOPHICAL
## TRANSACTIONS.

Monday, *October* 21. 1667.

(539)

*An Account*
*Of an Experiment made by M.*Hook, *of Preserving Animals alive by Blowing through their Lungs with Bellows.*

*This Noble Experiment came not to the* Publisher's *hands, till all the preceding Particulars were already sent to the Press, and almost all Printed off,* (*for which cause also it could not be mentioned among the* Contents:) *And it might have been reserved for the next opportunity, had not the considerableness thereof been a motive to hasten its Publication. It shall be here annexed in the Ingenious Author his own words, as he presented it to the* Royal Society, *Octob.* 24. 1667. *the Experiment it self having been* both *repeated (after a former successful trial of it, made by the same hand a good while agoe)* and *improved the week before, at their* publick *Assembly. The Relation it self followes ;*

I Did heretofore give this *Illustrious Society* an account of an Experiment I formerly tryed of keeping a Dog alive after his *Thorax* was all display'd by the cutting away of the *Ribbs* and *Diaphragme*; and after the *Pericardium* of the Heart also was taken off. But divers persons seeming to doubt of the certainty of the Experiment (by reason that some Tryals of this matter, made by some other hands, failed of success) I caus'd at the last Meeting the same Experiment to be shewn in the presence of this *Noble Company*, and that with the same success, as it had been made by me at first; the Dog being kept alive by the Reciprocal blowing up of his Lungs with *Bellowes*, and they suffered to subside, for the space of an hour or more, after his *Thorax* had been so display'd, and his *Aspera arteria* cut off just below the *Epiglottis*, and bound on upon the nose of the Bellows.

Fig. 1. Philosophical Transactions 1667;2: 539–40.

the Charter Book of the Royal Society clearly spells his surname 'Hooke' [3]. He was described as irascible and often defended his priority in experiments against other scientists. He is said to have frequently argued with Sir Isaac Newton and, although both initially had considerable respect for each other's ability, relations between them grew acrimonious [8]. After the great fire of 1666 Hooke presented a model for the rebuilding of London. Ultimately, Sir Christopher Wren's plan was adopted, but Hooke was appointed surveyor and assisted Wren. Hooke's relentless stream of innovation in so many subjects led him to experiment and invent, but he did not take the time to perfect his discoveries. Thus, others improved and perfected his ideas and gained the credit. It was said that 'his extraordinary ingenuity was marred by his extraordinary versatility' [8]. His temperament was described as 'melancholy, mistrustful and jealous' [8]. Hooke did not marry or have children. He died on 3 March 1702 and was buried in the Church of St. Helen, Bishopsgate (Fig. 1).

The work of Hooke and others within the Royal Society established the principles of artificial respiration in experimental animals and helped lay the foundation for its application in humans in the next century after the discovery of carbon dioxide and oxygen, and the establishment of societies to resuscitate the apparently drowned.

## References

[1] Baker AB. Artificial respiration, the history of an idea. Med Hist 1971;15:336–46.

[2] An account of an experiment made by M. Hook, of preserving animals alive by blowing through their lungs with bellows. Philos Trans 1667;2:539–40.

[3] Middleton WS. The medical aspect of Robert Hooke. Ann Med Hist 1927;9:227–43.

[4] Nichols R. Robert Hooke and the Royal Society. Sussex: The Book Guild Ltd.; 1999.

[5] Talbot JH. A biographical history of medicine. New York: Grune and Stratton; 1970. p. 139–42.

[6] Tomalin C. Samuel Pepys: the unequalled self. London: Penguin Books; 2003. p. 256, 427.

[7] Baskett TF. Anton von Leeuwenhoek. On the shoulders of giants: eponyms and names in obstetrics and gynaecology. London: RCOG Press; 1996. p. 121.

[8] Hunter M, Schaffer S, editors. Robert Hooke: new studies. Woodbridge: The Boydell Press; 1989. p. 1–19.

# John Mayow and oxygen

George L. Sternbach    Joseph Varon

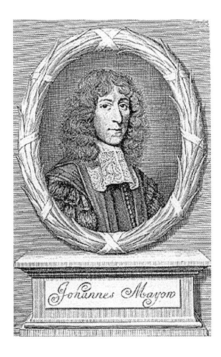

Johannes Mayow

The exact date and place of John Mayow's birth are uncertain. He was born sometime between 1640 and 1645, either in London or Cornwall [1,2]. He entered Wadham College, Oxford in 1658. It was an active time for science at Oxford. Robert Boyle, Christopher Wren, Richard Lower and Robert Hooke were all at the university during this period. Mayow studied law, earning a doctorate of civil law in 1670. There is no record that he ever received a medical degree [1,2]. Nevertheless, his scientific studies at Oxford, together with his degree in civil law rendered him capable of practicing medicine, which he did in both London and in the spa town of Bath.

Mayow's studies included the mechanics of respiration, the function of the intercostal muscles, the supply of nutrients to the fetus, and physical findings in rickets. His most important contribution to science was the determination that only a portion of air—the substance he termed "nitro-aerial" or "igneo-aerial"—was necessary for sustaining life. Mayow may have conducted his research in Boyle's laboratory. His equipment included an air pump similar to that used by Boyle in his gas experiments, but Boyle does not mention Mayow's work in his writings [3], and the time and place of the research are unknown [1].

Mayow published two books, both written in Latin, as was customary for medical works of the time. The first, *Tractatus duo Quorom prior agit de Respiratione*, was issued in 1668, and is considered by some to be his greatest work [2]. Six years later, a compilation of his work appeared. This was titled *Tractatus Quince Medico-Physici*. The studies in this text were arranged by the author in order of their importance. The first and longest, comprising 15 chapters, involved experiments on the chemical and physical properties of air, a component of which—the "nitro-aerial spirit" or "igneo-aerial particles"—was necessary to support a flame and to sustain life.

Using jars inverted over water into which animals and lighted candles had been placed, Mayow observed the nearly simultaneous extinction of the flame and vital functions of life as the critical component of air was consumed:

> "[A]nimals and fire draw particles of the same kind from the air...[L]et any animal be enclosed in a glass vessel along with a lamp so that the entrance of air from without is prevented...When this is done we shall soon see the lamp go out and the animal will not long survive the fatal torch." [1].

Mayow thus recognized the parallel between combustion and respiration. He realized that when substances burned in air, a chemical interaction took place with a particular constituent of that air:

"I take it for granted that the air contains certain parti-cles...which are absolutely indispensable for the produc-tion of fire, and that these in the burning of flame are drawn from the air and removed."

Moreover, it was not air as a whole that supported com-bustion, but only "its more active and subtle part". Simi-larly, the nitro-aerial constituent was extracted from air in the process of respiration, then carried to the tissues by ar-terial blood, which it made brighter and redder than venous blood. However, nitro-aerial particles could not be stored, and had to be replaced without interruption in order for life to be sustained.

Mayow's work was largely overlooked during his lifetime, and some have subsequently accused him of appropriating his ideas regarding respiration from Boyle and others [2]. Mayow died in 1679 in his 30s, thus precluding a prolonged career of scientific investigation. During the century that followed his death, his insight was eclipsed by the phlogiston theory, an erroneous concept that was nonetheless widely believed until disproved by the radical Unitarian minister Joseph Priestley in 1774.

Put forth in 1697 by the German chemist (and physician to King Frederick William I of Prussia) Georg Ernst Stahl, this theory held that "all combustible material contains some-thing (a phlogiston) that, on heating, is transformed into fire" [4]. Therefore, material was considered by this theory to contain the medium of its own combustion. The phlo-giston theory endured in the face of experimental evidence that the weight of metals that are burned increased during the process. Stahl explained this phenomenon by attributing negative weight to phlogiston [5].

In August 1774, Priestley discovered that a gas was lib-erated when he heated the mineral mercuric oxide. In the atmosphere of this gas, a candle burned more brightly, and a mouse could live longer than when sealed in a comparable volume of air. He reported his findings to the Royal Soci-ety, indicating that he had found a gas "much better than common air" [5].

In the course of his experiments, Priestley made some noteworthy observations. Intrigued by the salutary effects of the gas, he "gratified that curiosity by breathing it" himself. Announcing that "hitherto only two mice and I have had the privilege of breathing it", Priestley was careful not to overstate the effects:

"The feeling of it in my lungs was not sensibly different from common air, but I fancied that my breast felt pecu-liarly light for some time afterward. Who can tell but that, in time, this pure air may become a fashionable article of luxury."

Remarkably, he postulated a possible medical use, stating "it may be conjectured that it might be peculiarly salutary to the lungs in certain morbid cases." These insights appear sophisticated and prescient today. Priestley had not had ex-tensive training in chemistry, though. Unable to abandon the

phlogiston theory, he called the gas "dephlogisticated air" [6].

Later that same year, Priestley was invited to Paris by Antoine-Laurent Lavoisier, perhaps then the world's most eminent chemist. He presented his experimental findings at a distinguished gathering hosted by Lavoisier. As a conse-quence of this interaction, Lavoisier began his own exper-iments with the gas. He came to agree that air contained an element that supported life and combustion. Lavoisier initially called this element "eminently breathable air". Subsequently, incorrectly believing it to be a component of all acids, he chose to rename it "acidifying principle". He used the Greek root *oxus geinomais*, meaning "acid generator"—"oxygene" in French.

Although Lavoisier and Priestley are generally credited with the discovery of oxygen, the Swedish apothecary, Carl Wilhelm Scheele may have generated the gas through a vari-ety of chemical reactions as early as 1771 [6]. Scheele noted atmospheric air to be composed of one part "fire air" and three parts "vitiated air" (nitrogen) [7]. The publication of his findings having been delayed, he claimed to have written to Lavoisier in September 1774 describing the production of "fire air". Lavoisier subsequently denied ever receiving or even seeing Scheele's correspondence. It has been claimed that, among Nordic historians, Lavoisier "has never been forgiven for this rebuff" [6]. In 1775, Lavoisier announced to the French Academie de Sciences that he had identified that portion of atmospheric air essential for respiration. He made no reference to either Priestley or Scheele.

The work of Mayow, performed more than a century ear-lier, was now largely forgotten. However, his outlook on res-piration and combustion were nearer the modern one than was the phlogiston theory [3]. He had recognized these two processes to be analogous. With the passage of time, his standing among scientists has improved [1–3].

He is not, however, universally admired. According to critics, Mayow expanded his theory to cover, on the basis of little evidence, "a ridiculously wide range of phenomena" [8]. In addition to combustion and respiration, Mayow wrote about the influence of nitro-aerial spirit on "light, lightning, quicklime, and the thermal springs of Bath" [9]. He has been criticized of providing "a mass of speculations almost entirely unsupported by any kind of evidence" [9,10].

Should Mayow be credited as being the earliest to iden-tify oxygen? Has his discovery been overlooked because he applied to it the less euphonous name of "nitro-aerial particles"? Though he rightly concluded that only a fraction of air was essential for respiration, he did not recognize that this substance was a gas that could be isolated. His views on combustion and respiration were clearly ahead of their time, however. Had they been followed up, the correct un-derstanding of the function of oxygen might have emerged far earlier than it did [1,2].

Mayow's work was instrumental in understanding the need for oxygen in all animals for carrying on life processes. Despite his work and that of his successors, the vital role of oxygen in aerobic cellular metabolism is relatively recent. It was not until 1917 that J. S. Haldane described the "recuperative benefits of inspiring oxygen" [11]. Haldane suspected that even moderate increases in percent of oxygen in inspired air could reverse cyanosis and could be beneficial for inflammatory conditions of the lungs as well as for failure of the circulation. Since then, clinicians have developed a variety of oxygen delivery systems to assist patients [12]. Perhaps we should say: a variety of "nitro-aerial particles" delivery systems?

## References

[1] Partington JR. The life and work of John Mayow (1641–1679), Part 1. Isis 1956;47:217–30.

[2] John Mayow (1641–1679). J. Am. Med. Assoc. 1966;197:142–3 [editorial].

[3] Partington JR. The life and work of John Mayow (1641–1679), Part 2. Isis 1956;47:405–16.

[4] Lindahl SGE. Phlogiston-fire air-oxygen: the fascinating story of an 18th century discovery. Acta Anesthesiol Scand 2002;46:1.

[5] Comroe JH. Retrospecotscope: insights into medical discovery. Menlo Park, CA: Von Gehr Press, 1977. p. 117–8.

[6] Severinghaus JW. Priestley, the furious free thinker of the enlightenment, and Scheele, the taciturn apothecary of Uppsala. Acta Anesthesiol Scand 2002;46:2–9.

[7] Harken AH. Oxygen, politics and the American Revolution (with a note on the bicentennial of phlogiston). Ann Surg 1976;184:645–50.

[8] Guerlac H. The poets' nitre. Isis 1954;45:243–55.

[9] Patterson TS. John Mayow in contemporary setting. II. Mayow's views on combustion. Isis 1931;15:504–46.

[10] Patterson TS. John Mayow in contemporary setting. Isis 1931;15:47–96.

[11] Haldane JS. The therapeutic administration of oxygen. Br Med J 1917;i:181–3.

[12] Fromm RE, Varon J. State of the art: oxygen therapy. Hosp Physician 1993;29:19–26.

# THE 1700s

The second half of the 18<sup>th</sup> century has come to be known as *The Age of Enlightenment*. It was the time of musicians of genius like Beethoven and Mozart, the great poets such as Wordsworth, Coleridge and Burns, the artistry of Constable, the harnessing of steam by James Watt, and the mastery of language by Roget. Georgian architecture in Bath, Bristol, London and many other cities and the accompanying furniture and silver were in their hey-day. Humphry Davy experimented with nitrous oxide in Bristol and noted it gave a pleasurable feeling when it was inhaled and even observed that a person under the influence who struck his leg with some force on a bench appeared to experience no pain.
But did we learn? - not for another 45 years.

England was under the rule of George III, the so-called mad king, who nevertheless ruled over one of the most inspiring and important periods of history. France was in upheaval with the French Revolution. The consequences were to reverberate around Europe and even impinge on the lives of some of the Resuscitation Greats such as **Priestley** and **Lavoisier**. The United States of America gained its independence from Britain and Captain Cook discovered Australia.

At this time a spirit of philanthropy became widespread and there was a special interest in the management of the apparently drowned. With the prominence of seafaring, many young lives were lost through drowning and these were considered to be a potentially unnecessary tragic human loss and also an economic drain of valuable young manpower. Starting in Holland, perhaps because of the additional risk imposed by the canal network, **Humane Societies** were created across the United Kingdom, Europe and in the United States to encourage rescue from water and enhance the management of the apparently drowned. They were supported by the wealthy, and indeed also the rank and file as they could afford it. Many hospitals were built at the time catering for all and supported by generous endowments.
New techniques of resuscitation were important and many researchers became involved. **Munro** reported to **Dr Cullen and Lord Cathcart** that tracheal intubation with a curved silver catheter was perfectly feasible. **Benjamin Pugh** was able to do the same in a neonate. Between them, **Priestley, Scheele and Lavoisier** had isolated oxygen and shown that life depended on it. Mouth-to-mouth ventilation was considered feasible but undesirable and indeed unacceptable to some. In the course of his quest for knowledge of anatomy and its application to surgery **John Hunter** was able to demonstrate the possibility of lung ventilation using bellows and attempted to revive persons after judicial hanging in that way. **Charles Kite** made profound contributions to the management of the apparently drowned in his renowned essay on the subject. He emphasised the importance of detailed comprehensive records and presenting them at meetings. He introduced the application of electricity in cardio-respiratory arrest with apparent success. This was supported by **Herholdt** and **Rafn** in Denmark who called electricity "the best cardiacum".
But did we learn? – not for 150 more years.

# Benjamin Pugh: the air-pipe and neonatal resuscitation

Thomas F. Baskett

Benjamin Pugh, one of ten children, was born in Bishop's Castle, Shropshire in 1715. His uncle was a local surgeon and may have supervised Pugh's early training. He became an apothecary and surgeon having spent some time in London [1]. He moved to Essex in 1738 and established his practice in Chelmsford. There he married the widowed daughter of a local apothecary, which provided a substantial property inheritance upon the death of his father-in-law. From this, Pugh built his 'mansion house' on the site of 26 High Street, Chelmsford. Pugh was a successful practitioner and a respected and active member of community affairs. He served as a custodian of the local charity school and water charity, as well as being a member of the parish committe [2].

Pugh was one of the first to use inoculation against smallpox. He began this practice in 1746 and is said to have inoculated between 3000 and 4000 patients. He described his technique in correspondence in the *Gentleman's Magazine* [3]. Between July 1752 and April 1753, Pugh recorded 290 cases of smallpox in the Chelmsford area, 95 of them fatal [2].

Pugh's main fame rests with his publication *A Treatise of Midwifery* in 1754 (Fig. 1). As he said in the preface to his *Treatise*, his motive for publication was "...to recommend to public practice some instruments and other observations, and improvements in the art after 14 years practice, in which time I have delivered upwards of 2000 women with the greatest success..." [4]. Much of his rationale for publication was to publicise his new obstetric forceps. He may have been the first to design and use the pelvic curve on obstetric forceps. In the preface he claims: "The curved forceps I invented upwards of 14 years ago, made

me by a man of Mr. Archers, Cutler, now living in Chelmsford." He tried to publish his treatise four years earlier by filling a subscription. This is supported by an advertisement he placed in the *Ipswich Journal*, 16 April, 1748 for the sale of the *Treatise* and forceps [5]. However, this subscription was not filled: hence, the publication of his *Treatise* was delayed. The case can therefore be made that it was Pugh, rather than William Smellie and André Levret, who had primacy for development of the pelvic curve of obstetric forceps [6]. The design of these obstetric forceps is illustrated in his *Treatise*. Although it has received

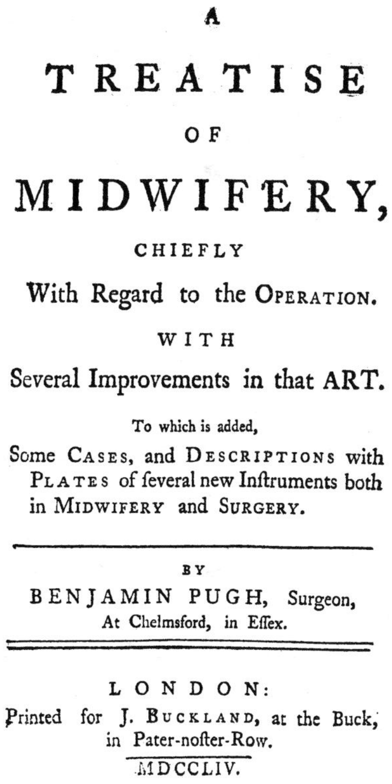

A

# TREATISE

OF

# MIDWIFERY,

CHIEFLY

With Regard to the OPERATION.

WITH

Several Improvements in that ART.

To which is added,

Some CASES, and DESCRIPTIONS with PLATES of several new Inftruments both in MIDWIFERY and SURGERY.

BY

BENJAMIN PUGH, Surgeon,
At Chelmsford, in Effex.

LONDON:
Printed for J. BUCKLAND, at the Buck,
in Pater-nofter-Row.
MDCCLIV.

Fig. 1. Title page of Benjamin Pugh's Treatise.

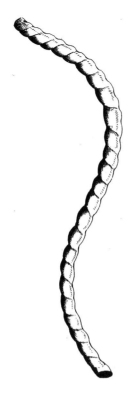

Fig. 2. Pugh's air-pipe.

less notice, Benjamin Pugh made a considerable contribution to neonatal resuscitation. In his *Treatise* he describes and illustrates his air-pipe (Fig. 2):

"The air-pipe, as a big as a swan's quill in the inside, ten inches long, is made of a small common wire, turned very close (in the manner wire-springs are made) will turn any way; and covered with thin soft leather, one end is introduced with the palm of the hand, and between the fingers that are in the child's mouth, as far as the larynx, the other end external."

Pugh initially advocated the use of his air-pipe in cases of breech extraction during delay in delivery of the after-coming head. He used the air-pipe in the manner quoted above as "I found many children were lost in this situation, for want of air..." Pugh then described an alternative method which he had developed making the use of his air-pipe rarely necessary:

"You must then introduce the fingers of your left hand into the vagina, under the child's breast, and put the first and second fingers into the child's mouth pretty far, so far, however, that you are able to press down the child's tongue in such a manner that by keeping your hand hollow, and pressing it upon the mother's rectum, the air may have access to the larynx, you will soon perceive the thorax expand, as the air gets into the lungs."

Pugh emphasised the risk of asphyxia to the fetus during delivery of the after-coming head of the breech saying "...every operator must know there is difficulty, and grave danger of losing the child by its stay in the passage; by my method of giving the child air, I have saved great numbers of childrens' lives, which otherwise would have died". Furthermore, Pugh goes on to give a remarkable early description of mouth-to-mouth respiration.

"If the child does not breath immediately upon delivery, which sometimes it will not, especially if it has taken air in the womb; wipe its mouth, and press your mouth to the child's, at the same time pinching the nose with your thumb and finger, to prevent the air escaping; inflate the lungs, rubbing it before the fire: by which method I have saved many."

It is interesting to compare Pugh's advice with extracts from the current International Liaison Committee on Resuscitation advisory statement on resuscitation of the newly born infant [7]. This report includes the following phrases "Assisted ventilation should be initiated after stimulation if the infant is apneic" and "to decrease the risk of infection to the rescuer, maternal blood and other body fluids should first be wiped from the face of the infant" and "Consensus continues to support initial attempts at ventilation via both the patient's mouth and nose, with the creation of a functional seal to ensure chest rise and ventilation..."

There is little reference to neonatal resuscitation in the obstetric texts of the 18th century, at which time it was considered fortunate if the mother survived. One exception was in the *Treatise on the Theory and Practice of Midwifery* by William Smellie, the celebrated Scottish obstetrician who, in 1752, outlined the standard approach to neonatal resuscitation of that era [8]: "...the child is kept warm, moved, shaken, whipd; the head, temples and breast, rubbed with spirits, garlick, onion or mustard applied to the mouth and nose..." He did, however, also advocate a form of artificial respiration "...the child has been sometimes recovered by blowing into the mouth with a silver cannula, so as to expand the lungs" [8]. Two years later, the same year as Pugh's published *Treatise*, Smellie published the second volume of his work and again proposed a method of artificial respiration for the newborn than "seemed to be dead, after all the common efforts were used for its recovery". He went on "Nevertheless, I inflated the lungs, by blowing into the mouth through a female catheter, and the child gave one gasp, upon which I repeated its inflation at several intervals, until the child began to breath and it actually recovered [9].

Smellie's description is less precise than Pugh's, who designed his own air-pipe and described placing this at the larynx to improve aeration, whereas Smellie seemed to improvise with a female catheter and only described blowing air into the mouth, as opposed to gaining access to the larynx.

In the preface to Pugh's Treatise, he clearly felt that it was the duty of the obstetrician to look after the safety of both the mother and the infant, "Consider there are two lives at stake, and no man of any goodness and humanity will do a bad thing" [4].

No other obstetric text of that time gave such an accurate description of mouth-to-mouth respiration in the newborn. The first account of mouth-to-mouth respiration was written in 1744 by the Scottish surgeon William Tossach [10]. However, it wasn't until the formation of the Societies for the Recovery of Persons Apparently Drowned, which evolved into the Humane Societies in the late 1700s, that coordinated efforts at resuscitation began. Long before mouth-to-mouth resuscitation was attempted in adults it seems that this method was tried instinctively in the newborn and there are accounts in the Hebrew Bible [10]. The Hebrew midwife Puah "breathed into the baby's mouth to induce the baby to cry" (Exodus 1:17).

Pugh retired from practice in 1779, his wife having died two years before. He spent some years traveling in Britain and the continent. He remarried and in 1788 bought Midford Castle, a moderate country estate outside Bath. Benjamin Pugh died on February 14, 1798 and was buried at St. Peter's Church, Freshford. Inside and above the entrance to the church there is a memorial plaque that reads as follows:

"Underneath lies the body of Benjamin Pugh, MD who departed this life the 14th day of February 1798 aged 84 years. He was a sincere friend and a punctual honest man. Requiem in pace."

After a long and productive life his obituary in *Gentleman's Magazine*, to which he had contributed a number of articles, read only: "At his seat at Midford Castle, in a very advanced age, Dr. Pugh" [11].

## References

[1] Wilkinson DJ. Benjamin Pugh and his air-pipe. In: Boulton TB, Wilkinson DJ, editors. Essays On the History of Anaesthesia. London: Royal Society of Medicine Press, 1996:1–3.

[2] Grieve H. The Sleepers and the Shadows. Chelmsford: A Town, its People and its Past, vol. 11. Chelmsford: Essex Record Office Publication No 128, 1994:137–8.

[3] Pugh B. Methods of inoculation. Gentleman's Magazine 1753;23:216–8.

[4] Pugh B. A Treatise of Midwifery. London: J. Buckland, 1754.

[5] Radcliffe W. Milestones in Midwifery. Bristol: John Wright and Sons, 1967:44.

[6] Baskett TR. On the Shoulders of Giants: Eponyms and Names in Obstetrics and Gynaecology. London: RCOG Press, 1996, p. 124, 214.

[7] Kattwinkel J, Niermeyer S, Nadkarni V, Tibbals J, Phillips B, Zideman D, et al. Resuscitation of the newly born infant: an advisory statement from the Pediatric Working Group of the International Liaison Committee on Resuscitation. Resuscitation 1999;40:71–88.

[8] Smellie W. A treatise of the theory and practice of midwifery. London: Wilson, 1752:226.

[9] Smellie W. A collection of cases and observations in midwifery, vol. II. London: Wilson and Durham, 1754:384.

[10] Eisenberg MS. Life in the Balance: Emergency Medicine and the Quest to Reverse Sudden Death. Oxford: Oxford University Press, 1997.

[11] Pugh B. (Obituary) Gentleman's Magazine. 1798;68:177.

# The humane societies

George L. Sternbach     Joseph Varon     Robert Fromm Jr     Peter J.F. Baskett

For centuries, mankind has shown a great interest in the treatment of drowning victims [1]. This interest has been nourished in part by examples of recovery by some who experienced seemingly fatal submersion. The latter half of the eighteenth century witnessed the formation of societies dedicated to resuscitation of victims of drowning and sudden death from other causes. Known as humane societies, these organizations maintained registries of drowning and resuscitation, accumulated books and manuscripts, published medical opinion on related subjects, and kept rescue equipment (including drags and hooks for recovering bodies submerged under water) in working order.

The first humane society was established in Amsterdam in 1767 as the Society for the Recovery of Drowned Persons. The canals of that city made drowning a particular hazard, with many lives lost. The Society published its first results in 1769 reporting on 19 lives saved in a period of 14 months [2]. None of the victims had shown any sign of life and those present considered most of them to be completely dead. In 1793 the Society reported that 990 lives had been saved over 25 years with over 50% survival rate during the last 9 years of the survey [3]. Rewards were offered by the Society to members of the public for each life saved.

Similar groups were formed the following year in Venice, Milan and Hamburg. In 1765 the authorities in the city of Hamburg issued orders to the military garrison that soldiers on duty should come to the rescue of anybody who had fallen into the water and admittance to the guard rooms was not to be refused to such victims as long as there was the slightest hope of recovery [4]. The city of Hamburg passed an ordinance in 1769 requiring the reading in churches of notices regarding assistance to "the drowned, the strangled, the frozen and those affected by noxious gases" [5].

Between 1767 and 1790 there had been 115 resuscitation attempts of which 75 were successful [6]. Societies were subsequently established in Vienna (1769), Paris (1771), Dresden (1773), London (the Royal Humane Society, 1774), St Petersburg (1774), Philadelphia (1780), New York (1784), Boston (1786) and Glasgow (1790).

In 1773, the Dutch Society published a brochure of its activities and successes. This was translated into English by Thomas Cogan, an English clergyman-physician who had studied medicine at Leiden. In the year of its founding, the Dutch Society had recommended the following methods as useful approaches to resuscitation: friction and rubbing of various parts of the body; stimulants applied to the nose or skin; blood-letting; induction of vomiting; application of heat to the victim; insufflation of tobacco smoke into the rectum or infusion of enemas containing tobacco extracts; and mouth-to-mouth artificial ventilation [7,8] Their admonition was: "keep the victim warm, remove swallowed or aspirated water, give mouth-to-

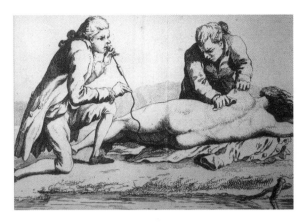

Fig. 1.

mouth respiration and perform insufflation of smoke of burning tobacco into the rectum" (see Fig. 1).

Because body warmth was equated with life, attempts to revive the dead by applying heat had been used since ancient times. The Royal Humane Society recommended that resuscitation efforts include the application of bottles of hot water or heated bricks onto the abdomen, in the axillae, between the thighs and to the soles of the feet [10].

Therapeutic use of tobacco smoke related to the American Indian belief that smoke contained the spirits of life. The chemical stimulation produced by tobacco was also considered to be beneficial to the body. Indians attempted to revive the dead by insufflating smoke into the rectum via an animal bladder. The Dutch version of this method, known as the Dutch fumigation technique, was widely practiced in Europe throughout the 18th century. This technique involved an instrument known as a fumigator, which was used to burn tobacco and pump the fumes into the victim's rectum. The machines for the administration of tobacco were distributed to barbers shops and other suitable retail outlets. In instances in which this instrument was not at hand, all passengers on a Dutch canal boat would be summoned to assist in administering this form of therapy to the drowned victim [10].

In 1774, 'The Institution for Affording Immediate Relief to Persons Apparently Dead from Drowning' was founded by Cogan and William Hawes, a London apothecary and friend and medical attendant of the writer Oliver Goldsmith. Hawes was enthusiastic about attempting the methods recommended by the Dutch Society. He had previously offered rewards to all boatmen between the Westminster and London bridges who would rescue and bring ashore the bodies of the drowned so he might apply these resuscitation measures. On April 18, 1774, he and Cogan assembled a group of 32 of their friends at the Chapter Coffee House, St Paul's Churchyard, London, to establish the Society. Goldsmith, who had studied medicine prior to embarking on his literary career, was listed as a founder, though he had died 2 weeks before. The organization's name was changed to 'The Humane Society' in 1776, and again to 'The Royal Humane Society' in 1787, after being granted royal patronage by George III.

Humane societies functioned as fora for the exchange of ideas regarding proper resuscitation techniques. Although drowning was the principal focus, attention was also given to strangulation and stifling in caves, wells and mines. The placing of the drowned victim over a barrel had long been a staple of resuscitation by sailors and others living near bodies of water. The Royal Humane Society dissented, however, and issued an injunction against the practice in 1774, and continued to do so every year thereafter until 1909 [5].

As noted above, the Dutch Humane Society advocated mouth-to-mouth ventilation as the preferred artificial respiration method. Conversely, mouth-to-mouth ventilation was widely denigrated in the venue of the Royal Humane Society. William Hunter considered it "a method practiced by the vulgar" [10] and Herholdt and Rafn considered that "insufflation of air by mouth is a very toilsome and loathsome act" '[11]. Mouth-to-mouth ventilation was condemned in part because of the belief that expired air acquired a poisonous quality by virtue of its passage through the lungs. Joseph Priestly had demonstrated that expired air contained a large quantity of phlogisticated air (nitrogen) and fixed air (carbon dioxide). The latter was thought in particular to produce harmful effects if re-inspired, the breath of the operator having "become noxious and unfit to enter any lungs again" [8].

In 1776, John Hunter presented to the Royal Humane Society the results of ventilation experiments he had performed while an assistant to his brother William in 1755. [12,13]. In so doing, he restored a method of ventilation initially recommended by Paracelsus in 1530. Hunter utilized a double-chambered bellows of his own design to ventilate experimental animals. With this apparatus, ventilation was carried out by placing the tip of the bellows into one nostril while the opposite nostril and mouth were occluded. The other chamber induced negative-pressure exhalation. He recommended the use of the bellows to support ventilation and suggested that dephlogisticated air (i.e. oxygen, an element described by Priestly in 1774) might be more efficacious in resuscitation than ordinary air [10]. As a consequence, the Royal Humane Society in 1782 recommended bellows ventilation in preference to the mouth-to-mouth method [5]. This bias against mouth-to-mouth ventilation was to persist for some time. In an 1812 report, the Society recommended that if bellows were not available, the rescuer should perform abdominal compressions to simulate respiratory movements [14].

John Hunter was one of the first to note the effects of respiration on cardiac function. Having observed the cardiorespiratory system in an open animal model being ventilated with the bellows, he found that when he "stopped the motion of the bellows, the heart became gradually weaker and less frequent in its contractions, till it ceased entirely to move. By renewing the action of the bellows the heart again began to move" [12,13]. He considered this condition to be analogous to the drowning victim deprived of respiratory function, and inferred that recovery of cardiac activity "must therefore depend immediately on the application of air to the lungs" [12,13].

Hunter also condemned blood-letting, emetics and fumigation as resuscitation techniques. In this he was well in advance of the thinking of his time. His advocacy of bellows ventilation led to its widespread utilization for the next half century, until the potential for barotrauma caused by pulmonary overinflation became realized. In 1837, use of the bellows was deleted from the list of methods recommended by the Society [13].

Although the Humane Society in Glasgow was not found until 1790, interest and practice in resuscitation was not wanting in Scotland. Tracheal intubation and artificial ventilation was described by W.A. Cullen in a letter to Lord Cathcard [15] (the President of the Board of Police who were responsible for drowning victims) in which he says "Dr Munro informs me, it is very practicable to introduce directly into the glottis and trachea a crooked tube such as a catheter used for a male adult," when blowing air into the mouth and nose is not satisfactory.

In France early edicts issued in 1770 by L'Academie des Science on the most suitable means for the rescue of drowned persons had been somewhat unfilled in practical terms until, following publication of the results from Holland, the Royal Lifeguards were instructed to assist drowning persons and both military and civilian personnel were offered rewards for lifesaving efforts. The results of these resuscitation efforts were given in the city of Paris annual report and showed that three out of four were rescued and revived.

The dependence of cardiac activity on respiration was challenged by Sir Benjamin Brodie in 1821 [7]. Brodie had, a decade before, found nicotine to be a potent cardiac poison, thereby dooming the practice of tobacco fumigation. He now delivered a series of lectures on asphyxia in which he contended that artificial ventilation was of benefit only to those drowning victims to whom it could be applied before the heart had stopped [13].

Brodie's influence was to be felt for some time. In 1855, the Society's recommendations for resuscitation from drowning contained no mention of artificial ventilation [14]. It was around this time that mechanical movement of the chest wall as a means of inducing respiration was popularized. One such method, introduced by Henry Silvester [16], was adopted by the Royal Humane Society in 1861. This technique attempted to imitate natural respiratory movements, and involved lifting the supine victim's arms above the head (inspiration), then lowering them and pressing them against the anterior thorax (expiration). This was to remain the Society's officially recommended method into the 20th century [14].

It was in the 1780s that Luigi Galvani observed the contractile effects that electrical current produced upon skeletal muscles [17]. Kite had described the application of electricity in resuscitation in 1788 [18] and Herholdt and Rafn describe "an electric shock applied across the chest, from the right to the left side, directly on the large blood vessels of the heart and lungs...is the best cardiacum in a drowned person" [19]. Electricity was utilized periodically in resuscitation from this point on, both as a general stimulant and to activate the phrenic nerve in order to induce diaphragmatic movement [20]. The Humane Society of New York pronounced electricity to be "a most powerful agent, a very proper remedy" in resuscitation [17]. The Society outlined a procedure for the use of electrical stimulation in resuscitation in 1795. In this method, it was recommended that after the patient was electrified for "four or five minutes, the hand of one of the attendants should be applied close to the body, so as to take strong sparks which should be drawn from the left side of the heart" [9]. This use of the patient as capacitor and the resuscitator as the ground did direct the exit of current via the heart, though the significance of ventricular fibrillation in cardiac arrest was not to be appreciated for more than a century. The use of electricity for purposes of defibrillation was not to follow for 50 years thereafter [21].

The American humane societies were closely modeled on the Royal Humane Society, but generally lacked that organization's scientific vitality. They functioned more as social and charitable clubs [22]. The Philadelphia Society was eventually renamed the Philadelphia Skating Club and Humane Society. American societies were ultimately absorbed into various philanthropic leagues during the nineteenth century.

By contrast, the Royal Humane Society continues to function to this day, though it no longer serves as an arbiter of resuscitation knowledge. It is concerned primarily with dispensing its awards. By offering prizes and monetary grants, the humane societies induced significant contributions to the fund of existing knowledge. An early recipient was James Parkinson, who had been a student of John Hunter. He was awarded the Royal Humane Society's silver medal for performing a rescue in 1777. E. Goodwyn was awarded the Society's Gold Medal for his excellent dissertation entitled 'The Connexion of Life with Respiration in 1788' [23]. Goodwyn showed that only small quantities of water entered the lungs during drowning, he investigated tidal and lung volumes and came to the conclusion that 100 cubic inches (163ml) should be inflated with each inspiration. He also demonstrated that blood changed in colour from "black" to "florid" as it passed through lungs and emphasised the importance of locating the hypothermia associated with near drowning [24].

Such presentations to individuals participating in the societies' work were frequently attended by considerable notoriety. One such event was the presentation by the Royal Humane Society of its Gold Medal to Czar Alexander I of Russia in 1806 [25]. The monarch had reputedly saved a Polish peasant from drowning in 1803. The Czar had arrived on the scene as the apparently lifeless body of a young man was being extracted from the Vilia River. He directed a resuscitation that proved successful after 3 h of effort. The details of the resuscitation methods are unknown, except that they included the ever-popular bleeding. His perseverence would have met with the Society's approval, inasmuch as it initially recommended an effort of at least 2 h duration [26].

Accolades also went to less exalted but no less worthy figures. In 1802, the Society presented its medal to Mrs Ann Newby, matron of the City of London Lying-in Hospital. In this position, she had achieved 500 successful neonatal resuscitations [14].

The humane societies stimulated research and new approaches to treatment. In so doing, they achieved many noteworthy advances in resuscitation. William Hawes petitioned parliament to establish schools where medical students would be taught the principles of resuscitation [5]. Lay populations had practiced resuscitation of the apparently dead for many centuries. The humane societies aided the medical profession in realizing that such resuscitation was a legitimate component of medical practice.

## References

[1] Varon J, Sternbach GL. Cardiopulmonary resuscitation; lessons from the past. J Emerg Med 1991;9:503–7.

[2] Geschichte und UrKunden der im Jahre 1767 3ur. Rethung der Ertrunken zu Amsterdam Errichteten Gesellschaft. Hamburg, 1769.

[3] Herholdt JD, Rafn CG. An Attempt at an Historical Survey on Life-Saving Measures for Drowning Persons and Information of the Best Means by Which They Can Again be Brought Back to Life. Printed at H. Tikiob's Bookseller with M Geest, 1794, p. 4.

[4] Herholdt JD, Rafn CG. An Attempt at an Historical Survey on Life-Saving Measures for Drowning Persons and Information of the Best Means by Which They Can Again be Brought Back to Life. Printed at H. Tikiob's Bookseller with M Geest, 1794, p. 4–5.

[5] Bishop RJ. A Short History of the Royal Humane Society to Mark its 200th Anniversary. London: The Royal Humane Society, 1976.

[6] Herholdt JD, Rafn CG. An Attempt at an Historical Survey on Life-Saving Measures for Drowning Persons and Information of the Best Means by Which They Can Again be Brought Back to Life. Printed at H Tikiob's Bookseller with M Geest, 1794, p. 7.

[7] Thangam S, Weil MH, Rackow EC. Cardiopulmonary resuscitation: a historical review. Acute Care 1986;12:63–94.

[8] Cary RJ. A brief history of the methods of resuscitation of the apparently drowned. Johns Hopkins Hosp Bull 1913;24:246–51.

[9] Lee RV. Cardiopulmonary resuscitation in the eighteenth century. J Hist Med Allied Sci 1972;27:418–33.

[10] Hermreck AS. The history of cardiopulmonary resuscitation. Am J Surg 1988;156:430–6.

[11] Herholdt JD, Rasn CG. An Attempt at an Historical Survey on Life-Saving Measures for Drowning Persons and Information of the Best Means by Which They Can Again be Brought Back to Life. Printed at H Tikiob's Bookseller with M Geest, 1794, p. 46.

[12] Proposals for Recovery of People Apparently Drowned. John Hunter Philosophical Transaction of the Royal Humane Society, 1776.

[13] Keith A. Three Hunterian lectures on the mechanism underlying the various methods of artificial respiration. Lecture I. Lancet 1909;1:745–9.

[14] Keith A. Three Hunterian lectures on the mechanism underlying the various methods of artificial respiration. Lecture II. Lancet 1909;1:825–8.

[15] Cullen WA. A letter to Lord Cathcart, President of the Board of Police in Scotland concerning the recovery of persons drowned and seemingly dead. London, 1776.

[16] Sylvester HR. The natural method of treating asphyxia. Medical Times & Gazette 1857;II:485.

[17] Bartecchi CE. Cardiopulmonary resuscitation — an element of sophistication in the 18th century. Am Heart J 1980;100:580–1.

[18] Kite C. An essay on the recovery of the apparently dead. London, 1788.

[19] Herholdt JD, Rasn CG. An Attempt at an Historical Survey on Life-Saving Measures for Drowning Persons and Information of the Best Means by Which They Can Again be Brought Back to Life. Printed at H Tikiob's Bookseller with M Geest, 1794, p. 64.

[20] Schechter DC. Application of electrotherapy to noncardiac thoracic disorders. Bull NY Acad Med 1970;46:932–51.

[21] Sternbach G, Varon J, Fromm RE Jr. Claude Beck and ventricular defibrillation. Resuscitation 2000 44;1:3–5.

[22] Eisenberg MS. Life in the Balance — Emergency Medicine and the Quest to Reverse Sudden Cardiac Death. New York: Oxford University Press, 1997.

[23] Goodwyn E. The connexion of life with respiration 1788. Philosophical Transaction of the Royal Humane Society, London.

[24] Baskett PJF. The History of Resuscitation in Cardiopulmonary Resuscitation 1989. Elsevier, Amsterdam, p. 3.

[25] Schechter DC. Role of the humane societies in the history of resuscitation. Surg Obstet Gynecol 1969;129:811–5.

[26] Schester NH. The Emperor of Russia and the Royal Humane Society. J Royal Coll Gen Pract 1971;21:634–44.

# Dr. William Cullen and Lord Cathcart

David J. Wilkinson

## Introduction

Early attempts at resuscitation of the dead or apparently dead, both animals and humans, have been recorded for centuries. Modern 'interpretation' of anecdotal records suggests successes for Elisha in the *Old Testament*[1] Vesalius and Hooke in the 16th and 17th centuries[2,3] and Bruhier and Jackson in the early 18th Century.[4,5]

It is generally accepted that the inception of a Society in Amsterdam for the recovery of drowned persons in 1767[6] provided the impetus for further research in the UK and Europe and subsequently around the world particularly after the translation and publication of their minutes by Johnson in 1773[7] and then again by Cogan in the same year.[8] Although the work of the Amsterdam Society was reported in France in 1768[9] and in the *Gentleman's Magazine* in London in 1771,[10] it was the creation of a London Society by Hawes and Cogan in 1774[11] that was to stimulate further research and the adoption of the continental methods of resuscitation.

## Dr. William Cullen

### Early career

William Cullen was born in Hamilton, Lanarkshire on 15 April 1710. His father, the factor to the Duke of Hamilton, arranged for his early education at the local grammar school and then in 1726, he attended Glasgow University for a general studies arts course. He was then apprenticed to an apothecary in Glasgow, John Paisley, and on completion of this apprenticeship he became a ship's surgeon in 1729 to a merchant vessel commanded by a relative sailing between London and the West Indies. After further time as an assistant apothecary in London and following the death of his father and elder brother, he returned to Scotland and started a general practice in Auchinlee, Shotts, Lanarkshire in 1732.

In 1734, he went to Edinburgh to study medicine for 2 years and then set up practice in Hamilton as a physician and surgeon. Between 1737 and 1740, William Hunter was his pupil and they remained lifelong friends. In 1740, Cullen took his MD in Glasgow and after marrying in 1741, Miss. Anna Johnstone, and becoming a town councillor and magistrate he eventually moved to Glasgow and settled there in 1744. He had 11 children.[12,13]

### University life

Cullen had devoted considerable time to the study of natural sciences while in practice in Hamilton and had sufficient a reputation that, on moving to Glasgow, he was able to lecture at the University on botany, material medica and chemistry. He was regarded as a good lecturer and in 1747 he was appointed the first Lecturer in Chemistry to the University. In 1751, he became Professor of Medicine in Glasgow but the Medical school did not develop

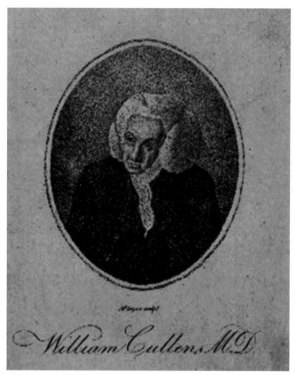

William Cullen from http://digitalgallery.nypl.org detail id 1219463.

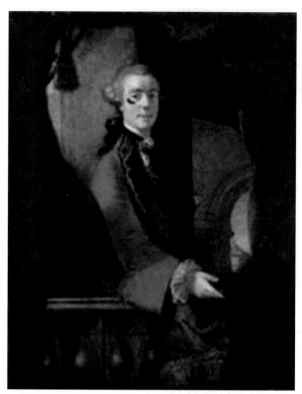

Lord Cathcart from www.tate.org.uk/britain/exhibitions/reynolds/roomguide2.shtm.

substantially and he found his private practice limited so in 1756 he moved to Edinburgh to take up a joint chair in chemistry which became his alone the following year. In 1766, he was appointed Professor of Medicine in Edinburgh where his popularity remained undiminished. His lectures were published in 1777 and were considered to be the basic text for medical teaching amongst the student body at that time. His teaching was also highly regarded as he lectured in English instead of Latin.[13] In his final years, his intellectual prowess and health decreased and he died on February 5th 1790.[14]

## Lord Cathcart

Charles Schaw Cathcart (21/3/1721—14/8/1776) was the 9th Lord Cathcart, taking the title after the death of his father, Charles, in 1740. A soldier of great distinction, like his father, he commanded the 20th regiment of foot under the Earl of Stair in 1742. He was aide-de-camp to the Duke of Cumberland and accompanied him in Flanders, Scotland and Holland. He was lucky to survive being shot in the face during the Battle of Fontenoy in 1745. He was also wounded at Culloden in 1746. He became a colonel in 1750 and a lieutenant-general in 1760. Highly regarded by the Duke of Cumberland, he was retained in his service as Lord of the Bedchamber. He had married Jean Hamilton in 1753 and had three children. After inheriting his mother's estates he sold the family home of Castle Sundrum in 1758.[15] In 1763, he was created a knight of the Order of the Thistle and between 1768 and 1772 was a special ambassador to the Russian Court of Catherine the Great based in St Petersburg. In 1773, he was elected Rector of Glasgow University, a position he held for 2 years.[16] In addition from 1773 until his death he was Lord High Commissioner in the General Assembly of the Kirk of Scotland. His other notable achievements were to be 1 of 16 representative peers of his country, its first Lord Commissioner of Police and the lieutenant-general of the forces stationed within its borders. He had two portraits painted by Sir Joshua Reynolds which, at the request of Cathcart, clearly showed the patch with which he covered his facial scar. There is a further portrait of him with the Duke of Cumberland at Culloden. He died in London in 1776.[17]

## Cathcart and Cullen

Where and when our two protagonists met is purely a matter for conjecture. As can be seen from their brief biographies both were influential men in Scotland who would have mixed in the same social circles. Although Cathcart was based in Glasgow and London while Cullen was resident in Edinburgh there could be little doubt that their paths would cross on occasion.

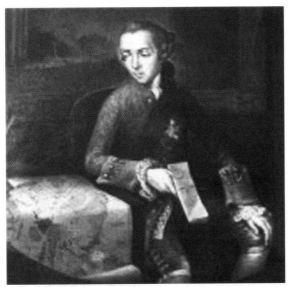

Lord Cathcart from www.sundrumcastle.com/clanappeal/chiefs.html.

## Pamphlet contents

There are four sections to the pamphlet published by Murray in London in 1776.[18] Firstly the letter to Lord Cathcart written by Cullen and dated 8 August 1774; this comprises the first 27 pages. The second is *an Extract from the Journals of the Board of Police concerning the recovery of persons drowned and seemingly dead*, dated 11 August 1774 and comprising 3 pages. The third section is a *Paper presented by Lord Cathcart and referred to in the preceding minute*, this is undated and comprises 13 pages. The final section are some 2 pages of advertisements for further books published by Murray (which has no further relevance for this paper).

## Cullen's letter

After the usual pleasantries, Cullen reviews the current understanding of human physiology in relation to drowning and states how in both man and animals *life does not immediately cease upon the cessation of the action of the lungs and heart and the consequent ceasing of the circulation of the blood.*[1] *Though the circulation of the blood is necessary to the support of life, the living state of animals does not consist in that alone, but especially depends upon a certain condition in the nerves, and muscular fibres by which they are sensible and irritable, and upon which the action of the heart itself depends. It is this condition, therefore, which may* be properly called the vital principle in animals; *and as long as this subsists, or though much weakened, as long as it can be again restored to its activity and vigour, while, at the same time, the organization of the parts remains entire, it is presumed, that the action of the heart and lungs, the circulation of the blood, and therefore all the functions of life, may also, though they have many of them long ceased, be again entirely restored.* He also noted that: *From the dissection of drowned men, and other animals, it is known, that very often the water does not enter the cavity of the lungs, nor even into the stomach, in any quantity to do hurt to the system; and in general, it is known, that, in most cases, no hurt is done to the organisation of the vital parts. It is therefore probable, that the death which ensues, or seems to ensue in drowned persons, is entirely due to the stopping of respiration, and to the ceasing, in consequence, of the circulation of the blood, whereby the body loses its heat, and with that the activity of the vital principle.*

Cullen then reviews the published success of the Amsterdam and Paris Societies for Resuscitation and cites a 75% success rate! He goes on to explain that the 'old' practices of hanging patients upside down, rolling them over casks or setting them on the crown of their heads were both unnecessary and positively dangerous and should never now be used. His basic treatment regime incorporates the careful transport of the patient in a slight head up tilt to a warm dry bed in the nearest available house, careful drying and massage of the skin with the use of a moderate fire or warm bricks placed at the feet, behind the knees and under the armpits to facilitate warming.

In an attempt to *restore the action of moving fibres. It is well known that the intestines are the parts of the body which, both from their internal situation and peculiar constitution, retain the longest their irritability; and therefore, that, in drowned persons stimulants applied may have more effect upon the intestines than on other parts.* This then, is the rationale behind the use of tobacco smoke enemas applied through a clyster pipe which should be in the position of every surgeon. Cold air or warm water (up to four pints) or even salt solutions (half an ounce of common salt to a pint of water) had been shown to be also effective.

*While these measures for recovering the heat of the body and the activity of the moving fibres are employed, and especially after they have been employed for some time, pains are to be taken to compleat and finish the business, by restoring the action of the heart and lungs.*

---

[1] The author has here changed the published letter f to s so as to make the document more readable; all other spellings in italics are taken from the original document unaltered.

For this Cullen cites the work of his colleague Monro who had performed experiments to find the best manner to inflate the lungs of drowned persons. He advocated expired air ventilation either to the patients mouth, nostril or through a wooden pipe fitted into the nostril. A pair of bellows could be used if preferred. He writes: *Dr. Munro finds, That a person of ordinary strength can blow into such a pipe, with sufficient force to inflate the lungs to a considerable degree; and thinks that the warm air from the lungs of a living person, will be most conveniently employed at first; but when it is not soon effectual, in restoring the respiration of the drowned person, and that a longer continuance of the inflation is necessary, it may be proper to employ a pair of bellows, large enough at once to contain the quantity of air necessary to inflate the lungs to a due degree.*

There is then a clear description of the use of cricoid pressure to prevent gastric distension during such lung inflations.

*If it should happen, that, in this practice, the air does not seem to pass readily into the lungs, Dr. Munro informs me, it is very practicable to introduce directly into the glottis a crooked tube, such as a catheter used for a male adult. For this he offers the following directions: The surgeon should place himself on the right side of the patient and introducing the forefinger of his left hand at the right corner of the patients mouth, he should push the point of it behind the epiglottis; and using this as a directory, he may enter the catheter, which he holds in his right hand, at the left corner of the patient's mouth, till the end of it is passed beyond the point of his forefinger; and it is then to let fall, rather than being pushed into the glottis; and through this tube, by a proper syringe applied to it, air may be with certainty blown into the lungs.*

Cullen observes that this technique had been proposed by Monsieur Le Cat in France but that he was unaware of any practical use of the technique in that country. Cullen also observed that bronchotomy may be required in some cases if a skilled operator is at hand but he doubted its efficacy. He believed that ventilation should continue for several hours before being abandoned.

Additional therapies which might be beneficial at a later stage included bleeding particularly from the jugular veins to relieve congestion once the circulation had been restored, the use of smelling salts and the administration of wine and brandy once a swallowing reflex was present. Forced emesis using direct pharyngeal stimulation or following the administration of ipecacuana might also be beneficial at a later stage. Finally Cullen observes that: *The directions proposed to be promulgated by advertisement in the several counties and Royal Boroughs in Scotland, of which your Lordship has been pleased to shew me a copy, appear to me very judicious, and perfectly adapted to the purpose intended.*

### Extract from the *Journals of the Board of Police*

This is, as it suggests, a very brief three page extract from the *Journals of the Board of Police* which is dated 11 August 1774. There were three people present at the meeting; Lord Cathcart (President), the Earl of Lauderdale and the Earl of Leven. Lord Cathcart presented a personal paper to the Board together with Cullen's letter and the Board then 'ordered' that: *The said paper and letter be printed; and that the clerk do send copies of it to all the Sheriffs of Counties, Magistrates of Royal Burghs, and Moderators of Synods and Presbyteries in Scotland; and that he do prepare a book for registering such communications as he may hereafter receive from any Sheriff, Magistrate, or Minister; and particularly such accounts of successful cases as may be transmitted to him.*

It was also 'resolved' by the Board that the following articles constitute a proper apparatus for the recovery of drowned persons which could be obtained from Lawrie Jnr & Co., druggists, at the head of Niddry's Wynd, Edinburgh at the following prices:

| | | | |
|---|---|---|---|
| 1 | A fumigator; consisting of a small set of bellows, a brass box and handle, a flexible tube and ivory pipe | 10s... | ...6d |
| 2 | A spare flexible tube and pipe | 2s | 0d |
| 3 | Four wooden pipes, for blowing into the nostrils | 1s | 6d |
| 4 | Two vials of flint glass, with ground stoppers, containing spirits for smelling | 1s | 6d |
| 5 | Two vials of flint glass, with ground stoppers, containing spirits to be applied to the wrists etc. | 4s | 0d |
| | All these included in a box, value, | 4s | 0d |
| | Separately, a pair of bellows for blowing into the lungs | 6s | 0d |

### Paper presented by Lord Cathcart

This is undated but bears an uncanny resemblance to the letter produced by Cullen. There is some extra detail of other resuscitation societies in Milan, Venice and Hamburg and a reference to the creation of the London Society, *'this summer'* (this would again put the date at 1774). He puts forward the case for such policies to be adopted in Scotland with great eloquence. *There is no country, which, from its situation, surrounded by the sea, and everywhere intersected by rivers, lakes, and bays, calls more loudly for effectual measures, for affording immediate relief to persons seemingly dead, from drowning, than Scotland; no nation more likely eagerly to adopt such measures, if proposed; nor any, where, from the nature of its government, such measures may so easily be carried into execution; and by the following steps: Let the Board of Police compose a proper advertisement, founded on the principles of those of other countries, containing the necessary advice to the public, and informing them of the reward offered by way of encouragement to those who shall follow it ...*

Cathcart explains that the adoption of this policy would be entirely optional on the various sheriffs, magistrates and clergy to whom the advertisement was to be sent but as there were few costs involved, except the initial purchase of the recommended equipment, he felt its adoption and implementation would not be a problem.

He provides an outline plan for the advertisement which has a series of recommendations:

(1) The patient should be transported with great care to a nearby house.
(2) The patient should be carefully dried and then gently warmed.
(3) The lungs should be inflated either with expired air mouth to nostril or with bellows; at the same time tobacco smoke should be blown into the rectum.
(4) If signs of life appear then the patient should be bled, given oral fluids and be encouraged to vomit.

Cathcart also outlines a set of rewards for initiating such resuscitation which were to be paid by the clerk of the county within two weeks of receipt provided such applications were supported by a certificate from a clergyman:

| | |
|---|---|
| (1) For the first person to alert a doctor or clergyman that someone had been taken out of the water | 2s—6d |
| (2) For the person who attempts resuscitation for at least 2 h | £2—2s—0d |
| (3) For that same person if resuscitation is successful | £4—4s—0d |
| (4) For any publican who allows a patient in | £1—1s—0d |

Cathcart also recommends that each parish should buy two sets of apparatus as previously described and that the notice should be fixed to every church door and market place in Scotland.

The techniques described in this pamphlet were very appropriate for the age and were a great improvement on many of the more injurious techniques described by previous authors. The adoption of expired air ventilation or the use of intubation and ventilation with or without bellows was sound and would have been quite practicable. Sadly there appears to be no information as to the implementation of these ideas. The pamphlet was published in London two years after it was written and there is no evidence that Cathcart's notice was distributed to every town or that the advice was adopted.

Cathcart died the year that the pamphlet was published and so perhaps did not have time to promote the ideas it contained. Cullen was 'busy' teaching at the University in Edinburgh and seems not to have taken the concept further. Professor Anne Crowther from the Centre for the History of Medicine at Glasgow University has suggested that "*the Board of Police was a group of sinecurists with no great reputation for practical activity*" and further that the implementation required the local clergy to invest in the basic sets of apparatus for which there might have been little enthusiasm.[19]

It would be interesting to know if local museums in Scotland have any records relating to these ideas and if there were any records anywhere of resuscitation attempts throughout Scotland as a direct result of the publication of Cathcart and Cullen's proposals.

## References

1. The Holy Bible. King James Version London 1611 11Kings 4:33—5.
2. Vesalius A. De Humani Corporis Fabrica Libri Septum. Basel; 1555.
3. Hooke R. An account of an experiment made by M Hook, of preserving animals alive by blowing through their lungs with bellows. Philos Trans R Soc 1667:2.
4. Bruhier d'Ablaincourt JJ. The uncertainty of the signs of death and the danger of precipitate internments and dissections demonstrated with proper directions both for preventing such accidents and repairing the misfortunes brought upon the constitution by them. London; 1746.
5. Jackson R. A physical dissertation on drowning; in which submersion, commonly call'd drowning, is shewn to be a long time consistent with the continuance of life ... to which is

subjoined, the proper measure for recovery and relief by a physician. London; 1746.

6. Historie en gedenkschriften van de maatschappy, tot redding van drenkelingen, opgerecht binnen Amsterdam MDCCLXVII. Amsterdam; 1768.

7. Johnson A. A short account of a Society at Amsterdam instituted in the year 1767 for the recovery of drowned persons; with observations shewing the utility and advantage that would accrue to Great Britain from a similar institution extended to cases of suffocation by damps in mines, choaking, strangling, stifling and other accidents. London; 1773.

8. Cogan T. Memoirs of the Society instituted at Amsterdam in favour of drowned persons for the years 1767, 1768, 1769, 1770, and 1771. London; 1773.

9. Histoire et memoires de la Societe, formee a Amsterdam en faveur des Noyes A⁰. MDCCLXVII. Amsterdam; 1768.

10. Anon. List of books with remarks. Gentleman's Mag 1771;16:512—4.

11. Wilkinson DJ. The development of resuscitation in the United Kingdom, in The History of Anaesthesia. Edited by Atkinson RS, Boutlton TB. RSM 1989:348—351.

12. http://www.glasgowguide.co.uk/info-fame_William_Cullen.html.

13. The compact edition of the Dictionary of National Biography, vol. 1. Oxford University Press; 1975. p. 483.

14. http://www.answers.com/topic/william-cullen.

15. http://www.sundrumcastle.com/clanappeal/chiefs.html.

16. http://www.en.wikipedia.org/wiki/Charles_Cathcart_9th_Lord_Cathcart.

17. The compact edition of the Dictionary of National Biography, vol. 1. Oxford University Press; 1975. p. 330.

18. Cullen W. A letter to Lord Cathcart, President of the Board of Police in Scotland, concerning the recovery of persons drowned and seemingly dead. London: Murray J; 1776.

19. http://special.lib.gla.ac.uk/teach/Cullen/letter.html; personal communication.

# The contributions of Lavoisier, Scheele and Priestley to the early understanding of respiratory physiology in the Eighteenth Century

David J. Wilkinson

## 1. Introduction

The mid Eighteenth Century was a time of great scientific experimentation and observation during which some of the basic aspects of respiratory physiology and metabolism began to be elucidated. This was the time when the fundamental elements of earth, air, fire and water proposed by Aristotle began to be reappraised. The Phlogiston theory was finally exploded and a basic understanding of elements, respiratory gases and metabolism began to emerge. It was also a time of radical social movements with political and religious unrest and revolution taking place. This scientific and social upheaval can be seen in the lives of three great chemists of that era: Scheele, Lavoisier and Priestley, all of whom added significantly to the pieces of the physiological jigsaw puzzle that was being put together at this time.

## 2. Joseph Priestley (1733–1804)

### 2.1. Early life

Priestley was born near Birstall in a small village called Fieldhead near Leeds on March 13 1733. (It is interesting to note that this was before the introduction of the Gregorian calendar which came into general usage in 1751 after which time he celebrated his birthday on the 24 March!) He was the oldest child and had three brothers and two sisters and when his mother, Mary Swift, died in 1739 his father, a cloth-dresser, brought up the five children single-handed. In 1742, Joseph went to live with his aunt, Sarah Keighley who arranged for his schooling. He was an avid scholar (perhaps because he was often ill, with one severe attack of tuberculosis) and was soon competent in maths, Latin,

Hebrew, Chaldee, Syriac and Arabic as well as English. He also taught himself the basics of algebra, geometry and mathematics.

### 2.2. Training as a Priest

When aged 19, Priestley entered Daventry School, Northamptonshire, (which was a Dissenting Academy i.e. their doctrines differed from the Church of England) to train for the church. He was thus trained as a Nonconformist clergyman which meant that he could only preach in a chapel and that he would be unable to serve in the army or attend a university. Although the school was recognised to have the highest academic standards, the young Priestley augmented his lessons with further studies of history, science, philosophy and Greek. His views began to become steadily more unorthodox despite their sincerity and his genuine piety. In 1755 he became an assistant minister to a Presbyterian congregation in Needham Market, Suffolk but his 'freethinking' views and poor public speaking ability related to a stammer plus his single marital status, soon upset the congregation and he was forced to leave. In 1758 he moved to Nantwich in Cheshire where he found more sympathetic parishioners and he soon started a day school with some 36 students.

### 2.3. Life as a teacher

While teaching in Nantwich he became more and more interested in science and was soon providing his students with air pumps and electrostatic generators to develop their interest too. Due to these successes he was appointed as a tutor in languages and literature at Warrington Academy in Lancashire in 1761. In the same year he published a textbook on "The rudiments of English Grammar" which was to remain popular for the next 50 years. 5 further books on the theory of language, biography, liberal education, history and general policy followed between 1762 and 1788. His teaching was based on his desire to prepare his pupils for the practicalities of life and the school at which he taught became one of the most popular in the UK at that time. In recognition of his accomplishments, Edinburgh University conferred a LL.D degree on Priestley in 1765. He taught new subjects at that time including modern history and science.

## 2.4. Family life

Whilst at Warrington, in 1762, he married the only daughter of an ironmaster of Bersham, near Wrexham in Wales. He had been introduced to the family through the son, William, who was a student at his school. This 18-year-old woman called Mary Wilkinson gave him a daughter and three sons and provided a stable home life. Priestley was a great family man, caring for his wife and children and enthusiastic to develop every aspect of his and their lives. He taught himself to play the flute and believed everyone should have musical skills. They were never a wealthy family but the house was always busy with often boarders being taken in to supplement their income.

## 2.5. Interest in science

Over the next few years Priestley began to become more and more interested in science. From 1765 onwards, he spent at least one month a year in London where he met and debated with the leaders in the field of science as well as leading political theorists including Richard Price and Benjamin Franklin. In 1766 he was elected to the Royal Society of London mainly as a result of his experiments in electricity and the following year he published his work on *"The history and Present State of electricity."* He produced two versions of this, one for the scientific elite and a simpler version for more general reading. He was the first to note that graphite was an electrical conductor. It is interesting to see that he was the first to describe the use of India rubber to erase pencil marks, something he discovered whilst publishing a book on perspective drawing that he had written because there was nothing available on the subject and he had taught himself the technique to illustrate his book on electricity.

In 1767 he became minister of Mill Hill chapel in Leeds where he could devote more time to his researches. His initial interest in gases was initiated by observations in the local brewery in Leeds where he observed the production of 'fixed air' (carbon dioxide) from the fermentation vats. At this time the world of chemistry recognised only three gases; air, carbon dioxide and hydrogen. In the next six years, Priestley was to isolate 4 further gases which he did through the development of a special pneumatic trough that collected the gases above mercury and thus 'saved' those that were water soluble. The pneumatic trough that collected gases over water had been described by Stephen Hales in 1727 in his book Vegetable Staticks. Priestley was able to isolate and describe nitrous air (nitric oxide), red nitrous

vapour (nitrogen dioxide), diminished nitrous air (nitrous oxide) and marine acid air (hydrogen chloride). In 1772 he published this work in the Philosophical Transactions where it was seen by Lavoisier. In that same year he published work on light and optics and described a technique of making stored water more palatable for drinking by adding carbon dioxide to it. He called the new drink a 'mephitic julep' and thus initiated the whole of the 'fizzy drink' industry.

In December 1772 Priestley moved again, this time to Calne in Wiltshire where he was appointed as librarian and tutor to the sons of the Earl of Shelbourne, William Fitzmaurice-Petty. The following year he was awarded the Copley medal by the Royal Society for his work on gases.

## 2.6. Priestley and oxygen

On August 1 1774 Priestley collected a colourless, odourless gas from the heating of red mercuric oxide with sunlight focussed through a 12 inch 'burning lens'. He had isolated oxygen. He called this 'dephlogisticated air' as it supported the vigorous burning of a candle flame and allowed a mouse to survive in a sealed container for an hour compared to the expected 15 min of life in a similar volume of air. Priestley wrote *"I have discovered an air five or six times as good as common air"*. Priestley inhaled the 'new gas' himself and remarked *" I fancied that my breast felt peculiarly light and easy for some time afterwards."* In 1775 writing of his discovery in the Philosophical Transactions he says *"this air is of exalted nature.....A candle burned in this air with amazing strength of flame; and a bit of red hot wood crackled and burnt with a prodigious rapidity, exhibiting an appearance something like that of iron glowing with a white heat and throwing sparks in all directions."*

On a tour of the continent the following year, Priestley met Lavoisier in Paris and told him of this development and the French scientist immediately set about his investigation of this 'new gas'. Priestley was unable to accept Lavoisier's later research that suggested the Phlogiston theory was not valid and he was to remain almost the last chemist to continue to uphold the theory until his death.

Priestley was able to show that green plants gave off dephlogisticated air in sunlight, an observation that would help elucidate photosynthesis over the next two decades by Ingenhousz and Senebier. Priestley wrote *"The injury which is continually done to the atmosphere by the respiration of such a large number of animals.....is, in part at least, repaired by the vegetable creation."*

Oxygen was not his only discovery at this time as he described ammonia, sulphur dioxide, silicon tetrafluoride and carbon monoxide in subsequent years.

## 2.7. Later life

In 1779 Priestley moved to Birmingham, partly at the suggestion of his brother-in –law, John Wilkinson and partly because his presence at Lord Shelbourne's house and within his social circle was becoming increasingly difficult. It was Priestley's political views that engendered this discomfort and he actively supported the American revolutionaries in their attempts to cede from the UK. Shelbourne retained his respect for Priestley and provided him with a significant pension of £150 a year for the rest of his life. In Birmingham, Priestley continued to preach and experiment, writing a large series of books and pamphlets on religion and theology. His viewpoint was rather radical for this era with his rejection of the Trinity and the factual base of the Bible. This was the doctrine of Unitarianism in which Christ is considered to be an ordinary man, the Trinity does not exist and the Virgin birth did not occur; Priestley had firmly adopted these tenets whilst preaching in Leeds. Priestley joined the Lunar Society, Birmingham's rival to the Royal Society that was so named as its members held monthly meetings and then walked home in the evening by the light of the full moon. Its members included Erasmus Darwin, Mathew Boulton, Josiah Wedgwood and James Watt and their remit was the use of science to enhance industry.

In 1780 Priestley was elected to the St. Petersburg Academy in recognition for his scientific contributions but he was now more involved with theological debate and investigation. Priestley's radical views were not however limited to religion and he was a great believer in the rights of the individual and the rights of people to have a voice in government. It was this background that caused him to support the French revolution openly, a stance that angered local residents who stormed his house in July 1791 and burnt it and his laboratory to the ground.

Having lost his library and all his papers, Priestley moved to Hackney in North London where he taught at the New College and preached at the Gravel Pit Chapel. By 1793, with the execution of Louis XVI and the declaration of war with France, Priestley found himself more and more isolated so that in April of 1794 he emigrated to the USA and took up residence in Northumberland, Pennsylvania where his three sons had elected to live the previous year. Although he continued to experiment and research he felt isolated from his English colleagues and refused offers of a Chair at the University of Pennsylvania. His wife and youngest son died within a year of each other in 1796 and Priestley found himself short of funds and under considerable attack for his radical political and religious views. There were moves to extradite him back to England as he never took American citizenship but thanks to 'friends in high places', and notably the patronage of Thomas Jefferson and John Adams, Priestley was allowed to stay. In 1796 he published a final scientific paper on why the phlogiston theory was still valid, an ironic statement at a time when almost the whole of the scientific world had abandoned it. He published some further religious books but his health was in considerable decline and died on February 6 1804.

His home is now a National Historic landmark museum and can be visited.

## 3. Antoine-Laurent de Lavoisier (1743–1794)

### 3.1. Early life

Lavoisier was born on 26 August 1743 in Paris. His father, a prosperous lawyer, was a prosecutor at the Parlement de Paris and he ensured that his son had an extensive education. He was enrolled at the College des Quatre Nations where his interest in science was encouraged and his interest in precise and logical thought emerged. He wrote "I was accustomed to the rigorous reasoning of mathematicians. They never take up a proposition until the one preceding it has been solved. Everything is connected, from the definition of the point and the line up to the most sublime truths of transcendent geometry." In June 1761 he left this college and started to study law and having graduated in 1764 he joined his father at the Parlement de Paris. Whilst he was taking his law degree he continued to follow his interest in science and spent time studying meteorology, botany, anatomy, electricity, mineralogy and geology. Each one of these was studied with the help of a specialist in that field. This broad education in both arts and science gave Lavoisier a unique grounding on which his subsequent career was based. He had a mind that could adapt itself to any problem e.g. in 1766 he was awarded a gold medal by the King for the design of a new form of street lighting for Paris.

### 3.2. Initial interests

His first major research work was on geology and mineralogy. In 1767 Lavoisier worked for 4 months with Jean Etienne Guettard who produced the prodigious Atlas mineralogique de la France. Lavoisier soon felt able to create a theory on how the earth had formed. He believed that the earth's crust was formed from two components, an old soil, made of granites that were poor in fossils and a second soil that was sedimentary and full of fossils. His observations could not always be fitted into this simple theory and he soon turned his mind to other matters.

Meteorology was to be a life-long interest, from the age of 20 until his death he collected basic barometric observations. His comparative work on temperature measurements led to the development of precise rules for the manufacture and graduation of thermometers. He was interested in weather forecasting and used a network of people across France to collect data on atmospheric pressure, wind directions and relative humidity. He wrote "With all this information it is almost always possible to predict one or two days in advance, within a rather broad range of probability, what the weather is going to be; it is even thought that it will not be impossible to publish daily forecasts which will be very useful to society"[1].

In 1768 he was elected to the Academy of Sciences, France's most elite scientific institution. Later in the same year he joined the private corporation that collected taxes for the French crown on a profit and loss basis. This was the Ferme Generale. This was to prove his eventual downfall as such work was denounced as traitorous to France by Citizen Jean-Paul Marat in the French revolution some 25 years later. It was to be beneficial in other ways as it was his future father-in-law, Jacques Paulze, who had a controlling share in the Ferme Generale and it was to him that Lavoisier first suggested investing his mother's inheritance in this corporation; and in so doing was to meet his future wife.

In 1775 he was appointed a commissioner of the Royal Gunpowder and Saltpetre Administration and moved into the Paris Arsenal. It was here that he developed his laboratory that was to attract visits from chemists from across Europe. During this time he developed a greater purity of saltpetre and also improved the method of granulating the various other constituents of gunpowder.

### 3.3. Family life

In 1771, Lavoisier married a beautiful 13 year old girl called Marie-Anne Pierrette Paulze (1758–1836). She was able to translate English documents for him (including Priestley's papers) and also illustrated his books having taken painting lessons from the French artist, David and then studying engraving. David's portrait of the couple in their laboratory hangs in the New York Metropolitan Museum of Art. Lavoisier had no children.

### 3.4. Chemistry

It was to chemistry that Lavoisier was naturally drawn although he continued to work in other disciplines. At this time chemistry was still bound by Aristotle's view that there were four elements in nature; fire, earth, water and air. It was believed that the principle goal of chemistry was to analyse individual substances, determine their properties, 'break them down' into their basic constituents and then see how they reacted with other compounds. It was recognise that there was a point at which substances could not be 'decomposed' further and that these should be regarded as principles or elements and were essentially the elements of Aristotle. It was not long before Lavoisier recognised the limitations of such a theory and noted that it was surprising that chemists who had identified so many 'elemental' substances were still bound by this theory of only four. He, himself, was able to demonstrate 33 substances that he considered were elements in that he was unable to break them down into simpler substances. One of these was something he called 'caloric' which could not be weighed as it was the heat or light emitted during some chemical reactions. It is perhaps ironic that he was a believer in caloric but was adamant in his opposition to the equally nebulous phlogiston.

It is difficult for modern science to understand the rationale for a large number of the then current theories of chemistry. There was a fully accepted belief for example that matter could be transmuted into other matter. The best example of this was the changing of water into soil by boiling.

Lavoisier was to demonstrate the inaccuracy of this theory by boiling pure water in a special container for 100 days after which time no earth had been created.

### 3.5. The chemistry of gases

In September of 1772 Montigny (1733–1777) who was a senior figure in both the French Academy and the Finance Ministry asked Lavoisier to look into a secret report he had received from England that scurvy could be treated by carbonated water. Priestley had reported to the Royal Society that a mixture of fixed air and water was very effective in this respect. While there was a strong tradition of pneumatic experimentation in England, the French regarded such work as uninteresting and believed that air was just a receptacle for exhalation! This simple request was to be the impetus for a huge development in the understanding of respiratory gases and basic physiology.

### 3.6. Phlogiston

Johann Becher (1635–1682) had proposed his theory of phlogiston and this was refined and developed by Georg Stahl (1660–1734). They believed that when substances were burnt they released phlogiston which was an element of their composition. The phlogiston could be seen during combustion as fire, flame or light. It was this loss of phlogiston that turned metals into oxides. When phlogiston was lost by a substance then it was taken up by the air but there was a limit to the amount of phlogiston that the air could take up and this explained why if something was burnt inside a closed container the fire sometimes went out before all the substance had been consumed. To create a metal from its oxide then phlogiston had to be returned to the compound and this was done by a process of reduction in the presence of carbon (usually charcoal). It was considered that different substances contained different amounts of phlogiston so that carbon, wood and fat contained a lot while stone contained very little.

Respiration was considered to be a form of combustion so that phlogiston was emitted by a creature during breathing. If air was removed from around a living creature then there was nowhere for the phlogiston to go and so respiration would cease and the creature died. The problem with this theory was that if oxidation caused the release of phlogiston then there should be a change in weight of the substance that could be measured. In fact oxidation increases the weight of the metal and this was either conveniently ignored or it was suggested that phlogiston had a negative weight. Lavoisier could not accept such a concept or indeed the whole theory of phlogiston. It was nonsense to him that phlogiston could have both positive weight and negative weight or sometimes no weight at all just to satisfy the results of experiments. He was able to demonstrate that the production of metal oxides that were heavier than their original metals was the result of a combination of the metal with air. In 1777 he wrote a paper on combustion in general that outlined his findings and then in 1783 he wrote Reflexions sur le Phlogistique in which he elaborated the inconsistencies within the whole Phlogiston Theory.

### 3.7. Oxygen

Carl Wilhelm Scheele (1742–1786), a Swedish Chemist from Stralsund, Pomerania in Germany, wrote a chemical treatise on air and fire which was published in Upsalla and Leipzig in 1777 [2]. He had been working as a Pharmacist in Stockholm while performing his experiments between 1772 and 1773. His work thus predated that of both Priestley and Lavoisier but it was not published until after them. He called oxygen 'fire air' and manufactured it in a variety of ways. His experiments with plants, bees and other insects which he isolated in containers of air demonstrated clearly the importance of oxygen to maintain life. He described nitrogen (vitiated air) that was inert with respect to combustion and respiration, oxygen (fire air) that made up one third of common air and carbon dioxide (aerial acid) that was released by combustion and respiration. He noted that plants would not grow well in pure oxygen and yet sadly could not work out the relationship between respiration in animals and plants from his experimental results. His observation that "it is the fire-air by means of which the circulation of the blood and of the juices in animals and plants is so fully maintained" was close but not quite close enough.

Lavoisier had communicated by letter with Scheele in 1774 and knew all about his work with bees and his concept of fire air. In March of 1775 Lavoisier performed his experiments on red oxide of mercury. He did this over a 12 day period and showed that by heating mercury he was able to form an oxide which on further heating reduced itself to the metal again with the liberation of gases. Lavoisier was able to collect these gases in a pneumatic trough and showed that this fixed air had remarkable properties. It would support respiration in animals and activated combustion. This was an 'air eminently respirable' or vital air. He had demonstrated that air was composed of two main parts; one of these would combine with metals to form calxes and was also responsible for acidity this he called 'air eminently respirable'. He wrote this up in Considerations Generales sur la nature des Acides in 1778. He repeated Scheele's work and was able to demonstrate that after an animal had died in a confined space and the carbon dioxide was absorbed by alkali the remaining portion (which he called foul air [nitrogen]) was identical to that found after metals were oxidised in air. He noted that this foul air could be turned in to common air again by the addition of 'air eminently respirable'. The following year he named this gas oxygen (which is Greek for acid-former) the other portion he named azote (Greek for no-life).

He was also able to show that the 'inflammable air' described by Cavendish, which he termed hydrogen (Greek for water-former) did exactly this when combined with oxygen it formed dew that appeared to be water.

### 3.8. Respiratory and metabolic experiments

In collaboration with Pierre Simon de Laplace, Lavoisier performed a series of experiments to clarify details of respiratory physiology. In 1780 they showed that a guinea pig could produce 3 g of carbonic acid in ten hours when breathing oxygen. They then surrounded another guinea pig in a cage with ice which in turn was surrounded by another outer wall of ice. They postulated that the heat produced by the animal would melt the inner portions of ice in a directly proportional manner while the outer layer of ice maintained a constant temperature for the experiment. In a 24 h period 370 g of ice melted. They stated that "*heat produced during respiration by the transformation of humid air into dry air is the principle cause of animal heat conservation and if other causes intervene the effect is negligible. Respiration is thus a very slow combustion phenomenon, very similar to that of coal, it is conducted inside the lungs, not giving out light since the fire matter is absorbed by the humidity of the organs of the lungs. Heat developed by this combustion goes into the blood vessels that pass through the lungs and which subsequently flow to the entire body. Thus air that we breathe is used to conserve our bodies in two fashions: it removes from the blood fixed air, which can be very harmful when abundant; and heat which enters our lungs from this phenomenon replaces heat lost in the atmosphere.*"

Lavoisier then collaborated with another chemist, Armand Seguin (1767–1835) to investigate the influence of muscular work on metabolism. They used measurements of carbon dioxide production together with changes in pulse rate to determine metabolic effects of cold, exercise and food in themselves. In one series of experiments they suggested that resting metabolism increased by 10% in a cold environment when no food had been taken, increased 50% with food intake, 200% with exercise and 300% with exercise and eating. The exact figures are quite interesting.

Seguin at 26C at rest consumed 24 litres of air per hour, at 12C this increased to 27 litres; after a good meal this rose to 38 litres. While carrying a 7 kg load a distance of 200 metres and fasted, Seguin consumed 63 litres per hour which rose to 91 litres after he did a similar exercise after a good meal.

This was a major linking of the effects of respiration and in particular oxidation (combustion in their view) with food intake, ambient temperature and exercise.

Lavoisier observed "we have succeeded in observing two laws of the utmost importance: the first is that the increase in the number of heartbeats is in quite direct proportion to the sum of the weights lifted to a determined height; the second is that the quantity of vital air consumed is in direct proportion to the product of the inspirations through heartbeats."

By 1790 Lavoisier was able to report to the Academy of Science that "the purpose of respiration is not to cool the blood, as was believed in ancient times. It is rather a slow combustion of carbon and hydrogen, similar in every way to that which takes place in a lamp or lighted candle and, in that respect, breathing animals are active combustable bodies that are burning and wasting away." He continued "it is the atmospheric air which furnishes the oxygen necessary for this combustion. The blood provides the fuel and its oxidation in the lungs explains the change in colour. This combustion produces carbonic gas and water. This combustion is also the source of body heat. Since air vital cannot be converted into carbonic acid except by the addition of carbon, and cannot be converted into water except by the addition of hydrogen and the double combination cannot occur unless the air vital loses a part of its specific caloric, the result is that the effect of respiration is to extract from the blood a portion of carbon and hydrogen and to replace it with a portion of its specific caloric. During circulation the caloric is distributed with the blood through the animal system, and maintains that almost constant temperature observed with all breathing animals."

Lavoisier was so close to the physiological truth and it was perhaps only his reliance on the concept of caloric as an element that prevented him from fully linking metabolic and respiratory physiology. He noted the link between nutrition and metabolism when he wrote "*This combustion* (as described above) *has a metabolic cost. Since it is the very substance of the animal, it is the blood which transports the fuel. If the animal did not habitually replace, through nourishing themselves, what they lose through respiration, the lamp would very soon run out of oil and the animal would perish, just as the lamp goes out when it lacks fuel.*"

He was open minded enough to realise that the carbonic acid might come from metabolism. He wrote "It is possible that a part of the carbonic acid is formed by digestion, that it is introduced into the circulation with the chyle and when it reaches the lungs is released from the blood as the oxygen combines with it through a superior affinity."

Lavoisier also realised that there was a cooling mechanism present in the body to overcome the production of too much heat (caloric). However he viewed it in an unusual manner. He believed that perspiration drew water from an organism and combined it with caloric to produce water vapour. This loss of caloric helped to maintain the temperature of an organism within narrow limits. He also noted that much caloric and water vapour was lost from the lungs during respiration.

### 3.9. Nutritional experiments

Lavoisier was aware that animal tissue contained nitrogen and showed by the study of plants that sugars and starches were made up of carbon, hydrogen and oxygen. In 1778 he reported to the French Academy of science that wheat and flour as well as barley and oats contained a variety of nutritious substances. He highlighted the potential value of gluten and suggested that starch was not the only valuable substrate for metabolism.

### 3.10. Observational base to chemistry

Lavoisier initiated the move from qualitative experimentation in chemistry to one based on quantitative work. He was a firm believer in the value of careful laboratory experimentation coupled with meticulous observation.

He said "*I have tried ... to arrive at the truth by linking up facts; to suppress as much as possible the use of reasoning, which is often an unreliable instrument which deceives us, in order to follow as much as possible the torch of observation and experiment*".

The main characteristic of his methodology was the use of very accurate weighing scales to weigh both the reagents and the products of his experiments. He thus showed that during any chemical reaction there was a conservation of this weight, the fundamental law of conservation of matter was thus described.

He published a book in 1789 Traite elementaire de chimie in 1789 [3] which is regarded as the first modern textbook of chemistry and also initiated a scientific journal on the subject, the Annales de Chimie, that reported the latest developments in experimental work.

### 3.11. Public health

Lavoisier was not content to spend all his time researching in the laboratory; he was equally active in trying to improve public health. He studied the provision of better water supply to Paris via the Yvette Aqueduct, advocated the cessation of dumping of cesspits into the Seine and lobbied for the removal of slaughter-houses to non-residential areas. He perfected a device to distil sea water into drinking water on board ships and experimented on ways to feed abandoned neonates with cow's or sheep's milk. He was able to show the dangers of mercuric poisoning in those working with felt and the dangers of carbon monoxide poisoning in workers spending time in cesspools or sewers.

In addition Lavoisier worked with a Commission that was attempting to close the grossly inadequate Hotel Dieu Hospital in Central Paris and replace it with four buildings placed more peripherally round the city. Despite royal support and the project development to the stage of designing the new hospitals, the whole concept was opposed by the Church and 15 years of constant effort came to nothing.

### 3.12. Early work with ether

Lavoisier joined the Royal Society of Medicine in Paris in 1782 and presented 2 papers to the members. The first advocated the inhalation of ether to relieve the pain of migraine and the second, presented in 1785, described the effects of large numbers of people staying in confined spaces such as hospitals or theatres and the effect that this had on the air they breathed.

### 3.13. Social reform

Lavoisier was a political liberal and felt very strongly that there should be greater social reform in France. In the late 1780's he served on a committee concerned with these social conditions and suggested sweeping tax reforms and new economic policies. He also served on another committee that tried to introduce reforms of the hospitals and prisons of France. Despite all of these efforts he remained a figure of affluence and was a constant target of Marat and radical journalists at the beginning of the revolution.

### 3.14. Death

He was beheaded during the French Revolution on 8 May 1794, despite his liberal political and social views, because of his involvement in taxation collection. Lavoisier had given himself up some five months previously once a warrant for his arrest had been issued by the Convention. He was tried with 32 colleagues all of whom were accused of misappropriation of funds, excessive profits, abusive distribution of bonuses, unjustified delays in payment to the public treasury and increasing profits by introducing excessive amounts of water into tobacco and then using these profits in a plot against the French people. 28 of the 32 were found guilty and executed on the same day. His father-in-law was beheaded immediately before him. All of their property was confiscated, probably the real reason behind the prosecution. A contemporary mathematician, Joseph-Louis Lagrange, is quoted to have said "*It took them only an instant to cut off that head but it is unlikely that a hundred years will surface to reproduce a similar one.*"

It is perhaps ironic to note that at the moment of Lavoisier's execution, Priestley was sailing away from Plymouth to New York to start his new life having been made an honorary citizen of France and remaining a staunch supporter of the Revolution.

## 4. Conclusions

There appears to be a great desire in history to define who was the first to do something. In reality it makes no great difference to today's work who was first to define oxygen in the Eighteenth century. What can be seen from the above lives is the ability of these three great men to set new paradigms and work to prove their theories. Some were more accurate than others but it is the ability to take that lateral step that sets these characters apart from their peers.

It could be considered that if Scheele first isolated oxygen then Priestley defined its properties and then Lavoisier showed it was an element but in fact they all added a significant set of pieces to the physiological jigsaw puzzle of which oxygen was just a part.

All three were great scientists and all have added to our knowledge in physiology. It is also interesting to note that all three have been recognised in the world of stamp collecting and all three can be found on postage stamps [4].

## 5. Bibliography

Lavoisier AL. Oeuvres, publiees par les soins de son Excellence le Ministre de l'Instruction Publique et des Cultes, sous la direction de M. Dumas et E Grimaux, Paris, Imprimerie Nationale. (6 vols) 1864–1893.

Useful web sites

http://historyofscience.free.fr/Lavoisier
http://www.chemherritage.org
http://www.jimloy.com/physics/phlogstn.htm
http://scienceworld.wolfram.com/biography/Lavoisier.html
http://en.wilkipedia.org/wiki/Karl_Wilhelm_Scheele
http://webserver.lemoyne.edu/faculty/giunta/scheele77.html
http://www.spaceship-earth.org/Biograph/Priestley.htm
http://www.woodrow.org/teachers/chemistry/institutes/1992/Priestley.html
http://www.phmc.state.pa.us/ppet/priestley

### References

[1] Lavoisier AL. Oeuvres. Volume 3; 771
[2] Scheele CW. Chemische Abhandlung von der Luft und dem Feuer. 1777 Leipzig.
[3] Lavoisier AL. Traite élémentaire de chimie, présente dans un ordre nouveau et d'après les découvertes modernes. 2 vols. Paris Chez Cuchet 1789. Reprinted and translated as Lavoisier AL. Elements of chemistry. 1965 Dover publications, New York.
[4] McKenzie A. A history of anaesthesia through postage stamps. 2000. Mclean Dubois, Edinburgh.

# John Hunter—Surgeon and Resuscitator

## Wendy Moore

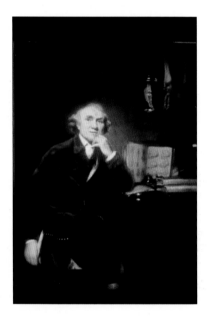

Fig. 1. John Hunter—a painting by Reynolds. Reproduced by kind permission of the President and Council of the Royal, College of Surgeons of England.

When the former king's chaplain, the Rev William Dodd, stepped up to the Tyburn gallows on 27 June 1777, the crowds wept. Details of Dodd's life and even more famous death are taken principally from Jessie Dobson [1]. Sentenced to hang for attempting to forge a cheque in the name of his ex-employer, Lord Chesterfield, the popular curate had evoked widespread sympathy for his plight. More than 23,000 people signed a petition calling for a reprieve and Dr Samuel Johnson, the celebrated lexicographer, had pleaded his case to George III.

All their efforts had been in vain and the royal pardon never came. But even as Dodd felt the rope tighten around his neck he had not given up hope of cheating death. If Dr Johnson could not save him from the noose, he fully believed that John Hunter could bring him back from the dead.

Not far away, in an undertaker's parlour in Goodge Street, Hunter and several medical friends stood ready. A bed had been prepared, a fire had been lit, medicines were lined up and a pair of bellows was placed at the ready. As minutes ticked by, Hunter waited anxiously for the arrival of the coach bearing the lifeless body of the curate that he fully intended to revive from the dead.

If anyone could do it, John Hunter could. From humble beginnings on his family's farm in lowlands Scotland, Hunter had risen to become one of the most popular and controversial surgeons of his day. Having skipped schooling, hated all learning and left formal education at the age of 13, the wayward youth had idled his days on the farmstead until a sudden impulse sent him to London at the age of 20 to work for his elder brother William at his new anatomy school in Covent Garden.

Working side-by-side with William for the next 12 years, John Hunter relentlessly explored human anatomy in the bodies of men, women and children bought or stolen from the gallows and the grave. He dissected more human bodies than anyone else of his time. Where human corpses failed to provide the answers, he resorted to animals in a tireless mission to understand all forms of organic life.

Keen to hone his skills on the living, Hunter spent a spell in the army – healing injured redcoats during the Seven Years War – before joining the staff of St George's Hospital in 1768. At a time when operations were crude, bloody and often fatal, Hunter forged a revolution by insisting surgery should be founded on the outcome of anatomical exploration, scientific experiment and meticulous observation. His 1000 or so pupils spread his doctrine throughout the British Isles and to America, so that today Hunter is justifiably known as the founder of scientific surgery—even if his ideals are still permeating into practice.

Fascination with the boundaries between life and death had always been one of Hunter's passions. At his country retreat and research laboratories in the sleepy hamlet of Earls Court, he had conducted experiments on hibernating animals and attempted to freeze fish then bring them back to life.

He even thought he might make his fortune by discovering the key to immortality through freezing then intermittently thawing volunteers. 'I thought that if a man would give up the last 10 years of his life to this kind of alternative oblivion and action, it might be prolonged to a 1000 years; and by getting himself thawed every 100 years, he might learn what had happened during his frozen condition,' he wrote [2].

Though recognising this particular technique had failed, he had not surrendered his interest in reviving the dead. And so when a group of philanthropists decided to draw up advice on ways to save people who drowned, Hunter was the obvious person to approach.

William Hawes, an apothecary in the Strand, and Thomas Cogan, a physician, had founded the Humane Society – later the Royal Humane Society – in 1774 based on a similar body in Amsterdam dedicated to rescuing victims of drowning [3]. The charity offered up to four guineas to anyone who succeeded in restoring life to any person 'taken out of the water for dead' within 30 miles of London. Well-meaning surgeons and physicians living near the Thames agreed to offer their aid free to help revive those who drowned.

However, since bloodletting and tobacco enemas were the commonest remedies for drowning, the demands on the charity's coffers were relatively few. So in 1776 Hawes asked John Hunter to draw up a rather more scientifically based regime for resuscitation.

Happy to oblige, Hunter not only prepared directions on attempted resuscitation for the charity, but presented his ideas to the Royal Society the same year [4]. It was a subject close to his heart, he explained, since inquiries into suspended animation had for many years 'been my business and favourite amusement'.

Based on experiments he had performed and the theories he had developed so far, Hunter argued that a person who drowned should not automatically be considered dead but 'that only a suspension of the actions of life has taken place'.

Naturally, given his belief in evidence of effectiveness, he rejected bloodletting and tobacco enemas, along with purging or vomiting remedies, as more like to 'depress life' than to restore it. Instead, he stressed that the first aim of any rescuer should be to throw air into the victim's lungs. For this he recommended a pair of double bellows, 'such as are commonly used in throwing fumes of tobacco up the anus' – though hopefully not the same ones – for pumping air into a person's mouth or nose.

Perhaps, he suggested, the newly discovered 'dephlogisticated air' – oxygen – which the chemist Joseph Priestley had described in 1775 might also prove effective. And if all else failed, Hunter suggested attempting to restart the heart with electric shocks. 'Electricity has been known to be of service, and should be tried when other methods have failed,' he advised. 'It is probably the only method we have of immediately stimulating the heart.'

In fact Benjamin Franklin, the American diplomat and scientist, had first suggested that electricity might be used to revive people apparently dead, although he never put his theory into practice. But Hunter may well have been referring to a case in 1774, when a 3-year-old girl who fell from a first storey window was revived with electric shocks to her chest, probably from a Leyden jar, in the first recorded example of successful defibrillation [5].

Finally, Hunter proposed that two people should work in tandem to effect resuscitation and at every attempted rescue 'an accurate journal' should be kept of the methods used and degree of success. As ever, he believed that continual reassessment of practice was the route to improvement.

Hunter's recommendations to act quickly, concentrate on restoring breathing and apply artificial respiration would become cornerstones in standard resuscitation practice—although simple mouth-to-mouth resuscitation would eventually be adopted from 1959 as the most successful method. His recommendation to use defibrillation to restart the heart or regulate its rhythm would only become widely adhered to in the 1950s.

But while effective methods of revival would take time to introduce, the society's laudable aims attracted numerous supporters. Among them was the Reverend Dodd, who made a donation in 1776, the same year Hunter produced his guidance. A year later, as he faced the gallows, Dodd had the chance to make an even greater contribution to the charity's cause. In death he represented the first opportunity for Hunter to test out his theories on revival.

Hunter's conviction that he could bring back Dodd from the dead was not entirely far-fetched. Since most hanged convicts died from a long and slow process of asphyxiation rather than a swift and irredeemable broken neck it was not unknown for hanged people to revive.

Several cases were recorded in the 18th century. In the most notorious, in 1740 a 17-year-old thief called William Duell swung on the gallows for half-an-hour before he was delivered to the barber-surgeons for customary dissection. Just as the surgeons were about to slice open his chest, the youth emitted a groan and sat up; having cheated death once, his sentence was commuted to transportation [6].

Hunter knew from his long experience of obtaining corpses from Tyburn that revival was theoretically possible and he had already outlined sound recommendations for achieving this. But as he famously told his favourite pupil, Edward Jenner, when he posed a query to the surgeon, 'why think, why not try the Expt' [7]. All he needed was a willing guinea pig.

The events that ensued in the undertaker's parlour in Goodge Street would remain secret for nearly two decades.

Hunter never referred in writing to what may well have been his most remarkable experiment.

Yet as soon as Dodd swung from the gibbet the speculation began. 'Experiments were said to have been tried to bring Dr Dodd to life,' reported the *Gentleman's Magazine*, 'according to the instructions formerly published by Dr [sic] Hunter, but without effect. He hung an hour, and it was full 40 min before he was put into a hearse' [8].

Later that year another magazine reported an Irishman's claim to have dined with Dodd in Dunkirk shortly after his supposed execution [9]. And even 20 years later, the *Gentleman's Magazine* was still appealing to its readers to throw light on events. According to one response, Hunter and his helpers tried to resuscitate the curate in a hot bath – and believed they would have succeeded had the crowd not delayed their efforts by half-an-hour too long. After it proved clear their plan had failed, the correspondent continued, the body was interred at St Laurence's Church in Cowley, West London [10].

But the obsession with Dodd did not end there. In 1794 a Scottish newspaper suggested Dodd was alive and well and living in Glasgow, 17 years after being brought back to life by John Hunter. Relating an account of his dramatic resurrection, the anonymous writer revealed:

'When he was turned off, he felt a sudden impulse of pain at first, by his body whirling round very swiftly, he was soon deprived of all sensation, and afterwards remained totally senseless, until he found himself in bed, surrounded by Doctor C, Mr H, Mr D and Mr W, whom he perceived to be in tears, which may be considered as an effusion of joy at his recovery, of which they at one time despaired' [11].

According to this precise description, Dodd's body had been conveyed to the undertaker's house where Hunter and his three medical friends were waiting. As soon as Dodd's body was bundled out of the hearse and into the house, Hunter and 'Mr D' stripped the corpse and rubbed the skin vigorously for 2 hours before at last they saw a sign of breathing. The next moment Dodd's skin broke out in a sweat, a groan emerged and the curate sat up. Now fully restored to 'sound health', Dodd was living at the house of a friend, the writer claimed.

So did the life-loving curate really breathe again after swinging at Tyburn? Had the remarkable surgeon actually defeated death?

Although Hunter would never commit to paper the events which followed Dodd's hanging, he did disclose details of the attempted revival to his closest friends in the coffee-house club which he hosted after weekly meetings of the Royal Society. Charles Hutton, professor of mathematics at the Royal Military Academy, Woolwich, and a Royal Society fellow, later recalled the evening – shortly after Dodd's execution – when Hunter was persuaded to reveal the story [12].

It was true, Hunter admitted, that he and several other Royal Society fellows had concocted a scheme to procure Dodd's body in order to attempt an experiment to bring him back to life. But the delays in obtaining his body meant by the time it arrived at the undertakers', they had all but given up hope of revival. Still they 'tried all the means in their power for the reanimation' but after labouring for a considerable time, the chaplain's body remained cold and lifeless. The experiment, according to Hutton, had 'entirely failed'.

Hutton's account, published in a newspaper in 1822 after all the participants in the experiment were long dead, certainly tallied with earlier descriptions of the attempted revival. Almost certainly, Hunter would have attempted inflating Dodd's lungs with bellows, as well as warming his body by the fire and rubbing his flesh, according to the guidelines he had submitted to the Humane Society. It is likely too that he would have employed electric shocks from a Leyden jar in his efforts to revive Dodd – in a scene evocative of the future *Frankenstein* novel. Yet all the evidence points to the conclusion that Hunter's ambitious experiment had indeed 'entirely failed'.

Nevertheless, speculation about Dodd's whereabouts would continue down the centuries – fuelled partly by the fact that while a memorial stone attests to his burial in St Laurence's churchyard, no record of his interment can be found in the parish register [13].

I am grateful for the help of Peter Baskett, Editor of *Resuscitation*, and to John Zorab, retired consultant anaesthetist, for help in my research.

The Knife Man by Wendy Moore is published on 1st February by Bantam Press, Price £18.99. Save £2.00 and order a copy at the special price of £16.99 including postage and packing. Please call Bookpost PLC on 01624 677237.

## References

[1] Dobson J, John Hunter and the unfortunate Doctor Dodd. In: Journal of the History of Medicine, vol. 10, 1955. p. 369–78; Rev W. Foster, Samuel Johnson and the Dodd Affair (Lichfield, Johnson Society, 1951) and accounts in the Gentleman's Magazine.

[2] Hunter J. In: James Palmer, editor. The Works, vol. 1. London: Longman, Rees, Orme, Brown, Breen; 1835. p. 284.

[3] Bishop PJ. A Short History of the Royal Humane Society. London: RHS; 1974.

[4] Hunter J. Proposals for the recovery of persons apparently drowned, read to the Royal Society. In: The Works, vol. 4, 21 March 1776. p. 165–75.

[5] Duda D, Brandt L, El Gindi M. The history of defibrillation. In: Atkinson R, Boulton T, editors. The History of Anaesthesia: Proceedings of the Second International Symposium on the History of Anaesthesia held in London, 20–23 April 1987. London and New York: Royal Society of Medicine; 1987. p. 464–8.

[6] Linebaugh P. The Tyburn riot against the surgeons. In: Douglas Hay, editor. Albion's Fatal Tree: Crime and Society in Eighteenth-century England. London: Allen Lane; 1975. p. 103.

[7] Hunter J. Selter to Edward Jenner, 2 August (no year). In: Cornelius EH, Harding Rains AJ, editors. Letters from the Past, from John Hunter to Edward Jenner. London: Royal College of Surgeons of England; 1976. p. 9.

[8] Gentleman's Magazine, vol. 47, 27 June 1777. p. 346.

[9] Dobson J, John Hunter and the unfortunate Doctor Dodd. Citing the London Review of English and Foreign Literature of September 1777.

[10] Gentleman's Magazine, vol. 60, 1790. p. 1010, 1066 and 1077–8.

[11] Dobson J, John Hunter and the unfortunate Doctor Dodd. Citing the Aberdeen Journal, 19 August 1794.

[12] Dobson J, John Hunter and the unfortunate Doctor Dodd. Citing a letter from Charles Hutton in the Newcastle Magazine, March 1822.

[13] Dobson J, John Hunter and the unfortunate Doctor Dodd. p. 376.

# Charles Kite: The clinical epidemiology of sudden cardiac death and the origin of the early defibrillator

Ana Graciela Alzaga    Joseph Varon     Peter Baskett

In the eighteenth century, drowning had the equivalent impact that sudden cardiac death has today. In the latter part of this century scientists throughout Europe established Humane Societies to develop resuscitation techniques and to keep registries on the successful and unsuccessful cases [1,2]. The first was the "Maatschappy Tot Redding Van Drenkelingen" in Amsterdam in 1767 [3]. Soon after, in 1771, a Humane Society was established in Paris followed by the Humane Society (later the Royal Humane Society – the Royal title being granted by King George III) in London founded in 1776 from the original concept started by Cogan and Hawes in 1774 as "An Institution for Affording Immediate relief to Persons Apparently Dead from Drowning" [1]. This Society established houses which would receive drowned victims between the Westminster and the London Bridges [1]. The members of this Society would apply resuscitation techniques suggested by their own and other Societies and their colleagues and maintained registries of the successful and unsuccessful cases [1].

Dr. Charles Kite was an active member of the London Humane Society and in 1778 he wrote "*An Essay on the Recovery of the Apparently Dead*" for which he was awarded the Silver Medal given by the Society [4–6]. In this essay, he differentiated suspended animation from irreversible death [4,5]. Kite described the importance of collecting the necessary information regarding each victim of drowning in an organised

table [4,5]. He mentioned in his essay a total of 442 cases of which 125 were successful and 317 unsuccessful [4]. In the Appendix to his essay, he included the contents of a resuscitation kit and described one of the first defibrillators [4,5].

Charles Kite was an English doctor and scientist from Gravesend in Kent. He had noticed the high incidence of drowned victims and recognized the need to prevent and treat people who were in "suspended animation" [4]. He believed that the "success in the recovery of the apparently dead, is related to the length of time that elapses before the proper remedies can be applied" [4]. Kite also believed that unsuccessful outcomes could be prevented "if proper and timely assistance could have been given" [4]. Nevertheless, he stated that "even putrefaction should not deter the enthusiast since it might inadvertently represent advanced scurvy" [4]. His motto was "*hac animas ille evocat Orco Pallentes*" meaning "here souls challenge the greenish death" [6].

## 1. The "Essay on the Recovery of the Apparently Dead"

Charles Kite followed John Hunter's recommendations which encouraged all who were involved in resuscitation to be "required to keep accurate journals of the means used, and the degree of success attending them; whence we may be furnished with facts sufficient to enable us to draw conclusions, on which a certain practice may hereafter be established" [1,7]. In 1788 he published in London "An Essay on the Recovery of the Apparently Dead" describing the epidemiology

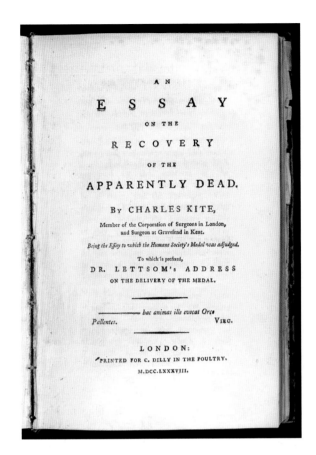

Fig. 1. Cover of Kite's *Essay on the recovery of the apparently dead.*

of drowning [4] (Fig. 1). His numerous contributions to the science of resuscitation included the proposal of considering "principally drowning, as the cause of suspended animation which most frequently occurs, and which was therefore the most important" [4]. Kite's principles for resuscitation attempts show parallels with the guidelines used nowadays and some would consider him to be the father of the clinical epidemiology of sudden death [5].

Kite's essay distinguished apparent death ("suspended animation") from real or irreversible death, which he "conceived to rest entirely to one circumstance, of the presence or absence of the principle of irritability" [4]. He understood that "the powers of life may be suspended by various causes" [4] (Table 1). An important development was the fact that he used electrical shocks to the body to determine if a patient was dead [4]. If no muscular contraction occurred, it was irreversible [4]. Indeed, in this essay he includes, the description

of the one of the first successful defibrillators and the contents of a portable resuscitation case [4,5].

Kite believed that the basis of resuscitation techniques was to remove the congestion about the heart and lungs and to excite the muscular fibres [4]. The lack of muscular activity was equivalent to death [4]. Among his recommendations, he included making "great noises" near the victim's ears which is similar to "shake and shout", artificial respiration with either warm air from the lungs or dephlogisicated air (oxygenated air) and placing the victim in a correct position—that is laying the person flat on the back [1,4] (See Table 2). Interestingly, he did not mention the use of chest or abdominal compressions, but did advocate cricoid pressure by an assistant to completely "stop up the gullet".

From an epidemiological standpoint, his essay was unique as he listed and published the information which was required to be collected in every episode of drowning or near-drowning such as: length of time in and under the water, season of the year, temperature of the air, and the times elapsed between entering the water and the application of resuscitation techniques [4] (Table 3). He organized large data collection as a "spreadsheet" including demographic information (age and sex), life situation, general health, circumstances before drowning [4]. This "spreadsheet", which extended to $3 \times 2$ feet ($39 \times 67$ cm) when unfolded, provided an ample opportunity to record the detailed information [4,5]. The information recovered was correlated with the outcome: data on the return of life, time of acquired external signs of life, and so on [4,5]. These recommendations are strikingly similar to those advocated in the Utstein style report [5,8]. Kite's essay was really the first formal study of prehospital sudden death [5].

In 1788, Charles Kite was awarded the Silver Medal by the Humane Society with the Latin words inscribed *Propter Erudituam Dissertationem de Resuscitatione* ("For Scholarly Dissertation on Resuscitation") "as attributed justly due to his industry, abilities, and philanthropy" and whose mind has been "enlarged by true science" [6]. He truly honoured the expression which represented the Society: "If one life be saved within the year, the Society will be established forever" [6].

## 2. A resuscitation kit

In the eighteen century, scientists had already arranged a kit containing vital instruments to perform artificial respira-

Table 1
The principal causes to which the death of drowned people have been attributed

| The principal causes to which the death of drowned people have been attributed, may be comprehended in the four following: |
|---|
| 1. That species of apoplexy which arises from an over distension of the stomach. |
| 2. The blood being rendered unfit for performing its offices, by want of the action of the air, in respiration. |
| 3. Water in the lungs: and, |
| 4. A contraction of the parts about the larynx, preventing the air from [assign into or out of the lungs], and producing death by |
|     a. The enclosed air being rendered highly phlogisticated. |
|     b. Suffocation, or a congestion of blood about the heart and lungs; or, |
|     c. Apoplexy. |

Table 2
Two indications in the recovery of persons apparently dead from drowning

In the recovery of persons apparently dead from drowning, there are two indications:
I. To remove the compression of the brain, and the congestion about the heart and lungs.
II. To excite the irritability of the muscular fibres.
   A. The removing the compression of the brain, and the congestion about the heart and lungs, may be effected by
      i. Bleeding
      ii. Artificial respiration
      iii. Proper position
   B. The exciting the irritability of the muscular fibres may be done by
      i. General stimulants; as
         a. The proper application of heat
         b. Electricity
         c. Frictions
         d. Gentle concussions
      ii. Local stimulants; as
         a. Aromatic and irritating medicines thrown into the stomach
         b. Aromatic and irritating medicines injected into the intestines
         c. Particular stimuli adapted to the different organs of the senses

Table 3
Sketch of a plan for obtaining accurate histories apparently dead from drowning

**Circumstances previous to the accident**
   1. Sex
   2. Age
   3. Constitution
   4. Situation in life
   5. General health
   6. Circumstances increasing the action of the heart and arteries
   7. Circumstances diminishing the energy of the vital powers
**At the time of the accident**
   8. In the water, (length of time, if he/she sunk, voluntary motion, if he/she floated on his /her back or belly)
   9. Under water, (length of time, if he/she sunk, depth, fresh/salt)
   10. Season of the year, and temperature of the air
**Circumstances and appearances as soon as taken up**
   11. The length of time that had elapsed between the taking up to the body and the application of proper remedies
   12. The manner in which, during that period, he had been treated
   13. Appearance of the body: face, eyelids, eyes, jaw, mouth, tongue, skin, stomach, abdomen, joints, limbs)
**The method of recovery**
   14. Every individual remedy to be expressed: order, length of time, benefit or disadvantage, remedies which seemed to work)
**At the return of life**
   15. The length of time the external signs of life appeared to be suspended
   16. The first symptoms of life
   17. The progressive order in which the other symptoms made their appearance
**Complaints after recovery**

tion for victims of near-drowning and inhalation exposures [5]. In 1775, Dr. Cogan, who was patronized by the Society, developed an apparatus to assist respiration for such victims [4,5]. Unfortunately, the major problem with this apparatus was its unpractical size [4,5].

Dr. Kite was the first clinician to recognize and document the importance of a portable "apparatus, comprehending a collection of all the articles and instruments which are a requisite on these occasions... if it could be comprised in a case..., it will prove a very considerable acquisition to the resuscitation art" [4]. He described in the Appendix of his Essay, a pocket case of instruments for the recovery of the apparently dead, "a collection which comprehends every article except an electrical machine" and the correct way to use these instruments [4] (Figs. 2 and 3).

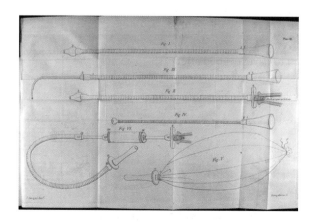

Fig. 2. Contents of the resuscitation kit.

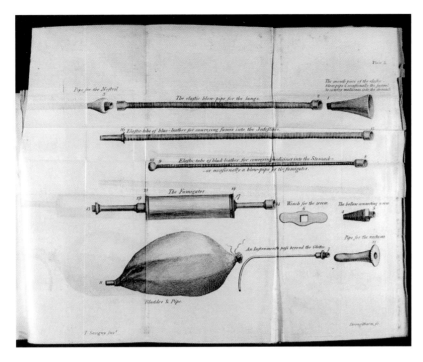

Fig. 3. Contents of the resuscitation kit.

## 3. Remarkable recovery from drowning

Dr. Kite describes in his book *Essays and observations, physiological and medical on the submersion of animals*, "one of the most remarkable cases" of a recovery from drowning he had ever participated in [9]. He narrates the case of a 35-year-old private in the militia who had been suffering with a fever for a week. He felt much better on the morning of February 12, 1793. He marched with the rest of the regiment and then crossed the river on the baggage wagon. It was a cold windy day and the water was "equally cold". He first fell ill with what was described as an epilepsy attack ("epilepsia febricola"), and became delirious and fell into the water. He remained in the water for 12 minutes, at least, with "his body entirely under water, and his head two feet beneath the surface". His body was "entirely passive"; "he made not the least attempt to swim".

When the boats that went to his rescue took him on board, he did not show "the least appearance of life". "His head was bloated and his face black". His clothes were removed and the "rubbing the water off the chest and upper part of the body" seemed to have a "good effect" since he made his first effort to breath, although without a pulse. He was then "immediately dried and warmed", and the breathing was repeated. An irregular pulse was perceived. He had a significant epistaxis. He "lay in a mild epileptic state for an hour and a half" but his heart beat regained strength. He was given an anodyne with antimony as a stimulant.

By the evening, he was completely alert and oriented and was able to sleep throughout the night. The next morning, he was completely recovered, his "intellects" were "very clear", with no complaints and felt better than the morning before.

This was one of the cases Dr. Kite considered to be "remarkable" since for a considerable amount of time his head was underwater, he had "an injury to the vessels of the head" evidenced by "the haemorrhage from the nostrils" and a "long obliteration and confusion of the senses" [9].

## 4. The defibrillator

Electricity was first generated by electrostatic machines and possibly the first was developed in 1705 by Hawksbee. Application of electricity to the chest had been suggested by Wilkinson [10]. Edward Nairn had also developed a machine in 1760.

Charles Kite includes in his essay the description of his own "defibrillator" (Fig. 4). This device was used to apply electric shocks to collapsed victims paying "singular attention to the powers of the electrical fire" [4]. This defibrillator included the same basic elements of a modern defibrillator: a capacitor (a means to store energy), a way to adjust the charge, and two electrodes to be applied across the chest (See Fig. 4).

Kite describes this device composed of "...two pieces of brass wire each 2 feet long, enclosed in glass tubes or wooden cases well varnished with knobs at one end, and rings at the other: the knobs are to be applied like common directors, to those parts between which we intend the fluid to pass; and one ring connected with a chain or metallic string, coming from the electrometer, and the other with a chain joined to the outside of the vial, which will be more convenient if suspended on the prime conductor. In the manner, shocks may be sent through any part of the body; and their direction constantly

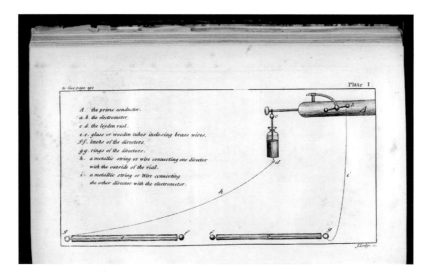

Fig. 4. Kite's defibrillator.

varied, without a probability of the assistants receiving any inconvenience..." [4,11].

Kite envisaged the application of electricity in resuscitation as Herholdt and Rafn [12,13] had described it as "an electric shock applied across the chest, from the right to the left side, directly on the large vessels of the heart and lungs... is the best cardiacum in a drowned person" therefore stimulating the phrenic nerve inducing diaphragmatic movement [4].

The application of successful "defibrillation" was recorded in 1774 when Catherine Sophie Greenhill, a 3-year-old, fell out of a second story window and was "taken up to all appearance dead" and 20 minutes after a doctor applied electricity in an attempt for resuscitation [4,5,13–16]. "On transmitting a few shocks through the thorax, he perceived small pulsations" and the girl began breathing. After 4 days of coma, the child was revived to perfect health. The girl probably had a brain contusion with undetectable, shallow respirations and the shocks stimulated her to produce perceptible vital signs [4]. Kite would recommend electric stimulation without question, "the most powerful stimulus we can apply" to awaken the body from suspended animation [4].

"These accounts establish facts of a very important and interesting nature. Do not they prove, clearly and indubitably, that animation is capable of being suspended longer than we are aware of? Do they not plainly point out, that electricity is the most powerful stimulus we can apply? Is not the superior advantage of this stimulus evinced in the most incontrovertible and unequivocal manner? And are we not justified in the presuming, that if it is able so powerfully to excite the action of the external muscles, that it will be capable of reproducing the motion of the heart, which is infinitely more irritable, and by that means accomplish our desideratum, the renewal of the circulation?" [4].

The Royal Humane Society described electricity as a "most powerful agent, a very proper remedy" in resuscitation [14]. It was recommended that after the patient was electrified for "4–5 minutes, the hand of one of the attendants should be applied close to the body, so as to take sparks which should be drawn from the left side of the heart" using the patient as a capacitor and the resuscitator as the ground to direct the exit of current via the heart [14].

Amazingly, electricity was not used for defibrillation until over a century later when Prevost and Battelli demonstrated electrical fibrillation and defibrillation in dogs [17]. Later it was developed by Hooker et al. [18], and Gurvich and Yuniev [19], before being introduced into clinical practice by Claude Beck in 1947 [20] and being applied externally by Zoll et al. [21] as Kite had done almost 200 years before.

## References

[1] Sternbach GL, Varon J, Fromm R, Baskett PJF. The Humane Societies. Resuscitation 2000;45:71–5.

[2] Schechter DC. Role of the humane societies in the history of resuscitation. Surg Gyn Obstet 1969:811–5.

[3] Meijer P. Historie en Maatschappy tot Redding van Drenkelingen. Amsterdam; 1768.

[4] Kite C. Essay on the recovery of the apparently dead. 1788: xxvi-274.

[5] Eisenberg MS. Charles Kite's essay on the recovery of the apparently dead: The First Scientific Study of Sudden Death. Ann Emerg Med 1994;23:1049–53.

[6] Kite C. Essay on the Recovery of the Apparently Dead. Dr Lettsoms Address pp iii, iv-v, xiv-xxv 1788.

[7] Hunter J. Proposals for the recovery of people apparently drowned. The Philosophical Transactions 1776;66:412–3.

[8] Cummins RO, Chamberlain D, Abramson NS, et al. Recommended guidelines for uniform reporting of data from out of hospital cardiac arrest: the Utstein Style. A Statement for health professionals from a task force of the American Heart Association, the European Resuscitation Council, the Heart and Stroke Foundation of Canada and the Australian Resuscitation Council. Resuscitation 1991;22;1–26.

[9] Kite, C. Essays and observations, physiological and medical on the submersion of animals. London, 1795. p. 377–85.

[10] Wilkinson J. Tutanem Nauticum (the Seamans Preservation) London, 1764.

[11] Stillings D. The first defibrillator? Med Progr Technol 1974;2:205–6.

[12] Herholdt JD, Rafn CG. An Attempt at an Historical Survey of Life Saving measures for Drowning and Information of the Best Means by which They can be Brought Back to Life. Printed at H Tikiob's, Bookseller, Copenhagen, 1796. p. 63–7.

[13] Baskett PJF, Herholdt JD, Rafn CG. Two unsung heroes from Denmark. Resuscitation Greats Resuscitation 2003;58:283–5.

[14] Reports of the Humane Society. London, 1774.

[15] Struve CA. A practical Essay in the art of recovering suspended animation. Pub Murray and Highly. London, 1802.

[16] Wilkinson DJ. The History of Trauma Anaesthesia. In: Grande CM, Baskett PJF, Bircher NG, Capan LM, Carli PA, Cicala RS, Cullen BF, Dick WF, Grenvik ANA, Stene JK, editors. Textbook of Trauma Anesthesia and Critical Care. Mosby Baltimore, 1993. p. 11–2.

[17] Prevost JL, Battelli F: On some effects of electrical discharges on the hearts of mammals. Compt Rend Acad Sci, Paris 1899;129:1267.

[18] Hooker DR, Kouwenhoven WB, Langworthy OR. Effect of alternating electrical current on the heart. Am J Physiol 1933;103:444–54.

[19] Gurvich NL, Yuniev SG. Restoration of a regular rhythm in the mammalian fibrillating heart. Am Rev Sov Med 1946;3:236–9.

[20] Beck CS, Pritchard H, Feil SH. Ventricular fibrillation of long duration abolished by electrical shock. JAMA 1947;135:985–6.

[21] Zoll PM, Linenthal AJ, Norman LR, et al. Termination of ventricular fibrillation in man by externally applied electric countershock. New Engl J Med 1956;254:727–32.

# JD Herholdt and CG Rafn: two unsung heroes from Denmark

Peter J.F. Baskett

The Scandinavian Society of Anaesthesiologists was founded in 1950 and, to celebrate its 10th anniversary, it gave a gift to all Scandinavian anaesthesiologists of a quite remarkable book in the Danish language by JD Herholdt and CG Rafn. Moreover, as a typical kindness to others outside Scandinavia, the book was translated into English and distributed to fortunate colleagues [1]. The driving force for this initiative was Henning Poulsen from Aarhus, the President of the Scandinavian Society at the time. He sought professional translators from his own university and the help of the renowned anaesthesiologist from Newcastle-upon-Tyne, MH Armstrong Davidson. The project was achieved with the financial support of Leo Pharmaceutical Products. So, a largely forgotten, but vital work, was brought to the attention of scientists of the 20th century.

The book rejoices in the wonderful title "An Attempt at an Historical Survey of Life-saving Measures for Drowning Persons and Information of the Best Means by Which They Can Be Brought Back to Life" (Fig. 1).

In that period scientific authors displayed a natural modesty. Not for them the snappy, and perhaps, arrogant title such as "Epinephrine beats vasopressin in raising coronary artery perfusion" but the rather diffident "An Attempt at an Historical Survey......". The book is small and comprises just 88 pages. It was published originally in 1796 and yet contains an enormous amount of information, and more importantly, wise comment—much of which was visionary and subsequently has been proven to be of key relevance to resuscitation of the submerged victim as practiced today.

Who then were Herholdt and Rafn?

John Daniel Herholdt was born in Aabenraa, Denmark in 1764. Having trained at the Theatrum Anatomico-Chirurgicum in Copenhagen, he became a surgeon in the Danish navy. A Latin scholar, he won the annual medical essay prize at the University of Copenhagen, although he had not matriculated there. Nevertheless,

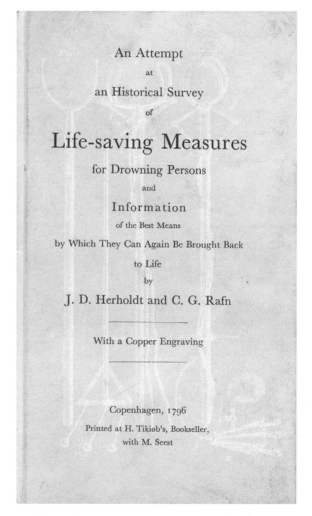

Fig. 1.

his application for the post of Professor of Anatomy was rejected. However, in 1805 he was appointed Professor Extraordinarius, and Professor of Medicine and Medical Physiology in 1818, and Rector of the University for two terms in 1819–1820 and 1834–1835. He died in 1836, aged 71.

Herholdt's publications, as was common in those days covered when scientists were versatile, covered a wide field. Many of them, such as this book, took the form of surveys or reviews with perspicacious comments, and many of them were written with his good friend Rafn.

Carl Gottlob Rafn was born in 1769 in Viborg, Denmark. He studied medicine, veterinary medicine and botany at the University of Copenhagen but did not sit the final examination. Instead he chose the field of administration, becoming Assessor in the Ministries of Agriculture and Commerce, a member of the Royal Inspectorate of Factories, Commissioner in the Ministries of Production and Fisheries, and the Director of the Royal Aquavit Distillery (probably a highly sought-after post!).

Unlike today's administrators and managers, Rafn made considerable scientific contributions which exerted considerable beneficial influence in his fields of interest which included medicine, veterinary medicine, botany, chemistry and mineralogy. Rafn died in 1808. His short life spanned just 38 years. His scientific contributions are certainly impressive for one who died so young.

Herholdt and Rafn formed a mutually supportive partnership. "Herholdt dealt with the theoretical aspect—and Rafn with the practical. The professor of medicine and physiology, and the practical scientifically trained, versatile government official, supplemented each other in a way which could well serve as a model" [2].

In their book Herholdt and Rafn devote the first 17 pages to a "Survey of the Progress in Life-saving Measures especially during Recent Times". This is a most valuable historical survey of the large number of humane initiatives being taken throughout the world towards the end of the eighteenth century. The survey is laced with personal comment, sometimes passionate and vehement, revealing their own compassion for their fellow human being.

They praise the people of Amsterdam, "the Lover of Mankind", who had formed a society in 1767,— "Maatschappy ter Redding der Drenkelingen"—to give instruction in life-saving measures after submersion (with rewards of 6 Ducats or a Gold Medal to encourage rescue attempts). This society was the first of the many humane societies to spring up around the world during the ensuing decades. The project in Holland spread from Amsterdam to Rotterdam where it was required that the owner of any house, including an inn, should allow the rescuer and the victim to enter to receive assistance, with a penalty of 25 Gulden for refusal. Fourteen months after its foundation the society reported that 19 persons, who had no signs of life when taken from the water, had been saved [3]. These results stimulated generous donations from worthy citizens and businesses sufficient to ensure the financial security in perpetuity. The Dutch society published its results again in 1793 and successful resuscitations by then had amounted to 990 cases. During the first 19 years of the report one victim in three survived; during the final nine years leading up to 1793, over 50% were resuscitated successfully.

"This Society worked not only in the Netherlands, but also influenced Foreign Nations by arousing their desire for Emulation. Soon did Lover of Mankind see similar Measures being furthered in Germany, France, England, and Italy, in North America, the East Indies, and indeed even in Algeria. Yet in particular did Hamburg distinguish itself".

As early as 1762, the Hamburg city authorities had a plan for rescuing victims of submersion with a reward system, but there was considerable prejudice and aversion to touching a person who had "died an unnatural death". The authorities dealt with this problem by ordering the troops based in the local garrison to rescue anybody who had fallen into the water and to attempt resuscitation "as long as there was the slightest hope of recovery". A society akin to the Netherlands society was formed in 1768 but progress was slow and it was to be over a decade before things improved. Between 1790 and 1793 115 awards were given for attempted rescues which had been successful in 75 cases. The average cost per life was 10 Rd. "We find that this price must be said to be very low compared to the Real Worth of the life of a Man, a Fellow Citizen".

Similar initiatives started in Paris in 1770, again with a reward system, and a reported success rate of 75% in 1776. That year "The English have also shown that they appreciate the worth of the lives of their Fellow Human Beings" for the London (later Royal) Humane Society was established in London and was highly successful— "so efficacious that even the citizens of Hamburg, whose Measures are so excellent, admitted that they were decidedly superior in all respects to theirs". It was AA Johnson who brought the ideas from Amsterdam and he believed that the resuscitation principles could be applied to other emergencies occurring in Great Britain [4]. However, it was William Hawes, one of the founder members of the London Humane Society, who was the driving force behind the organisation [5]. He was editor of the Transactions of the Society for many years. He also did a phenomenal amount of fund raising and arranged annual sermons which referred to work on resuscitation. He produced an action card and requested that "this always be at hand, as by the resuscitation process immediately employed, an immense number of lives will be restored" [6]. Although there is no mention of a financial reward system (only the award of a medal in special cases), the Royal Humane Society in 1794 was able to report on 3000 rescue attempts with a successful outcome in 2000 victims.

The system had also spread to Scotland at the instigation of William Cullen in a letter to Lord

Cathcart, President of the Board of Police in Scotland, setting out the recommended methods of resuscitation [7]. Citing Dr Monro, Cullen reports that "Dr Monro informs me, it is very practical to introduce directly into the glottis and trachea a crooked tube, such as a catheter used for a male adult". Precise directions for tracheal intubation followed. The Glasgow Humane Society was started in 1790 and remains active to this day [8]. Indeed members of one family have provided a rescue service on the River Clyde for almost a century. The Parsonage family, notably Ben and George, have worked on the Clyde during most of the 20th century, until recently in rowing boats (Fig. 2).

Herholdt and Rafn provide the best resume of the activities of the humane societies for they were writing contemporaneously. They describe the spread of societies in Vienna, Saxony, Milan, Padua, the East Indies and America. "But we must add the curious Item that the inhabitants of Algeria, these rough, unenlightened, barbaric people—whose Mullah, Ismael, with his own hand killed 80 of his kinsmen—these people, who generally hold Human Life so cheap and are so indifferent to Human Misery, not only were touched by the news of the Progress and great Usefulness of the English Life-saving Measures, but even more, they at once established similar Public Measures, which now

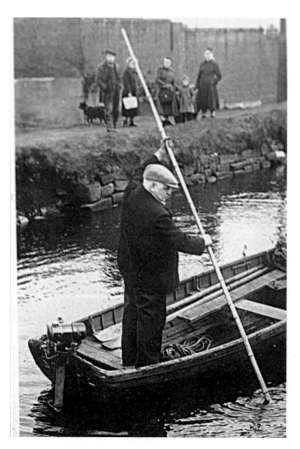

Fig. 2.

afford hope of Rescue, even for Danish citizens, who might be so unlucky as to fall into the water in Algeria".

With considerable feeling and passion Herholdt and Rafn berate the authorities in Denmark in their next paragraph.

"Less safe is the Danish citizen in the bosom of his own fatherland, whose sad lot it was, for a long time, to be less forward both in the Sciences and in Institutions for promoting the Public Weal. His country had unfortunately as yet done very little for the recovery of Fellow Citizens whose lives by accident become a Prey to Water". Despite pleas to the Government by the famous and venerated Achivator, Professor PG Hensler, little was done that proved effective for some years. At the time of writing in 1796, Herholdt and Rafn felt bitter at the lack of progress and paint a vivid literary picture.

"Consequently, public Life-saving measures are still lacking everywhere in the Danish States. Not even in our Capital of Copenhagen, which is surrounded by water and intersected by so many canals, has taken the least measures for the rescue of the many People who, according to the reports of the Gazettes, are found dead in the water every week".

"Much, nay everything! is lacking both for him who desires to rescue his brethren from the water, and for the doctor, who by his Art, endeavours to bring him back to life. Therefore large Crowds of People so often throng together, with no avail, on the banks of the water in which such a Drowning Person fights against death. In vain does the Victim utter the most heart-rending cries for Help. Because of the lack of implements the Spectators usually find that all help is impossible no-one ventures to place his own life in such evident jeopardy. The consequence is that the Distressed Person sinks lifeless to the bottom and is not rescued until the last Spark of Life has left his body".

Herholdt and Rafn feel that further efforts and initiatives are urgently required in Denmark and make proposals.

"Accordingly, these Means ought to be provided at the Public Expense and be available for the Doctor in the vicinity of every Canal and in any place where a Human Being is exposed to the risk of dying in water. The Private Physician does not always himself own the Apparatus for this purpose, and even if he has this, he cannot always carry it about with him; nor can it be had at the Apothecaries"

There is clearly a feeling of disgrace and disgust in the minds of the authors at the situation in Denmark at the time as they conclude this section of the book. This forms the prologue for the second part of the book which is a "Survey of the Most Beneficial and most Convenient Means for the Recovery of Apparently Drowned Persons".

Here the science takes over from the passion.

All of the methods of resuscitation in vogue at the time are reviewed. Although the is clearly aimed at the authorities of the time to exhort them to improve the situation in Denmark, the critical and perspicacious comments on each technique and theory offers us a glimpse of the considerable insight and foresight of this remarkable pair of scientists.

Great attention is paid to rescuer techniques using ingenious devices, the "Seeker" and "Catching Forceps" designed in Hamburg and "made of brass instead of iron they would be more costly, but also more durable, as this metal does not rust so easily". The victim rescued from the water is placed in a wicker basket or a special wicker and leather boat cunningly designed to allow the rescuer to carry it on land or walk on ice with safety (Fig. 3).

Graphic descriptions of the process of drowning pay testimony to the authors personal clinical experience. By reasoned argument they eliminate some of the theories of the time; that drowned persons died of apoplexy or pulmonary collapse. They argue cogently that death is due to hypoxia. It is noteworthy that oxygen had been discovered just over 20 years earlier. Priestley had described "dephlogisticated air" in 1772 [9], but it is likely that the original discoverer was Scheele but he did not publish until 1777 [10]. It was Lavoisier who coined the term oxygen in 1774 [11].

The process of dying during drowning is attributed by Herholdt and Rafn to respiratory obstruction and failure, followed by cardiac failure and cerebral damage.

"It is clear that the entire Plan of Treatment must aim at (1) removing all Hindrances to the Vital Functions... (and supporting) especially (2) the Respiration and (3) the Circulation of the Blood and (4) the suppressed energy of the Nerves". Exactly as we advocate today.

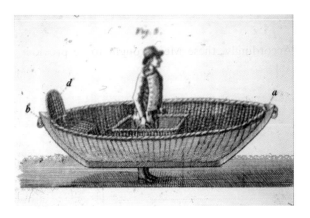

Fig. 3.

They exhort the rescuer not to give up too early for "an Asphyxiated Person, even when left to himself, may thus awaken from his slumber". "This truth, substantiated by reliable experiments, cannot be brought too strongly to the notice of the Practicing Physician. Suppose that a drowned Fellow Citizen awoke either spontaneously or by being moved in the Coffin after the Physician had definitely proclaimed his certain Death. Woe unto him, especially if he had not done everything in his power! Self Reproach, Disgrace and Deserved Contempt would follow him even unto the Grave". No doubt hypothermia at work here!

"Above all the Arrested Respiration should be started again" Herholdt and Rafn did not think much of the methods involving manual compression of the chest, even though these methods were advocated over a century later with what was to turn out to be misplaced enthusiasm [12-14].

Rather they preferred methods of insufflation of air into the lungs directly. Acknowledging that Mouth to Mouth ventilation is physiologically sound as "some oxygen invariably remains unconsumed when a Healthy Person takes a deep breath and at once expels that air again" they do not like the practical aspects very much.

"But as the insufflation of Air by mouth is a very Toilsome and Loathsome Act, and since accordingly an otherwise delicacy of feeling prohibits both the Physician and other People of Propriety from using this method, especially in adults and People of advanced years who have been drowned, it is of little use. So far, we have heard of only a few examples where well known men have overcome the unpleasant feeling associated with this act and in Honourable Enthusiasm used their own mouths for that purpose". This echoes the attitudes prevailing in some quarters today.

Instead of mouth to mouth ventilation they advocate the bellows method of John Hunter using "pure atmosphere" [15]. Inflation was through both nostrils but if this did not work well they advised that the jaw be depressed and the tongue forward or the trachea be intubated "by the introduction of a curved tube, similar to a male catheter, into the windpipe" in the manner described by Monro. They conclude that "this procedure is not difficult to perform". Herholdt and Rafn also remind us that it was Monro who devised the concept of cricoid pressure. "The cartilaginous rings of the windpipe (cartilage cricoidea) were pressed back against the neck bones in order to close the gullet".

Tracheotomy is identified as the only method of securing the airway when the "jaws of the victim are firmly locked together or when air cannot be forced through the nose into the lungs". Recommending that the procedure should only be done by a doctor they state "for the reassurance of the common people we may add that tracheotomy is far less dangerous that previously believed".

Condemning the practice of blood letting by scientific argument, they take the famous Hr Hensler to task for advocating this technique—"Is it not due to his Authority that many Danish Physicians still have far too unlimited confidence in this Remedy, and that in our Country, hardly any Drowned Person, of whose possible recovery there was the slightest hope, is buried here nobody is saved!—until without much hesitation, Blood Letting has been carried out one or more times? Is it not due to his treatise that Blood Letting on the Order of a responsible Person is sometimes performed on the lifeless Drowned Person?

Addressing the matter of stimulation of the circulation, Herholdt and Rafn had appreciated the risk of hypothermia and give a lucid review of the rewarming methods available and come down in favour of warm dry clothes and a warm bath at normal body temperature rather than the application of hot stones, ashes, sand or even horse dung advocated in some quarters.

Perhaps the most remarkable visionary statement in this book is the following:

"Among all means of resuscitation, nature has none which can be applied so directly to the heart or produce such a rapid and potent effect as— Electricity".

"All other so-called Cardiac Stimulants are of no other Use than this; either they bear witness to the obscure and incorrect concepts of our forefathers; or they exert an effect quite different from what has been believed, on quite different Organs, perhaps even scarcely by sympathy on the Heart".

"An Electric Shock applied across the chest, from the right to the left side, directly on the large blood vessels of the Heart and Lungs—such a shock of suitable strength, applied when the lungs are filled with pure Atmosphere or Vital Air, is the best Cardiacum in a Drowned Person"

The application of electric shocks to the chest had been mentioned by Kite at the Royal Humane Society in 1788, some 8 years previously [16], but it was not until 1802 that a case of recovery after application of an electric shock to the chest of a three year old child who had fallen from a second storey window was reported by Struve [17]. It is uncertain whether the child recovered in spite of, or because of, the electric shock!

It was over a century later that Prevost and Battelli added science to inspired conjecture and showed that application of an electric shock was effective in reversing ventricular fibrillation and that direct current was more effective than alternating current [18]. Herholdt and Rafn may not have understood the mechanism of defibrillation precisely but they certainly had identified

the correct priority with remarkable foresight and vision. It took over one and a half centuries for the rest of the medical world to appreciate that they were correct in their hypothesis.

Herholdt and Rafn conclude their book by setting out a simple sequential algorithm for rescuing and treating the victim of submersion and a list of equipment required. They are set out with a clarity and brevity that is an example to us all.

Henning Poulsen, in his Foreword to the reprint published in 1960, writes: "Together they (Herholdt and Rafn) stand as a token of the valuable centuries-old tradition within Scandinavian medical science. They took up vital problems for critical analysis and evaluation, and reported their findings in a clear and objective fashion, and also ensured that their patients themselves would derive benefit from the experience gained. They pointed the way forward towards the methods used today in anaesthesiology and resuscitation" [19].

That statement still holds true 40 years on.

Perforce, much of the contents of this lucid book is anecdotal but today's anecdotes provide the inspiration for tomorrow's evidence based medicine.

## References

[1] Herholdt JD, Rafn CG. An Attempt at an Historical Survey of Life-saving Measures for Drowning Persons and Information of the Best Means by Which They Can Again Be Brought Back to Life. Copenhagen: Printed at H Tikiob's Bookseller with M Seest; 1796.

[2] Poulsen H. 1960 Foreword p. VII. In a Reprint of An Attempt at an Historical Survey of Life-saving Measures for Drowned Persons and Information of the Best Means by Which They Can Be Brought Back to Life. Copenhagen: Printed at H Tikiob's Bookseller with M Seest; 1796.

[3] Geschichte und Urkunden der im Jahre 1767 zur Rettung der Ertrunkenen zu Amsterdam errichteten Gesellschaft. Hamburg; 1769.

[4] Johnson AA. A short account of a society in Amsterdam instituted in the year 1767 for the recovery of drowned persons showing the utility and advantage that would accrue to Great Britain from a similar institution extending to cases of suffocation by damp in mines, choking, strangling and other accidents. London; 1778.

[5] Hawes W. The Transactions of the Royal Humane Society. Vol 1. London; 1796 .

[6] Hawes W. The Pocket Companion. Trans. R. Soc. London; 1806.

[7] Cullen WA. A letter to Lord Cathcart, President of the Board of Police in Scotland, concerning the recovery of persons drowned and seemingly dead. London; 1776.

[8] Parsonage G. Rescue his business, the Clyde his life. Glasgow Cities Libraries Publications Board, The Mitchell Library, North Street, Glasgow G3; 1990.

[9] Priestley J. Experiments and observations on different kinds of air. Phil Trans 1772;61:216.

[10] Scheele CW. Discovery of Oxygen. (1772). Alembic Club Reprint No 8. Edinburgh. Clay; 1894.

[11] Priestley J. Discovery of Oxygen. (1775). Alembic Club Reprint No 7. Edinburgh. Clay; 1894.

[12] Silvester HR. A new method of resuscitating stillborn children and of restoring persons apparently dead or drowned. Brit Med J 1858;2:576.

[13] Schafer EA. Description of a simple method of performing artificial respiration in the human subject. Medico-Chirurgical Trans. Royal Med. and Chir. Soc. London 1904;87:609.

[14] Neilsen H. A method of resuscitation. Ugeskr. Laeg. 1932;94;1201-3

[15] Hunter J. Proposal for the recovery of people apparently drowned. Phil Trans R Soc London 1776.

[16] Kite C. An essay on the recovery of the apparently dead. London; 1788.

[17] Struve CA. A practical essay on the art of recovering suspended animation. Translated from the original text in German of 1797. London: Murray and Highley; 1802.

[18] Prevost JL, Battelli F. On some effects of electrical discharges on the hearts of mammals. Compt Rend Acad Sci (Paris) 1899;129:1267.

[19] Poulsen H. 1960 Foreword p. VIII. In a Reprint of An Attempt at an Historical Survey of Life-saving Measures for Drowned Persons and Information of the Best Means by Which They Can Be Brought Back to Life. Copenhagen: Printed at H Tikiob's Bookseller with M Seest; 1796.

# The 1800s

To some extent the 1880s was a period of consolidation, building on the scientific foundations of the previous two hundred years. The experimental groundwork for the intravenous injection of drugs and blood was laid in the 17th century by Sir Christopher Wren (1632-1723) and Richard Lower (1631-1691). Wren, assisted by Robert Boyle, first injected opium into the veins of dogs in 1656. Richard Lower was the first to perform direct transfusion of blood from one animal to another in 1665. Shock associated with blood loss was observed by the ancients, most commonly associated with the trauma of battle. As Hippocrates said: 'He who desires to practice surgery must go to war'. It was in the military arena that tourniquets were developed to arrest blood loss from severed limbs. **Frederich von Esmarch** introduced the principle of triage and a field pressure dressing during the Franco-Prussian war. However, it was to be in the obstetrical arena that the first transfusion of human-to-human blood was successfully carried out by **James Blundell** for severe postpartum haemorrhage. Intravenous crystalloid solutions were to come later. The innovative and courageous introduction of intravenous saline by **William O'Shaughnessy** and **Thomas Latta** during the cholera epidemic in England in 1831 was successful and appropriately reported in the *Lancet,* but forgotten for the next fifty years until it re-emerged as the standard treatment for severe dehydration and hypovolaemia. Lactated Ringer's solution was developed by **Sydney Ringer** for physiological experiments in 1883 and adapted for intravenous infusion in the early 20th century.

The mid 19th century saw the start of the manual methods of artificial respiration and these were to hold sway for the next century. Ironically they were to be replaced by mouth-to-mouth respiration, which had originally been advocated and accepted in the latter part of the 18th century. The reason for fall from favour of the mouth-to-mouth techniques was a combination of things: the demonstration of carbon dioxide in expired air, the germ theory of disease and aesthetic distaste. **Marshall Hall** developed his ready method of manual resuscitation in 1856. Variations on this theme were soon developed by others in the 19th century, including **Henry Silvester** and **Benjamin Howard**. Further modifications were applied by **Frank Eve, Edward Schafer** and **Holger Neilsen** in the early 20th century.

Stimulated by events in war and civilian disasters the organization of emergency and resuscitation services continued in the 19th century. During the Napoleonic wars two French surgeons, **Dominique Larrey** and **Pierre Percy** organized triage and horse drawn 'flying ambulances' on the battlefield. Following the disastrous fire at the Ring Theatre in the city of Vienna **Baron von Mundy** organized the volunteer ambulance service of Vienna. **Jean-Henri Dunant** from Geneva founded the International Red Cross after observing the plight of the wounded on the battlefield of Solferino, ultimately paving the way for the Geneva Convention.

# Claude Bernard: On the origin of carbon monoxide poisoning

George L. Sternbach    Joseph Varon

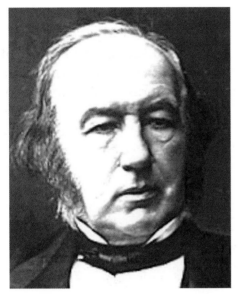

## 1. History

Although it was Claude Bernard who first published an accurate description of the physiology of carbon monoxide poisoning, [1] this is not the work for which he is best known. The nineteenth century French physician and scientist is renowned for a wide variety of physiological and biological discoveries, the most important of which pertain to the glycogenic function of the liver, the role of the pancreas in digestion, muscle physiology and vasomotor nerve function [2]. He is recognized as establishing physiology as an important area of medical study, and his magnum opus, *Introduction to the Study of Experimental Medicine* is considered a classic in scientific literature [3].

Born in 1813 in the village of Saint-Julien in the Beaujolais region, Bernard began his career as an apprentice in a pharmacy. He was an indifferent trainee, and a year and a half of service managed mainly to induce in him a distrust of the haphazard empirical methods then prevalent in medicine. Years later, a testimonial from the pharmacist indicated that he had "conducted himself honorably and faithfully" but excluded to mention that he showed any special talent for pharmacy [4]. Among his tasks was the compounding of "theriaque", a widely-used panacea composed of opium, squills, spikenard and myrrh dissolved in honey and wine. Bernard soon discovered that any available excess medicinal powders were also often appended to the mixture.

His real interest lay in becoming a playwright. Having had a play produced in the provinces, Bernard proceeded to Paris to have his literary work reviewed by Saint-Marc Girardin, an influential critic and professor of literature at the Sorbonne. The latter was unimpressed, allegedly advising Bernard, "You have done some pharmacy, study medicine. You have not the temperament of a dramatist" [4]. Following this advice, Bernard entered the Medical College of France, from where he graduated in 1843.

While at medical school, he became a disciple of Francois Magendie, a vigorous proponent of the experimental method. Bernard never practiced clinical medicine, turning instead to laboratory investigation and teaching. His wife and daughters eventually abandoned him when he refused to give up experimental medicine in order to pursue a more lucrative clinical practice [5].

Upon Magendie's death in 1855, Bernard replaced him as lecturer at the College of France. He began to compile his lectures beginning in that year, and by 1879, this comprised a body of work of fourteen volumes. In 1857, Bernard published a volume entitled *Lecons sur les Effets des Substances Toxiques et Medicamenteuses* (Lectures on the effects of toxic and medicinal substances), this constituting the series of lectures he had delivered the year before. These being his first lectures as Magendie's successor, he opened his introduction with a tribute to his mentor.

In the sixth lesson in this volume (based on a lecture initially delivered on February 29, 1856), Bernard began to direct attention to carbon monoxide, declaring it to be "an eminently toxic gas" [1]. His experiments with carbon monoxide had begun in 1846, though its deadly effects had been known since the ancient Greek and Roman empires, when the gas has been used in judicial executions [6].

One of the most useful concepts that Bernard developed was the use of toxic agents in physiological investigation. He showed that poisons did not act by producing a general effect on the organs of the body, but induced specific unique changes in physiological function. Bernard viewed experimentation using poisons as akin to using chemical scalpels, "destined, so to speak, to dissect one by one the properties of the anatomical elements of the living organism" [1,7]. In addition to carbon monoxide, the *Lecons* address poisoning with curare, snake venom, cyanide and strychnine.

It was his experiments with curare, the exotic poison with which South American head-hunters tipped their spears and arrows, that first brought Bernard to a broader reading public [3]. Curare had been an object of his investigations since 1844 [7]. He showed that this agent paralyzed the motor nerves, which led to death by asphyxia through impairment of the respiratory muscles. In the case of poisoning with carbon monoxide, the result was also asphyxia, but through a quite different method. Bernard noted that "carbon monoxide gives the blood a nice gleaming arterial color" [1]. Carbon monoxide, in Bernard's lyrical phrasing, "poisons by preventing the arterial blood from becoming venous" [1].

He demonstrated this feature in both in vitro and in vivo animal experiments. In addition, he presented the cases of two young women who had been overcome by fumes from a furnace fuelled with coke. As Bernard put it, referring back to the toxic reactions he had observed in experimental animals, "you see the same phenomena in the house of man" [1]. He found that the scarlet colouration was most pronounced in the red corpuscles of the blood.

Through his experimentation with carbon monoxide, Bernard arrived at the fundamental facts that oxygen is not carried loosely in solution by the blood, but is fixed, and that it was the red blood cells that were responsible for the blood's respiratory function (hemoglobin had yet to be described as the blood's oxygen-carrying element). In carbon monoxide poisoning, the ability of the blood to provide oxygen to the tissue became impaired. Bernard identified carbon monoxide as a "poison that troubles the blood by displacing oxygen", the delivery of oxygen by the blood being "indispensable for life functions" [1].

## 2. Discussion

Carbon monoxide (CO) remains the leading cause of injury and death due to poisoning worldwide [8,9]. This colourless, odourless and toxic gas is a product of incomplete combustion of any carbon-containing fuel. The sources of CO are plentiful, and with the exception of carbon dioxide, CO is the most abundant pollutant present in the lower atmosphere [10]. CO poisoning undoubtedly has been recognized for many millennia, with poisoning occurring soon after our ancestors attempted to build fires in non-ventilated shelters.

Since the description of Claude Bernard many advances in our understanding of the pathophysiology and epidemiology have been achieved. The true incidence of CO poisoning worldwide is unknown, as many non-lethal exposures go undetected [8]. It has been estimated that more than one-third of all cases of CO poisoning are undiagnosed. Every year between 10 000 and 40 000 persons will seek medical attention in an emergency department or will miss at least one day of normal activity due to CO poisoning [9,10]. From 1979 to 1988, of the 11 547 unintentional CO deaths, 57% were caused by motor vehicle exhaust; and of these 83% were associated with stationary vehicles [11]. Most motor-vehicle-related CO deaths occur in garages, even when the garage doors or windows have been open, suggesting that passive ventilation may not be adequate enough to reduce the risk in semi-closed spaces. Worldwide, smoke inhalation from all types of fires is the second leading cause of CO poisoning. Indeed, most immediate deaths from building fires are due to CO poisoning and therefore fire fighters are at a high risk.

Various mechanisms of CO toxicity have been proposed since the initial description of Bernard and include; (i) a decrease in the oxygen-carrying capacity of blood; (ii) alterations in the dissociation characteristics of oxyhemoglobin, further decreasing oxygen delivery to the tissues; (iii) a decrease in cellular respiration by binding with cytochrome $a_3$; and (iv) binding to myoglobin, potentially causing myocardial and skeletal muscle dysfunction.

The most well understood mechanism by which CO toxicity occurs is competitive binding to the hemoglobin heme groups [13,14]. This effect is augmented by the characteristic allosteric properties of the hemoglobin molecule. The hemoglobin's tetrameric structure undergoes a conformational change when CO is bound at one of the four heme sites, with a resulting increase in the affinity of the remaining heme groups for oxygen. This not only shifts the oxygen-hemoglobin dissociation curve to the left, but distorts its sigmoidal shape towards a hyperbola. The result is an "impaired" hemoglobin that is poorly equipped to release oxygen at the tissue level. This diminished oxygen delivery will be then sensed by the central nervous system, stimulating ventilatory effort and increasing minute ventilation. The latter will increase uptake of CO and raise COHb levels, and will result in a respiratory alkalosis, further shifting the oxygen-hemoglobin dissociation curve to the left.

As CO exposure continues, central respiratory depression arises, possibly resulting from cerebral hypoxia. CO can also cause tissue hypoxia as well as tissue injury by impairing perfusion. Animal models of CO intoxication, as well as human experience, indicate that myocardial depression, peripheral vasodilation, and ventricular arrhythmia causing hypotension may be important in the genesis of neurological injury.

The clinical features of acute CO exposure and poisoning are more dramatic than those resulting from chronic exposure. At low COHb levels in patients with chronic cardiopulmonary problems, such as angina and chronic obstructive pulmonary disease, the symptoms may be exacerbated, since cardiac myoglobin binds with great affinity and rapidly reduces myocardial oxygen reserve. Chest pain due to myocardial ischemia may occur, as can cardiac dysrhythmias. Subacute or chronic CO poisoning presents with less specific symptoms (e.g. nausea, vomiting, headache) and patients may initially be misdiagnosed as having other illnesses such as gastroenteritis [8].

The clinical presentation of acute CO poisoning is variable, but in general, the severity of observed symptoms correlates roughly with the observed level of COHb. However, clinicians must be careful when using these values in terms of diagnostic value, as the nonspecificity of these presenting symptoms makes definitive diagnosis difficult. In addition, there have been several reports of levels near zero with patients showing neurological deficits ranging from partial paralysis to coma [15-17]. Therefore, COHb levels should not be used alone to determine the risk of morbidity or mortality.

A history of potential CO exposure is the most reliable indicator of poisoning. However, if the history of exposure is not evident, then a high index of suspicion is needed to make the diagnosis. Any patient at a fire scene should be immediately evaluated for CO poisoning. Confirming the diagnosis may be difficult in some patients, as the COHb may be low or undetectable because of the time between exposure and presentation at the emergency department [15-17]. The normal COHb levels is 1-3%, a result of endogenous production of CO by the heme catabolism and low-level environmental CO exposure. Cigarette smokers increase their COHb level by an average of 5% per pack smoked

per day, and otherwise healthy smokers tolerate COHb levels of 10% without having symptoms.

In addition to supportive care, the mainstay of therapy for CO poisoning is the administration of supplemental oxygen, ventilatory support and monitoring for cardiac dysrhythmias. Most clinicians agree that 100% oxygen should be administered prior to laboratory confirmation when CO poisoning is suspected. The goal of this therapy is to improve the oxygen content of the blood by maximizing the fraction dissolved in plasma ($PaO_2$). Once oxygen treatment begins, observation must continue long enough to prevent delayed sequelae as carboxymyoglobin unloads.

Other modes of therapy of severe CO poisoning have been under investigation for several decades [18-22]. Hypothermia, was used in the 1950s and 1960s in the management of these patients. However, at the beginning of the 1970s controlled studies showed no benefit in improving survival after severe CO poisoning [19].

Whether or not to use hyperbaric oxygen (HBO), and, if so, when to use it, are matters that have been debated since it emerged in 1960. HBO was first used successfully in Glasgow [20]. Since then, the clinical use of HBO for CO poisoning has occurred with increasing frequency. Indeed, over 2500 CO-intoxicated patients are treated in North American chambers each year [23]. Practice guidelines have been developed on the basis of clinical experience and inferences of efficacy in uncontrolled studies. Results of past controlled trials comparing HBO therapy and normobaric oxygen therapy have been inconclusive due to methodological difficulties.

## 3. Conclusions

Carbon monoxide poisoning remains a common clinical entity. Our understanding of this disorder has dramatically increased since the first documented description by Claude Bernard. However, the basic principles of initial recognition and basic management remain unchanged.

## References

[1] Bernard C. Lecons sur les Effets des Substaces Toxiques et Medicamenteuses. Paris: J-B Bailliere et Fils, 1857.
[2] Silverman BD. Claude Bernard. Clin Cardiol 1996;19:916-8.
[3] Virtanen R. Claude Bernard and his Place in the History of Ideas. Lincoln, NB: University of Nebraska Press, 1960.
[4] Olmstead JMD. Claude Bernard, Physiologist. New York: Harper & Brothers, 1938.
[5] Haas LF. Claude Bernard (1813-78). J Neruol Neurosurg Psych 1996;61:345.
[6] Conzi F. Claude Bernard's Des Fonctions du Cerveau: an ante literam manifesto of the neurosciences. Nature Rev Neurosci 2002;3:979-85.

[7] Varon J, Marik PE, Fromm RE, Gueler A. Carbon monoxide poisoning: a review for clinicians. J Emerg Med 1999;17:87–93.

[8] Gasman J, Varon J, Gardner J. Revenge of the barbecue grill-Carbon monoxide poisoning. West J Med 1990;153:656–7.

[9] Thom S, Keim L. Carbon monoxide poisoning: A review. Epidemiology, pathophysiology, clinical findings, and treatment options including hyperbaric therapy. Clin Toxicol 1989;27:141–56.

[10] Jaffe LS. Sources, characteristics and fate of atmospheric carbon monoxide. Ann NY Acad Sci 1970;174:76–88.

[11] Hampson N, Norkool D. Carbon monoxide poisoning in children riding in the back of Pickup trucks. J Am Med Assoc 1992;267:538–40.

[12] Guy C, Salhany J, Eliot R. Disorders of hemoglobin-oxygen release in ischemic heart disease. Am Heart J 1971;82:824–32.

[13] Rodkey F, O'Neal J, Collison H. Relative affinity of hemoglobin S and hemoglobin A for carbon monoxide and oxygen. Clin Chem 1974;20:83–4.

[14] Petersen J, Stewart R. Absorption and elimination of carbon monoxide by active young men. Arch Environ Health 1970;21:165–71.

[15] Norkool DM, Kirkpatrick JN. Treatment of acute carbon monoxide poisoning with hyperbaric oxygen: a review of 115 cases. Ann Emerg Med 1985;14:1168–71.

[16] Myers RAM, Thom S. Carbon monoxide and cyanide poisoning. In: Kindwall. EP, editor. Hyperbaric Medicine Practice. Flagstaff, AZ: Best Publishing, 1995:343–72.

[17] Myers RAM. Do arterial blood gases have value in prognosis and treatment decisions in carbon-monoxide poisoning. Crit Care Med 1989;17:139–42.

[18] Dolan M. Carbon monoxide poisoning. Can Med Assoc J 1985;133:393–9.

[19] Pearce E, Zacharias A, Alday J, Hoffman B, Jacobson J. Carbon monoxide poisoning: experimental hypothermic and hyperbaric studies. Surgery 1972;72:229–39.

[20] Smith G, Ledingham IM, Sharp GR. Treatment of coal-gas poisoning with oxygen at 2 atmospheres pressure. Lancet 1962;1:816–8.

[21] Pace N, Strajnan E, Walker E. Acceleration of carbon monoxide elimination in man by high pressure oxygen. Science 1950;111:652–4.

[22] Goulon M, Bariois A, Rapin M, Nouailhat F, Grosbuis S, Labrousse J. Intoxication oxycarbonee et anoxie aigue par inhalation de gaz de charbon et d'hydrocarbures. Ann Med Interne (Paris) 1969;120:335–45.

[23] Weaver LK, Hopkins RO, Chan KJ. Hyperbaric oxygen for acute carbon monoxide poisoning. New Engl J Med 2002;347:1057–67.

# Larrey and Percy—A tale of two Barons

David Baker , Jean-Bernard Cazalaà, Pierre Carli

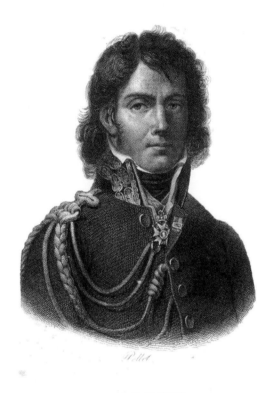

LARREY.

Fig. 1. Dominique Jean Larrey (Musée de l'histoire de la médecine de Paris).

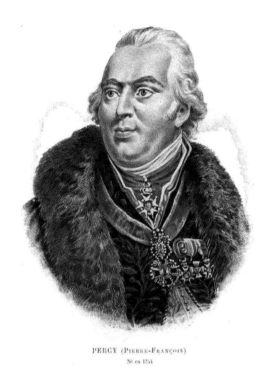

PERCY (Pierre-François)
Né en 1754

Fig. 2. Pierre Francois Percy (Musée de l'histoire de la médecine de Paris).

The wars of the late 18th and 19th centuries produced casualties on a scale that is usually assumed to have started during the First World War. This was a result of a deadly combination of close engagement of mass formations of troops (a practice dating from medieval times) with increasingly concentrated and accurate firepower from rifled musketry and cannon. Thus Napoleon Bonaparte would lose over 40,000 dead and wounded in 2 days at the battle of Wagram (1809) while the murderous engagement at Antietam in the American civil war in September 1862 produced 1-day losses of 25,000 men, which rivaled even the fatalities of the British on the Somme during 1st July 1916.

Into the grim conditions of warfare at the end of the 18th century stepped two eminent French military surgeons who were to change the fate, not only of those wounded in battle,

71

but also of those injured in accidents and mass disasters up to the present time. Dominique Jean Larrey (Fig. 1) is familiar to many English-speaking doctors for his groundbreaking contributions to triage and the rapid evacuation of the wounded from the battlefield. His contemporary and compatriot Pierre François Percy (Fig. 2) (whose name is immortalized to this day in the newest of the Parisian military hospitals) is less familiar outside France but his contribution to casualty management was no less than that of Larrey.

Dominique Jean Larrey was born near Bagnères de Bigorre in the Pyrénées on the 6th July 1766. Orphaned at the age of nine he followed the career of his uncle, a surgeon at Toulouse. After studying in Lyon he went to Paris in 1786 shortly before the French Revolution with the intention of continuing his surgical studies but instead he joined the Royal French Navy and saw service in North America in the frigate Vigilante. He did not remain in the navy (he suffered from chronic seasickness) but returned instead to continue his studies at the Hôtel-Dieu hospital, beside the cathedral of Notre Dame in Paris.

In 1792, at the outbreak of the War of the Monarchist Coalition against the newly declared French Republic he joined the Army of the Rhine as an assistant surgeon and served in Corsica and Spain before becoming Professor of Surgery at the great military hospital of Val de Grace in Paris. The French Army was becoming reformed and highly effective under the leadership of the 26 year-old General Bonaparte with whom Larrey soon became a favourite. Larrey accompanied him on his campaigns to Egypt, Palestine and Syria and undertook a complete re-organization of the field medical services, which hitherto had been rudimentary in common with other armies at that time. Larrey was appointed Surgeon in Chief to the French Army in 1805 and took part in increasingly bloody campaigns in Germany and Poland as well as the ill-fated expedition to Russia in 1812. In 1815 Larrey was wounded and captured during the Battle of Waterloo. He avoided being executed by the Prussians after being recognized by their Commander-in-Chief, Blucher, whose son's life Larrey had saved some years earlier. Larrey had been created Baron by Napoleon in 1810 and it is a mark of the esteem in which he was held in France that his title was confirmed by the restored Monarchy in November 1815. Larrey's busy medical life was to continue for another 27 years. After the restoration he was appointed Inspector General of the Medical Service and held surgical posts at the Garde Royale and the Hôpital des Invalides in Paris as well as organizing the medical service of the newly-created Belgian Republic in 1831.

Pierre François Percy (1754–1825) was born at Montagney in Haute Saône on the 28th October 1754 a decade before Larrey. The son of a surgeon, he qualified from the University of Besançon and entered the French Army a year later. His active military career was to span three decades, first in the service of Louis XVI and then for Napoleon where, as Inspector General of the Medical Services, he introduced a major re-organization. Percy was surgeon to the Grande Armée in 1803 at the time of the aborted invasion of England and the victory at Trafalgar forced Napoleon to pursue campaigns on the mainland. Percy took part in some of the bloodiest battles of the wars including Austerlitz (1805), Jena (1806), Eylau (1807) Wagram (1809) and the Spanish campaign of 1808–1809. After the battle of Eylau Percy wrote graphically of the plight of the wounded for whom there was practically no organization, a fact which came to the attention of Napoleon who ordered radical changes in the provision of surgical care. After Wagram, Percy, because of his age and health, withdrew from active campaigning and devoted his time to administration of the army health services and to teaching in the University of Paris. Percy was not so gifted in diplomacy as Larrey and did not fare so well after the restoration in 1815. He was, however, created a member of the newly formed Academy of Medicine in 1820.

Before the Napoleonic Wars the plight of battle wounded was dire. Left on the battlefield or removed to the rear of the action by their comrades using commandeered farm carts or whatever else was available they often waited several days for rudimentary surgical treatment which consisted either of amputation or the probing of wounds to try and locate a musket ball or piece of shrapnel. Penetrating wounds of the head, abdomen and thorax were usually fatal. Transportation was slow and agonizing and perhaps the major contribution of both Barons was the realization that this had to be improved.

From the outset of his career Percy tried to organize a means of bringing surgeons further forward into the battlefield and evacuating the wounded. His first idea was to transform captured Bavarian artillery wagons into an 'ambulance' drawn by six horses, a vehicle known as the 'Wurst' (sausage). This idea did not prove to be a success and further attempts to provide rapid transport were blocked by the military administration who did not feel it was appropriate to give horses to medical officers ('who might become insolent to authority as a result and in any case should go by foot').

Percy finally did succeed in creating the first formation of medical attendants (or brancardiers). This was the first time personnel had been dedicated solely to the care of the wounded. These men used collapsible stretchers made from two lances. They wore large shako hats in which were stored basic dressings which could be transported to the point of wounding. Larrey, however, was the first to conceive and introduce special horse-drawn wagons to remove the wounded from the field as quickly as possible. His 'flying ambulances' are justly famous for the effective transport service they provided from the battlefield but, more importantly their creation underlined the understanding (long before Trunkey's 'Golden Hour') that the quicker a wounded man could receive attention the better his chances of survival. The other important development in military medicine at the time was the concept of triage. It was Percy who first specified the idea that evacuation from the battlefield should be based upon the seriousness of the wound and chances of survival if treated early. Evacuation was therefore not based upon wealth or rank. The palpably Republican notion of triage at

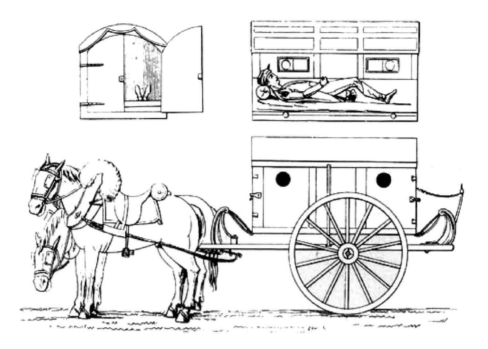

Fig. 3. Plan of the flying ambulance; the central section was carefully sprung on the chassis to provide a less painful ride for the wounded (D. Larrey, Mémoires de chirurgie et campagnes. Paris, Rémanences, 1982, 5 volumes).

that time laid the basis of a system that is used in military and civil disaster medicine to the present day.

Larrey's creation of the flying ambulance (Figs. 3–5) and the impact it had on the prognosis of the wounded lead to him being appointed Baron by Napoleon in 1810. Apart from his organizational achievements, Larrey made many notable contributions to the military surgery of the time. He stipulated that surgery must be carried out within 24 h of wounding to have a good chance of success. Most field surgery at that time involved amputations and Larrey laid down rules for these. Immediate amputation was indicated if the limb was shattered, or there were comminuted fractures, and if there was major muscle or arterial loss. Larrey operated quickly; he could remove a leg in 1 min and an arm in 17 s. Despite this speed he developed an inverted cone approach that allowed

skin flaps to fall together and be dressed with adhesive bandages that permitted the stump to drain. Larrey stopped the historic use of salves and ointments and washed wounds with water at the point of collection by the flying ambulance.

Larrey, who unlike Percy was a major believer in amputation (he performed more than 200 in one day at the Battle of Borodino in Russia (7 September 1812) noted that delayed treatment lead to increased pain during operation, haemorrhage and subsequent infection. Percy had a more conservative approach to amputation. He always attempted, despite the difficulties and lack of resources, to sew and cauterize. If amputation were necessary Percy stipulated that no operation should last more than 20 s.

Percy was no less a skilled surgeon that Larrey but his contribution to re-organization of the medical service was per-

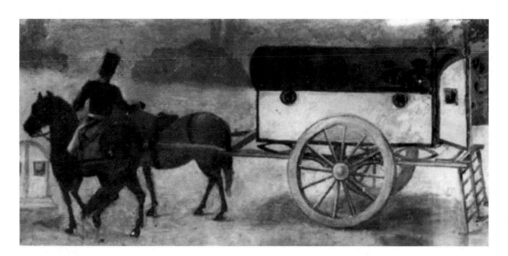

Fig. 4. Larrey's 'flying ambulance' (D. Larrey, Mémoires de chirurgie et campagnes. Paris, Rémanences, 1982, 5 volumes).

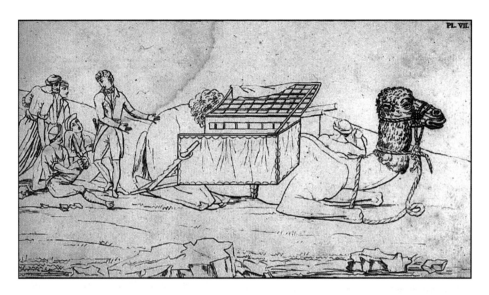

Fig. 5. Camel ambulance in Egypt (D. Larrey, Mémoires de chirurgie et campagnes. Paris, Rémanences, 1982, 5 volumes).

haps his greatest achievement. An insight into his approach is given by the following quotation from his writings

'the art of healing men is a little like that of destroying them; timid actions gain nothing and if victory often follows the audacity of brave soldiers success also crowns the efforts of enterprising surgeons.'

Apart from their surgical advances Larrey and Percy also made contributions to early anaesthesia. In his memoires, Larrey noted the lack of sensation produced by cold while amputating during the winter retreat from Russia in 1812 and advocated this technique to reduce pain. Percy, writing in the Panckouke medical dictionary (Paris, 1820) described how he had used intravenous injections of opium in cases of tetanus.

'An aqueous extract of opium, introduced in small doses into the crural and medial veins is of great value in cases of traumatic tetanus. We tried this technique seven times in cases of this infamous condition and definitely saved three patients. These experiments done openly and with the consent of Russian officers on their soldiers at the Hopital des Abattoirs, established at Menilmontant in 1814 (at that time a village near Paris but now part of the 20th arrondissement of that city).'

Percy also used extracts of Datura Stramonium (thorn apple) . . . 'a distillate of Datura Stramonium or 24 grains of this plant in half and ounce of warm water forced into the veins induces a sort of universal paralysis, which helps to treat tetanus.' Percy was thus among the first to have induced sedation intravenously with a therapeutic objective.

Percy died in Paris in 1825 while Larrey died at Lyon on the 25th July 1842, active to the end of his days. Napoleon had finally died in exile on St. Helena in 1821. In his will he left 100,000 francs to Larrey, his surgeon of the Imperial Guard and wrote;

'-he was the most courageous and virtuous man I have ever known. . .'

Both Larrey and Percy were great Frenchmen of their era who made a lasting contribution to military medicine. It would be several decades before their lessons were taken up by English speaking nations, notably by Letterman in his re-organization of medical services during the American Civil War. Their contribution to reducing the suffering of the wounded was recognized by both Napoleon and ordinary soldiers alike and is remembered to this day in French- and English-speaking countries alike. They well deserve to be remembered among the ranks of Resuscitation Greats.

# Czar Alexander I, Emperor of Russia (1777–1825)

John Zorab    Diana Coke

---

*Death may usurp on nature many hours*
*And yet the fire of life kindle again*
*The overpress'd spirits. I heard*
*Of an Egyptian, that had nine hours lien dead,*
*who was by good appliances recovered.*

Shakespeare, Pericles, Act III, Sc. II.

His Imperial Majesty, Alexander I, Czar of all the Russias, Alexander Pavlovich (Alexander I) (Fig. 1) was the grandson of Catherine the Great (1762–96) and became Emperor of Russia in 1801. Catherine had been a remarkably perceptive woman, with an interest in medical advances. For example, being aware that she had never had smallpox she resolved to be inoculated at a time when this procedure had only just been introduced. An English inoculator, Thomas Dimsdale, was summoned to St. Petersburg in 1768 and the Empress and her son were successfully inoculated. Voltaire, with whom she had a regular correspondence, reported that "she had been inoculated with less fuss than a nun taking an enema" [1]. Furthermore, in 1774, a Humane Society had been formed in St. Petersburg on the lines of a similar society in Holland, and in the same year that the Humane Society in London was founded, to become the Royal Humane Society in 1787 [2]. This, then, was the climate in which Alexander I was raised. He had both liberal and radical ideas and, at one time, after the defeat of Napoleon in 1814, was the most powerful man in Europe.

The following account was written by James Grange, a governor of the Royal Humane Society (RHS), in a letter to Dr. William Hawes, the RHS Founder and Treasurer, the account having been told to Mr. Grange by Dr. Weilly, surgeon to His Imperial Highness. It was published, together with illustrations, in the Annual Report of the Society for 1807. The correspondence with the Czar was published in the 1815 Annual Report. These extracts are reproduced here with the kind permission of the RHS.

*London, March 24, 1806.*

*Dear Sir,*

*Agreeably to your request that I would commit to writing the Narrative that formed part of our late conversation, I have now the renewed pleasure to inform you that H.I.M., the Emperor Alexander, in one of his journeys through Poland, and by his own humane perseverance and personal exertion, restored to life a peasant of that country, who had been drowned a considerable time. This very interesting occurrence came to my knowledge during my late stay at St. Petersburg and took place between Konna and Wilna (in Lithuania) on the banks of the little river Wilna from whence the last-mentioned town derives its name.*

*The Emperor … had considerably preceded his attendants; and being led, by the winding of the road, within a short distance of the above-mentioned river, and perceiving several persons assembled near the edge of the water, out of which they appeared to be dragging something, instantly alighted; and, on approaching the spot, found it to be the body of a man, apparently lifeless (Fig. 2). Prompted by humanity alone, and without any other assistance than that of the ignorant boors around him (to whom he was not otherwise known, than that his uniform indicated an officer of rank), he had him conveyed to, and laid on the side of a bank, and immediately proceeded, with his own hands, to assist in taking off the wet clothes from the apparent corpse, and to rub his temples, wrists, etc. which H.I.M. continued for a considerable time, using every other means (though destitute of every*

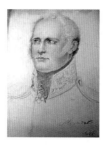

Fig. 1. His Imperial Majesty, Alexander I (by Agostino Aglio, from www.antiqnet.com by courtesy of Greg Page-Turner).

*medical assistance), that appeared at the moment most likely to restore animation, but all without effect.*

*In the midst of this beneficent occupation, the Emperor was joined by the gentlemen of his suite among whom were Prince Wolkonsky and Co. Liewen (two Russian noblemen) and Dr Weilly, His Majesty's head surgeon, an English gentleman who always travels with, and indeed never quits His Majesty at any time. Their exertions were immediately added to those of the Emperor; and on the Doctor's attempting to bleed the patient, His Majesty held and rubbed his arm and gave every other assistance in his power; however that, and all other means that they could devise, proved equally ineffectual; so much so that after above three hours fruitless attempts to recover him, the Doctor declared, to the extreme chagrin of*

*the Emperor (who, was by this time very anxious about it,) to be his opinion that life was quite gone, and that it was useless proceeding any further.*

*Fatigued as he was with such continued exertion, the Emperor could not, however, rest satisfied without entreating Dr Weilly to persevere, and to make a fresh attempt to bleed him. The Doctor, although (as he has declared to me himself, and from whose own mouth I have these particulars) he had not the slightest hope of being more successful in this than in former ones, proceeded, nevertheless, to obey the positive injunctions of H.I.M.; when the whole of them (the noblemen, etc.), making a last effort in rubbing, etc. the Emperor had, at length, the inexpressible satisfaction of seeing the blood make its appearance, accompanied by a slight groan.*

*The emotions of H.I.M. on this occasion, the Doctor informed me, are not to be described and, in the plenitude of his joy, he exclaimed, in French: "Good God, this is the brightest day of my life" ("Grand Dieu! Voici le jour le plus brillant de mon existence") and the tears which instantaneously sprang into his eyes indicated that these words came from the heart.*

*It is useless to say, my dear Sir, that their exertions were, as you may suppose, redoubled and finally crowned with complete success; but I must not forget to add (as in justice to H.I.M. no trait, however trifling, ought to be omitted, which reflects such honour on his feelings as a man), that, on Dr Weilly's looking about for something to stop the blood with, and tie up his arm, the Emperor without any hesitation, instantly took out his handkerchief, tore it in pieces, and with his own hands bound the poor fellow's arm with it (whose gratitude and astonishment, when informed as to whom he was indebted for his life, you may easily conceive); and remained with him till he saw him quite recovered and conveyed to a place where proper care would be taken of him; besides ordering him a considerable present of money, and having since otherwise provided for him and his family.*

*The accompanying snuff box, on which this interesting event is faithfully, though roughly delineated (the poor inhabitants of that part of Poland being no great artists), was sketched at a neighbouring town, for the purpose of commemorating his restoration; and is one of four presented, on the occasion, to the principal actors in it, namely, H.I.M. and the three gentlemen above-mentioned who are (though not very correctly, it is true) represented on it (Fig. 3).*

*Knowing my attachment to everything in the least connected with that truly amiable and good Prince, or his actions, Dr Weilly was kind enough, at my request, to present me with it; and although I would not part with it on any other account, I think it cannot be better disposed of, than by taking the liberty of offering it to you, Sir, to the end that so striking an example of humanity, perseverance and philanthropy in so exalted a character may not be entirely lost to the world and to posterity.*

*Requesting you to excuse the hasty, imperfect way in which I have endeavoured to narrate this very affecting transaction (to which I feel myself totally incompetent to do adequate justice), allow me to assure you, Sir, of the*

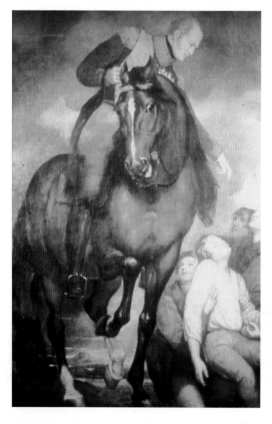

Fig. 2. His Imperial Majesty, Alexander I gazing at the apparently lifeless body of the Polish peasant being taken from the river (from the painting by James Northcote and by courtesy of the Royal Society of Medicine).

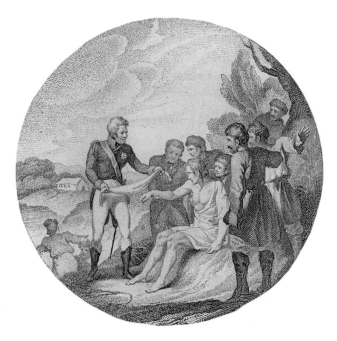

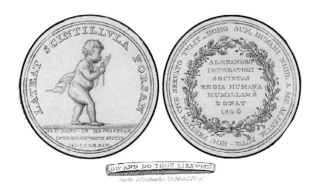

Fig. 4. The obverse and reverse of the Gold Medal presented to His Imperial Majesty, Alexander I (by courtesy of the Royal Humane Society).

Fig. 3. A drawing depicting the event in the 1807 Annual Report (by courtesy of the Royal Humane Society).

*sentiments of respect and esteem with which I beg leave to subscribe myself, dear Sir,*

*yours most faithfully,*

*JAMES GRANGE.*

Dr. Weilly gave his snuff box to Mr. Grange who, subsequently, gave it to the Royal Humane Society but no trace of it has been found [3]. Fortunately, a depiction of the event was included in the 1807 Annual Report Fig. 3. However, the story does not end there. Following receipt of this account by the RHS at its meeting on Tuesday, 15th April, 1806, the following motion was put:

"That it be recommended to the managers of this Society that the Gold Medal be voted to, and that H.I.M. Alexander, Emperor of all the Russias, be humbly requested graciously to accept the same, being the highest tribute in its power to offer, in testimony of the sincere respect entertained by the RHS for the character of H.I.M. by whose noble, unwearied and persevering efforts, Life was, under divine Providence, restored to one of his subjects who otherwise, would have been prematurely consigned to the grave"!

Several other meetings, with related motions, were held to accept and confirm the above resolution and it was agreed that the Most Noble the Marquis Douglas, His Majesty's representative at the court of St. Petersburg should present the Gold Medal of the Society to His Imperial Majesty (Fig. 4). It was also agreed that His Imperial Majesty should be invited to become an honorary member of the Society. The following answer (in French), in the Emperor's own hand, acknowledged the receipt of the Medal and the consent of His Imperial Majesty to become an Honorary Member:

*St. Petersburg, Feb. 28, 1807.*

*MR. PRESIDENT,*

*The Marquis of Douglas and Clydesdale, his Britannic Majesty's Ambassador at my Court has conveyed to me the very flattering compliment paid by your Society to an action, the notice of which must appear unimportant among the records you preserve of the highest services rendered to humanity. Yet, while I cannot consider so simple an action as entitling me to what you have conferred, I accept the distinction with pleasure and gratitude. It is impossible to deny myself the satisfaction of being enrolled among the Members of a Society, of which the objects and the zeal are so interesting to humanity, and so congenial to the dearest feelings of my heart. I beg you will express to the Society the sincere regard and interest I take in its prosperity; and accept the esteem with which I am,*

*Mr. President,*

*Your most affectionate,*

*ALEXANDER.*

*To the President of the Royal
Humane Society of Great Britain.*

As can be seen from the letter from His Imperial Majesty above, the Medal was graciously accepted with unassuming modesty. The letter is dated February 28, 1807, so the presentation was, presumably, some time before that. The next related episode did not happen until June 1814, when the Allied Sovereigns met in London following the defeat of Napoleon. The Czar was among them. In her article, Schuster mentions that the drawing shown in Fig. 3 was exhibited as a transparency among the new gas illuminations and, on the following Sunday, the Czar received 30 members of the Royal Humane Society at Pulteny's Hotel in Piccadilly, and Dr. Pettigrew, Honorary Secretary of the RHS, presented him with an "Address" shown above.

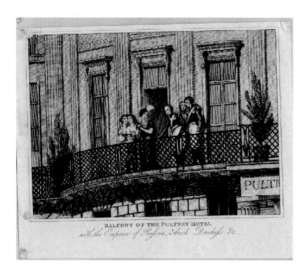

Fig. 5. The balcony of Pulteny's Hotel, Piccadilly, London with His Imperial Majesty, Alexander I bowing to the crowd. Copyright of the British Museum. 1880-11-13-2019 (Crace Collection).

There is a little water colour sketch in the British Museum that shows the Czar on the balcony of Pulteny's hotel, Piccadilly, acknowledging the crowd below (Fig. 5).

*Sunday, 19th June, 1814*

*To His Imperial Majesty, Alexander, Emperor of all the Russias*

*May it please your Imperial Majesty:*

*The Vice Patron, President, Vice President, Directors, and Governors of the Royal Humane Society, instituted for the recovery of the apparently drowned or dead, humbly approach Your Imperial Majesty to offer their respectful and cordial welcome to Your Imperial Majesty, on your happy arrival in Great Britain.*

*In common with all their fellow subjects, they feel that lively interest and high exultation so naturally the consequence of the mighty efforts and glorious victories of the brave armies of Your Imperial Majesty, and Your Illustrious Allies: victories, by which Nations, oppressed by a most hateful tyranny, have been emancipated; and by which the latent spark of Liberty has been fanned to the flame which now re-animates the world. But the Royal Humane Society, which the beloved Sovereign of Britain has so long patronized, feels, in its approach to Your Imperial Majesty, peculiar emotions, in the remembrance, that, it addresses a Monarch whose powerful arm maintained the cause of freedom against confederated hosts, has yet deigned his own assiduous exertions in rescuing a subject (though of the meanest class) from premature death: a Monarch, who can adopt with eminent propriety, and whose generous tears on a successful result confirmed a right to, the claim of the worthy sage of Antiquity: "Homo sum, humani nihil a me alienum puto."*

*The Royal Humane Society is impressed with the sincerest gratitude for the condescension with which Your Imperial Majesty has been pleased to accept the Medal of the Society, the highest token of admiration and respect in its power to offer, and for the gracious manner in which Your Imperial Majesty has been pleased to consent to be an Honorary Member of the Royal Humane Society.*

*The Vice Patron, President, Vice Presidents, Directors, and Governors, in order further to testify their respectful veneration for Your Imperial Majesty, humbly beg leave to present, personally, to Your Imperial Majesty's acceptance, the Diploma by which the Royal Humane Society has had the honour to enroll Your Imperial Majesty among its Members.*

*That Your Imperial Majesty may long reign over a brave, united, and an unconquered people, and be gratified with the effects of a Peace so gloriously achieved in the effusions of emancipated millions, is the fervent prayer of,*

*Sire, Your Imperial Majesty's*

*Most obedient, humble servants,*

*The Members of the Royal Humane Society.*

## References

[1] Alexander JT. Catherine the great: life and legend. Oxford: Clarendon Press; 1989.

[2] Bishop PJ. A short history of the Royal Humane Society. London; 1974. p. 2.

[3] Schuster N. The Emperor of Russia and the Royal Humane Society. J R Coll Gen Tractit 1971;21:634.

# James Blundell: the first transfusion of human blood

Thomas F. Baskett

In August, 1825, James Blundell, obstetrician and physiologist of Guy's Hospital, was summoned by a surgeon colleague, Mr Waller, to a woman dying from postpartum haemorrhage in the Finsbury Square district of London. The case was recorded by Mr Waller and was the first successful human blood transfusion [1].

The vein in the bend of the arm was laid bare, and an incision of sufficient extent to admit the pipe of the syringe was made into it. . . . The syringe used by Dr B. was similar to the common injecting syringe, and contained two ounces. . . . The blood was drawn from the patient's husband into a tumbler, and Dr B. stood ready with his syringe to absorb it instantly, in fact, while it was flowing: it was then immediately introduced into the orifice in the vein, and cautiously injected. No effect appeared to be produced by the first injection of two ounces, but towards the end of the second there was an approach to syncope; the pulse fell a little; there was sighing. . . [1]

James Blundell was unusually well prepared for this challenge as 7 years before he had been stimulated to investigate the feasibility of blood transfusion after attending a woman who died from postpartum haemorrhage [2].

Reflecting afterwards on this melancholy scene, for there were circumstances which gave it a peculiar interest, I could not forbear considering, that the patient might very probably have been saved by transfusion; and that, although there was little opportunity for operating in the usual manner, the vessels might have been replenished by means of the syringe with facility and promptitude. As it seemed doubtful, however, whether the blood would remain fit for the animal functions after its passage through the instrument, the following experiments were instituted with a view to ascertain the point. . . [2]

As a result of this 'melancholy scene' Blundell carried out extensive studies with transfusion in animals and after a series of logical experiments reached the following conclusions: haemorrhagic shock could be corrected by transfusion of blood from animals of the same species; blood from different species was not suitable, and for humans only human blood would be safe. He also discovered that both venous and arterial blood were effective for resuscitation, and that blood could be passed from donor to recipient through a syringe without losing its effectiveness [2]. He found that a small amount of air mixed with the blood would be tolerated but that large amounts could be fatal [2,3].

Although Blundell was the first to transfuse human blood he was not the first to experiment with transfusion in humans. After William Harvey's discovery of the circulation of blood, Sir Christopher Wren (1632–1723), architect of St. Paul's Cathedral, and the celebrated chemist, Robert Boyle, injected opium and other substances via a goose quill into the blood stream of a dog [4]. In February 1665, Richard Lower (1631–1691), a physiologist from Cornwall, first documented the direct transfusion of blood from one animal to another [5]. The first transfusion performed on a human was by Jean Baptiste Denis (1620–1704), physician to Louis XIV, in Paris in July 1667 [6]. He transfused blood directly from the carotid artery of a sheep to a young man with a fever who was hypovolaemic from repeated therapeutic venesections. The patient survived and recovered. After initial enthusiasm there were several fatal cases of animal to human transfusion and the procedure was banned in Europe and fell into disuse, to be revived by Blundell more than 150 years later.

In his textbook *The Principles and Practice of Obstetricy* Blundell, with his creative use of the English language, in a section entitled '*Is the system on the rally or the decline?*' outlined the assessment of a woman in hypovolaemic shock following postpartum haemorrhage [7]:

Now sometimes, you find the patient is evidently improving from half hour to half hour; her hands and feet are warmer—her pulse is stronger—her countenance is brighter—her mind is livelier—in a word, there are all those appearances of amendment which, after you have been in practice a little, you expect to meet with when the strength is rising. On the other hand, however, you are sometimes meeting with different cases, in which, although the haemorrhage is stopped, the patient is evidently on the decline. After floodings, women sometimes die in a moment, but more frequently in a gradual manner; and over the victim, death shakes his dart, and to you she stretches out her helpless hands for the assistance which you cannot give, unless by transfusion. I have seen a women dying for two or three hours together, convinced in my own mind that no known remedy could save her: the sight of these moving cases first lead me to transfusion [7]

Blundell was a thoughtful and cautious physician. He acknowledged that there were potentially serious risks to 'the operation', as he called it, and felt "...therefore it seems right, as the operation now stands, to confine transfusion to the first class of cases only, namely those in which there seems to be no hope for the patient unless blood can be thrown into the veins" [8]. Over a decade there were only ten documented cases of Blundell using human blood transfusion. The first was in August 1818 in a man terminally ill with cancer of the stomach, who lived for 56 h after 12 ounces of blood was transfused by syringe [9]. Another unsuccessful case in which Blundell transfused human blood, for reasons other than haemorrhage, was in a woman with puerperal sepsis. He transfused six ounces of blood but the woman died of her infection without apparently suffering any ill effects from the transfusion [10]. Of the other eight cases, all haemorrhagic shock, six were due to postpartum haemorrhage. The first two of these cases failed but were obviously in women who were moribund from postpartum haemorrhage [10]. The next four cases of postpartum haemorrhage that Blundell treated were successful, starting with the one noted above in August 1825 [1,10–13]. Testimonials following transfusion from two of the patients were included in the case reports: "I am as strong as a bull" [11] and "she felt as if life were infused into her body" [13]. In the first two successful cases of transfusion for postpartum haemorrhage the donor was the husband and in the third and fourth cases the attending surgeons donated their own blood. The volume transfused ranged from 4 to 14 ounces. Blundell transfused two other patients with haemorrhage: one man with a 'burst artery' in severe hypovolaemic shock received 16 ounces, which failed to revive him; and a young boy who was hypovolaemic following amputation of his leg and was successfully restored by transfusion [10].

Blundell was very aware that any delay in transmitting the blood from the donor risked clotting. He developed an elaborate system with a funnel and syringe, the Gravitator, to overcome this problem [8] (Figs. 1 and 2).

Two other obstetricians in the mid 19th century also played significant roles in the evolution of human blood transfusion. John Braxton Hicks (1823–1897), also of Guy's Hospital in London, was the first to use phosphate of soda mixed with the donor blood to prevent coagulation. Although technically successful, the first four cases in which he used this approach died-albeit of very severe obstetric haemorrhage [14]. Another London obstetrician, James Hobson Aveling (1828–1892), invented a simple device for direct blood transfusion from a donor. He carried this with him for 8 years, "...until at length the opportunity for using it arrived". The occasion, in 1872, was a woman with postpartum haemorrhage who was given about 250 ml of her coachman's blood and survived [15]. Aveling's device consisted of two silver canulae, inserted into the donor and recipient respectively, connected by rubber tubing with a compressible bulb in the middle to promote and sustain flow [15].

James Blundell was born in London on December 27, 1790. There are no details of his forebears except that he must have come from a wealthy family as he received a classical education from a private tutor. His initial medical training was taken at the United Hospitals of St. Thomas' and Guy's following which he went to Edinburgh to take his MD, presenting a study of the differences in the senses of hearing and music as his graduation thesis in 1813 [10,16]. A year later he returned to London as a lecturer in physiology and midwifery at the combined schools of St. Thomas' and Guy's. In this position he assisted his uncle, Dr John Haighton, who was the professor of physiology. In 1823, after his uncle's death, he took over these lectures completely and attracted the largest audience throughout London for his obstetrical classes. His lectures were published in the *Lancet* at a time of legal controversy between its editor and Sir Astley Cooper, the most prominent surgeon at Guy's Hospital—causing Blundell to be censored by the hospital authorities. Later, in 1834, Blundell resigned from the hospital when, without consulting him, they appointed another physician to assist him with his midwifery lectures. In addition to the publication of his lectures in the *Lancet* Blundell published the essence of his lectures in his classic text *The Principles and Practice of Obstetricy* in 1834 [7] (Fig. 3). The breadth of his knowledge based on his experiments and clinical experience is evident in this book. He foresaw many of the developments in obstetrics, gynaecology and abdominal surgery. All of his

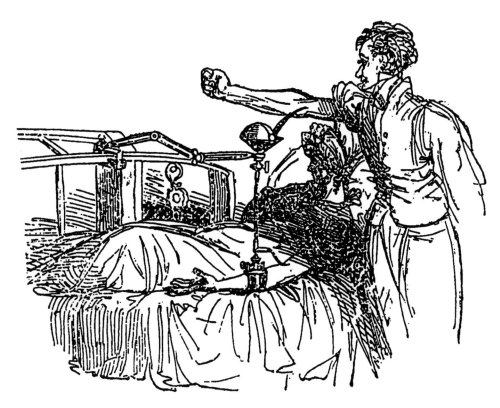

Fig. 1.

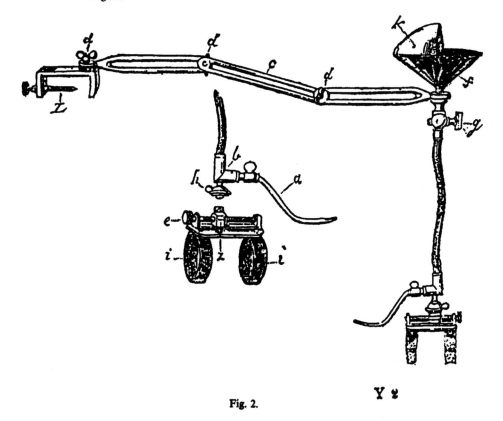

Fig. 2.

Figs. 1 and 2. James Blundell's transfusion gravitator (*Lancet* 1828;2:321).

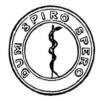

THE

PRINCIPLES AND PRACTICE

OF

OBSTETRICY,

AS AT PRESENT TAUGHT

By JAMES BLUNDELL, M.D.

PROFESSOR OF OBSTETRICY AT GUY'S HOSPITAL.

———

In Five Parts:

I. THE ANATOMY OF THE FEMALE SYSTEM.
II. THE PHYSIOLOGY OF THE FEMALE SYSTEM.
III. THE SIGNS AND DISEASES OF PREGNANCY.
IV. THE ART OF DELIVERY.
V. THE AFTER-MANAGEMENT OF THE PUERPERAL STATE, THE
DISEASES OF PUERPERAL WOMEN, AND STRICTURES
ON THE DISEASES OF INFANTS.

———

TO WHICH ARE ADDED,

NOTES AND ILLUSTRATIONS.

By THOMAS CASTLE, M.D. F.L.S.

MEMBER OF TRINITY COLLEGE, CAMBRIDGE,
ETC. ETC.

London :

PRINTED FOR E. COX, ST. THOMAS'S STREET,
SOUTHWARK.

———

MDCCCXXXIV.

Fig. 3.

statements were backed up by his own experiments and clinical observation. He was criticised for his experiments in abdominal surgery with living animals. In response to his critics Blundell replied: "Is not pain daily and hourly inflicted on the inferior animals to contribute to the support or pleasure of man; and shall it be fastidiously objected to when inflicted for the purpose of advancing physiological and medical knowledge?" [16] And in more dramatic tone: "Strike gentleman, but hear!...which will you sacrifice, your women or your cats?" [17] From these animal experiments Blundell showed that opening the peritoneum was not necessarily followed by overwhelming infection and that certain

organs could be removed without fatal results. He was one of the first in Britain to successfully carry out a vaginal hysterectomy for malignant ulceration of the cervix [16]. Blundell was the first to advocate tubal ligation: "I would advise an incision of an inch in length in the linea alba above the symphysis pubis; I would advise further, that the fallopian tube on either side should be drawn up to this aperture; and lastly, I would advise, that a portion of the tube should be removed, an operation easily performed, when the woman, would forever after, be sterile" [7].

Blundell also had some sensible advice about neonatal resuscitation, in particular urging the physician not to give up too early:

Never hastily despair of the means of resuscitation. Many a foetus has been laid aside as dead which, by a diligent use of resuscitants, might have been saved...the bud of life may appear withering, dying, nay dead—when unexpectedly, nature, from her deep and hidden recess, comes forth and raises the sinking embryo to vigorous life [7].

Concerning artificial respiration Blundell felt "The only mode of performing this operation effectually is by means of a small instrument, the tracheal pipe, which I think every accoucheur should carry along with him to a labour". Blundell described his own technique as follows:

I pass the fore-finger of my left hand down upon the root of the tongue and into the rima glottidis, and then using the tube with the right hand, I slide it along the surface of the finger, used as a director, till reaching the rima I insert the tube at the moment when the finger is withdrawn from it, afterwards feeling on the front of the neck whether the instrument is lying in the trachea or the oesophagus. This done, you may take the child into your hands, and from your own lungs you may inflate the lungs of the foetus, emptying them afterwards by means of double pressure of the hand, on the thorax I mean, and the abdomen, the latter pressure being necessary in order to urge upwards the diaphragm. Operating in this manner, you may execute the artificial respiration with the best success. Five-and-twenty, or thirty respirations there ought to be in a minute, the new-born child breathing faster than an adult [7].

After resigning from the hospital, Blundell (Fig. 4) continued his private practice for a number of years. He tended to rise late, see consultations in the afternoon and travel to see patients in their homes late in the evening in his yellow coach with a special light that allowed him to read between houses [17,18]. He retired

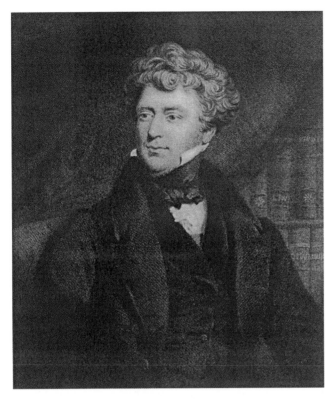

Fig. 4. Portrait of James Blundell.

from practice in his late 50s and lived comfortably on the considerable fortune from his earnings and family bequest. He remained a bachelor in Piccadilly, devoting the remaining years of his life to study of the classics and his collection of rare books on obstetrics and gynaecology which were left to the Obstetrical Society of London. He died at his home on January 15, 1878 at the age of 87.

## References

[1] Waller C. Case of uterine hemorrhage, in which the operation of transfusion was successfully performed. Med Phys J 1825;54:273–7.

[2] Blundell J. Experiments on the transfusion of blood by the syringe. Med Chir Trans 1818;9:56–92.

[3] Blundell J. Lectures on the theory and practice of midwifery. Delivered at Guy's hospital by Dr James Blundell. Lecture 28: After-management of floodings, and on transfusion. Lancet 1827;8(1):673–81.

[4] Wren C. An account of the rise and attempts of a way to conveigh liquors immediately into the mass of blood. Phil Trans 1665;1:128–30.

[5] Lower R. The method observed in transfusing the blood out of one live animal into another. Phil Trans 1665;1:353–7.

[6] Boulton TB. Classical file: James Blundell, MD, FRCP, and the introduction of the transfusion of human blood to man. Surv Anesthesiol 1986;30:100–6.

[7] Blundell J. The principles and practice of obstetricy. London: E. Cox, 1834:247, 337, 580, 838.

[8] Blundell J. Observations on transfusion of blood by Dr Blundell. With a description of his gravitator. Lancet 1828;2:321–4.

[9] Blundell J. Some account of a case of obstinate vomiting in which an attempt was made to prolong life by the injection of blood into the veins. Med Chir Trans 1818;10:310–2.

[10] Jones HW, Mackmull G. The influence of James Blundell on the development of blood transfusion. Ann Med Hist 1928;10:242–8.

[11] Doubleday E. Case of uterine hemorrhage successfully treated by the operation of transfusion. Med Phys J 1825;54:380–6.

[12] Medical Society of London Report. November 14, 1825. Lancet 1825;9: 295.

[13] Blundell J. Successful case of transfusion. Lancet 1829;1:431–2.

[14] Hicks JB. Cases of transfusion with some remarks on a new method of performing the operation. Guy's Hosp Rep 1869;14:1–14.

[15] Aveling JH. Immediate transfusion in England: seven cases, and the author's method of operating. Obstet J Gr Brit Irel 1873;5:289–311.

[16] Blundell J. Lancet 1878;1:255–6 (Obituary).

[17] Baskett TF. On the Shoulders of Giants: Eponyms and Names in Obstetrics and Gynaecology. London: RCOG Press, 1996:22–3.

[18] Blundell J. BMJ 1878;1:351–2 (Obituary).

# William O'Shaughnessy, Thomas Latta and the origins of intravenous saline

Thomas F. Baskett

In the port of Sunderland, in northeast England, on October 26, 1831 the second pandemic of Indian cholera claimed its first of 23 000 victims in Britain [1]. At that time the mode of transmission or the specific treatment of cholera was unknown. The standard method of management, as it was for most conditions at that time, was blood-letting with or without emetics. The most thoughtful entrant into the debate on treatment was a 22-year old recent medical graduate of Edinburgh University, William O'Shaughnessy. His first contribution was a paper read before the Westminister Medical Society on December 3, 1831 and published shortly thereafter in the *Lancet* [2]. Pointing out the high mortality rate in Sunderland with conventional treatment he wondered if 'The habits of practical chemistry which I have occasionally pursued,...might lead to the application of chemistry to its cure' [2]. The end result of cholera was, as O'Shaughnessy wrote, 'The universal stagnation of the venous system, and rapid cessation of the arterialisation of the blood, are the earliest, as well as the most characteristic effects. Hence the skin becomes blue...' [2]. In this context 'arterialisation' was used interchangeably with 'oxygenation'. O'Shaughnessy therefore felt that if 'we could bring certain salts of highly oxygenated constitution fairly into contact with the black blood of cholera, we would certainly restore its arterial properties, and most probably terminate the bad symptoms of the case' [2]. After experimentation in dogs O'Shaughnessy felt that the nitrate and chlorate of potash dissolved in water 'heated to a blood warmth' were the best oxidising agents.

Within a few days O'Shaughnessy 'proceeded to Sunderland for the purpose of making myself practically acquainted with the celebrated disease therein prevailing...' [3]. Shortly after his arrival in Sunderland, O'Shaughnessy sent a letter to the *Lancet* including this graphic description of terminal cholera [3].

'On the floor, before the fireplace...lay a girl of slender make and juvenile height; with the face of a superannuated hag. She uttered no moan, gave expression of no pain,...The colour of her countenance was that of lead—a silver blue, ghastly tint; her eyes were sunk deep into the sockets, as though they had been driven in an inch behind their natural position; her mouth was squared; her features flattened; her eyelids black; her fingers shrunk, bent, and inky in their hue. All pulse was gone at the wrist, and a tenacious sweat moistened her bosom. In short, Sir, that face and form I never can forget, were I to live to beyond the period of man's natural age'.

O'Shaughnessy was convinced that this was the dreaded Indian cholera and much more severe than previous epidemics of so-called English cholera. This Indian cholera was, he said 'sudden, deadly, overwhelming, collapsed, the living death...' [3].

In a letter to the *Lancet* dated December 29, 1831, O'Shaughnessy outlined the results of his experiments on blood drawn from 'the worst cases of the cholera' and found it 'unchanged in its anatomical or globular structure' [4] (Fig. 1). His main findings were that the blood had lost a large proportion of its water and 'neutral saline ingredients'. In a later report, O'Shaughnessy noted 'a material diminution of water in the blood...and a notable decrease in the quantity of soluble salts, amounting, as far as regards the serum, to a mean loss of one-third of these substances...' [5]. After this chemical analysis, O'Shaughnessy changed his recommendation from potassium salts to 'the injection into the veins of tepid water holding a solution of the normal salts of the blood' [6].

Although O'Shaughnessy carried out detailed analysis of the blood, emesis and diarrhoea of cholera patients, along with experiments of intravenous infusions in dogs, he never applied the treatment to humans. However, shortly after these publications in the *Lancet*, Thomas

## EXPERIMENTS ON THE BLOOD IN CHOLERA.

*To the Editor of* THE LANCET.

SIR,—Having been enabled to complete the experimental inquiries on which I have some time back been engaged in Newcastle-upon-Tyne, I beg you will have the kindness to give insertion to the annexed outlines of the results I have obtained :—

1. The blood drawn in the worst cases of *the* cholera, is unchanged in its anatomical or globular structure.

2. It has *lost a large proportion of its water*, 1000 parts of cholera serum having but the average of 860 *parts of water*.

3. *It has lost also a great proportion of its* NEUTRAL *saline ingredients*.

4. *Of the free alkali contained in healthy serum, not a particle is present in some cholera cases, and barely a trace in others.*

5. Urea exists in the cases where suppression of urine has been a marked symptom.

6. *All the salts deficient in the blood, especially the carbonate of soda, are present in large quantities in the peculiar white dejected matters.*

There are other results of minor consequence, to which I will not at present allude, neither shall I *on this occasion* offer any observation on the practical inference to which my experiments may lead. In a few days a detailed report shall be published, in which the mode of analysis, &c. will be minutely described. It will be found, I regret to say, in every essential particular, to contradict that recently given by Hermann. All my experiments, however, have been publicly performed, and can be authenticated by numerous witnesses, a precaution I thought it necessary to adopt, lest it might be supposed that I impugned, without sufficient foundation, the accuracy of the Moscow professor.

May I add, that until the publication of my report, I shall deem the suspension of discussion on the results now introduced as a matter of personal courtesy and obligation.     I am, Sir,
Your obedient servant,
W. B. O'SHAUGHNESSY, M.D.
London, 29 December, 1831.

Fig. 1. O'Shaughnessy [4].

Latta of Leith acknowledged and successfully applied O'Shaughnessy's advice in human sufferers. Using O'Shaughnessy's principles Latta 'attempted to restore the blood to its natural state, by injecting copiously into the larger intestine warm water holding in its solution the requisite salts, and also administered quantities from time to time by the mouth' [7]. He found this gave no benefit and 'at length resolved to throw the fluid immediately into the circulation' [7]. As Latta said: 'having no precedent to direct me, I proceeded with much caution'. He did not have long to wait until a woman moribund from cholera and unresponsive to all other treatment presented [7]:

'She had apparently reached the last moments of her earthly existence, and now nothing could injure her—indeed so entirely was she reduced, that I feared I should be unable to get my apparatus ready ere she expired. Having inserted a tube into the basilic vein, cautiously, anxiously, I watched the effect; ounce after ounce was injected, but no visible change was produced. Still persevering, I thought she began to breath less laboriously; soon the sharpened features and sunken eye and fallen jaw, pale and cold, bearing the manifest impress of death's signet, began to glow with returning animation; the pulse which had long ceased, returned to the wrist, at first small and quick, by degrees it became more and more distinct, fuller, slower and firmer, and in a short space of half an hour, when six pints had been injected, she expressed in a firm voice that she was free from all uneasiness, actually became jocular, and fancied all she needed was a little sleep; her extremities were warm, and every feature bore the aspect of comfort and health. This being my first case, I fancied my patient secure, and from my great need of a little repose, left her in charge of the hospital surgeon; but I had not been long gone, ere the vomiting and purging recurring, soon reduced her to her former state of debility. I was not apprised of the event, and she sunk in five and a half hours after I left her. As she had previously been of a sound constitution, I have no doubt the case would have issued in complete reaction, had the remedy, which already had produced such effect been repeated'.

A classic and acutely observed description of the first resuscitative effect of intravenous saline in a case of profound dehydration and hypovolaemic shock (Fig. 2). Three weeks later, on June 16, 1832, Latta wrote a letter to the editor detailing three further cases he had treated with intravenous saline, one of which was successful [8]. These cases represented a spectrum of humanity and included: 'a prostitute of the very lowest order...; a middle-aged female brought to the hospital *in articulo mortis*...; a middle-aged man, of sober industrious habits...' [8].

In his first case, Latta prepared the intravenous injection as follows: 'I dissolved from two to three drachms of muriate of soda and two scruples of the subcarbonate of soda in six pints of water, and injected

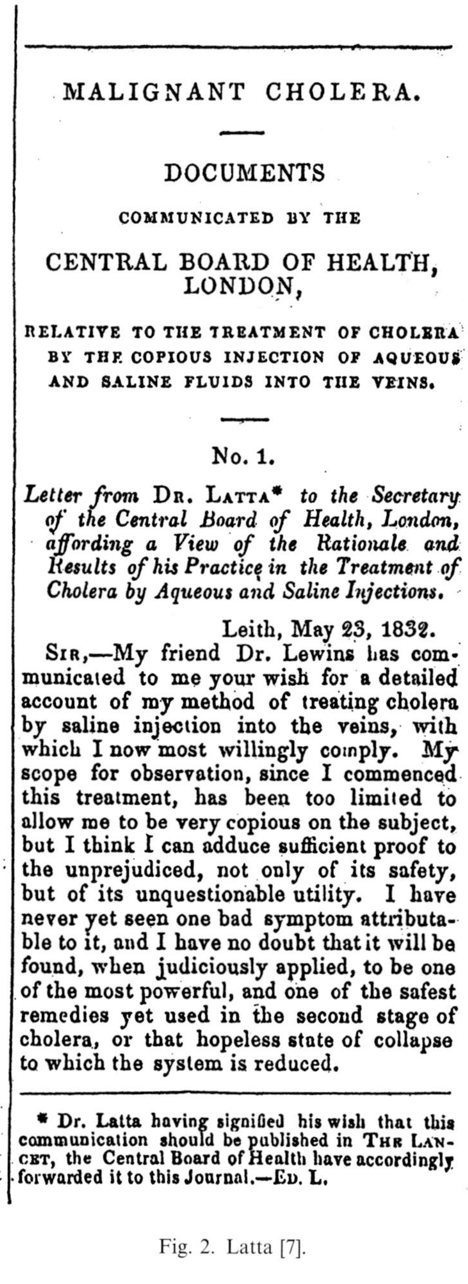

## MALIGNANT CHOLERA.

### DOCUMENTS

COMMUNICATED BY THE

### CENTRAL BOARD OF HEALTH, LONDON,

RELATIVE TO THE TREATMENT OF CHOLERA BY THE COPIOUS INJECTION OF AQUEOUS AND SALINE FLUIDS INTO THE VEINS.

#### No. 1.

*Letter from Dr. Latta\* to the Secretary of the Central Board of Health, London, affording a View of the Rationale and Results of his Practice in the Treatment of Cholera by Aqueous and Saline Injections.*

Leith, May 23, 1832.

Sir,—My friend Dr. Lewins has communicated to me your wish for a detailed account of my method of treating cholera by saline injection into the veins, with which I now most willingly comply. My scope for observation, since I commenced this treatment, has been too limited to allow me to be very copious on the subject, but I think I can adduce sufficient proof to the unprejudiced, not only of its safety, but of its unquestionable utility. I have never yet seen one bad symptom attributable to it, and I have no doubt that it will be found, when judiciously applied, to be one of the most powerful, and one of the safest remedies yet used in the second stage of cholera, or that hopeless state of collapse to which the system is reduced.

---

\* Dr. Latta having signified his wish that this communication should be published in THE LANCET, the Central Board of Health have accordingly forwarded it to this Journal.—ED. L.

Fig. 2. Latta [7].

it at temperature 112 F' [7]. This has been calculated as equivalent to 58 meq/l sodium; 49 meq/l chloride; 9 meq/l bicarbonate [6]. Latta noted that the body temperature in patients with cholera was very low and he therefore added a warm vapour bath to his treatment. He felt that by placing the patient in the warm bath at body temperature the necessary volume of 'saline fluids' might be reduced and that he could give the intravenous saline at 'body heat, 97–98 F' rather than heating it to 112 F as he had done with his first case [9,10]. He also increased the 'saline matter' in the solution by one-third [10]. Latta further advised that as soon as the patient was resuscitated with intravenous saline 'mild, warm stimulants, such as weak gin-toddy mixed with some

astringent, should be freely and assiduously administered' [7].

Dr Jachnichen, a German physician appointed to the Institute of Artificial Mineral Waters in Moscow, is reputed to have given six ounces of intravenous water to a woman suffering from cholera in 1830 [6]. This is not substantiated by a report on cholera in Moscow from Jachnichen in 1831 [11] in which he notes that his chemist colleague Mr Hermann felt that the blood of cholera victims lacked 'essigsäure' which translates to 'vinegar' or 'acid'. He went on to write: 'I suggested the injection of $H_2O$ at 30 F into the veins and after Mr Hermann found free acid I suggested an equivalent of acid with the $H_2O$ into the veins of the sick one. But the honorable colleagues felt this procedure was too daring and the success highly doubtful. And even if it was theoretically sure of success the responsibility seemed too large to assume alone'. From this report and another to the *Gazette Médicale de Paris* it seems unlikely that Dr Jachnichen used intravenous treatment and certainly not intravenous saline [12].

Intravenous saline infusion for cholera was not widely accepted, although the Central Board of Health in Britain did ask a number of physicians to test this new method of treatment [13]. Of the first 25 reported cases treated with intravenous saline only eight recovered [6]. However, the treatment tended to be given only to moribund patients and once rehydrated the diarrhoea would often reoccur, and the saline infusions were usually not maintained long enough to sustain fluid balance. During 1832 the cholera pandemic subsided in Britain, but with no clear support for intravenous rehydration. It was not used in subsequent epidemics in the United States and Europe in the mid 19th century [13]. The reintroduction of intravenous saline for cholera and other conditions of severe dehydration and hypovolaemia was not fully established until the 1880s after work by Peter Little and Robert Barnes in England and Emil Schwarz of the Physiological Institute in Halle [13].

William Brooke O'Shaughnessy was born in Limerick, Ireland in 1809 and graduated in medicine from Edinburgh University in 1830. He was only 22 years old when he carried out his original observations on the blood of cholera patients. In 1832, he was appointed as cholera inspector for the Camberwell and Newington districts of London. The following year he moved to Bengal as an assistant surgeon with the East India Company. He was active and published widely on both medical and chemical subjects and was appointed professor of chemistry in the Medical College in Calcutta. By 1839 he became interested in the electric telegraph and in 1853 was appointed Director General of the Indian Telegraph Company. Despite enormous difficulty, he established 4000 miles of telegraph lines between Calcutta, Agra, Bombay and Madras, which was said to have influenced the outcome of the Indian mutiny. O'Shaughnessy was knighted for his services in 1856 and retired from his work in India, returning to England in 1861. He later transposed his name to Sir William O'Shaughnessy-Brooke. He died at Southsea in January 1889 [14].

Thomas Aitchison Latta was the fourth son of Alexander Latta of Jessfield near Leith, Scotland. His exact date of birth is unknown but was probably in the late 1790s [15]. His father died in 1807 but his older brother, Alexander, who qualified in medicine from Edinburgh University in 1805, looked after young Thomas who later followed him to the medical school at Edinburgh and graduated MD in August, 1819. As a medical student he accompanied William Scoresby (1789–1857) on a whaling expedition to Greenland to study icebergs. He even had the courage to publish his own observations, some of which were at odds with those of Scoresby [16]. In 1822, he established his general practice in Leith. He died on October 19, 1833 of 'pulmonary consumption'.

Ironically, William O'Shaughnessy received recognition and a knighthood for his work on the electric telegraph but his obituary makes no reference to his work on cholera [14]. Thomas Latta, the young general practitioner, had the courage and prepared mind to grasp the significance of O'Shaughnessy's observations and put them into practice. A fellow practitioner in Leith, Robert Lewins, embraced Latta's treatment and was so impressed that he wrote in a letter to the *Lancet* 'a method of medical treatment which will, I predict,...entitle Dr. Latta's name to be placed amongst the numbers of those, alas! how few, who have really contributed to the improvement of the healing art' [17]. It was not to be and Thomas Latta died unheralded 1 year after his pioneering efforts. It would be another half century before the groundwork of O'Shaughnessy and Latta led to the almost ubiquitous use of intravenous saline in hospital medicine, while the originators were largely forgotten.

## Acknowledgements

Thanks to Katharina Kieser, MD for the translation of Ref. [11].

## References

[1] van Heyningen WE, Seal JR. Cholera: the American scientific experience 1947–1980. Boulder, Colorado: Westview Press, 1983:1–25.
[2] O'Shaughnessy WB. Proposal of a new method of treating the blue epidemic cholera by the injection of highly-oxygenised salts into the venous system. Lancet 1831;1:366–71.
[3] O'Shaughnessy WB. The cholera in the North of England. Lancet 1831;1:401–4.
[4] O'Shaughnessy WB. Experiments on the blood in cholera. Lancet 1831;1:490.
[5] O'Shaughnessy WB. Chemical pathology of cholera. Lancet 1832;2:225–32.
[6] Cosnett JE. The origins of intravenous fluid therapy. Lancet 1989;1:768–71.
[7] Latta TA. Relative to the treatment of cholera by the copious injection of aqueous and saline fluids into the veins. Lancet 1832;2:274–7.
[8] Latta TA. Letter detailing three cases. Lancet 1832;2:370–3.
[9] Latta TA. Saline venous injection in cases of malignant cholera performed while in the vapour-bath. Lancet 1832;2:173–6.
[10] Latta TA. Saline venous injection in cases of malignant cholera performed while in the vapour-bath. Lancet 1832;2:208–9.
[11] Jähnichen. Die Cholera in Moskau. Helk 1831;19:385–454.
[12] Jachnichen. Mémoire sur le cholera-morbus qui règne en Russie. Gaz Méd (Paris) 1830–31;1–2:85–8.
[13] Astrup P, Bie P, Engell HC. Salt and water in culture and medicine. Copenhagen: Munksgaard, 1993:165–90.
[14] O'Shaughnessy WB. Obituary. Br Med J 1902;1:40.
[15] Masson AHB, Latta TA. Pioneer in saline infusion. Br J Anaesth 1971;43:681–6.
[16] Latta TA. Observations on icebergs, made during a short excursion in Spitzbergen. Edin Phil J 1820;3:237.
[17] Lewins R. Correspondence. Lancet 1831–32;2:370.

# Johann Friedrich August von Esmarch — a pioneer in the field of emergency and disaster medicine

Christian W. Beyer, Wolfgang F. Dick

A full appreciation of the contributions made by Friedrich von Esmarch to emergency and disaster medicine needs to include his endeavours in medical fields like clinical therapy (where he initiated fundamental changes), medical education and research in trauma and disaster medicine. This is in addition to the political, cultural and scientific environment that influenced his work.

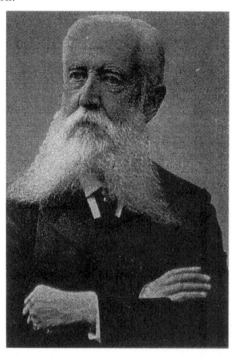

Esmarch was born on 9 January 1823 in northern Germany, into a family of physicians, judges and lawyers with a long academic tradition. His father was a highly respected surgeon, who encouraged his gifted son to follow in his footsteps. von Esmarch began his medical studies at the University of Kiel in 1843, to graduate only 3 years later from the University of Göttingen. His career advanced at a rapid pace and he received an appointment as professor and chairman of the department of surgery at the University of Kiel. In 1867 von Esmarch married, an aunt of Emperor Wilhelm II, who raised him to the rank of a peer in 1887 in recognition of his outstanding achievements in the field of medicine. von Esmarch founded the German Society of Surgeons and was named president in 1894. On 23 October 1908 he died from the effects of an influenza infection.

In the early 19th century the focus of surgical interventions was primarily on the body surface and the extremities. From the beginning of his medical career von Esmarch showed a passionate interest in trauma care, placing the emphasis on reconstructive surgery instead of the conventional practice of limb amputation in battle victims. The political climate of the time favoured decisions made on the battlefield over diplomatic solutions and his work as a surgeon in the campaigns against Denmark, led by Bismarck in 1848 and 1864, provided him with ample experience in the treatment of war injuries. In contrast to the rapid progress in war technologies with all their horrible consequences, improvements in the military medical service sadly lagged behind and the soldiers received inadequate treatment under unacceptable conditions which had remained unchanged over the preceding centuries.

Common consequences of surgical interventions were wound infections, frequently leading to the death of a patient due to massive septic shock. In the 1850s the causes of wound infections were still largely unknown by the practising physicians. von Esmarch's observation that the cooling of wounds resulted in a reduction in local inflammation and pus-formation and thus to an improvement in the patient's outcome led him to introduce cryotherapy into clinical practice. In 1862 he published his findings, introducing his new therapeutic principle with detailed instructions on the application of the new method in surgical practice.

At his department in Kiel he not only educated his residents in current concepts of medical care, but also emphasised the importance of regular postgraduate medical education, as well as the need for accurate patient information and consent for medico-legal reasons. A number of von Esmarch's publications are still of relevance today, especially with regard to malpractice regulations. Other concepts introduced by him include the need for accurate documentation on patient charts and the collection and recording of data as a basis for scientific research. He encourged the development of official instructions and regulations to ensure standardised medical therapy and quality control.

von Esmarch was an absolute perfectionist, hard to please, even to himself. None of his students reportedly ever received a grade higer than a B in an examination, and it was not unusual that examinations had to be repeated. His list of publications is impressive, ranging from topics on the resection of gun wounds (1851) to the use of cryotherapy in surgery (1862), artificial exsanguination (1873) and a manual of war surgery (1877), to name just a few.

August Bier, one of his colleagues and a famous surgeon himself, praised von Esmarch as being a genius with the ability to see the underlying relationships in apparently simple and natural processes and to evaluate their importance. He felt that von Esmarch was worthy to be called a genius even if he had achieved nothing else in his medical career than the development of a method designed to avoid major blood loss in the course of surgical procedures on extremities, artificial exsanguination. Yet, his significant contributions to surgery were evenly matched by his outstanding achievements in resuscitation and disaster medicine.

His battlefield experience convinced von Esmarch of the need for a system to enable analysis of the most effective use of medical resources, known today as triage. The introduction of this principle was unprecedented at a time when the decision as to whether treatment was to be provided depended on military rank instead of the severity of the injury. It was von Esmarch's conviction that the well-organised administration of medical resources and personnel on the battlefield, including ambulance carriages, movable pharmacies and soup kitchens was of equal importance in providing the wounded soldiers with medical care to the treatment itself. The introduction of mobile hospitals and hospital trains were further innovations in support of his scheme and may be regarded as precursors of today's MASH hospitals. von Esmarch gave detailed instructions for the equipment for these units, ranging from the installation of stretchers in 4th class carriages which were not fitted with seats to the manufacturing methods to be used in the construction of these units. Interestingly, the first of these trains which transported wounded soldiers back to Berlin from the French battlefields in 1870 was sponsored by a private initiative and not by the German army. Based on the recommendation of von Esmarch, from 1873 soldiers were required to carry first aid packets, which were fitted out according to his proposals and included, for example elastic suspenders that could be used as tourniquets. von Esmarch was also among the first physicians to emphasise the importance of first aid by non-health care professionals.

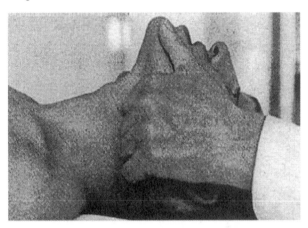

While the delivery and improvement of medical treatment under battle conditions constitute a significant contribution to medical science, the achievements of von Esmarch in times of peace are of no lesser importance.

While Langenbeck's introduction of ether (1847) to anaesthetise a patient undergoing a surgical procedure represented a major improvement of surgical conditions, it nevertheless involved the risk of possible harm to the patient from asphyxia, due to inadequate control in the deep stages of anaesthesia. von Esmarch identified a backward movement of the mandible and tongue as a cause of occlusion of the airway in the unconscious state as the cause of this not infrequently encountered problem. He devised a simple but effective measure designed to ensure an open airway under the described conditions, consisting of an overextension of the neck and forward movement of the mandible. Until today this procedure, the 'Esmarch manoeuvre' represents an elementary intervention in resuscitation procedures.

Later in his career the focus of von Esmarch's interest was again on emergency and disaster medicine. In the course of a lecture held in 1875 he stated that the expansion of disaster situations must be expected to be in proportion to technological progress. He continued to say that it would therefore be essential for medicine to have accurate algorithms and logistics at its disposal, which enable the provision of medical care without a waste of resources. He concluded his lecture with instructions on the development of a logistic structure enabling the timely availability of equipment in disaster situations. These instructions still form the basis of algorithms used today to ensure the placement of equipment at specific intersection points or railway junctions for rapid transfer to disaster scenes.

In a lecture given by von Esmarch in 1899 he left the following testimony of his humanistic attitude and goals:

"If someone were to draw up a record of the triumphs of the 19th century, the efforts made to relieve the injuries, pain and harm suffered by the wounded soldier as a result of technological warfare would hardly be a part thereof. Although perhaps later generations will assess these efforts made in an attempt to change the miserable conditions on the battlefield as one of the most commendable acts of the outgoing 19th century".

## Bibliography

Schmauss A.K. Johann Friedrich August von Esmarch – Leben und Werk. ZBL Chirurgie 1983;108:1577–83.

Schober K.L. Fr. von Esmarch Die Anwendung der Kälte in der Chirurgie ZBL. Chirurgie 1978;103:1632–34.

Paul U. Friedrich von Esmarch. ZBL Chirurgie 1980;105:549–50.

Pagel. Ärzte des 19. Jahrhunderts. Urban and Schwarzenberg, München.

von Esmarch F. Über Resektionen nach Schußwunden; Beobachtungen und Erfahrungen aus den Schleswig-holsteinischen Feldzügen von 1848–1851. Kiel, 1851:1851.

von Esmarch F. Die Anwendung der Kälte in der Chirurgie. Berlin: Archiv für klinische Chirurgie; Bd.1 S, 1861:275–333.

von Esmarch F. Über künstliche Blutleere bei Operationen. Leipzig: Volkmanns Sammlung klinischer Vorträge, Chir. Bd. 1, Nr. 58,' S. 1873:373–384.

von Esmarch F. Handbuch der kriegschirurgischen Technik. Leipzig und Kiel, 1877.

# Bernhard Schultze and the swinging neonate

Thomas F. Baskett        Fritz Nagele

The 19th century was an era of rapid development in obstetrics and gynaecology in Germany and among several prominent investigators and teachers was Bernhard Sigmund Schultze (1827–1919). Schultze made many contributions in the field of obstetrics, several of which were outlined in his extensive obstetric atlas [1]. He is remembered eponomously for his description of the Schultze method of placental separation in the third stage of labour. Schultze felt that when the placenta completely separated from the uterine wall after delivery of the infant it descended into the vagina with the smooth, shiny fetal surface presenting. This was in contrast to the description by Matthews Duncan who described separation as occurring with the placenta sliding down from the uterine wall so that the rough maternal surface of the placenta presented [2]. Several generations of medical students have learned to remember the distinction between these two methods of placental presentation as 'shiny Schultze' and 'dirty Duncan'.

Schultze is less well known for his considerable contribution to neonatal resuscitation. In 1871, he published his 179 page monograph *Der Scheintod Neugeborener* [3] (Fig. 1). In this book, he describes a method of artificial respiration for asphyxiated infants which he endorsed based on 12 years practice with the technique, "Which I recommend warmly, because—if applied in time—it is rarely unsuccessful". Schultze described that he had previously used 'insufflation of air' for neonatal resuscitation and developed his technique when this was ineffective. "At the beginning I used it in cases, in whom insufflation of air was unsuccessful, and when in such cases—after much loss of time—I was able to resuscitate the by then even more asphyxiated infant, I now use this method right from the beginning in all cases of profound asphyxia".

## Der Scheintod Neugeborener.

Sendschreiben

an

## Herrn Dr. C. Ludwig
Professor der Physiologie in Leipzig

von

## Dr. B. S. Schultze
Professor der Geburtshülfe in Jena.

Jena,
Mauke's Verlag
(Hermann Dufft).
1871.

Fig. 1.

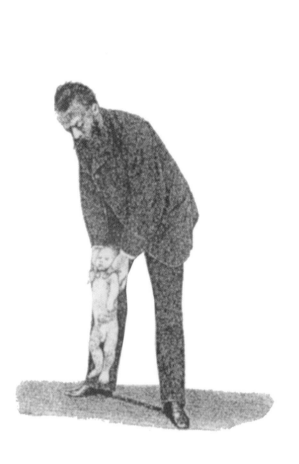 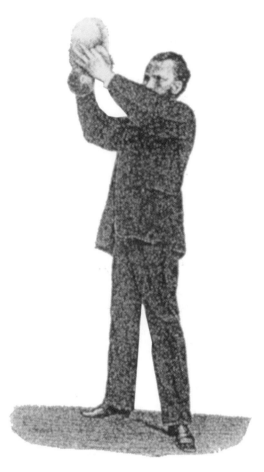

Fig. 2.

At the beginning of the chapter on treatment in his book, Schultze gives four indications for his technique of artificial respiration.

1. The deeply depressed medulla olongata, which does not react any longer to the extreme stimulus of oxygen deficiency by inspiration movements.
2. This oxygen deficiency combined with the accumulation of carbonic acid in the blood stream, both of which increased steadily as long as circulation exists.
3. The reduction of the circulation resulting in cardiac contractions becoming rare and weak, and its sequelae which are vital in maintaining this critical situation, namely the overfilling of the heart and the thoracic blood vessels.
4. Accumulation of amniotic fluid, meconium, and mucus within the airways.

Scultze went on to give a detailed description of his technique with two accompanying figures depicting himself carrying out the manoeuvre.

"The objective of this method is to simultaneously move the ribs and the diaphragm of the thorax in a passive way in order to alternately provide expansion and compression of the thoracic cavity......The child is taken with both hands at the shoulders such that both thumbs overlie the anterior surface of the thorax, the forefingers reach behind to the axillary fossae, and the other three fingers obliquely and lengthwise rest on the posterior surface of the thorax. In so doing, the head, which usually flops backwards, is comfortably supported by the palms. The obstetrician with legs astride and the upper part of the body bent forward, takes the floppy infant in the above way with the arms stretched downwards (Fig. 2(1)). Without delay the obstetrician swings the infant from this position upwards. When the arms of the obstetrician reach a position slightly above horizontal, they slow and stop gently to avoid over-twisting the child; the body should sink down slowly, and due to the weight of the pelvis and abdomen is strongly compressed; at this moment the entire weight of the baby lies on the obstetrician's thumbs positioned at the thorax (Fig. 2(2)). Utmost care must be taken not to compress the baby's thorax at the start when grasping it in the above way. Applying the grip, the body of the child rests exclusively on the forefingers of the obstetrician positioned in the base of the axillary fossae; there must be no lateral pressure to the thorax by the obstetrician's palms and the thumbs must not press the thorax anteriorly. When swinging the baby up, the flexion of the spine should not be at the thoracic level, but almost exclusively at the lumbar part of the spine; while the thumbs continue to keep minimal pressure on the thorax and only provide support to the infant's body as it slowly sinks down. Lifting the infant to the horizontal level should be performed with vigorous drive of the arms at the shoulder joints, then by slowing down the arms and with careful control of the elbows and shoulders, the physician regulates the gradual flexion of the infant's lower trunk. This gradual flexion of the infant's pelvis over the abdomen results in a significant compression of the thoracic viscera, the diaphragm, and the entire chest wall. As a result of this passive expiratory movement, aspirated fluids often come out of the respiratory tract. The flexion of the child having been completed slowly but steadily, the obstetrician again moves his arms down between his legs. In so doing the infant's body is stretched with the acceleration and the thorax, without any pressure, due to its elasticity will now expand......The weight of the infant moving down, will also elevate the ribs, move the diaphragm down resulting in a passive but massive inspiration. After an interval of some seconds, the child is again moved up and, while flexing its entire weight on the thumbs positioned on the anterior thoracic wall, the next mechanical expiration takes place.

This swinging up and down of the infant is repeated eight to ten times. At inspiration, the passage of air through the glottis causes an audible sound. If, at expiration, aspirated fluids continue to be expelled from the mouth and nose it is to be prolonged. If spontaneous inspiration starts (which is most likely following artificial expiration), it is enhanced by immediately swinging down the infant, thereby adding to the effects of passive inspiration. The other possibility in this situation is to stop artificial respiration, and to put the infant in a warm bath in order not to interrupt spontaneous respiration by artificial effects.

Having said this, it becomes evident that this method of artificial respiration by swinging the infant is very effective, it reduces the difference of the tension between arterial and venous blood columns and therefore effectively launches the entire circulation".


Schultze may have been influenced to try this technique as an extension of that proposed by Silvester who, in 1858, stressed that the essential part of resuscitation was to induce expiration and inspiration by alternative compression and relaxation of the chest [4].

Schultze's technique was also described in a popular United States obstetrical text in the late 19th century [5]. However, the section on neonatal resuscitation also states, 'the simplest and most effective method of inflating the lungs is by direct insufflation—the mouth-to-mouth method'. A standard British text of the early 20th century describes the Schultze method, as well as the Silvester technique, in the section on neonatal resuscitation [6]. They added the very practical advice to first carefully dry the infant's body so that the swinging neonate did not become the flying neonate. Both of these editions advise that the Schultze technique was best for milder cases of neonatal asphyxia, asphyxia livida, as opposed to the more profound asphyxia pallida as recommended by Schultze himself. The method was advocated in most of the standard German textbooks for half a century-from the 1870s to the 1920s [7–10].

Bernhard Sigmund Schultze was born in Freiburg on 29th December, 1827 (Fig. 3). His father and older brother were distinguished anatomists at Greifswald and the younger Schultze soon emulated them in this field. Like many of the great anatomists of his era, he was a skilled artist and did the illustrations for all his own papers and books. In 1853, he moved to Berlin to

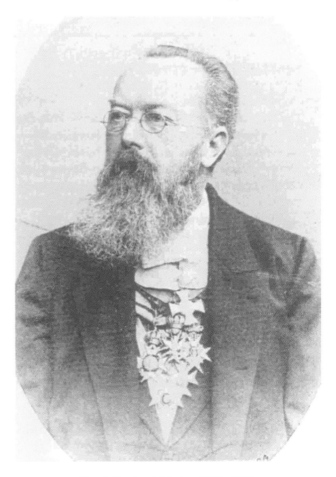

Fig. 3. Bernhard Schultze (1827–1919).

93

study obstetrics and by 1858 had established such a reputation that he was appointed to the Chair of Obstetrics and Gynaecology in Jena, where he remained until he retired in 1902. He was a prodigious and productive teacher and investigator. His textbook of midwifery ran to 15 editions in his lifetime. From the publication of his monograph on resuscitation of the newborn in 1871, he was considered an authority on the subject, which he continued to study for the next 50 years. He actively continued his research after retiring from the chair at Jena in 1902 and, although at the end of his days he was almost totally blind and deaf, he continued to publish extensively and refine his technique of neonatal resuscitation. His last paper was published one day before his death at the age of 91. His obituary, written by the eminent gynaecologist Otto Küstner, said, "He passed away not like an old, tired man who had done his work and was now relaxing, but death took him out in the middle of his productive activity" [11]. He died in Jena on April 17, 1919. He had four sons and one daughter.

## References

[1] Schultze BS. Wandtafeln zur Schwangerschafts und Geburtskunde. Leipzig: Gunther, 1865.

[2] Duncan JM. On the mechanism of the expulsion of the placenta. Edin Med J 1871;16:899–903.

[3] Schultze BS. Der Sheintod Neugeborener. Jenna: Mauke's Verlag, 1871.

[4] Silvester HR. A new method of resuscitating still-born children, and of restoring persons apparently drowned or dead. Br Med J 1858;17:576–9.

[5] Chapin HD. In: Jewett C, editor. The Practice of Obstetrics by American Authors. New York: Lea Brothers, 1899:15–7.

[6] Berkeley C, Bonney V. The Difficulties and Emergencies of Obstetric Practice, 3rd ed. London: Churchill, 1921:729–30.

[7] Spiegelberg O, editor. Lehrbuch der Geburtshülfe. Lahr: Verlag Schauenburg, 1878:674–6.

[8] Olshausen R, Veit J, editors. Lehrbuch der Geburtshilfe. Bonn: Verlag Cohen, 1899:851–2.

[9] Stoeckel W, editor. Lehrbuch der Geburtshilfe, 2nd ed. Jena: Verlag Fischer, 1923:809–10.

[10] Zagermeister W, editor. Lehrbuch der Geburtshilfe. Leipzig: Verlag Hirzel, 1927:774.

[11] Küstner O. Bernhard Sigmund Schultze-Jena. Zentrabl für Gynäk 1919;21:393–8.

# John Snow and resuscitation

David A.E. Shephard    Thomas F. Baskett

## 1. Introduction

John Snow's work on resuscitation is less well known than his contributions to the scientific foundations of anaesthesia [1]. However, together with his understanding of the physiopathology of respiration, it was not the least of the reasons for his fundamental contributions to anaesthesia. His initial work on resuscitation with asphyxiated still-born infants, was published in 1841 [2], but, as his anaesthesia textbook of 1858 shows, he maintained an interest in resuscitation for the rest of his career [3].

## 2. Snow's career

John Snow (Fig. 1) was born on March 15, 1813 in the ancient English city of York [4]. His early medical training included a short period at the medical school in Newcastle, an apprenticeship to a doctor in the same city, and assistantships to two physicians back in Yorkshire. In 1836, deciding that he should take further training, he set out, on foot, for London, where he enrolled as a student in the Hunterian School of Medicine and then at Westminster Hospital. To break into London's medical hierarchy, he climbed the rungs of the academic medical ladder with characteristic thoroughness. In 1838 he passed the examinations for membership in the Royal College of Surgeons and for the licentiateship of the Society of Apothe-

caries; in 1843 he obtained the diploma (MB, BS) of London University; in the following year he was awarded the MD of London University; and to cap it all, in 1850 he became a licentiate of the Royal College of Physicians of London, which was as far as the current regulations would permit this

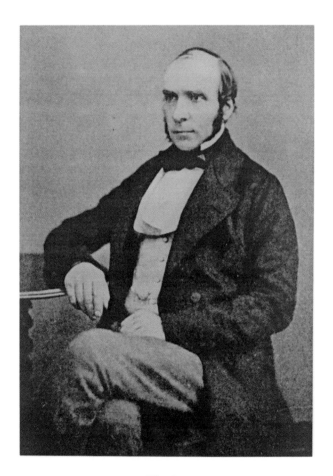

Fig. 1.

Yorkshire lad to go. By then, however, he was well known, both in London and other parts of Great Britain. A regular participant in the meetings of the Westminster Medical Society (which merged with the Medical Society of London in 1850)[5], beginning in 1847 he published classic texts in both anaesthesia and the epidemiology of cholera that eventually brought him renown. On the Inhalation of the Vapour of Ether in Surgical Operations... appeared in 1847 [6]; a series of papers 'On Narcotism by the Inhalation of Vapours' was launched in 1848 [7]; the first edition of On the Mode of Communication of Cholera followed in 1848 [8]; and the better known second edition of this monograph came out in 1854 [9]. Success bred further success: in 1853 and 1857 he anaesthetised Queen Victoria in labour, and in 1854 he was elected president of the Medical Society of London and of the Physiological Society. Just before he died on June 16, 1858, he completed his great text On Chloroform and Other Anaesthetics... [3].

ON
ASPHYXIA, AND ON THE RESUSCITATION OF STILL-BORN CHILDREN.

By John Snow, M.R.C.S.*

*(For the London Medical Gazette.)*

Respiration, in a limited sense, signifies the mutual change which takes place between the oxygen of the air and the blood; and this is not strictly a vital process, but only an operation of organic chemistry, since it continues after death as well as before, when the mechanical advantages for access of air remain the same. The celebrated Spallanzani, in his work on Respiration, has shown that snails and other animals, which respire chiefly by the surface of the body, continue after death to absorb to some extent the

* Read at the Westminster Medical Society on October 16, 1841.

Fig. 2.

## 3. Resuscitation of the stillborn

On October 16, 1841, when Snow read his paper on asphyxia and the resuscitation of stillborn children before the Westminster Medical Society he was on the threshold of a remarkable career (Fig. 2) [2]. He began his paper by discussing respiratory physiology and the effects of asphyxia, making the basic premise that "respiration seems essential to the life of the whole animal kingdom and when it is arrested from any cause the state called asphyxia is induced". Snow then addressed two questions that were moot at that time: first, whether 'insensibility' resulted from circulation of blood that was venous or from 'stoppage' of the circulation; and second, whether the carbon dioxide resulting from respiration was formed in the lungs by 'direct union' of oxygen in the air and carbon in the blood or whether oxygen was absorbed in the blood united with the carbon in the capillary circulation. He answered the first question by concluding that "blood which has totally lost its arterial properties, is unable to maintain sensibility or even vitality"; the second, by stating that carbon dioxide was indeed formed in the tissues. Snow's account of the context of the physiological knowledge of his time remains of interest today for, as Calverley noted, "it orients the reader to the knowledge of respiratory physiology and resuscitation that would have been available to a clinician at the time of the discovery of anaesthesia" [10].

Snow then turned to practical considerations. In reviewing the influence of temperature on the effects of asphyxia, he observed that lower temperatures enhanced survival, but also noted that the Royal Humane Society advocated warmth under these circumstances. Snow's recommendation was that heat should be avoided until respiration had been reestablished, when it would be 'a useful auxiliary to restore sensibility and renovate the patient'.

Snow's main purpose in presenting his paper of 1841, however, was to describe a device that would serve as 'a useful auxiliary' in resuscitating the asphyxiated stillborn (Fig. 2). His own experience in general practice had shown him that a 'very considerable' number of the newborn die at birth, and he reminded his audience that the literature indicated that one-twentieth of infants delivered were stillborn, many of whom were asphyxiated. Measures such as exposure of the baby's skin to cool air or cold water and immersion of the infant in warm water were sometimes beneficial, but more important, Snow believed, was artificial respiration. In these babies, he wrote, 'the great object... is to establish respiration; and if the patient cannot be roused to perform natural breathing, artificial respiration must be had recourse to as quickly as possible'. He dismissed both the standard recommendations of 'breathing into the lungs of the child', which he felt might injure or suffocate the infant, and using the bellows which might damage 'the texture of the lungs by over distension', and more to Snow's point, was marred by 'the difficulty of expelling the air from the lungs after it has been injected....' Snow had a better solution: a modification of a device that was "superior" to the bellows and one that had, in fact, been demonstrated before the Westminster Medical Society three years earlier by a Mr Read of Regent Circus, and Dr James Johnston. Their instrument was designed for use in adults, and its possible use for stillborn infants then seemed to Snow to have 'insurmountable difficulties'. Read, however, made some improvements, and showed Snow what he had done. Snow thereupon suggested that 'he should make a little instrument on exactly the same plan, adapted to the size of new-born children'. It was this new instrument that Snow described on that October evening in 1841:

It consists of two syringes, one of which, by a tube adapted to the mouth, and closing it withdraws air from the lungs, and the other syringe returns the same quantity of fresh air through a tube fitted to the nostrils. The two pistons are held in the same hand and lifted up and pressed down together, the cylinders being fixed side by side and each having two valves. When the pistons are raised, one cylinder becomes filled with air from the lungs, and the other with fresh air from the atmosphere, which can be warmed on its way by passing through a tube and metal coil placed in hot water. When the pistons are depressed, the latter cylinder is emptied into the lungs, and the air in the former is ejected into the atmosphere. In this way a constant current of air to and from the lungs is maintained, as in maternal respiration.

Snow emphasized two other points. One was to clear the airway before initiating artificial respiration. He recommended that 'the exhausting syringe be used first to remove any mucus there may be about the fauces; then, since the lungs are empty, a little air may be injected with the other syringe, before beginning with the pistons raised to work the two syringes together'. Snow, observing that 'the danger of asphyxia to the child is frequently foreseen', implied that physicians should have appropriate equipment ready in cases of abnormal labour and of haemorrhage. He also recommended that supplemental oxygen be used. Oxygen could 'be generated, in great purity in a few minutes, from chlorate of potash by means of a spirit-lamp and a small retort..., after which it could be mixed with air 'in one of the bags belonging to the instrument'. If all other means failed Snow supported the use of electricity, in 'the form of galvanism...', saying there was 'no harm in administering slight shocks after these other means have failed'. He claimed the main intention was to stimulate respiratory movements as he believed 'that oxygenating the blood in the lungs is the most efficient means to restore the action of the heart....'

There is no evidence that Snow used the double-syringe apparatus on any infants. His paper was evidently presented as the theoretical basis for neonatal resuscitation. Even so, Snow's place in the annals of neonatal resuscitation is secure. As Calverley observed, Snow was 'the first to recommend consideration of both the use of supplemental oxygen and the aspiration of material from the mouth and upper airway before initiating ventilation-the two cardinal principles of modern practice' [10].

### 4. Resuscitation in anaesthesia

In his paper on resuscitation of the stillborn, Snow described an experiment he performed on a guinea pig that he had drowned. After an hour he applied artificial respiration via the divided trachea, and observed that 'rhythmical contractions of the heart continued for three-quarters of an hour'. He was therefore familiar with artificial respiration as a means of resuscitation in anaesthesia, both in his research and in the advice he gave clinicians in administering anaesthesia. For example, in an experiment to determine the effects of chloroform in a rabbit he observed that with 10% chloroform the right heart became distended with blood and that "the action of the heart was quite reestablished by the artificial respiration"; he also noticed that the lungs "became paler, as the artificial respiration was continued..." [11] (Fig. 3). And clinically, as he wrote in 1855, 'I still consider, as I have all along, that artificial respiration, promptly and efficiently applied, is the best means of affording the patient a chance of recovery from an overdose of chloroform' adding that he knew 'from experiments that it will not answer if the heart is completely paralysed' [12].

Snow noted the means of resuscitation, including artificial respiration, that had been used in the first 50 cases of cardiac arrest reported in patients who had received chloroform [3]. The techniques of resuscitation included use of the 'tracheal tube', administration of oxygen, mouth-to-mouth or mouth-to-nostril ventilation, compression of the ribs and abdomen, and introduction of galvanic current. Of the techniques of artificial respiration, Snow favoured the Marshall Hall method, which

ON

# CHLOROFORM

AND

# OTHER ANÆSTHETICS:

THEIR

## ACTION AND ADMINISTRATION.

BY

## JOHN SNOW, M.D.

LICENTIATE OF THE ROYAL COLLEGE OF PHYSICIANS.

EDITED,

## WITH A MEMOIR OF THE AUTHOR,

BY

### BENJAMIN W. RICHARDSON, M.D.,

LICENTIATE OF THE ROYAL COLLEGE OF PHYSICIANS.

### LONDON:

### JOHN CHURCHILL, NEW BURLINGTON STREET.

MDCCCLVIII.

Fig. 3.

consisted of 'placing the patient on the face and making pressure on the back; removing the pressure, and turning the patient on his side and a little beyond...' and repeating these manoeuvres 'in about the time of natural respiration' [13].

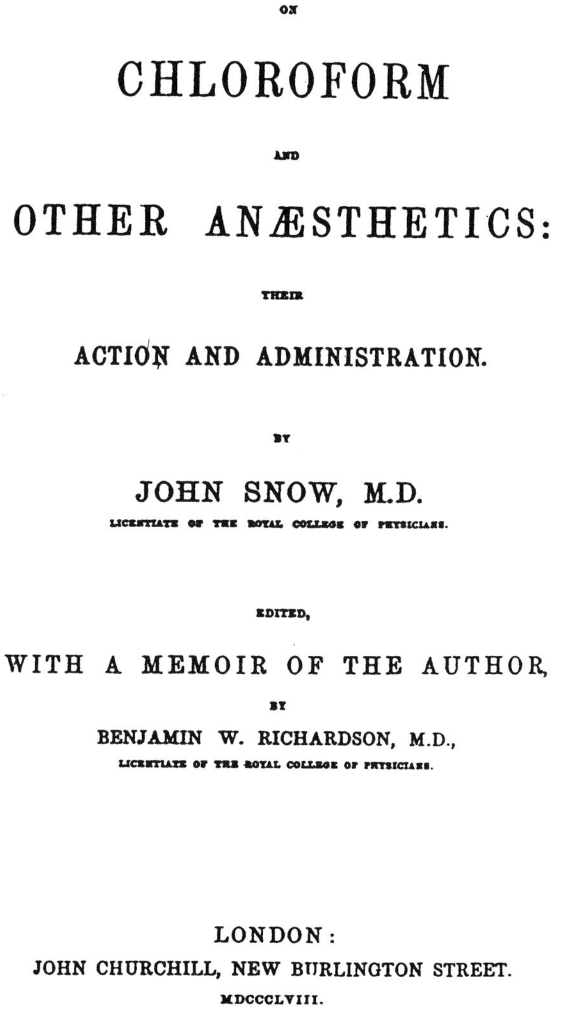

## 5. Comment

Snow's profound knowledge of resuscitation was based on his knowledge of the physiopathology of respiration and of the pharmacological effects of chloroform and other anaesthetic agents, as well as his wide knowledge of medicine. Interest in resuscitation, especially of the drowned, had grown following the founding of societies in the latter part of the 18th century to foster this interest in Holland and in England [14]. Among those with an interest in resuscitation was John Hunter, who invented a double chambered bellows-one chamber to fill the lungs and the other to empty them [15]. Snow's work on resuscitation was therefore a continuation of the studies in this field. It added to the knowledge on resuscitation, although Snow approached it from a different perspective. His work also foreshadowed other advances, particularly in neonatal resuscitation, with the studies of other anaesthetists such as Virginia Apgar [16].

## References

[1] Shephard DAE. From empirical craft to scientific discipline: the contributions of Claude Bernard and John Snow to the foundations of anaesthesia. In: Fink BR, Morris LE, Stephens CR, editors. The History of Anesthesia: Third International Symposium. Park Ridge, IL: Wood Library-Museum of Anaesthesiology, 1992:360–6.

[2] Snow J. On asphyxia and on the resuscitation of stillborn children. Lond Med Gaz 1841;29:222–7.

[3] Snow J. On Chloroform and Other Anaesthetics: Their Action and Administration. London: John Churchill, 1858.

[4] Shephard DAE. John Snow: Anaesthetist to a Queen and Epidemiologist to a Nation — A Biography. Cornwall, PE: York Point Publishing, 1995.

[5] Hunt T. The Medical Society of London, 1773–1973. London: The Medical Society of London and William Heinemann Medical Books, 1973:17.

[6] Snow J. On the Inhalation of the Vapour of Ether in Surgical Operations: Containing a Description of the Various Stages of Etherization, and a Statement of the Results of Nearly Eighty Operations in which Ether has been Employed. London: John Churchill, 1847.

[7] Ellis RH, editor. Snow J. On Narcotism by the Inhalation of Vapours. London: Royal Society of Medicine Services, 1991 (facsimile edition).

[8] Snow J. On the Mode of Communication of Cholera. London: John Churchill, 1848.

[9] Snow J. On the Mode of Communication of Cholera, 2nd edn. London: John Churchill, 1855.

[10] Calverley RK. Classical file. Surv Anesthesiol 1992;36:17–8.

[11] Snow J. On Chloroform and Other Anaesthetics: Their Action and Administration. London: John Churchill, 1858:117–8.

[12] Snow J. The breathing and the pulse under the influence of chloroform. Assoc Med J 1855;3:313–8.

[13] Snow J. On Chloroform and Other Anaesthetics: Their Action and Administration. London: John Churchill, 1858:26–61.

[14] Mushin WW, Rendell-Baker L. The Origins of Thoracic Anaesthesia. Park Ridge, IL: Wood Library-Museum of Anesthesiology, 1991.

[15] Hunter J. Phil Trans Lond 1776;66:412.

[16] Apgar V. A proposal for a new method of evaluation of the newborn infant. Curr Res Anesth Analg 1953;32:260–7.

# Joseph O'Dwyer and laryngeal intubation for croup

## Thomas F. Baskett

After medical qualification in 1866, Joseph O'Dwyer's first appointment was as sanitary superintendent at the Charity Hospital on Blackwell's Island, New York. Shortly after taking up his duties an outbreak of cholera hit the island which O'Dwyer managed to contain in the calm methodical fashion that was to be a hallmark of his medical career.[1] In 1873, the New York Foundling Asylum opened its hospital near Lexington Avenue, New York, with Joseph O'Dwyer one of the newly appointed physicians. This hospital looked after the orphans and the poor children of New York City. It was here that O'Dwyer was to encounter the ravages of diphtheria in young children and its lethal accompaniment—-diphtheritic croup. Until his death some 25 years later the management of croup, and more specifically the maintenance of an airway in the more extreme cases, was to become an obsessional focus of O'Dwyer's work. Before the introduction of antitoxins, diphtheria in its most severe form was accompanied by inflammation of the larynx which created a pseudo-membrane thick enough to physically block air entry. The word croup probably derives from the Anglo-Saxon 'kropan' meaning to cry aloud. In such cases tracheotomy to by-pass the laryngeal obstruction was the only treatment. However, when the child reached this stage the mortality was usually about 90%.

Infants and children up to the age of four were most often seriously affected by the laryngeal form of diphtheria. Tracheotomy was only considered in extreme cases when the child was on the verge of suffocation. For the first seven years of the New York Foundling Hospital's existence (1873—1880) tracheotomy was performed many times but without survival in a single case[2] (Figure 1). By 1880 O'Dwyer had applied his mind to an alternative to tracheotomy and how to provide a channel from the oropharynx through the swollen larynx that would remain in place until the disease had run its course. Unknown to O'Dwyer, a Dr. E. Bouchut in Paris in September 1855, had proposed inserting a hollow tube from the oropharynx through the larynx for just this purpose. He presented this idea to his medical peers in Paris but it was rejected. However, he subsequently did achieve three successful recoveries from croup out of ten cases that he treated with his tube.[3]

In 1880 William MacEwan, a surgeon in Glasgow, reported three successful cases of oro-tracheal intubation for cases (non diphtheria) of acute swelling of the base of the tongue and larynx.[4] O'Dwyer began his research in 1882 with the aid of Dr. William Northrup in the pathology department. Between them they fashioned a small bi-valve

# FIFTY CASES OF CROUP IN PRIVATE PRACTICE TREATED BY INTUBATION OF THE LARYNX, WITH A DESCRIPTION OF THE METHOD AND OF THE DANGERS INCIDENT THERETO.

By JOSEPH O'DWYER, M.D.,

VISITING PHYSICIAN TO THE NEW YORK FOUNDLING ASYLUM.

In estimating the value of any method in the treatment of disease, we are compelled to rely chiefly upon statistics, unsatisfactory though they often may be. A plausible theory is very seductive, but it will not cure disease. Theories, indeed, may and often do lead up to the adoption of certain methods of treatment, but there their office ends, and henceforth the therapeutic measures based upon them must be judged by a comparison of their results with those of the older established methods.

These are the considerations which have led me to prepare the following table, giving a summary of the results obtained in my first fifty cases of intubation of the larynx in private practice.

**Figure 1** Medical record (New York).[2]

speculum which was introduced with the valves held together by a spring which, after insertion, was released so that the valves parted creating a passage for air.[1] It was first used on 21 October, 1882 on a four year old girl. It relieved the obstruction for eight hours but the child died subsequently. This first case did however show that the presence of the foreign body airway could be tolerated in these cases. After three years experience, and only one successful recovery, O'Dwyer abandoned the use of the bi-valve speculum. He became aware of the work of Bouchut in Paris.[1] O'Dwyer then produced a new tube, flattened laterally with a collar at its upper end and about one inch in length. The tube was placed directly, with one finger covered by a metallic shield inserted first as a guide. During the insertion, which usually took 10—15 s, the child was restrained. O'Dwyer described his technique as follows[2]:

'The child is held upright on the lap with its head on the left shoulder to prevent interference with the gag, the arms are secured by the sides, either by wrapping a towel or sheet around the body, or by being grasped firmly below the elbows... The operator, holding the introducer in the right hand, inserts the index finger of the left hand well back towards the oesophagus, and in bringing it forward raises the epiglottis and locates the cavity of the larynx. To the uneducated finger, the cavity of the larynx is a better landmark than the epiglottis... In the beginning of the operation the handle of the introducer is held close to the patient's chest, and elevated as the tube approaches the glottis. Very little force is necessary to overcome any form of acute stenosis of the larynx and if the tube does not enter easily it should be withdrawn and another attempt made.'

O'Dwyer first used this tube in April 1884 which restored the airway but the child died 16 h later. In the second case the tube was tolerated for 2 1/2 days but was then coughed out and required reinserting. During this reinsertion the child shut her teeth firmly upon O'Dwyer's finger which could not be released for 15 min, until chloroform was administered to the child.[2] However, the second insertion of the tube was tolerated and the child made a full recovery. This traumatic episode prompted O'Dwyer to use a mouth gag for future insertion and removal of tubes. O'Dwyer's attempts at intubation were beset with many problems including, difficulty in removal because the pseudo-membrane grew over the tube, and pressure necrosis causing epiglotic and cricoid lacerations. Much research was carried on during this time by Northrup and O'Dwyer: in the postmortem room they carefully studied the anatomy of the normal and diphtheritic larynx, creating moulds made of putty.[1,2] These studies led to modifications of the tubes over the years. Initially O'Dwyer had the tubes made by a German craftsman in New York However, he was unreliable and fond of drink so O'Dwyer often had to go to an adjacent bar to find him and stand over him while he manufactured the tubes.[1,3] Later he was able to find a reliable firm, George Tiemann and Company, to make the tubes to his specification. During these years of experimentation with intubation O'Dwyer continued to perform the traditional tracheotomy on many cases of croup. As he wrote[2]:

'From Jan 1880 to Dec 1885, or during the experimental stages of intubation, I operated on sixty-five cases of croup, sixty of them being in the New York Foundling Asylum and had but nine recoveries, or not quite 14%'.

Over the years O'Dwyer modified his instruments which included an introducer, an extractor, a mouth gag and five intubation tubes of varying length and diameter to accommodate different sized children. By the 1890s these instruments were sold as a set and carried by many general practitioners in their medical bag (Figure 2). Once O'Dwyer had perfected his tube he had a 24% survival rate in 50 cases during 1886.[2] The children who had recovered had retained the tube for an average of 5 days. By 1887 the recovery rate was approximately 50%. This was similar to the improved recovery rate with tracheotomy at the same time. The advantage of the tube was that it required less maintenance then a tracheotomy and subsequent stenosis was not a problem.

## MOUTH AND THROAT INSTRUMENTS.

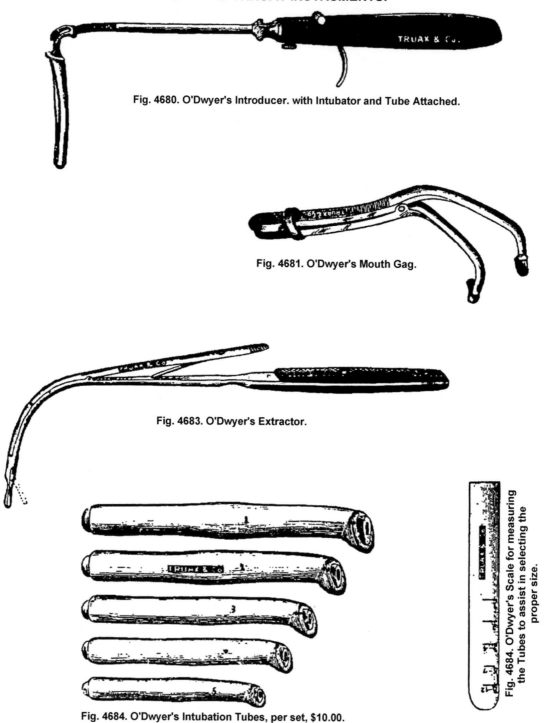

Fig. 4680. O'Dwyer's Introducer. with Intubator and Tube Attached.

Fig. 4681. O'Dwyer's Mouth Gag.

Fig. 4683. O'Dwyer's Extractor.

Fig. 4684. O'Dwyer's Intubation Tubes, per set, $10.00.

Fig. 4684. O'Dwyer's Scale for measuring the Tubes to assist in selecting the proper size.

**Figure 2**  O'Dwyer's laryngeal intubation set. As advertised in the price list of physician's supplies. Chicago: Charles Truax, Green and Co.; 1893. p. 1294.

O'Dwyer was well aware of the controversy between those who advocated tracheotomy and those who favoured intubation. He made a plea for the collection of statistics to aid the rational selection of treatment[2]:

'With a view to obtaining more reliable statistics on this subject, if all those who practise intubation of the larynx in the treatment of croup will report the results whether good or bad, and at the same time give the results that they have had

102

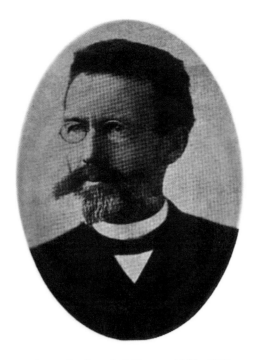

**Figure 3**  Joseph O'Dwyer, 1841–1898.

*with tracheotomy, in a few years a sufficient number of cases will have been accumulated to give something like a true estimate of the percentage of recovery from both operations, and render a fair comparison of their merits possible.'*

In the later years of his career O'Dwyer used his laryngeal tubes for cases of chronic stenosis of the larynx, which could follow the operation of tracheotomy.[5] Dilatation, often resulting in permanent cure, was achieved by the serial insertion of tubes of increasing size.

An off-shoot of O'Dwyer's work with laryngeal intubation in adults was to lead to the development of intra-laryngeal intubation for anaesthesia in thoracic surgery.[6] In 1887 Dr. George Fell of Buffalo, New York reported a series of cases with opium poisoning which he successfully treated by assisted respiration using foot-bellows attached to a length of tubing to either a tracheotomy tube or a tightly applied face mask.[7,8] O'Dwyer adapted Fell's apparatus and attached the foot-bellows to one of his adult intra-laryngeal tubes thereby obviating the need for tracheotomy and improving the integrity of the airway, compared to a face mask.[9,10] It was Rudolph Matas, the surgeon of New Orleans, who modified the Fell–O'Dwyer apparatus for the provision of anaesthesia in thoracic surgery.[6]

Joseph O'Dwyer was born in Cleveland, Ohio on 12 October, 1841 (Figure 3). When he was a young boy his family moved to Canada and he was raised and went to school in London, Ontario As a boy he suffered a pulmonary haemorrhage, presumably from tuberculosis.[1] As part of his fresh air cure, which was successful, he spent three years with a surveying team in the woods of Michigan. In 1864 he attended the New York College of Physicians and Surgeons and graduated MD in 1866. During his first job at the Charity Hospital on Blackwell's Island O'Dwyer contracted typhus fever after examining a patient with the disease. He made up his will, left letters for his family and friends and, anticipating death, took to his bed. The disease did affect him severely but he made a full recovery. In 1869, O'Dwyer opened a medical practice in New York City.[3] He developed a large obstetrical practice and in the coming years attended more than 3000 confinements. In 1873 he joined the staff of the New York Foundling Hospital and expended much of his effort on the treatment of children. O'Dwyer was a introspective, thoughtful man who apparently dwelt on his medical failures. He became a chronic insomniac. In a memorial address his close friend and longtime colleague William Northrup noted, that due to O'Dwyer's worry about the children under his care '...his whole tranquility of mind was destroyed, and sleep was gained only with greatest difficulty... it broke his health and it made him prematurely old.'[1] On 7 January 1898, at the age of 57, Joseph O'Dwyer died at his home on Lexington Avenue in New York City.

## References

1. Northrup WP. Memorial address on Joseph O'Dwyer, MD. Med Rec 1898;53:361–4.
2. O'Dwyer J. Fifty cases of croup in private practice treated by intubation of the larynx with description of the method and the dangers incident thereto. Med Rec 1887;32:557–61.
3. Gelfand C. Diphtheria: Dr. Joseph O'Dwyer and his intubation tubes. Caduceus 1897;3:1–34.
4. MacEwen W. Clinical observations on the introduction of tracheal tubes by the mouth instead of performing tracheotomy or laryngeotomy. BMJ 1880;2:122–4.
5. O'Dwyer J. Intubation in the treatment of chronic stenosis of the larynx. BMJ 1894;2:1478–81.
6. Hamilton GR, Baskett TF. Rudolph Matas and the development of intralaryngeal intubation and artificial respiration in thoracic surgery. Resuscitation 2001;51(3):221–4.
7. Fell GE. Cases of opium poisoning treated by forced respiration. Trans Int Cong Med 1887;1:237.
8. Duncum BM. The development of inhalation anaesthesia. London: RSM Press; 1994. p. 609–11.
9. Northrup WP. Apparatus for prolonged artificial forcible respiration. BMJ 1894;2:697–8.
10. Keys TE. The history of surgical anesthesia. Reprint of 1945 edition. Park Ridge, IL: Wood Library Museum of Anesthesiology; 1996. p. 65–7.

# Friedrich Trendelenburg (1844–1924)

Wolfgang F. Dick

Friedrich Trendelenburg is regarded to be one of the 'greats' in surgery of the 19th and 20th century. 1999 marks the 75th year of the death of Trendelenburg who was born 155 years ago, in May 1844, as the son of a distinguished professor of philosophy and Rector Magnificus of the University of Berlin, and his wife Ferdinandie.

Despite his limited spare time, Trendelenburg's father was able to teach his children mathematics and Latin while the mother instructed the children in literature and the English language. Friedrich's knowledge of Latin was such that later he was able to write his doctoral dissertation in that language. On finishing grammar school, Trendelenburg first went to Edinburgh and Glasgow to begin his studies. One of his mentors in Glasgow was the anatomist Allen Thomson, who advised him on the course of his studies in anatomy and physiology. Trendelenburg left Scotland after 15 months with many fond memories, and he maintained life-long friendships with a number of the people he met there.

In October 1863, he returned to Germany and matriculated at the University of Berlin. Although he attended lectures in philosophy, he became more and more interested in anatomy, the history of medicine, and experimental chemistry. He was fascinated in particular by lectures held by the physiologist Du Bois-Reymond. On returning from service in the war of Schleswig-Holstein, he attended the surgeon Langenbeck, who played a key role in his further development and his decision to become a surgeon, by inspiring him with great interest and enthusiasm.

He travelled widely between semesters to improve his French, and to visit the university hospitals of Halle, Leipzig, Jena and Göttingen.

In 1866 he began his service in a military hospital in Görlitz where he was assigned to treat wound infections and hospital gangrene. When he was in Görlitz he witnessed the outbreak of a cholera epidemic and was horrified by the suffering inflicted on the patients, most of whom died a painful death.

Trendelenburg underwent medical training at a time when anaesthesia was not yet available and the surgeon, to quote Langenbeck, 'had to move as fast as possible without delays, any of which would have been an act of cruelty', and 'the best surgeon was the one who performed the intervention most rapidly, but nevertheless with the greatest accuracy'. The German–French War forced Trendelenburg to return once again to the battlefield where sadly he had to put into practice what his university teachers had taught him by treating endless numbers of wounded soldiers. Eventually he was allowed to leave the army with an honourable discharge in 1871.

After the war, Trendelenburg was given the opportunity to work with Langenbeck at the University Hospital in Berlin and to prepare for a university career. He soon met and became engaged to Charlotte Fabricius, the daughter of one of the Directors of the Prussian Ministry of Finance. As it was unacceptable for a young married assistant to work at the clinic, he resigned from his post at the university and went to head the Department of Surgery at the Freidrichshain Hospital before marrying Charlotte. He held this position only for a short time before accepting the appointment to the Chair of the Institute of Surgery at the University of Rostock. Unfortunately, there was a persistent shortage of patients at this University Hospital. This eventually caused Trendelenburg to leave Rostock and to accept a full professorship at the University of Bonn.

Nevertheless, the situation in Rostock had allowed him sufficient time for scientific research which lead him to re-invent a technique known in the Middle Ages as the head-down position. This position facilitates pelvic interventions by lowering the head of the patient at an angle of 15–20°. Trendelenburg first used the position in the transvesical approach in the repair of vesico-vaginal fistula and designed an operating table with shoulder blades to stabilise the patient in this position. The re-invented manoeuvre has become known worldwide as the Trendelenburg position. The head-up position, although never described by Trendelenburg, is not infrequently referred to as the 'anti-Trendelenburg position'. Further scientific endeavours begun in Rostock were related to the investigation and observation of the venous circulation and studies on the prevention of venous thrombosis, i.e. by ligation of the long saphenous vein.

Trendelenburg moved his, by then large, family to Bonn and began to work at the university hospital there. His clinical and teaching activities involved a large number of surgical patients and five times the number of students at Rostock. He started his daily work between 0600 and 0700 h in the morning by going on rounds. This was followed by morning lectures and operations, at times six or more major interventions per day. The afternoon was taken up by consulting hours, and the evening by a surgical course. During his time in Bonn he first described abdominal wall tension as being a reaction to abdominal diseases and injuries. In addition to a great variety of methodological and scientific improvements and inventions, he perfected his surgical skills by performing urological procedures for traumatic injury.

Apart from his numerous clinical and scientific activities he found the time to spend with his family and, like his own father, he enjoyed drawing with his younger children and to instruct his older children in the English language. But he had to move his family once again after 13 successful and happy years in Bonn, when he was offered and accepted a chair of the medical faculty in Leipzig in 1885. In connection with his university post he was awarded the title of Royal Privy Councillor, Senior Officer of Health by King Albert of Saxony.

Being himself a scientifically and clinically active academic teacher and surgical chief, he expected all his residents and staff members to come forward with one 'decent' scientific publication per year. His own scientific endeavours were now primarily focused on the area of thrombosis and embolism, and it was in those years that he first described an operation for the treatment of pulmonary artery embolism, a procedure which is still performed today under the name of 'Trendelenburg operation'. At the German Congress of Surgery in 1924, Trendelenburg was delighted to witness Martin Kirschner present the first case of long-term survival after Trendelenburg's embolectomy.

In 1898 Trendelenburg was elected President of the German Society of Surgery, and in 1897 and 1906 he was Dean of the Medical Faculty. In the same year he was invited to give lectures at the American Congress of Surgery in New York and was awarded an Honorary Doctorate by the University of Aberdeen.

In his early sixties Trendelenburg developed respiratory and cardiac symptoms which forced him to retire earlier than he had foreseen. In 1911 he resigned from his post and was bestowed the title Privy Senior Officer of Health, which made him one of the highest ranking Officers at the Royal Court.

In his memoirs Trendelenburg wrote, 'it has given me great pleasure to take advantage of the leisure of old age to write a book that does not create anything new, but attempts to put old accomplishments into perspective'. Trendelenburg finished his modest memoirs of a full personal and scientific life in the spring of 1924. He died a peaceful death in December of the same year.

Friedrich Trendelenburg was one of the most important German surgeons, who showed great interest in the emerging field of anaesthesia as well as in the observation of vital functions at a time when little knowledge was available in these fields. In his work, he observed ether to be less dangerous than chloroform, and found it to affect cardiac function only to a limited extent. He described his experiences of resuscitation in cardiac arrest following the administration of chloroform, and used tracheostomy and artificial ventilation long before the description of tracheal intubation by Franz Kuhn. Trendelenburg's most significant and valuable contributions to anaesthesia and emergency medicine include an inflatable cuff for the tracheostomy tube, the Trendelenburg position for the prevention of aspiration or air embolism during central venous cannulation, and the improvement of spinal anesthesia. He has one of the largest lists of eponymous credits to his name. In addition to his position there are a sign, gait, test and four operations.

His personality, his comprehensive knowledge, not only of medicine but also of languages, philosophy, and history, distinguish Friedrich Trendelenburg as one of the greatest physicians and surgeons of the past two centuries. Anaesthesia and particularly emergency medicine are greatly indebted to Friedrich Trendelenburg for a large number of developments and inventions that are still used today.

## Acknowledgements

Quoted with the kind permission of Professor Dr med. C. Schwokowski, Leipzig, from his article Friedrich Trendelenburg 1844–1924 — Lebensweg cines Heroen der Chirurgie. In: Christian Schwokowski (Hrsg.), Friedrich Trendelenburg, 1844–1924. Steinkopff, Darmstadt; 1998: 1–18.

## Further Reading

Perthes G. Friedrich Trendelenburg, DMW 1975;51:279–280.

Sauerbruch F. Friedrich Trendelenburg, Disch Zschr f Chir 1925;190:1–1V.

Trendelenburg F, Jr. Unser Elternhaus Familienchronik, im Besitz der Familie Trendelenburg.

Trendelenburg F. De Veterum Indorum Chirurgia. Med. Inaugural-Diss., Berlin, 1867.

Trendelenburg F. Verletzungen und chirurgische Krankheiten des Gesichts, In: Bruns P v (Hrst) Dtsch Chir, Lief 33, Enke, Stuttgart, 1886.

Trendelenburg F. Über Blasenscheidenfisteloperationen und über Beckenhochlagerung bei Operationen in der Bauchhöhle, Klin Vortr 1890;355:3373–3392.

Trendelenburg F. Über die Unterbindung der Vena saphena magna bei Unterschenkelvarizen, Bruns Beitr Klin Chir 1891;7:195–210.

Trendelenburg F. Operationsstuhl zur Beckenhochlagerung, Bruns Beitr Klin Chir 1892;8:225–230.

Trendelenburg F. Über den Gang bei angeborener Hüftgelenksluxation, DMW 1895;21:21–24.

Trendelenburg F. Über die chirurgische Behandlung der puerperalen Pyämie, MMW 1902;49:513–516.

Trendelenburg F. Erinnerungen an Bernhard v. Langenbeck, DMW 1902;28:233–236.

Trendelenburg F. Über die operative Behandlung der Embolie der Lungenarterie, Arch Klin Chir 1908;86:686–700.

# Marshall Hall and his ready method of resuscitation

Thomas F. Baskett

By the late 18th century Royal Humane Societies had been established in Britain, Europe and the United States. These societies promoted the organization of local facilities and guidelines for resuscitation "of the apparently dead", particularly those who drowned. The techniques that were advocated mostly involved warming, physical stimulation with massage and shaking, and the application of stimulants via the stomach and rectum [1]. In 1856, Marshall Hall challenged the rationale of the Royal Humane Society's advice [2]. Hall pointed out that "The remedy for the suspension of respiration is, on every principle of common sense, the restoration of respiration" [2]. He criticized the Royal Humane Society's rules for treating asphyxia which started with the advice to "convey the body carefully...to the nearest house" [2]. Marshall Hall pointed out that the "...loss of time necessary for this purpose is—loss of life!" and drew special attention to the position of the patient during resuscitation. In correspondence 1 month before his first full paper on the subject Hall pointed out "In the *supine* position, the tongue *falls* backwards and closes the glottis, all inspiration is, therefore, impossible. In the *prone* position, the tongue *falls* forwards, and leaves the glottis freely patent. Inspiration is, therefore, possible" [3]. Marshall, therefore, advised that the patient be placed in the prone position and noted that in this posture "...the thorax and abdomen will be compressed with a force equal to the weight of the body, and expiration will take place". He then proposed "Let...the body be now turned gently on the side (through rather more than the quarter of a circle) and the pressure on the thorax and abdomen will be removed, and inspiration—effectual inspiration—will take place! The expiration and inspiration are augmented by timeously applying and removing alternately pressure on the spine and ribs" [2]. As he enthusiastically observed "Nothing can be more beautiful than this life-giving—(if life can be given)—this

breathing process" [2]. In the first full paper describing his technique Hall included a diagram of the appropriate position of the patient and rescuer (Fig. 1). An earlier brief report of experiments on a cadaver carried out at St. George's Hospital, London, in front of witnesses had shown that the movements of the body from the prone position to the side at a rate of "...sixteen times a minute, and no more, respiration is efficiently performed, and this without bellows, syringe or any

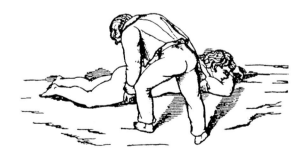

### ASPHYXIA,

#### ITS RATIONALE AND ITS REMEDY.

#### By MARSHALL HALL, M.D., F.R.S.

THE term Asphyxia, which ought to be exchanged for Apnœa, designates that condition of the animal system which results from the suspension of respiration.

Respiration involves two processes—the inhalation of oxygen, and the exhalation of carbonic acid.

The *remedy* for the suspension of respiration is, on every principle of common sense, the restoration of respiration. This view might be considered, irrespective of physiological inquiry and proof, as self-evident; but that proof is amply supplied by physiology.

Of the two functions suspended, it is certain, from physiological inquiry, that the retention of the carbonic acid is by far the more fatal, and that, in a word, asphyxia is the result of carbonic acid retained in the blood, which becomes, in its excess, a blood-poison.

If this view be correct, it is evident that restored respiration is to the blood-poison in asphyxia what the stomach-pump is to poison in the stomach; and that it is *the* special remedy, the *sine quâ non*, in asphyxia.

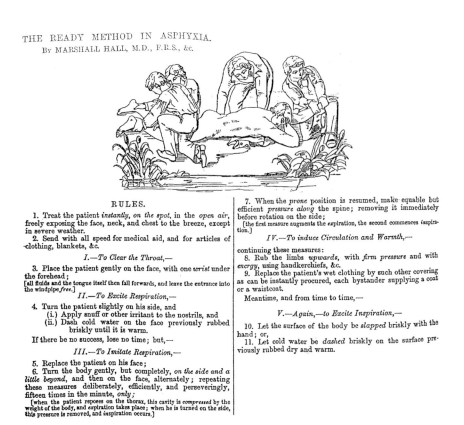

RULES.

1. Treat the patient *instantly, on the spot,* in the *open air,* freely exposing the face, neck, and chest to the breeze, except in severe weather.
2. Send with all speed for medical aid, and for articles of clothing, blankets, &c.

*I.—To Clear the Throat,—*

3. Place the patient gently on the face, with one *wrist* under the forehead;
[all fluids and the tongue itself then fall forwards, and leave the entrance into the windpipe *free*.]

*II.—To Excite Respiration,—*

4. Turn the patient slightly on his side, and
  (i.) Apply snuff or other irritant to the nostrils, and
  (ii.) Dash cold water on the face previously rubbed briskly until it is warm.
If there be no success, lose no time; but,—

*III.—To Imitate Respiration,—*

5. Replace the patient on his face;
6. Turn the body gently, but completely, *on the side and a little beyond,* and then on the face, alternately; repeating these measures deliberately, efficiently, and perseveringly, fifteen times in the minute, *only;*
[when the patient reposes on the thorax, this cavity is *compressed* by the weight of the body, and *expiration* takes place; when he is turned on the side, this pressure is removed, and *inspiration* occurs.]

7. When the *prone* position is resumed, make equable but efficient *pressure along* the spine; removing it immediately before rotation on the side;
[the first measure augments the *expiration,* the second commences *inspiration*.]

*IV.—To induce Circulation and Warmth,—*

continuing these measures:
8. Rub the limbs *upwards,* with *firm pressure* and with *energy,* using handkerchiefs, &c.
9. Replace the patient's wet clothing by such other covering as can be instantly procured, each bystander supplying a coat or a waistcoat.
Meantime, and from time to time,—

*V.—Again,—to Excite Inspiration,—*

10. Let the surface of the body be *slapped* briskly with the hand; or,
11. Let cold water be *dashed* briskly on the surface previously rubbed dry and warm.

Fig. 2. Lancet 1856;2:458–9. (2nd paper, October 25th, 1856 with revised rules for resuscitation).

apparatus..."[3]. Hall had first pointed out the advantage of the prone position during resuscitation in a letter to his friend and colleague, M. Flouriens, Editor of the *Comptes Rendu* in Paris [4], which was later translated in an editorial note in the *Lancet* in February 1856 [5]. Soon after Hall's publication with his full set of rules for resuscitation in the April edition of the *Lancet* [2] a number of individual reports describing the success of this technique appeared in the correspondence columns of that journal [6]. In the 25 October 1856 edition of the *Lancet*, Hall published an up-to-date and slightly revised set of rules for resuscitation and entitled his technique "The ready method in asphyxia" [7] (Fig. 2). The term "ready method" was used to emphasize that this technique could, and should, be carried out at any site without delay and without additional apparatus or personnel. This term was suggested by his house surgeon, Charles Hunter, working at St. George's Hospital, London at the time Marshall Hall was carrying out his experiments on cadavers [3,8].

Perhaps because he was so critical of the Royal Humane Society's current advice Hall's method was not approved by them. It was, however, adopted by the National Lifeboat Institution and strongly endorsed by the editor of the *Lancet* in glowing terms [6]:

"Anything more simple, philosophical, or beautiful than the process described, could not have been

designed. It is proposed to call the plan the "Ready Method" of treating the drowned; but we think that title may lead to an uncertainty of action, and to some confusion in practice. Infi-

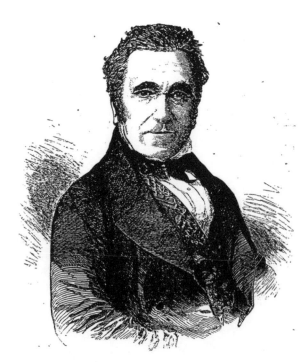

Fig. 3. Marshall Hall, 1790–1857.

nitely preferable, in our opinion, would be the title, "*Marshall Hall's Method*". This designation is due to the distinguished discover, and the method would thus be benevolently associated with his name to the end of time".

Hall was later to publish a modification of his technique for the treatment of stillborn children [8]. He argued that because of physiological adaptation in the fetus "the new-born foetus can long survive the absence of respiration". He did not advocate mouth-to-mouth respiration fearing that this "...may tear the delicate tissues of the foetal lungs". As in the adult, he relied upon postural and mechanical means to promote air exchange [8]:

"We must, on the contrary adopt some measure of *drawing* the air into the lungs. This is effectually accomplished by first placing the little patient briskly in the prone position, to clear the fauces; then pressing gently on the back; and then removing that pressure, and turning it gently on the side and a little beyond".

He also advocated gentle stimulation of the limbs and sprinkling the infant alternately with hot and cold water. He finished his advice with the extortation "Continue these measures, or renew them, from time-to-time even for hours. The embers of life may not be entirely extinct!" This technique was still advised as one of the standard methods of neonatal resuscitation in a British text of midwifery in 1926 [9].

Marshall Hall was born on 18th February, 1790 at Basford, outside Nottingham (Fig. 3). He was the sixth of eight children. His father was a cotton manufacturer and chemist who was among the first to use chlorine in the bleaching of cotton. In 1809, Marshall Hall went to Edinburgh to study medicine and graduated in 1812 [10,11]. This was followed by 2 years as resident house physician at the Royal Infirmary, Edinburgh. During this time he made a careful study of the diagnosis of disease, upon which subject he was, in 1817, to publish his first book [12]. Following his 2 years at the Royal Infirmary he made a tour of hospitals and medical schools in Paris, Berlin and Gottingen. Much of this traveling was on foot and he covered 600 miles during the month of November 1814 [11]. He returned to establish his practice in Nottingham. He made a particular study of infectious diseases, especially puerperal fever, and was one of the first to speak out against excessive blood letting in fevers which was prevalent at that time [11,13]. After establishing himself as a successful provincial physician, Hall moved to London in 1826. As his practice in London became well established he lived in Manchester Square and later at 38 Grosvenor Square. His lectures and academic pub-

lications led, in 1832, to his election as a Fellow of the Royal Society [14]. It was in 1833 that he published his work on the reflex function of the nervous system for which he is best known [13,15,16].

By 1853, Hall was sufficiently independent to end his clinical practice and sail to the United States for a prolonged visit with his wife [17]. Ever observant he utilized the voyage to make a number of observations and publish a paper on sea sickness [18]. He traveled and lectured throughout the United States, Canada and Cuba. Hall spoke out on broader issues: against corporal punishment of soldiers, the problems of sewage disposal, and in favor of the abolition of slavery [11,17].

Hall's work on resuscitation was carried out late in his career. By November 1856 he was troubled with a sore throat and difficulty in swallowing and moved to Brighton. He died from cancer of the oesophagus on 11th August, 1857 [11,14,17].

Hall's method was not accepted by the Royal Humane Society and was later challenged by Silvester who claimed that his own technique moved much more air into the patient's lungs [19]. Eventually a committee of the Royal Medical and Chirurgical Society studied the two techniques and recommended Silvester's method [1,11]. This was endorsed by the Royal Humane Society and remained a popular method for the next 75 years.

## References

[1] Eisenberg MS. Life in the balance. New York: Oxford University Press, 1997:74–7.
[2] Hall M. Asphyxia, its rationale and its remedy. Lancet 1856;1:393–4.
[3] Hall M. On a new mode of effecting artificial respiration. Lancet 1856;1:229.
[4] Hall M. De la position la plus favorable à donner aux individus asphyxiés sur lesquels on tente la respiration artificielle. Compt Rend 1855;61:949 (correspondence).
[5] Editorial Note, Lancet 1856;1:144.
[6] Editorial and correspondence, Lancet 1856;2:654–6.
[7] Hall M. The ready method in asphyxia. Lancet 1856;2:458–9.
[8] Hall M. The asphyxia of still-born infants, and its treatment. Lancet 1856;2:601–2.
[9] Berkeley C, Dupuis GM. An atlas of midwifery. Toronto: MacMillan Company Limited, 1926:142.
[10] Biographical sketch of Marshall Hall, MD, FRS, Lancet 1850;2317–22.
[11] Green JHS. Marshall Hall (1790–1857): a biographical study. Med Hist 1958;2:120–33.
[12] Hall M. On diagnosis. London: Longman, 1817.
[13] Talbott JH. A biographical history of medicine: excerpts and essays on the men and their work. New York: Grune and Strutton, 1970:464–7.
[14] Hall M. Proc R Soc London 1857;9:52–6 (Obituary).
[15] Hall M. Reflex function of the medulla oblongata and medulla spinalis, Phil Trans R Soc London 1853:635.

[16] Keith A. Marshall Hall and the bearing of his discoveries on orthopaedic practice. In: Menders of the maimed. New York: Robert E. Krieger Publishing, 1975:78–90.

[17] Hall C. Memoirs of Marshall Hall, MD, FRS, by his widow. London: Richard Bentley, 1861:502–13.

[18] Hall M. Sur la physiologie du mal-de-mer. Compt Rend 1853;36:600.

[19] Silvester HR. The Marshall Hall method of treatment in asphyxia. Lancet 1858;1:616.

# Silvester's technique of artificial respiration

Thomas F. Baskett

The widespread acceptance of manual methods of artificial respiration followed upon the introduction of a simple technique published in 1856 by Marshall Hall, a senior and widely respected London physician.[1,2] In essence Hall's technique involved alternate rotation of the patient's body from a prone position to the side. As a later modification he added expiratory pressure to the thorax when the patient was in the prone position.[3] About the same time in London a young recently qualified physician, Henry Robert Silvester, turned his attention to the technique of artificial respiration. He was prompted to do so when Hall's technique was used on a stillborn male infant without success. He changed the position of the infant, put him on his back and raised both arms upward to cause expansion of the chest and inspiration, after which he folded the arms on the chest and applied expiratory pressure. The infant recovered.[4] He referred to this technique as the ''natural method'' and outlined the rationale in a more detailed publication in the *British Medical Journal* in 1858.[5] (Figure 1) In this paper he pointed out that the current methods of artificial respiration involved alternate compression and relaxation of the chest. He felt this was inadequate because *''there is no elevation of the ribs, such as takes place in natural deep inspiration, in which they are made to rise above their ordinary or quiescent level, and the cavity of the chest greatly increased in size''*.[5]

Silvester questioned the technique of Hall and, using fresh cadavers with a glass tube filled with fluid inserted into the trachea, demonstrated that the movement of fluid in and out of the trachea, and by inference the movement of air, was limited.

He outlined the rationale for his own technique as follows:[5]

''The new method which I venture to bring forth before the profession is a simple imitation of natural deep respiration, and is effected by means of the same muscles as are employed by nature in that process. In ordinary deep inspiration *we lift the ribs and sternum by pectoral and other muscles which pass between the chest and the shoulders, and thus produce the threatened vacuum which inflates the lungs. In my method we lift the ribs and sternum by the pectoral and other muscles which pass from the shoulder to the parities of the thorax, by steadily extending the arms up by the side of the patient's head; by elevating the ribs the cavity of the chest is enlarged, a tendency to a vacuum is produced, and a rush of air immediately takes place into the lungs. Expiration is brought about by simple compression of the side of the chest by the patient's*

**Figure 1**  BMJ 1858;2:576.

arms... *The arms of the patient are to be used by the operator as handles to open and close the chest.''*

Silvester performed the same experiments on cadavers using his technique and found that the excursion of fluid in the tube attached to the trachea was much greater than with Marshall Hall's technique. Silvester's specific description of his technique was as follows[5] (Figure 2):

''1. To adjust the patient's position. Place the patient on his back, with the shoulders raised and supported on a folded article of dress. 2. To maintain a free entrance of air into the windpipe. Draw forward the patient's tongue and keep it projecting beyond the lips. If the lower jaw Be gently raised the teeth may be made to hold the tongue in the required position. Should it be found necessary, the tongue may be so retained by passing a handkerchief under the chin and fastening it over the head. 3. To imitate the movements of respiration. Raise the patient's arms upwards by the sides of his head, and then extend them gently and steadily upwards and forwards for a few moments.

(This action enlarges the capacity of the chest by elevating the ribs, and induces inspiration.) Next, turn down the patient's arms and press them gently and firmly for a few moments against the sides of the chest. (This action diminishes the cavity of the thorax, and produces a forcible expiration.) Repeat these measures alternately, deliberately and perseveringly 15 times in a minute.''

Silvester also encouraged additional measures advocated by the Royal Humane Society, namely providing warmth and massage to the limbs to stimulate the circulation. He also pointed out that his technique, unlike that of Marshall Hall, could be carried out with the patient in a warm bath - particularly in the case of a stillborn infant. Silvester was careful not to condemn too harshly the technique of the widely respected Marshall Hall or the principles laid down by the Royal Humane Society. He supported the use of his method in the following diplomatic terms: '*The process is moreover, of universal application; it is easy of performance, entirely in harmony with that of Nature and does not prevent or supercede the use of those means in which confidence has hitherto been placed.*'[5]

Following the publication of Silvester's technique the medical profession was divided in its support between the methods of Hall and Silvester.[6] Over time a variety of physiological experiments were carried out in both the living and the dead to evaluate the efficacy of the different methods of respiration with mixed results.[7,8] In an effort to provide some clarity the Royal Medical and Chirurgical Society formed a committee on suspended animation to investigate the subject of resuscitation. The committee reported in 1862 and favoured the method of Silvester over that of Hall.[9] Silvester's technique gained wide acceptance, particularly in Europe and also in the United States. The director of the University Hospital in Groningen, Dr. Van Eysselsteijn, noted that Silvester's

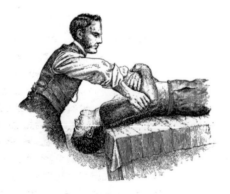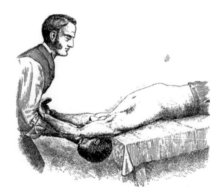

**Figure 2**  Silvester's technique. From: Hewitt FW. Anaesthetics and Their Administration. London: MacMillan and Co. Ltd.; 1907. pp. 556—7.

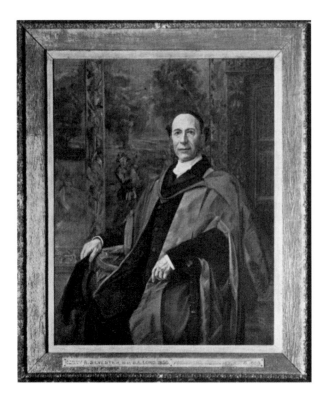

**Figure 3** Henry Robert Silvester, 1828—1908.

method had become the standard in Holland.[10] In Britain opinion was divided between proponents of Hall's and Silvester's techniques.

Abraham Lincoln was the most famous person to receive Silvester's method of artificial respiration.[11] The army surgeon, Charles Augustus Leale, who attended Lincoln on that Good Friday, 14 April 1865, immediately after the assassin's bullet struck the President, used Silvester's technique for artificial respiration, possibly followed by mouth-to-mouth resuscitation. The President was revived but died the next day.

Henry Robert Silvester was born in London in 1828 (Figure 3). He attended the King's College in London and qualified in medicine as a member of the Royal College of Surgeons in 1853, followed by his MD from the University of London

in 1855. He became an associate physician at the Kings's College in London and consultant physician to the Clapham General Dispensary. In 1861 he was appointed an honorary assistant to the Royal Humane Society.

In the years after its introduction Silvester defended his method of artificial respiration. He was to criticise the Schafer method in which the rescuer was positioned astride the prone patient saying: 'The posture of the operator "athwart the patient" in respect of the female patient, was, moreover undesirable.'[6] Among other interests Silvester gained some short lived notoriety by proposing a technique of hypodermic inflation of air to render men and animals unsinkable. In 1883 he received the Fothergill Gold Medal from the Royal Humane Society. He died in London in March 1908.

## References

1. Hall M. On a new mode of effecting artificial respiration. Lancet 1856;1:229.
2. Baskett TF. Marshall hall and his ready method of resuscitation. Resuscitation 2003;57:227—30.
3. Hall M. Asphyxia, its rationale and its remedy. Lancet 1856;1:393—4.
4. Silvester H. Dr. Marshall Hall's "ready method". Med Times Gaz 1857;15:503.
5. Silvester HR. A new method of resuscitating still-born children, and of restoring the persons apparently drowned or dead. BMJ 1858;2:576—9.
6. Karpovich PV. Adventures in artificial respiration. New York: Association Press; 1953. pp. 34—40.
7. Schafer EA. The relative efficiency of certain methods of performing artificial respiration in man. Proc Roy Soc Edin 1904;25:39—50.
8. Gordon AS, Fainer DC, Ivy AC. Artificial respiration: a new method and comparative study of different methods in adults. JAMA 1950;144:1455—64.
9. Report of the Committee on Suspended Animation. Medico-Chirurg. Trans 1862;45:449.
10. Van Eysselsteijn G. Artificial respiration as practised in Holland. Lancet 1909;1:474—5.
11. Sternbach GL, Varon J, Fromm RE. Charles Augustus Leale and the resuscitation of Abraham Lincoln. Resuscitation 2000;45:3—5.

# Janos Balassa and resuscitation by chest compression

Thomas F. Baskett        Mihaly Kis

Early efforts at resuscitation in the 18th century involved restoration of the airway followed by artificial respiration [1]. With the development of anaesthesia, cardiac arrest was recognized as a specific entity, particularly following the use of chloroform. This provided the impetus for attempts to maintain artificial circulation by cardiac massage [2]. In 1874, Moritz Schiff, a professor of physiology in Florence, Italy, carried out experiments on animals reviving them with open cardiac massage after an overdose of chloroform. In 1880, the Swiss surgeon, Paul Neihans made an unsuccessful attempt at open cardiac massage in man [1]. Professor R. Boehm at the University of Dorpat, used external cardiac massage in 1878 to resuscitate cats after cardiac arrest, induced by chloroform. In some cases, he was able to sustain the circulation until spontaneous cardiac activity returned [3]. In his textbook of general surgery published in 1883, the German surgeon Franz Koenig described his technique of external chest compression as a means of artificial ventilation, which he had successfully used to resuscitate six patients with an absent pulse, induced by chloroform anaesthesia [1,4]. Dr Friedrich Maass, an assistant of Koenig, successfully revived two patients using external cardiac compressions following chlorform-induced cardiac arrest in 1891.

An often-overlooked earlier contribution to the use of chest compression in cardiopulmonary resuscitation was that of the Hungarian surgeon Janos Balassa in 1858 [5,6]. Summoned to the house of an 18-year-old woman Balassa found her *in extremis* with asphyxia, secondary to laryngeal oedema associated with ulcerative tuberculous laryngitis. She had stopped breathing and was pulseless when Balassa performed an emergency tracheotomy followed by anterior chest compressions for 6 min before her ultimate recovery. He reported this case in the Hungarian Medical Weekly of 24 October 1858 (Fig. 1) as follows [7]:

"An 18-year-old girl, her extremities in cold sweat, her pulse barely palpable and thread-like, her struggle for breath terrifying, her appearance shocking, the situation had reached dangerous heights ... from the darkened little room, we helped the patient into the nearby window; however, as soon as we sat her down she immediately fell lifeless, her head rolled back, her frantically labouring shoulders and arms went limp, her blue face the picture of death, her chest became immobile, her carotid pulse and heart beats ceased. With the last painful breath with a terrible swoop, a corpse became of the living, about whom – it seemed – all experimentation, and effort was without hope and yet with a death so fresh, it was not unreasonable to try everything to bring back the lost breath and lost life. Therefore, I immediately stabbed the laryngeal scalpel into the crico-thyroid ligament and inserted a Thompson tracheostomy instrument, using the forceps-like arms of the instrument, I expanded the wound downwards and to either side. After removing the laryngeal scalpel, I immediately inserted the Gorgelat-type double valve into the trachea and fixing this with the fingers of my left hand; with my right, I began to apply a rhythmic pressure to the chest simulating breathing. Meanwhile, the air was free to enter into the lungs with a shrill whistling sound. Efforts had been progressing for close to 6 min without the slightest sign of life, and just as I was beginning to despair and begin to contemplate stopping, a spontaneous fast sigh-like inspiration gave me joy. This was followed with the help of my hands a second and third breath, and from the hard death struggle, life began to smile at us. The breathing became regular, heart rate and pulse returned, the dark blue discoloration of the face began to dissipate and the mask of death turned into the pleasant facade of life; after about 15 min, I called by the name the still unconscious patient, and she with a weak smile and the opening of her eyes gave us the sign of her return to consciousness. At this profound moment, all those who witnessed it experienced a deep stirring of emotion .... Today is day number 15 postoperation, and the patient has for the

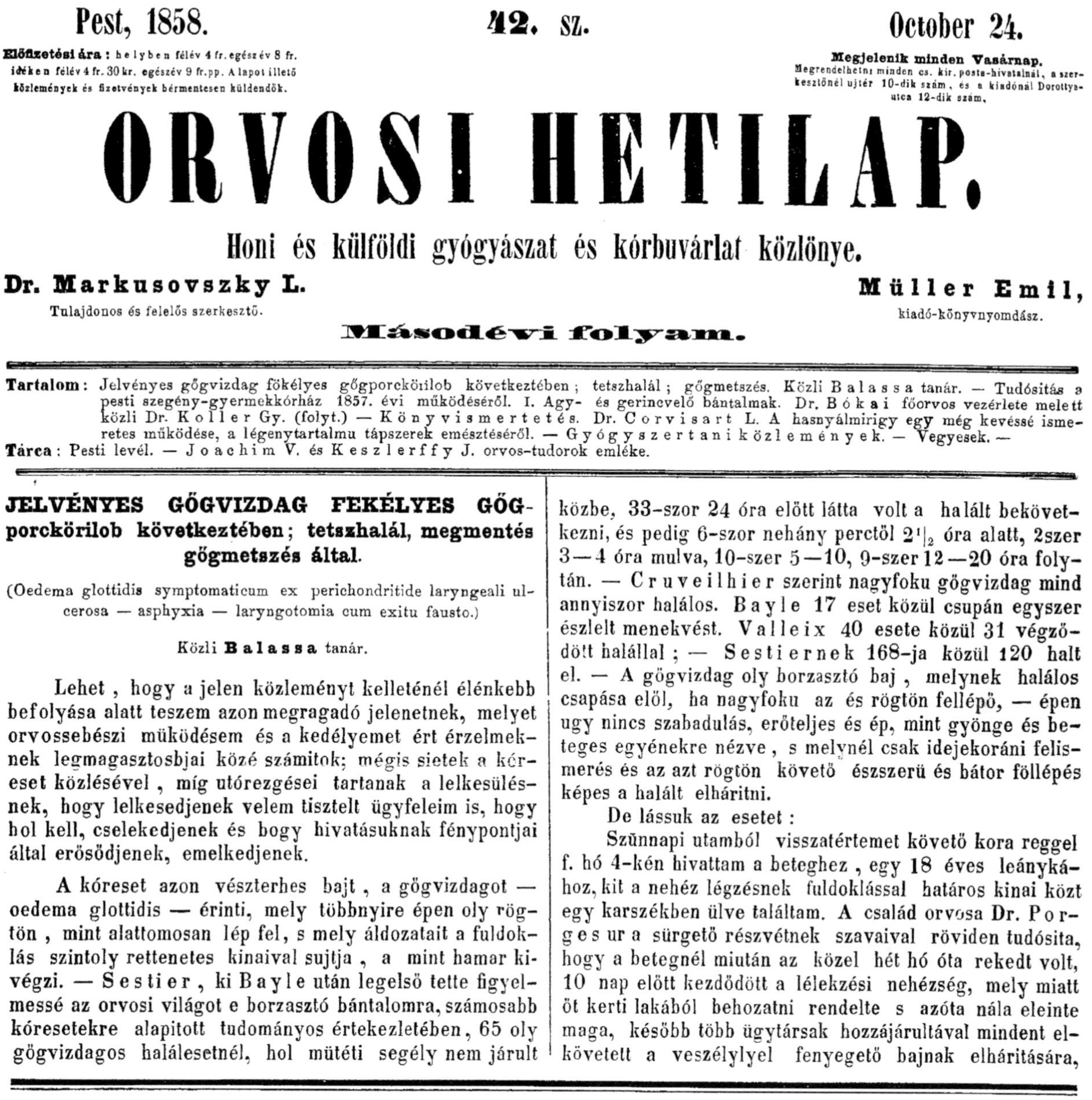

Pest, 1858.

42. SZ.

October 24.

Előfizetési ára : h e l y b e n félév 4 fr. egész év 8 fr.
idéken félév 4 fr. 30 kr. egészév 9 fr.pp. A lapot illető
közlemények és fizetvények bérmentesen küldendők.

Megjelenik minden Vasárnap.
Megrendelhetni minden cs. kir. posta-hivatalnál, a szer-
kesztőnél ujtér 10-dik szám, és a kiadónál Dorottya-
utca 12-dik szám.

# ORVOSI HETILAP.

### Honi és külföldi gyógyászat és kórbuvárlat közlönye.

**Dr. Markusovszky L.**
Tulajdonos és felelős szerkesztő.

**Müller Emil,**
kiadó-könyvnyomdász.

### Másodévi folyam.

**Tartalom :** Jelvényes gőgvizdag fökélyes gőgporckörilob következtében ; tetszhalál ; gőgmetszés. Közli B a l a s s a tanár. — Tudósitás a pesti szegény-gyermekkórház 1857. évi működéséről. I. Agy- és gerincvelő bántalmak. Dr. B ó k a i főorvos vezérlete mellett közli Dr. K o l l e r Gy. (folyt.) — K ö n y v i s m e r t e t é s. Dr. C o r v i s a r t L. A hasnyálmirigy egy még kevéssé isme-retes működése, a légenytartalmu tápszerek emésztéséről. — G y ó g y s z e r t a n i k ö z l e m é n y e k. — Vegyesek. —
**Tárca :** Pesti levél. — J o a c h i m V. és K e s z l e r f f y J. orvos-tudorok emléke.

---

**JELVÉNYES GŐGVIZDAG FEKÉLYES GŐG-porckörilob következtében ; tetszhalál, megmentés gőgmetszés által.**

(Oedema glottidis symptomaticum ex perichondritide laryngeali ul-cerosa — asphyxia — laryngotomia cum exitu fausto.)

Közli **Balassa** tanár.

Lehet , hogy a jelen közleményt kelleténél élénkebb befolyása alatt teszem azon megragadó jelenetnek, melyet orvossebészi működésem és a kedélyemet ért érzelmek-nek legmagasztosbjai közé számitok; mégis sietek a kór-eset közlésével , míg utórezgései tartanak a lelkesülés-nek, hogy lelkesedjenek velem tisztelt ügyfeleim is, hogy hol kell, cselekedjenek és hogy hivatásuknak fénypontjai által erősödjenek, emelkedjenek.

A kóreset azon vészterhes bajt , a gőgvizdagot — oedema glottidis — érinti, mely többnyire épen oly rög-tön , mint alattomosan lép fel, s mely áldozatait a fuldok-lás szintoly rettenetes kinaival sujtja , a mint hamar ki-végzi. — S e s t i e r , ki B a y l e után legelsö tette figyel-messé az orvosi világot e borzasztó bántalomra, számosabb kóresetekre alapitott tudományos értekezletében , 65 oly gőgvizdagos halálesetnél, hol mütéti segély nem járult

közbe, 33–szor 24 óra elött látta volt a halált bekövet-kezni, és pedig 6–szor néhány perctöl 2¹|₂ óra alatt, 2szer 3—4 óra mulva, 10-szer 5—10, 9-szer 12—20 óra foly-tán. — C r u v e i l h i e r szerint nagyfoku gőgvizdag mind annyiszor halálos. B a y l e 17 eset közül csupán egyszer észlelt menekvést. V a l l e i x 40 esete közül 31 végző-dött halállal ; — S e s t i e r n e k 168-ja közül 120 halt el. — A gőgvizdag oly borzasztó baj , melynek halálos csapása elöl, ha nagyfoku az és rögtön fellépő, — épen ugy nincs szabadulás, erőteljes és ép, mint gyönge és be-teges egyénekre nézve , s melynél csak idejekoráni felis-merés és az azt rögtön követő észszerü és bátor föllépés képes a halált elháritni.

De lássuk az esetet :

Szünnapi utamból visszatértemet követő kora reggel f. hó 4-kén hivattam a beteghez , egy 18 éves leányká-hoz, kit a nehéz légzésnek fuldoklással határos kinai közt egy karszékben ülve találtam. A család orvosa Dr. P o r-g e s ur a sürgető részvétnek szavaival röviden tudósita, hogy a betegnél miután az közel hét hó óta rekedt volt, 10 nap elött kezdődött a lélekzési nehézség, mely miatt öt kerti lakából behozatni rendelte s azóta nála eleinte maga, később több ügytársak hozzájárultával mindent el-követett a veszélylyel fenyegető bajnak elháritására,

Fig. 1. Janos Balassa's original article in the *Hungarian Medical Weekly: Orvosi Hetilap* [7].

---

last number of days been out of her bed from morning to night."

From this description, it seems clear that Balassa, after restoring the airway by tracheotomy, used rhythmic ante-rior chest compressions in an attempt to simulate respira-tion. However, it is likely that he also produced cardiac com-pression providing full cardiopulmonary resuscitation for 6 min before the patient revived. Safar et al. showed that anterior chest wall compressions produce adequate circula-tion but limited pulmonary ventilation [8]. Perhaps Balassa provided enough tidal volume and exchange via the unob-structed tracheotomy, which was his intention, and inadver-tently also maintained the circulation with cardiac compres-sions.

Janos Balassa (Fig. 2) was born in 1814 in the village of Szentlorinc, Hungary [5]. He started his medical studies at the University of Pest and finished in Vienna, qualifying M.D. in 1838. In 1843, at the age of 29, he was appointed professor of surgery at the University of Pest. He was a par-ticipant in the uprising against Austria in 1848 and served in the medical corps. After the defeat of the revolution, he was arrested and removed from his university appointment. He was restored to his full position in 1851. Balassa was the premier surgeon of his time in Hungary. After the failed revo-lution, the resources for the medical faculty at the University of Pest were extremely limited, and Balassa performed his work under very difficult circumstances. He was a contem-porary and friend of Ignac Semmelweis, who graduated from

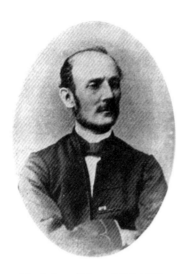

Fig. 2. Janos Balassa (1814–1868).

Vienna 6 years after Balassa and who was appointed Professor of Obstetrics at the University of Pest in 1855. Balassa applied Semmelweis's antiseptic principles to surgery with great success. He wrote the first article in the first edition of the *Hungarian Medical Weekly* in 1857 on the topic of bladder calculi, suggesting that the primary cause of urinary stones was nutritional. In addition to his many surgical contributions, Balassa introduced ether anaesthesia to Hungary in 1847 [5,9].

Janos Balassa died in 1868 at the age of 54 from peritonitis associated with a perforated appendicitis. One of his contemporaries, Lumnitzer Sándor, said in 1872: "his personality and the importance of his life's work has placed him as among the greatest practitioners of medical sciences [9]."

### References

[1] Hermreck AS. The history of cardiopulmonary resuscitation. Am J Surg 1998;156:430–6.
[2] DeBard ML. The history of cardiopulmonary resuscitation. Ann Emerg Med 1980;9:273–5.
[3] Juvin P, Desmonts JM. Cardiac massage: a method rescued from oblivion. Anesthesiology 1998;89:771–6.
[4] Böhrer H, Goerig M. Early proponents of cardiac massage. Anaesthesia 1995;50:969–71.
[5] Husveti S, Ellis H. Janos Balassa: pioneer of cardiac resuscitation. Anaesthesia 1969;24:113–5.
[6] Koetter KP, Mallick WH. Janos Balassa and Rudolf Eisenmenger: forgotten pioneers of resuscitation. Anesthesiology 1999;90:1490–1.
[7] Balassa J. Jelvenyes gogvizdag fekelyes gogporckorilob kovetkezteben: tetszhalal megmentes gogmetszes altal (oedema glottidis symptomaticum ex perichondritde laryngeali ulcerosa–asphyxia–laryngotomia cum exitu fausto). Orvosi Hetilap 1858;2:653–8.
[8] Safar P, Brown TC, Holtey WJ, Wilder RJ. Ventilation and circulation with closed-chest cardiac massage in man. JAMA 1961;176:574–6.
[9] Kudasz J. Remembering Janos Balassa. Orvosi Hetilap 1965;106: 2401–4.

# Charles Augustus Leale and the resuscitation of Abraham Lincoln

George L. Sternbach    Joseph Varon    Robert E. Fromm Jr

When Abraham Lincoln was assassinated in Ford's theater on April 14, 1865, the first physician to reach his side was 23 year old Charles Augustus Leale, Assistant Surgeon, United States Volunteers (Fig. 1). He had been specifically assigned to the theater that night during the performance of 'Our American Cousin' due to the presence of the presidential party.

Seated in the dress circle, Leale had observed Lincoln's entry into Box 78. He was impressed with the President's stoic gravity.

> I was looking at him as he took his last walk. The memory of that scene has never been effaced [1].

After the shot rang out, Leale witnessed John Wilkes Booth vaulting to the stage, then made his way to the President's box. Documenting what followed, he was to pen one of the most remarkable accounts in the annals of resuscitation.

Leale was assigned to duty at the US Army General Hospital, Armory Square, in Washington, DC. Having had extensive experience there with severely wounded officers, he could recognize a fatal wound when he encountered one:

> As I looked at the President, he appeared to be dead. His eyes were closed and his head had fallen forward.... I placed my finger on the President's right radial pulse but could perceive no movement of the artery.... I lifted his eyelids and saw evidence of brain injury. I quickly passed the separated fingers of both hands through his blood matted hair to examine his head and I discovered his mortal wound.... The assassin of President Lincoln had evidently planned to shoot to produce instant death, as the wound he made was situated within two inches of the physiological point of selection, when instant death is required.... The history of surgery fails to record a recovery from such a fearful wound, and I have never seen or heard of any other person with such a wound.... who lived even for an hour [2].

Leale's first action was to reduce intracranial pressure:

> The President had been shot in the back part of the head, behind the left ear. I easily removed the obstructing clot of blood from the wound, and this relieved the pressure on the brain [2].

The next steps related to clearing of the upper airway:

> As the President did not then revive, I thought of the other mode of death, apnoea, and assumed my preferred position to revive by artificial respiration. I knelt on the floor over the President, with a knee on each side of his pelvis and facing him. I leaned forward, opened his mouth and introduced two extended fingers of my right hand as far back as possible, and by pressing the base of his paralyzed tongue down-

117

ward and outward, opened his larynx and made a free passage for air to enter the lungs [2].

Two other physicians had by then entered the box, Drs Charles A. Taft and Albert F.A. King. Leale soon engaged their help:

I placed an assistant at each of his arms to manipulate them in order to expand his thorax, then slowly to press the arms down by the side of the body, while I pressed the diaphragm upward [2].

This form of artificial ventilation was a variant of the Silvester technique, a procedure recommended by the Royal Humane Society in 1861 as an effort to imitate natural respiratory movements [3]. Mouth-to-mouth ventilation, a method with roots in antiquity, had nonetheless been the object of much controversy within the medical community for a number of years [3]. Leale used this next:

I leaned forcibly forward directly over his body, thorax to thorax, face to face, and several times drew in a long breath, then forcibly breathed directly into his mouth and nostrils, which expanded his lungs and improved his respirations [2].

An additional action was to engender controversy more than a century later:

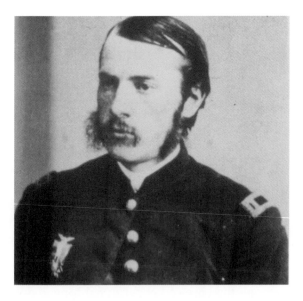

Fig. 1. Charles Augustus Leale.

I also with the strong thumb and fingers of my right hand by intermittent sliding pressure under and beneath the ribs, stimulated the apex of the heart [2].

The result was 'a feeble action of the heart and irregular breathing' [2]. Several authors have subsequently credited Leale with having thus performed external cardiac massage [1,2], though others disagree [4]. In any event, the resuscitation efforts appeared to have had the desired effect:

After waiting a moment I placed my ear over his thorax and found the action of the heart improving. I arose to the erect kneeling posture, then watched for a short time, and saw that the President would continue independent breathing and that instant death would not occur [2].

At this point, Leale deemed Lincoln stable to be transported, and he oversaw his removal to a boarding house across the street. There, several more senior physicians, including Joseph K. Bames, Surgeon-General of the United States Army, arrived and assumed charge of the case. Leale's prognosis proved to be correct some 9 h later, but he remained at the President's side until the end. John H. Littlefield's painting, 'Death-bed of Lincoln' depicts him at Lincoln's right hand at the moment of demise.

Born in New York City in 1842, Charles Augustus Leale received his Doctor of Medicine degree from Bellevue Hospital Medical College just 2 months before Lincoln's assassination. While there, he had received special instruction in diseases of the heart from Austin Flint. Following his involvement in the treatment of Lincoln, he served as executive officer of Armory Square Hospital, receiving an honorable discharge from the United States Volunteers in 1866, with the rank of brevet captain. He went on to a long and distinguished medical career that included much charitable and benevolent work [5]. Leale subsequently wrote an account of the resuscitation for the National Library of Medicine [2], but though he survived to the age of 90, he was always reticent to discuss the events of April 14, 1865 [6].

The autopsy of Abraham Lincoln was performed on the following day in an upper story guest room of the White House. Leale declined an invitation to be present, having already been sufficiently traumatized by the previous night's events. Four days later, he joined the Surgeon-General and other physicians who had attended Lincoln in a position of honor in the funeral procession to the Capitol rotunda, where the body lay in state. He kept his blood-stained shirt cuffs for the remainder of his life.

But was what he did really cardiac massage? The first known written description of closed-chest cardiac compression was by the Hungarian surgeon Janos Balassa in 1858 [7]. Balassa successfully resuscitated an 18 year old woman suffering from airway compromise due to tuberculous laryngeal edema. He performed a laryngotomy after the patient had suffered a cardiorespiratory arrest. Following this, he initiated rhythmic compression of the central portion of the anterior chest wall, continuing for 6 min until spontaneous cardiac activity was restored.

Balassa published an account of the case in the Hungarian medical weekly, but there is no indication that this method was widely known as a consequence in the United States. Although Leale had studied under one of the great masters of American cardiology, there is nothing in Austin Flint's writings to suggest that he advocated closed-chest cardiac massage as a method to main- tain an artificial circulation. It is likely that Leale used his method to stimulate the heart (just as he wrote), rather than to institute an artificial vascular pump. The concept of chest compressions to produce circulation in humans would have to await the 20th century. When Kouwenhoven, Jude and Knickerbocker presented their seminal work on closed-chest cardiac massage, they cited no historical antecedent prior to 1878 [8].

# References

[1] Brooks SM. Our Murdered Presidents: The Medical Story. New York: Frederick Fell, Inc, 1966.
[2] Montgomery JW. Resuscitation of President Lincoln. J Am Med Assoc 1961;176:160–2.
[3] Sternbach GL, Varon, J. The humane societies, Resuscitation (in press).
[4] Pearson JW. Historical and Experimental Approaches to Modern Resuscitation. Springfield, IL: Charles C. Thomas, 1965.
[5] The National Cyclopaedia of American Biography, vol. II. New York: James T. White and Co., 1921.
[6] Shutes MH. Lincoln and the Doctors: A Medical Narrative of the Life of Abraham Lincoln. New York: The Pioneer Press, 1933.
[7] Husveti S. Janos Balassa, pioneer of cardiac resuscitation. Anaesthesia 1969;24:113–5.
[8] Kouwenhoven WB, Jude JR, Knickerbocker GG. Closed-chest cardiac massage. J Am Med Assoc 1960;173:1064–7.

# Benjamin Howard and the direct method of artificial respiration

Thomas F. Baskett

One of the earliest advocates of manual artificial respiration was Leroy-d'Etiolles who proposed simultaneous pressure upon the abdomen and the chest for expiration, with the inspiratory phase accomplished by the recoil of the compressed part.[1] This paper, read before the French Academy of Sciences in 1829, initially did not lead to the adoption of manual artificial respiration. However, by the middle of the 19th century the manual techniques of Hall[2] and Silvester[3] were widely adopted and recommended by the Humane Societies. In 1869, Benjamin Howard, Professor of Clinical and Operative Surgery at the Long Island College Hospital, New York, entered the debate. He published a five page booklet *Plain Rules for Restoration of Persons Apparently Dead from Drowning*.[4] In this article, Howard laid out six rules covering the essential elements of appraisal, airway clearance and maintenance, and his manual technique of artificial respiration. He included figures which, in addition to the practicalities of the resuscitation technique, showed a high level of sartorial elegance in the rescuers (Figure 1). He ended the booklet with this plea:[4]

'By an hour's practice upon a friend, any reader may acquire as much skill for such emergencies as a physician need possess, and at this small cost may perhaps obtain the life-long satisfaction of having restored one or more valuable lives otherwise irrecoverably lost'.

Howard travelled widely and lectured as well as giving practical demonstrations of his 'direct method' of artificial respiration. One of these lectures was published in 1877 in the *Lancet* giving more widespread dissemination of his technique to the medical profession.[5] In this lecture delivered at King's College Hospital in London on 7 July 1877, Howard outlined the essential points for artificial respiration:[5]

'1. A clear passage through the lips to the lungs.
2. The greatest possible expansion of the thorax.
3. The greatest practical diminution of the thorax—
   -the two latter occurring with regular alteration and rhythm.'

He began with review of the method of Marshall Hall, a man whom he obviously held in high regard: 'I will begin with a demonstration of the method of Marshall Hall, reverence for whose memory and greatness make any criticism which may follow an uninviting and reluctant task'.[5] Howard pointed out that in Hall's method, the compression of the chest would be minimal as most of the patient's weight rested on the shoulder and hip. While acknowledging the contribution of Silvester's technique,

**RESTORATION OF PERSONS APPARENTLY DROWNED.**

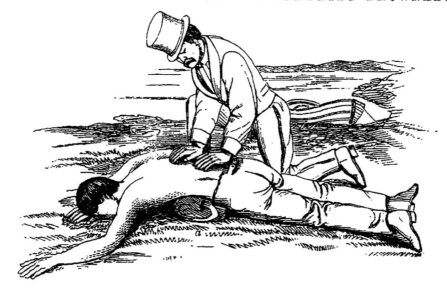

MODE OF FORCING AND DRAINING OFF WATER AND OTHER ACCUMULATIONS FROM THE STOMACH, THROAT, AND MOUTH, ACCORDING TO RULE 2, PREPARATORY TO PERFORMING ARTIFICIAL BREATHING.

*a*, Patient's clothing rolled tightly.

(b)

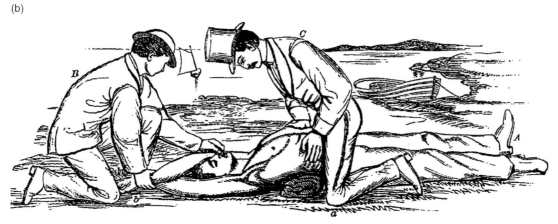

MODE OF PERFORMING ARTIFICIAL BREATHING ACCORDING TO RULES 3 AND 4.

**Figure 1** Howard's direct method of artificial respiration as illustrated [4].[4]

Howard had a number of criticisms about the limitations of this method, particularly in producing adequate compression of the thorax by the rescuer positioned at the patient's head. He felt that the compression of the lower ribs from this position did not allow adequate force as the direction of the compression was downwards, rather than the optimum upwards and inwards.

Howard went on to demonstrate his own technique which involved initially placing the victim face down over a bolster made of the patient's clothes and situated at the level of the epigastrium. The lower part of the chest was then compressed forcibly a few times to promote drainage of water from the lungs and stomach. The patient was then turned onto his back with the bolster just below the shoulder blades such that the epigastrium and lower thorax were the highest part of the body. He described the main elements of his technique as follows:[5]

'Seize the patient's wrists, and having secured the utmost possible extension with them crossed behind his head, pin them to the ground with your left hand, so as to maintain it. With the right thumb and forefinger armed with the corner of a

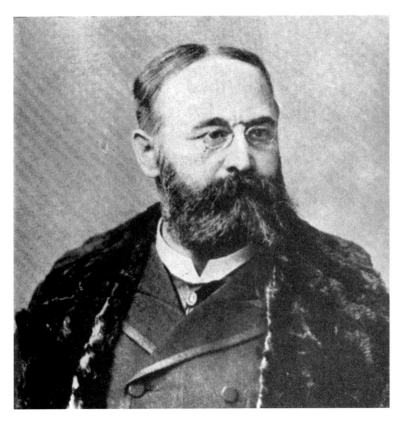

**Figure 2** Benjamin Howard, 1836–1900.

dry pocket-handkerchief, withdraw the tip of the tongue, holding it out of the extreme right corner of the mouth (This is the easiest, least barbarous and firmest way of holding the tongue). If a boy be at hand both wrists and tongue may be confided to his care'.

Howard pointed out the importance of keeping the tongue 'immovably fixed forward'. He also noted that the backward curvature of the neck, because of the bolster placed beneath the patient's shoulder blades, precluded closure of the epiglottis. After emphasizing these important aspects of airway maintenance, Howard went on to describe his technique of artificial respiration:[5]

'To produce respiration, you now kneel astride the patient's hips, rest the ball of each thumb upon the corresponding costo-xyphoid ligaments, the fingers falling naturally into the lower intra costal spaces. Now, resting your elbows against your sides and using your knees as a pivot, throw the whole weight of your body slowly and steadily forward until your mouth nearly touches the mouth of the patient, and while you might slowly count one–two–three; then *suddenly*, by a final push, spring yourself back to your first erect position on your knees; remain there while you might slowly count one–two; then

repeat; and so on about eight or ten times a minute .... This method is called the ''direct method'' because by it a few things needed to be done are, simply, done. The tongue needs holding forward, it is held; the ribs, pressing—they are pressed. It is so simple that a Harbour policeman, after a single lesson, has done it as well as I or any other always distant physician could do it'.

Howard emphasized that the method was not fatiguing as 'the force employed is the weight of the operator, who remains in an easy position with alternations of complete rest'.

Benjamin Howard (1836–1900) was born in Chesham, Buckinghamshire, England in 1836 (Figure 2). As a young boy he immigrated with his parents to the United States where he received most of his education.[1] He became Professor of Clinical and Operative Surgery at the Long Island College Hospital, New York and was a Fellow of the New York Academy of Medicine. He was also a member of the Royal College of Surgeons of England. After the publication of his booklet, *Plain Rules for Restoration of Persons Apparently Dead from Drowning* in 1869, Howard travelled widely and lectured in many centres in the United States and Britain.[6] He generally gave a lecture along with a practical demonstration of his method of artificial respiration. During one such session in Dublin he over-enthusiastically applied too much pressure during the demonstration and broke the ribs of his physician volunteer.[1,7] Benjamin Howard died in the United States in 1900.

## References

1. Karpovich PV. Adventures in Artificial Respiration, 27. New York: Association Press; 1953. p. 39–41.

2. Hall M. The ready method in asphyxia. Lancet 1856;2: 548–9.

3. Silvester HR. The Marshall Hall method of treatment in asphyxia. Lancet 1858;1:616.

4. Howard B. Plain rules for restoration of persons apparently dead from drowning, as taught under the auspices of the Metropolitan Board of Health of the City of New York. New York: E.B. Treat and Co.; 1869.

5. Howard B. The more usual methods of artificial respiration. With demonstrations of the ''direct method'' of the author. Lancet 1877;2:194–6.

6. Eisenberg MS. Life in the Balance. New York: Oxford University Press; 1997. p. 78–80.

7. Schafer EA. Artificial respiration in man. In: The Harvey lectures. Philadelphia: J.B. Lippincott Co.; 1909. p. 223–243.

# Jean-Henri Dunant
# The Founder of the Red Cross organisation

## Martin von Planta

### Early life

Henri Dunant was born on the 8th of May 1828 in Geneva as first son of the merchant Jean-Jacques Dunant and his wife Antoinette Dunant-Colladon (Figure 1). The family followed the pietistic Calvinistic faith, which explains the humanistic life Dunant led. His many socially motivated activities may be highlighted by the foundation of the worldwide YMCA movement in 1855. His professional formation was as a bank clerk in the private bank of Lullin and Sautter in Geneva.

In 1853 Dunant visited for the ''Compagnie genevoise des colonies suisses de Sétif'' Algeria, Tunisia and Sicily. In 1856 he founded his own colonial company (Société financière et industrielle des moulins des Mons-Djémila) and in 1859 took on an additional French citizenship. To regulate the finances of his business affairs, Dunant visited the emperor Napoléon III who was then in Lombardy waging war against Austria. The French headquarters were located in Solferino.

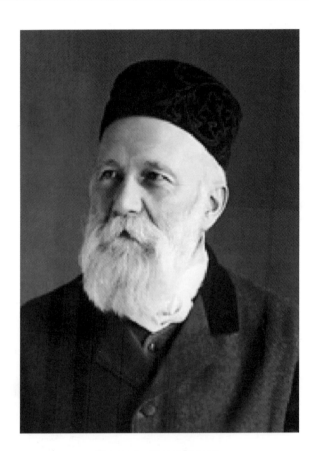

**Figure 1**  Henri Dunant.

## The battle of Solferino

On the evening of the 24th of June 1859 Dunant reached the battlefield where thousands of wounded and dying soldiers were uncared for. Deeply moved by this experience, Dunant organised voluntaries from the local population — mostly women and girls — for rudimentary first aid and set in the local church an improvised hospital up. Dunant soon recognised that knowledgeable help, medical equipment and transport facilities were sorely missing. In this dire situation no difference was made between Austrian or French soldiers and Dunant bought medical supplies out of his own pocket. Still, too many died because structured help was inadequate and human and logistic resources of the improvised medical troops were rapidly exhausted. Furthermore, water and food were unhygienic resulting in further disease and death.

After his return to Geneva, Dunant wrote his experiences from Solferino down in a book in 1862 which he distributed, at his own expense, to European political and military leaders and where he postulated the concept of medical help independent of the nationality of the wounded.[1]

## The founding of the Red Cross

The book of Dunant's experiences was rapidly recognised in its importance and awakened humanistic spirited personalities throughout Europe. It was mainly Gustave Moynier, the President of the Humanistic Society of Geneva who realised that the ideas postulated in Dunant's book would bear impact on the conduction of further conflicts. Thus, on the 17th of February 1863 the Red Cross organisation was founded in Geneva by five men (Figure 2): Henri Dunant the idealistic visionary, Gustave Moynier the practical organiser, two doctors with experience in wartime surgery: Louis Appia and Théodore Maunoir and the first commander of the young Swiss Federation army: General Guillaume-Henri Dufor as first president.

The organisation constituted itself as the permanent international committee of the Red Cross (ICRC) and formulated the principles according to which wounded troops and its medical helpers were to be treated:

1. Neutralisation of victims and medical personnel,
2. Creation of legally protected areas for care of patients (which in turn lead later to the human rights),
3. Creation of national committees for the care of patients (currently more than 60 organisations worldwide).

The continuing work of the first Red Cross committee resulted in 1864 in the first Geneva Convention on human rights. As a uniform symbol for the protection of patients and medical personnel a Red Cross on a white background (a reversal of the Swiss flag) was chosen.

Soon after the founding act, differences concerning the conduct of the Red Cross affairs arose between Dunant and Moynier. Dunant continuously pleaded for the protection by neutralisation during

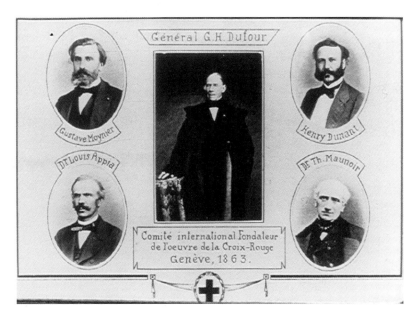

**Figure 2** Contemporary illustration of the five founders of the Red Cross.

warfare of hospitals, patients and medical personnel in all of Europe, an idea deemed unrealistic by Moynier.

## Bankruptcy and social disgrace

The Algerian business side of Dunant's life was going downhill with war, a cholera epidemic, an earthquake and a draught in 1865 in Algeria. In 1867 he went bankrupt and was condemned for criminal insolvency resulting in social disgrace and the withdrawal from the Red Cross committee. Dunant left Geneva and continued to live in Paris where he followed his humanistic ideals being active throughout Europe. In the pursuit of these activities he continued to spend his own monies and went deeper into poverty. After many travels and visionary social activities he ended up in 1887 in the village of Heiden in obscurity.

## Rehabilitation

In September 1895 Georg Baumberger, a journalist from St. Gallen, wrote an article on the founder of the Red Cross organisation which was widely reprinted in Europe.[2] Dunant crossed the threshold from obscurity into international reputation while the International Red Cross in Geneva continued to ignore him. His financial situation improved with the Binet-Fendt award by the Swiss government, a yearly stipend from the Czar's widow Maria Feodorowna. The Austrian pacifist Baroness Bertha Sophie Felicita von Suttner (born Countess Kinsky von Chinic und Tettau) who received herself the Nobel prize for peace, corresponded with Dunant in 1905 and through that contact he realised that women were more apt in promoting durable peace than men. He promoted these ideals in numerous articles and enhanced his reputation such that members of the Nobel committee became aware of him.

## Nobel price for peace in 1901

After many intricate political manoeuvers Dunant was awarded the first Nobel prize for peace in 1901 together with the French pacifist Frédéric Passy (Figure 3). Passy was the founder and president of the first French peace society (since 1889 called Société française pour l'arbitrage entre nations). Dunant and Passy received the prize for creating the Red Cross and initiating the Geneva conventions.[3]

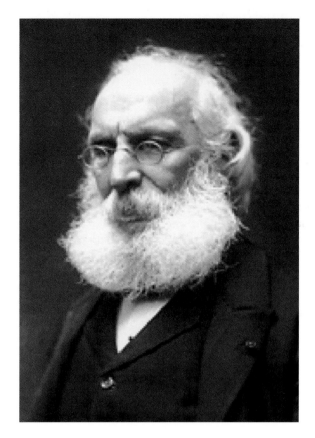

**Figure 3** Frédéric Passy.

The following telegram reached Dunant on December 10th wherein the Oslo committee announced his decision with the following wording:

''An Henry Dunant, Heiden. Das Nobelkomitee des norwegischen Parlaments hat die Ehre, Ihnen mitzuteilen, dass es den Friedensnobelpreis 1901 je zur Hälfte an Sie, Henri Dunant, und an Frédéric Passy verliehen hat. Das Komitee sendet seine Ehrerbietung und seine aufrichtigen Wünsche.''

The Norwegian military doctor Hans Daae played a pivotal role in the selection process of the awardees. Daae also preserved the prize money in a Norwegian bank and thus protected it from Dunant's creditors. Dunant himself never touched the prize money during the remainder of his life.

## Late life

The Nobel prize was followed by other distinctions such as an honorary doctor's degree from the medical faculty of the Heidelberg university without alleviating his poor economic situation. Thus, this did not change Dunant's depression, fear from persecution by creditors, and his arch enemy Moynier, with whom he could not make peace again. He died on the 30th of October 1910 lonesome and without heirs. His ashes rest on the cemetery of Sihlfeld in Zurich.

## Influence of Dunant's ideas

The tragedy of Dunant's life may lie in his visions for a more peaceful world and protection of wounded soldiers. These ideas were apparently ahead of their time and came into reality much later but they are still valid today. However, the impact of his fundamental humanistic ideas changed the conduct of warfare and the treatment of prisoners of war. Medical troops are nowadays an integral part of any structured army and still receive the protection that Dunant foresaw. Let us hope that this also remains true in future conflicts!

## References

1. Dunant JH: A translation from the French of the first edition of Un Souvenir de Solférino, published in 1862. A memory of Solferino. London, Cassell, 1947.
2. Baumberger G. In: Bärtsch A, Durand R, Müller G, et al., editors. Die Ostschweiz ISBN 2-88163-012-X. Croix-Rouge genevoise and St. Gallen: Société Henry Dunant; 1993, 21 avril, 172 p.
3. Nobel Prize committee: www.nobelprize.org/nobel_prizes/peace. Accessed 15.11.06.

## Further reading

1. Boissier P. History of the international committee of the Red Cross. Vol. I: from Solferino to Tsushima. Geneva: Henry Dunant Institute; 1985, ISBN 2-88-044012-2.
2. Moorehead C. Dunant's dream: War, Switzerland and the history of the Red Cross. London: Harper Collins; 1998, ISBN 0-00-255141-1.
3. Bennett A. The Geneva convention: the hidden origins of the Red Cross. Gloucestershire: Sutton Publishing; 2005, ISBN 0-75-094147-2.

# Moritz Schiff and the history of open-chest cardiac massage

Federico Vallejo-Manzur    Joseph Varon    Robert Fromm, Jr.    Peter Baskett

Open chest cardiac massage is still practiced in some instances of cardiac arrest. The historical development of this technique is frequently attributed to Moritz Schiff [1], one of the most distinguished physiologists of the latter half of the 19th century [2]. In 1874, Schiff was in charge of the physiology laboratory at the Institute of Advanced Studies in Florence in Italy. Doctor G. Hake joined him while he was investigating the comparative effects of ether and chloroform and in one of their articles published in *The Practitioner* in 1874, Hake described how Schiff practiced open-chest cardiac massage after cessation of heart function produced while using chloroform [3] and Green addressed the matter again later in 1906 [4].

"The heart is in a vital state favorable to its renewed action when paralyzed by the influence of chloroform on the vaso-motor nerves, is demonstrated by Professor Schiff's practice of artificial circulation. He lays open the thoracic cavity, and, compressing the passive heart with his fingers, imitates in it the periodic movements of the organ. The circulation is restored, the nerves of the heart recover their force, and the organ finally resumes its spontaneous action. Before long, signs of returning sensibility become apparent, the reflex action of the eyelid return and the animal is now capable of being brought back to the cerebral consciousness." [3].

Another method practiced by Schiff and described by Hake to revert the hypotensive effect of chloroform were compressions of the thoracic aorta or compressions of the abdomen restoring the pulse and raising the blood pressure to normal levels.

"When by action of chloroform the pressure has gone down nearly to zero, and there is no pulsation visible, compression of the thoracic aorta between the crura of the diaphragm, or compressions of the abdomen restores to the pulse, its strength and frequency, and causes the pressure in the manometer to rise to a considerable height, very often to 100 or 120 millimeters." [3].

Following the initial description of the techique by Schiff, the first attempt of open cardiac massage was attributed to Niehans in 1880. Zesas who had assisted Neihans during the operation, did not record this incident until 1903 [5].

" A 40-year-old man was operated for a goiter. Before the start of the operation, cardiac arrest. After unsuccessful attempts with artificial respiration, a resection of the ribs was carried out and the heart exposed. The heart, indeed, became firmer after massage, fibrillated; normal contractions, though, no longer occurred." [5].

Although the technique had been followed appropriately it was unsuccessful. In 1898, Tuffier conducted open chest cardiac massage in a patient with what was thought to be a pulmonary embolism, obtaining return of spontaneous circulation [6]. However, this patient expired after a second arrest [7].

"It was hard for us to let die of mechanical accident a young man of whom all the rest of the organ systems appeared normal while we may have had a means, for which it is true we had only experimental approval, to bring him back to life. My hesitation was of short duration. I rapidly made an incision in the left third intercostal space and, taking off the pericardium with the index finger, I exercised rhythmic compressions of the ventricular region for one or two minutes: the heart undulated at first irregularly then truly contracted. The pulses returned, the patient took some deep inspiration, his eyes opened wide, his pupils contracted..." [6].

Years later, Batelli in 1901, and Boureau and Pruss in 1902, published a series of animal experiments on the resuscitation of the heart by opening the thorax and direct cardiac massage [8,9].

Kristian Ingelsrud, in 1901 was the first clinician to achieve a successful outcome after open chest cardiac massage for the emergency treatment of cardiac arrest. This incident was reported by Keen in 1904 [10]. A year later in 1902, Gray reported another successful case [11]. Green, in 1906 reported 40 patients treated with open cardiac massage for cardiac arrest with nine survivors [4]. The use of open chest cardiac massage was uncommon until 1924 when Lee and Downs reported 99 cases with an overall survival of 25%. [12]. This made open chest cardiac massage the preferred method used for cardiovascular collapse in the first half of the last century [13]. Beck, using internal defibrillation in 1947, made open chest cardiac massage no longer a rare occurrence [14]. By 1953, Stephenson had accumulated 1200 cases of patients treated with open chest cardiac massage for cardiac arrest, of which 336 (28%) of the patients were discharged home with reasonable neurological function [15].

When Kouwenhoven, Jude and Knickerbocker describe closed chest cardiac massage in the early 1960s, with a 70% long-term survival rate [16], the use of open chest cardiac massage declined [17,18].

More recently several studies have demonstrated the haemodynamic and survival superiority of open chest cardiac massage compared to closed chest cardiac massage, and there has been a resurgence of interest in the application of this life saving technique [19–22]. Indeed, the American Heart Association in association with the International Liason Committee on Resuscitation recommends that open-chest CPR be considered in certain situations such as penetrating traumatic cardiac arrest [23]. Resuscitation teachers such as Safar has suggested that open chest cardiac massage should be instituted when advanced life support does not restore spontaneous circulation within 5–10 min [24].

Newer techniques involving 'minimal invasive surgery' have been recently developed for the treatment of cardiac arrest victims [25]. These newer techniques also have demonstrated their superiority when compared with closed cardiac massage in animal models [26]. It is possible that there will be a resurgence of open-chest cardiac massage in years to follow.

## References

[1] Pike FH, Guthrie CC, Stewart GN. Studies in resuscitation: I. The general condition affecting resuscitation, and the resuscitation of the blood and of the heart. J Exp Med 1908;10:371–418.
[2] Obituary—Moritz Schiff. Lancet 1896;2:1198–9.
[3] Hake TG. Studies on ether and chloroform from Prof. Schiff's physiological laboratory. The Practitioner 1847;12:241–50.
[4] Green TA. Heart massage as a means of restoration in cases of apparent sudden death. Lancet 1906;2:1708–13.
[5] Zesas DG. Zur Frage der Hermassage beim Chloroformkollaps. Centralblatt fur Chirugie 1903;17:588–9.
[6] Tuffier T, Hallion M. De la compression rhythmic du Coeur dans la syncope cardiaque par embolic. Bull Mem Soc Chir 1898;24:937–9.
[7] Paradis N, Martin G, Rivers E. Use of open chest cardiopulmonary resuscitation after failure of standard closed chest CPR: illustrative cases. Resuscitation 1992;24:61–71.
[8] Battelli F. Functions du Coeur et du systems Nerueux Central. J Physiol Pathol Gen 1900;25:443–56.
[9] Prus J. Veber die wiederbelebung un todesfallen in folge von erstickung, chloroform-vergiftung und electrishem schlage. Wien Klin Wochenschr 1900;21:482–7.
[10] Keen WW. Case of total laryngectomy and abdominal hysterectomy in both of which massage of the heart for chloroform collapse was employed with notes of 25 other cases of cardiac massage. Ther Gaz 1904;28:212–30.
[11] Gray HMW. Subdiaphragmatic transperitoneal massage of the heart as a means of resuscitation. Lancet 1905;2:1708–9.
[12] Lee WE, Downs TM. Resuscitation by direct massage of the heart in the cardiac arrest. Ann Surg 1924;80:555–61.
[13] Bircher N, Maryland B, Safar P. Manual open-chest cardiopulmonary resuscitation. Ann Emerg Med 1984;13:770–3.
[14] Beck CS, Mautz FR. Ventricular fibrillation of long duration abolished by electric shock. J Am Med Assoc 1947;135:525–37.
[15] Stephenson HE, Reid C, Hinton JW. Some common denominators in 1200 cases of cardiac arrest. Ann Surg 1953;137:731–44.
[16] Kouwenhoven WB, Jude JR, Knickerbocker GG. Closed-chest cardiac massage. J Am Med Assoc 1960;173:1064–7.
[17] Arai T, Dote K, Tssukahora I, Nitta K, Nagaro T. Cerebral blood flow during conventional, new and open-chest cardiopulmonary resuscitation in dogs. Resuscitation 1984;12:147–54.
[18] Varon J, Marik PE, Fromm RE. Cardiopulmonary resuscitation a review for clinicians. Resuscitation 1998;36:133–45.
[19] Hosler RM. Advantages of open and closed chest resuscitation. J Intern Coll Surg 1966;6:687–92.
[20] Del Guerico RM. Open chest cardiac massage: an overview. Resuscitation 1987;15:9–11.
[21] Rubertsson S, Grenvik A, Wiklund L. Blood flow and perfusion pressure during open-chest versus closed-chest cardiopulmonary resuscitation in pigs. Crit Care Med 1995;23:715–25.
[22] Boczar ME, Howard MA, Rivers EP, Martin GB, Horst HM, Lewandowski C, et al. A technique revised: hemodynamic comparison of closed-and open chest-cardiac massage during human cardiopulmonary resuscitation. Crit Care Med 1995;23:498–503.
[23] The American Heart Association in collaboration with the International Liason Committee on Resuscitation. Guidelines 2000 for Cardiopulmonary Resuscitation and Emergency Cardiac Care—An International Consensus on Science. Resuscitation 2000;46:291.

[24] Safar P, Bircher NG. Cardiopulmonary Cerebral Resuscitation. London: Saunders, 1988:212–9.

[25] Buckman RF, Badellino MM, Mauro LH, Aldridge SC, Milner RN, Malaspina PJ, et al. Open chest cardiac massage without major thoracotomy: feasibility and systemic blood flow. Resuscitation 1995;29:237–48.

[26] Pavia EF, Kern KB, Hilwig RW, Scalabrini A, Ewy GA. Minimally-invasive direct cardiac massage versus closed-chest cardiopulmonary resuscitation in a porcine model of prolonged ventricular fibrillation cardiac arrest. Resuscitation 2000;47:287–99.

# Sydney Ringer and lactated Ringer's solution

## Thomas F. Baskett

Along with the use of normal saline, Ringer's lactate is the most commonly administered intravenous crystalloid solution for perioperative care and circulatory resuscitation. It all started when an assistant in Sydney Ringer's laboratory used tap water instead of distilled water to make up the saline solution for Ringer's experiments on the effect of various constituents of the blood on the contractility of the frog's heart [1]. When Ringer performed the same experiment with saline made with distilled water he found that, in contrast to the earlier experiments with saline made with tap water, distilled water saline did not sustain contractility of the heart muscle. He wrote:

'I discovered, that the saline solution which I had used had not been prepared with distilled water, but with pipe water supplied by the New River Water Company. As this water contains minute traces of various inorganic substances, I at once tested the action of saline solution made with distilled water and I found that I did not get the effects described in the paper referred to. It is obvious therefore, that the effects I had obtained are due to some of the inorganic constituents of the pipe water.' [2]

Ringer analyzed the water of the New River Water Company and found, in keeping with its chalky origins, that it contained traces of calcium salts in addition to sodium, potassium, chlorine and magnesium (Fig. 1) [2]. This finding stimulated Ringer to conduct a further series of experiments in an attempt to isolate the individual constituents that were most important in sustaining the physiological activity of the frog heart muscle. Ringer noted: 'When the circulating fluid is composed of saline solution the ventricle grows weaker and weaker and contractility ceases in about 20 min [2]. He found that 'Calcium bicarbonate, or calcium chloride in physiological doses, or even in smaller quantities

than are present in the blood, restore good contractions...' [2]

Ringer summarized the results of his experiments as follows:

'A mixture containing 100 cc saline, 5 cc sodium bicarbonate solution, 5 cc calcium chloride solution with 1 cc potassium chloride solution also makes an excellent artificial circulating fluid, for with this mixture the heart will continue to beat perfectly. The heart's contractility cannot be sustained by saline solution nor by saline containing potassium chloride, nor with saline solution containing bicarbonate of soda, nor by saline solution containing bicarbonate of soda and potassium chloride; but after contractility has ceased, the addition of a lime salt will restore good contractility. The addition too of a calcium salt to any of the above solutions will sustain contractility. I conclude therefore that a lime salt is necessary for the maintenance of muscular contractility. But whilst calcium salts are necessary for the proper contraction of the heart, yet if unantagonized by potassium salts the beats would become so broad and the diastolic dilatation so prolonged that much fusion of the beats would occur and the ventricle would be thrown into a state of tetanus.' [2]

Ringer's solution, with its additional salts of sodium, potassium and calcium became ubiquitous in physiological laboratory experiments. By the early 20th century, as knowledge developed on the diffusion and dissociation of ions, the fundamental physiological importance of electrolytes to cellular activity was recognized [3]. As intravenous crystalloid solutions were developed, Ringer's solution was adapted for this purpose. There have been a number of modifications of the constituents of Ringer's lactated solution, most notably by Hartmann and Darrow [4–6]. The current constituents of Lactated Ringer's Injection USP are sodium 130 mmol/l, potas-

## A FURTHER CONTRIBUTION REGARDING THE INFLUENCE OF THE DIFFERENT CONSTITUENTS OF THE BLOOD ON THE CONTRACTION OF THE HEART. By SYDNEY RINGER, M.D., *Professor of Medicine at University College, London.* (Plate I.)

AFTER the publication of a paper in the JOURNAL OF PHYSIOLOGY, Vol. III., No. 5, entitled "Concerning the influence exerted by each of the Constituents of the Blood on the Contraction of the Ventricle," I discovered, that the saline solution which I had used had not been prepared with distilled water, but with pipe water supplied by the New River Water Company. As this water contains minute traces of various inorganic substances, I at once tested the action of saline solution made with distilled water and I found that I did not get the effects described in the paper referred to. It is obvious therefore that the effects I had obtained are due to some of the inorganic constituents of the pipe water.

Water supplied by the New River Water Company contains 278·6 parts of solids per million.

They consist of:

| | | |
|---|---|---|
| Calcium | 38·3 | per million. |
| Magnesium | 4·5 | ,, |
| Sodium | 23·3 | ,, |
| Potassium | 7·1 | ,, |
| Combined Carbonic Acid | 78·2 | ,, |
| Sulphuric Acid | 55·8 | ,, |
| Chlorine | 15 | ,, |
| Silicates | 7·1 | ,, |
| Free Carbonic Acid | 54·2 | ,, |

This water is faintly alkaline to test-paper from bicarbonate of lime. Saline made with this water I found at first rounds the top of the trace of each contraction and later greatly prolongs diastolic dilatation, and that these effects are completely obviated by about 1 c.c. of 1 % solution

Fig. 1.

sium 4 mmol/l, calcium 1.4 mmol/l, chloride 109 mmol/l, lactate 28 mmol/l, at a pH of 6.5.

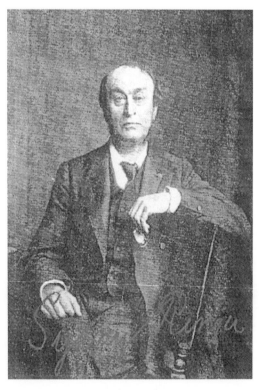

Fig. 2.

Sydney Ringer was born in Norwich in 1835, the middle of three sons (Fig. 2). His older and younger brothers both became very successful businessmen in the Far East [7,8]. Their father died when the boys were young but in a Quaker family education was paramount and, with the help of family and friends, Sydney Ringer received a good private education. After an initial apprenticeship to a local doctor, Ringer entered the Faculty of Medicine at University College, London in 1854—graduating MB in 1860. He was to spend his whole career associated with University College and its hospital, initially as a resident medical officer and later as an assistant physician, during which time he attained his MD and MRCP [9,10]. In 1866 he was appointed a full physician at the hospital. From 1864–1869 he was also an assistant physician at the Children's Hospital at Great Ormond Street. Ringer was a busy and successful clinical consultant and for many years also held the professorship of Materia Medica and Therapeutics. He later occupied the chairs of medicine and of clinical medicine. As part of this mandate he prepared and published *A Handbook of Therapeutics.* It became a standard text after he produced the first of 13 editions in 1869. The emphasis in his lectures and book was on clinical pharmacology. Indeed, in addition to Ringer's study of physiological solutions, he investigated the effect of a number of drugs and agents on the heart: including ether, chloroform, pilocarpine and atropine [11].

Ringer was said to have been '...extremely generous and kindly in assisting the original work of younger men, and was always ready to afford any real worker any assistance in his power...' [12]. As a newly qualified doctor, William Osler spent some months in London, mainly working at the University College Hospital and met Ringer several times: 'Last night I dined at Dr Ringer's. Everything was in grand style and the people very nice' [13]. Ringer was granted space for his research in the physiological laboratory of University College, where he was to carry out productive investigations for 30 years. An austere man of self-discipline and routine he had an early breakfast each morning, walked to the laboratory from his home in Cavendish Place and put in time there before his clinical duties. He usually returned to the laboratory in the late afternoon before returning home. Ringer was elected a Fellow of the Royal Society in 1885 and retired from his clinical and laboratory duties in 1900, after 40 years service to the hospital and university.

His wife came from an ancient Yorkshire family and they had two daughters, the eldest of whom died young. In her memory the Ringers restored the old village church of Lastingham in Yorkshire. He retired to Lastingham and following his wife's death became quite withdrawn. He suffered a stroke on 13 October 1910, lapsed into unconsciousness and died the following day.

He was buried beside his wife and daughter at Lastingham on the edge of the Yorkshire moors. In 1912 his surviving daughter endowed a lecture in his name to be given biennially at the University College Hospital [12,14].

Nowadays if Sydney Ringer was admitted to hospital during his final illness he would almost certainly receive an intravenous infusion of Ringers' lactate.

## References

[1] Ringer S. Concerning the influence exerted by each of the constituents of the blood on the contraction of the ventricle. J Physiol 1880-1882;3:380–93.

[2] Ringer S. A further contribution regarding the influence of the different constituents of the blood on the contraction of the heart. J Physiol 1883-1884;4:29–42.

[3] Astrup P, Bie P, Engell HC. Salt and water in culture and medicine. Copenhagen: Munksgaard, 1993:182–4.

[4] Hartmann AF, Senn MJE. Studies in the metabolism of sodium r-lactate II. Response of human subjects with acidosis to the intravenous injection of sodium r-lactate. J Clin Invest 1932;11:337–44.

[5] Darrow DC, Yannet H. The changes in the distribution of body water accompanying increase and decrease in extracellular electrolytes. J Clin Invest 1935;14:266–75.

[6] Maltby JR. Lactated Ringer's injection USP, Hartmann's compound sodium lactate solution BP. In: Maltby JR, editor. Notable Names in Anaesthesia. London: RSM Press, 2002:176–9.

[7] Starling EA. Obituary: Sydney Ringer, 1835–1910. Proc Roy Soc Lond 1912;84:1–3.

[8] Talbott JH. A biographical history of medicine. New York: Grune and Stratton, 1970:89–90.

[9] Lee JA. Sydney Ringer (1834–1910) and Alexis Hartmann (1898–1964). Anaesthesia 1981;36:1115–21.

[10] Sykes AH. Sharpey's fibres. York: William Sessions Ltd, 2001:130–1.

[11] Ringer S, Moshead EA. On the relative paralysing action of atropia and pilocarpine on the heart. J Physiol 1879-1880;2:235–9.

[12] Ringer S. Obituary. BMJ 1910;2:1384–6.

[13] Bliss, M. William Osler: A Life in Medicine. Toronto: University of Toronto Press; 1999. p. 72, 74, 78, 97.

[14] Ringer S. Obituary. Lancet 1910;2:1386.

# John Alexander MacWilliam

## Fernando Eugênio dos Santos Cruz Filho    Douglas Chamberlain

At the end of the 19th century, a brilliant and incisive Scottish physician called John Alexander MacWilliam[a] (1857–1937) concluded that ventricular fibrillation was an important mechanism for sudden cardiac death in man.[1] But he made other fundamental contributions to cardiovascular medicine that are less well known. That his recognition has been muted can be ascribed to one undeniable fact: many of his writings on sudden death and on resuscitation were too far ahead of their time.

MacWilliam was born in Kiltarlity, a small town in the highlands of Scotland, and graduated in 1880, with first class Honours at the University of Aberdeen.[2] In 1882 he was awarded an MD with highest honours for a thesis on the structure of cardiac and diaphragmatic fibers in various animals. After spending time in Edinburgh, he carried out research in the famous School of Physiology at Leipzig which set the course for his future career. This prestigious school produced many famous physicians whose names are still honoured today, including Pavlov, Fick, Schenov, Bowditch, and Kroenecker.

MacWilliam was strongly influenced by the work of Carl Ludwig in Leipzig. One of Ludwig's most important contributions to science was the invention of the kymograph in 1847, which opened the door to modern physiological research and made his laboratory one of the major centres for this discipline. At this time, Ludwig and Kroenecker were interested in the concept that disorders of heart rhythm could cause death to animals. In 1850, Hoffa and Ludwig produced a lethal arrhythmia in cold-blooded animals by delivering electric shocks to the heart that produced a tetanus-like state.[3]

After returning to Aberdeen in 1886, MacWilliam overcame considerable technical difficulties to show that the hearts of mammals as well those of as cold-blooded animals were vulnerable to electrical stimuli. This led directly to his observations on what we now know as ventricular fibrillation. It was also in 1886 that an important Chair in Aberdeen fell vacant. MacWilliam, then only 30 years old but already with an established reputation, was duly appointed to be Professor of the Institutes of Medicine which was the term then used for the science of physiology.[2]

134

In 1887, he published his landmark paper entitled *'Fibrillar contraction of the heart'*[4] that described the behaviour of the myocardium after induction of this malignant rhythm. He also postulated that it may be factors of a transient nature that cause the breakdown of the electrical stability of the heart. At the beginning of the article he mentioned that many years earlier Ludwig and Hoffa had shown that faradic currents to the ventricles of a dog's heart could abolish the normal beat—and continued:

''The ventricular muscle is thrown into a state of irregular arhythmic (sic) contraction, whilst there is a great fall in the arterial blood pressure. The ventricles become dilated with blood as the rapid quivering movement of their walls is insufficient to expel their contents; the muscular action partakes of the nature of a rapid incoordinated twitching of the muscular tissue.''

At about the same time in 1887, Waller,[5] a London physiologist and formerly MacWilliam's fellow, was attempting to study the electrical activity of the human heart. However, the lack of instruments available at the time limited progress; the capillary galvanometer proved a disappointment in this regard. It was not until 1897 that the string galvanometer was developed by Einthoven, the professor of physiology in Leiden.[6] This sensitive instrument was able successfully to record the electrical activity of the heart on a moving photographic plate. More than 14 years elapsed after MacWilliam's description of fibrillar contraction by the time Hoffman recorded and published the first tracing of what was then believed to be the first recording of human ventricular fibrillation (although a more modern interpretation would categorize it as a paroxysm of polymorphic ventricular tachycardia).[7]

Electricity had become important by this time, and was being distributed and used widely in Europe and North America[8] by the last two decades of the century. Inevitably, electrocution was becoming a relatively common tragic accidental event[9] that was a cause of concern to both to physicians and to electrical companies; some companies such as Consolidated Edison of New York were later to fund and sponsor important research in this area.[10]

In 1889, MacWilliam postulated in another landmark paper entitled *'Cardiac Failure and Sudden Death'*[1] that sudden death in man was due to ventricular fibrillation and described some of the degenerative cardiac diseases that may be found in this setting, namely:

''... degenerative changes of fatty or fibroid nature in the muscular walls, aortic regurgitant disease

with its more or less effective compensatory changes in the organ, and diseased conditions (atheromatous, calcareous, or sclerotic) of the coronary arteries. But sudden stoppage of the heart's action has often been observed apart from the occurrence of gross structural lesions, associated with no very obvious or extensive alteration in the cardiac tissues... not infrequently the cardiac substance has exhibited no pronounced morbid change.''

MacWilliam therefore anticipated the relatively recent notion that sudden cardiac death could occur without structural heart disease or extrinsic cause; the concept of purely electrical vulnerability would have to wait for many years of development in the science of electrocardiography. His work was also crucial in the rejection of the accepted wisdom of the time that cardiac arrest was inevitably due to 'silent standstill in diastole': a similar outcome as that seen in a motionless heart could be the result of the chaotic activity that he had described[1]:

''... Instead of quiescence, there is a tumultuous activity, irregular in its character and wholly ineffective as regards its results...''

He recognized, more than a century before the clinical implications of ventricular fibrillation were fully accepted, its relationship to myocardial ischaemia[1]—at a time when the pathophysiology of coronary artery disease was poorly understood:

''In the great majority of cases where sudden death is caused by cardiac failure, there is, no doubt, an altered and impaired state of nutrition in the cardiac tissues sometimes rendered palpable by degenerative changes recognizable with the microscope or pointed by the presence of disease in the coronary arteries.''

But MacWilliam had not lost sight of the importance of asystole. At the International Medical Congress in Washington of 1887[11] — the same year that he described fibrillar contraction — he foresaw the therapeutic use of electrical impulses to stimulate beating in the arrested heart:

''The question of the effects of electrical stimuli upon the mammalian heart is one of obvious importance, both in its purely physiological and its clinical aspects, bearing as it does on the possibility of restoring the cardiac beat after it has been arrested by causes of a temporary nature.''

Thus, he anticipated the clinical use of pacing as an adjunct to other means of resuscitation and gave details of how it might best be accomplished[12]:

"In order to do this in man one electrode should be applied in front over the area of cardiac impulse, and the other over the region of the fourth dorsal vertebra behind, so that the induction shocks may traverse the organ. The electrodes should be of considerable extent... and they and the skin should be well moistened with salt solution."

During a meeting of the influential Royal Society of Medicine of London, he also described the other mainstays – with electricity—of successful resuscitation – the combination of cardiac compression and artificial respiration. In a presentation 'On the rhythm of the mammalian heart'[13] he stated:

"The conditions of fibrillar contraction or heart-delirium induced in the ventricles of excitable hearts by the application of interrupted currents and other means can be recovered from even after long periods (three-quarters of an hour &c) under the combined influence of artificial respiration, rhythmical compression of the ventricles, and the administration of pilocarpin."

His interest in resuscitation centred principally around the use of anaesthetic agents, especially with chloroform which was known to be related to sudden unexpected death—although the mechanisms were poorly understood. Their perils joined those of electricity in capturing the interest of physicians and scientists.

MacWilliam was also a pioneer in research on the relation of the autonomic nervous system to sudden cardiac death. In 1845, Weber and his colleagues had reported that the vagus nerve not only controlled motor activity but also exerted an inhibitory effect on the muscular contraction of the frog.[14] Developing this basic notion, MacWilliam, in two presentations in 1888 on the rhythm[13] and on the inhibition[15] of the mammalian heart demonstrated that vagal stimulation could reduce both the heart rate and its power of contraction. Vagotomy, on the other hand, accelerated the heart rate but only when the cardiac inhibitory centre was active. He concluded correctly that the effect of the vagus on the heart was part of a complex system that we now call autonomic control.

Although the 1887 paper on fibrillar contraction[4] had postulated that factors of a transient nature might seriously disrupt the electrical stability of the heart, he later realized the importance of the autonomic nervous system in this context. Thus, in 1923 MacWilliam wrote a review[16] with a prescient description of the role of exercise and autonomic interaction in the genesis of ventricular fibrillation. He described not only the excitatory causes of ventricular fibrillation but also defined factors that could trigger them:

"The ever-recurring reports of sudden death during or shortly after exertion, in persons who up to the fatal issue had been able to pursue their usual avocations, emphasize the importance of the conditions attendant on muscular effort—those involving an increased demand on the powers of the heart and more or less stress on the organ. This is brought about in various ways: by the augmentation of rate and force and irritability through the agency of the nerves (diminution or suspension of vagus control and excitation of cardiac sympathetic augmentor fibres), increased arterial pressure presenting greater resistance to the pumping out of the ventricular contents, increased diastolic filling due to more rapid influence from the venae cavae, etc."

The interaction of central nervous system and cardiac physiology was also beautifully described in his article 'Blood pressure and heart action in sleep and dreams'[17] of 1923. It provides further prescient insights into the interaction between the autonomic nervous system and the cardiovascular system as physiological variables that influence metabolic demands. The description of how variation in pulse rate and systolic and diastolic pressures accompany changes in activity resemble the diaries completed during present-day ambulatory monitoring. MacWilliam's description of the physiological phases of sleep are particularly impressive. He classified sleep into two distinct phases: the undisturbed sound phase that is accompanied by a fall in blood pressure, heart rate, and respiratory rate; the restless phase during which the individual experiences vivid dreams accompanied by muttered speech, groaning, and facial and finger movements associated with an increase in blood pressure and heart rate (which we now call Rapid Eye Movement or REM sleep). To his surprise these changes were more marked than those that occur during moderate exercise. He documented increases in systolic blood pressure of up to 72 mmHg and diastolic pressure up to 30 mmHg. He recognized too that such perturbations during this phase could cause angina attacks which might well be fatal:

"In a heart susceptible to fibrillation a sudden call on the heart during muscular exertion and excitement in the waking state is often fatal; in the disturbed conditions of sleep and dreaming a similar mechanism is sometimes brought suddenly and strongly into action – diminution of vagus control and especially under emotional stress, stimulation of the cardiac sympathetic together with a high blood pressure – conditions which favour ventricular fibrillation."

He concluded the article with a touch of finesse found only in a researcher whose science has a very human dimension:

''In the light of these observations it is easy to understand how in certain circumstances death may come like a thief in the night to a susceptible person living with circulatory conditions that approach the danger line...''

MacWilliam deserves the greatest recognition for his elegant and unique experimental studies of ventricular fibrillation and sudden death which gave a major boost to the emerging science of physiology. The impact, however, could and should have been greater. In particular, clinical medicine was slow to benefit from his and other work that had great relevance to sudden death—already becoming recognized as a major and seemingly intractable problem.

Unfortunately, he had faced much scepticism during his lifetime; his innate modesty would have been a handicap in countering it. It was Maclean, in his 1937 appraisal of MacWilliam's achievements, who suggested that the world of scientific medicine was not ready for his ideas[2]; the history of medicine is replete with examples of major advances that were ignored because their time had not yet come. But Macleod, the Nobel laureate for his work on the isolation of insulin and a former pupil of MacWilliam, had been less forgiving of MacWilliam's contemporaries[18]:

''Failure of others to grasp the significance of fibrillation as a common cause of sudden death from cardiac failure in man is difficult to understand, since MacWilliam very clearly pointed out this application of his observations... in 1889.''

Although, the possibility of reverting experimental ventricular fibrillation by electric shock was recognized in 1899[19] and its clinical potential was suggested in 1913,[9] it took 60 years after the description of fibrillar contraction before Beck et al.[20] performed the first successful ventricular defibrillation to counter an arrest that had occurred following the closure of a patent ductus arteriosus. In 1923, at the age of 66, MacWilliam reviewed his work on ventricular fibrillation that had been published decades earlier[16]; in this paper he expressed disappointment that potential applications of physiology to medicine received so little attention.

Nearly 100 years after his classic paper on ventricular fibrillation was published, an automated external defibrillator was produced[21] and shown to be effective in clinical value. The scene was set for public access defibrillation[22] which enables modestly trained or even untrained laypersons to reverse cardiac arrest. Both this and the development of the implantable defibrillator[23] may have been beyond MacWilliam's dreams and the expectations of others of his time who had sought to counter sudden death. But it is their mission that has been accomplished. The plea of so many who face the grief of death, voiced by the unknown Lucy in Shakespeare's *King Henry VI*[24]:

'O, that I could but call these dead to life!'

is now regularly answered. John Alexander MacWilliam's contributions towards making this possible, ignored for too long, deserve even now to be more widely acknowledged.

## References

1. McWilliam JA. Cardiac failure and sudden death. Br Med J 1889;i:6–8.
2. MacLean H, John Alexander MacWilliam. Aberdeen Univ Rev 1937;24:127–32.
3. Hoffa M, Ludwig C. Einige neue versuche über Herzbewegung. Z Rat Med 1850;9:107–44.
4. McWilliam JA. Fibrillar contraction of the heart. J Physiol 1887;8:296–310.
5. Cope Z. Augustus Desiré Waller (1856–1922). Med Hist 1973;17:380–5.
6. Einthoven W. Un nouveau galvanomètre. Arch Néerland Sci Exactes Naturelle, serie 2 1901;6:625–33.
7. Hoffman A. Fibrillation of the ventricles at the end of an attack of paroxysmal tachycardia in man. Heart 1912;iii:213–8.
8. Jarvis CM. The distribution and utilization of electricity. In: Singer C, Holmyard EJ, Hall AR, Williams TI, editors. A history of technology, vol. 5. New York: Oxford University Press; 1958. p. 208.
9. Jex-Blake AJ. The Goulstonian lectures on death by electrical currents and by lightning. Br Med J 1913;I:425–30, 492–8, 548–52, 601–3.
10. Eisenberg MS. Cardiac arrest. The science and practice of resuscitation medicine. In: Paradis NA, Halperin HR, Nowak RM, editors. The quest to reverse sudden death: a history of cardiopulmonary resuscitation,. Baltimore: Williams and Wilkins; 1996.
11. MacWilliam JA. On the electrical stimulation of the mammalian heart. In: Trans Int Med Congress, Ninth Session, vol. III. 1887. p. 253 (citation from Fye WB. Ventricular fibrillation and defibrillation: historical perspectives with emphasis on the contributions of John MacWilliam, Carl Wiggers, and William Kouwenhoven. Circulation 1985;71:858–65).
12. McWilliam JA. Electrical stimulation of the heart in man. Br Med J 1889;i:348–50.
13. MacWilliam JA. On the rhythm of the mammalian heart. Proc R Soc London 1888;44:206–8.
14. Ernst Heinrich Weber (1795–1878). Leipzig physiologist (editorial). J Am Med Assoc 1967;199:272–3.
15. MacWilliam JA. Inhibition of the mammalian heart. Proc R Soc 1888;44:208–13.
16. MacWilliam JA. Some applications of physiology to medicine. II. Ventricular fibrillation and sudden death. Br Med J 1923;ii:278–82.

17. MacWilliam JA. Some applications of physiology to medicine. III. Blood pressure and heart action in sleep and dreams. Br Med J 1923;ii:1196—200.

18. Macleod JJR, John Alexander MacWilliam. Aberdeen Univ Rev 1928;15:224.

19. Prevost J-L, Battelli F. La mort par les courants électriques— -courants alternatifs a haute tension. J Physiol et Pathol Gen 1899;ii:427—42.

20. Beck CS, Pritchard WH, Feil HS. Ventricular fibrillation of long duration abolished by electrical shock. JAMA 1947;135:985—6.

21. Diack AW, Welborn WS, Rullman RG, Walter CW, Wayne MA. An automatic cardiac resuscitator for emergency treatment of cardiac arrest. Med Instrum 1979;13:78—83.

22. Weisfeldt ML, Kerber RE, McGoldrick RP, Moss AJ, Nichol G, Ornato JP, et al. Public access defibrillation: a statement for healthcare professionals from the American Heart Association Task Force on automatic external defibrillation. Circulation 1995;92:2763.

23. Mirowski M, Mower MM, Staewen WS, Tabatznik B, Mendeloff AI. Standby automatic defibrillator. An approach to prevention of sudden coronary death. Arch Int Med 1970;126:158—61.

24. Shakespeare W. Henry VI, Part 1 Act 4, Scene 7.

# Rudolph Matas and the development of intralaryngeal intubation and artificial respiration in thoracic surgery

Gillian R. Hamilton    Thomas F. Baskett

Rudolph Matas, professor of surgery in New Orleans in the early 20th century, is often referred to as 'the father of modern vascular surgery' in acknowledgement of his technique of treating traumatic arterial aneurysms by endoaneurysmorrhaphy. The first case which took place on April 1, 1888 involved a healthy 26-year-old man who developed a large and expanding brachial artery aneurysm 2 months after a gun shot wound [1]. Matas initially carried out the technique pioneered by John Hunter involving simple ligation of the artery above and below the aneurysm. However nine days later the aneurysm returned, so Matas made a large incision over the brachial artery and ligated any vessels he found entering the aneurysm. He then opened the aneurysm sac and discovered other vessels feeding the aneurysm which he ligated from within the aneurysm wall. The patient recovered, retained his arm, and a new improved method of dealing with such aneurysms was created (Fig. 1).

Less well known is the fact that Matas made two important contributions in the area of resuscitation. The first of these occurred in July 1888; Matas amputated the leg of a patient and a few hours later found him in hypovolaemic shock with a shallow, intermittent pulse and a great thirst. Based on his knowledge of the treatment of patients with cholera, Matas 'ordered 2 pints of distilled water, with a drachm of common salt dissolved in each pint to be brought at once' [2]. Intravenous saline solution had first been used in 1832 by Doctor Thomas Latta of Leith, Scotland to replace losses of salt and water in cholera patients [3] In subsequent years intravenous saline was used intermittently during cholera epidemics in New Orleans.

Immediately after the intravenous infusion of the two pints the patient made noticeable improvement, but died within 36 h. At the time, Matas speculated: 'It is, I believe, historically correct to state that no attempt prior to July 1888 had been made to infuse intravenously a saline solution for the relief of acute anaemia' [2]. Surprisingly, Matas did not continue his study of this treatment, although in 1906 he developed a clamp for controlling the rate of infusion of intravenous fluids to replace the old technique of raising or lowering the height of the fluid reservoir.

Matas's other contribution in the field of surgical resuscitation was in his understanding and promotion of positive pressure artificial respiration via direct laryngeal intubation for thoracic surgery. In May 1898, in a presentation to the Louisiana State Medical Society, later published in the *Annals of Surgery*, Matas reviewed the problems of thoracic surgery in relation to acute pneumothorax comprehensively [4]. As he said: 'Until the risk of seriously interfering with respiratory function by inducing acute collapse of the lung is clearly eliminated, or is reduced to a safe minimum, the analogy between the pleura and the peritoneum from the surgical point of view will never exist' [4]. In his review of the existing literature he said: 'The procedure that promises the most benefit in preventing pulmonary collapse in operations on the chest is the artificial inflation of the lung and the rhythmical maintenance of artificial respiration by a tube in the glottis directly connected with a bellows'. He went on to outline the work of Dr George Fell of Buffalo, New York who, in 1887, reported the treatment of cases of opium poisoning by forced respiration using foot-bellows connected

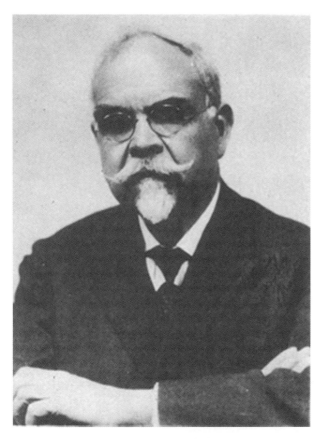

Fig. 1. Rudolph Matas, 1860–1957.

Fell–O'Dwyer apparatus for artificial respiration in many cases, mostly acute opium poisoning, but not for anaesthesia [7]. He did, however, demonstrate that the technique could be used for 24 h and longer without any injurious effect on the larynx, and thus further endorsed the apparatus for maintaining artificial respiration.

In 1896, Tuffier and Hallion, working in Paris, addressed the problem of thoracic surgery specifically in a number of animal experiments using intralaryngeal cannulae and continuous ventilation to prevent the lung collapsing during anaesthesia and thoracic surgery in dogs [8]. They felt their experiments were so successful that the technique could be safely adapted for use in humans [9].

With this background, Matas built up the case for using artificial respiration electively in anaesthesia required for thoracic surgery [10]. He acknowledged the contribution of Doyen in Paris in developing a compound bellows and intralaryngeal cannulae, although there was no reference to his clinical application of this apparatus [11]. At the end of this extensive review Matas described briefly a case report of a thoracic operation performed by a colleague in New Orleans using this technique, noting: 'The pleura was opened freely, but the collapse of the lung which would have inevitably followed, and the bad symptoms that were beginning to be noticed, were immediately corrected by the Fell–O'Dwyer apparatus' [4].

In his later, 1902 publication, Matas went on to the outline the application of artificial respiration in surgical practice and the extensive experiments he had undertaken to produce a modified device which replaced the bellows in Fell–O'Dwyer's apparatus with a graduated pump. As he said: 'It would now appear from all that has been said and done that no further discussion could be called for, at least on the value of a reliable

to a tracheotomy tube [5]. Dr Joseph O'Dwyer of New York refined the tracheal tube [6] and later combined this with Fell's apparatus to produce forced artificial respiration without requiring tracheotomy. While these techniques were used in humans they were not used for anaesthesia or thoracic surgery. At the Presbyterian Hospital in New York, Dr William Northrup used the

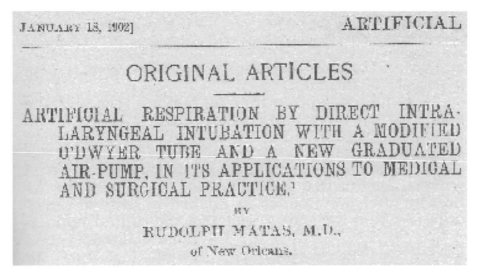

Fig. 2. American Medicine 1902;3:97–103.

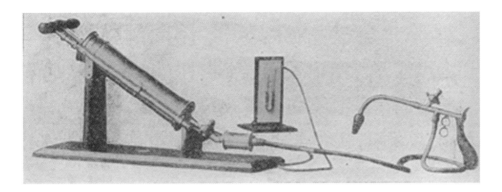

Fig. 3. Matas' modified apparatus for artificial respiration during thoracic surgery.

apparatus for maintaining artificial respiration in the course of intrathoracic operations.'[12] He did note that further refinement of the technique was required: '...with the view of elevating this mode of treatment to a higher plane of scientific accuracy' [12] (Figs. 2 and 3).

Matas was the first surgeon in the United States to use spinal anaesthesia, following the example of the German surgeon August Bier [13]. Matas used a saline solution, often containing both cocaine and morphine with the intention that the latter would prolong the effect of the cocaine and provide additional sedation [14,15] He was, therefore, probably the first to inject an opiod by the spinal route.

Rodolphe Matas, later anglicised to Rudolph, was born September 12, 1860 in Bonnet Carré just outside New Orleans. His Catalonian parents emigrated to the United States in 1856 shortly after their marriage in Gerona. His father studied both pharmacy and medicine at the then newly formed New Orleans College of Medicine, receiving his degrees in pharmacy in 1858 and medicine in 1859—each academic course apparently lasting 5 months. At the time of Rudolph's birth his father was the physician to a large plantation estate at Bonnet Carré [16]. His father soon forsake medicine for a variety of commercial and entrepreneurial activities. When Rudolph was 2 the family moved to Paris and then to Barcelona. When the family returned to New Orleans in 1867 the 7-year-old Rudolph was already fluent in Catelan, Spanish, French and English. Shortly thereafter the family moved to Brownsville, Texas and later across the border to Matamoras in Mexico. Rudolph continued his schooling in these two areas [17,18]. In 1877 he was accepted at the University of Louisiana's Medical College, later to become Tulane University. He graduated MD in 1880 before reaching his twentieth birthday. He developed a busy general practice in New Orleans and two years later was appointed editor of the *New Orleans Medical and Surgical Journal*. He also became a demonstrator in the department of anatomy and quickly developed the surgical side of his practice, so that his operation on the aneurysm, sometimes called the Matas

Operation, was developed only eight years after he qualified. In 1894 at the age of 34 he was made professor and head of department of surgery at Tulane, which position he held for the next 33 years.

Due to his father's nomadic commercial interests, Matas' homelife was rather unstable. About the time he became a medical student his father and mother separated. His mother and sister moved back to New Orleans but ultimately, in 1886, they both returned to Spain and Matas was only to see his mother on one more occasion. While Dr Matas' professional career developed successfully, his personal life was complex and difficult. He fell in love with Mrs Adrienne Landy, a divorceé with two sons. Indeed, she and her husband had been separated before the birth of their second son, who was delivered by Dr Matas in 1883. The son, Lucian, was later to join Matas in the practice of surgery. However, Matas' Catholic upbringing meant that his marriage to a divorced woman would not be sanctioned by the church until her ex-husband remarried. This did not happen until 1894 at which time the ever patient Matas proposed to Adrienne and they married shortly thereafter. In 1902 Adrienne gave birth to a son but he was to die within a few hours of birth. A desperately saddened Matas arranged for a photograph to be taken of the infant son in the arms of the delivery nurse, which he witheld from his wife [19]. Matas and his wife were very happy together but he was to suffer a tragic loss again when she died of influenza in December 1918. As he wrote to a friend: 'The hours pass, the sun sets, and with the darkness I feel the chill that tells me she has gone forever' [16].

Rudolph Matas received almost all the surgical honours possible, both nationally and internationally. He served as President of the American College of Surgeons and the American Association for Thoracic Surgery. He received six honorary degrees and was recognised with honorary fellowship or medals by surgical colleges in twelve countries. He was a prolific writer but notoriously late for publication dead lines. By invitation he produced the definitive chapter on aneurysms to be published in the first volume of a surgical text: it was eventually published in the fifth volume 3 years later. He was also a long-winded talker and time constraints meant nothing to him. Although his voice was described by students as 'high-pitched: and 'bleating'' his reputation ensured that he gained everyone's attention. Apparently it was not uncommon for him to rise to comment on a presentation given by a colleague and spend 30–40 min discussing a 15 min paper. Such was his reputation that the moderator rarely interrupted him.

Matas suffered an infectious complication not unknown to surgeons of the pre-antibiotic era. While removing a ruptured tubo-ovarian abscess in July 1908 the pus splashed onto his surgical gown. At the end of the operation he rubbed his perspiring face with the hem of his gown. He subsequently developed a gonococcal infection in his right eye which, despite numerous attempts to control the infection, resulted in the loss of his eye by enucleation in October of that year. He adjusted and carried on with surgical practice into his 80th year. He continued to write and a colleague recalls a visit to his home: 'I had the impression we were walking through caverns of books. There were books every where: on tables and desks, on shelves reaching to the ceiling, even on the floors' [16]. At the age of 92 Matas had to have an iridectomy and cataract extraction on his remaining eye. Unfortunately this was unsuccessful and he was left almost completely blind. Despite having lost his main joy in life, the ability to read, he wrote to a friend: 'While no one can be very cheerful living in the penumbra of a ghost world, I am not rehearsing the lamentations of Job...' His final year was spent in hospital where he died on 23 September 1957, shortly after his 97th birthday. The nearly 100 years of his life spanned the introduction of anaesthesia to cardio-pulmonary by-pass surgery. His 60-year surgical career began with Lister's principles of antisepsis and ended with the advent of penicillin.

In 1937 the library of the medical school of Tulane University was dedicated to Rudolph Matas. In his will Matas left an endowment to the library of 1 million dollars along with his own substantial book collection.

# References

[1] Matas R. Traumatic aneurism of the left brachial artery. Med News (Phil) 1888;53:462–6.

[2] Cohn I. Rudolph Matas: A Biography of One of the Great Pioneers in Surgery. New York: Doubleday & Co, 1960:228–30.

[3] Latta T. Relative to the treatment of cholera by the copious injection of aqueous and saline fluids into the veins. Lancet 1831;2:274–7.

[4] Matas R. On the management of acute traumatic pneumothorax. Ann Surg 1899;29:409–34.

[5] Fell GE. Cases of opium poisoning treated by forced respiration. Trans Int Cong Med 1887;1:237.

[6] O'Dwyer JP. Chronic laryngeal stenosis treated by intubation. B Med J 1894;2:1478.

[7] Northrup WP. Apparatus for prolonged artificial forcible respiration. Br Med J 1894;2:697–8.

[8] Tuffier MT, Hallion L. Études experimentale sur la chirurgie du poumon. Compt Rend Soc Biol 1896;3:951, 1047, 1086.

[9] Duncum BM. Appendix E: intubation and the growth of endotracheal anaesthesia. In: The Development of Inhalation Anaesthesia. London: RSM Press, 1994:597–620.

[10] Keys TE. Endotracheal anaesthesia. In: The History of Surgical Anesthesia. Park Ridge, IL: Wood Library, 1996:63–9 Museum Edition.

[11] Doyen EL. La Chirugie du Poumon. Rev Théap Med Chir 1898;15:129–33.

[12] Matas R. Artificial respiration by direct intralaryngeal intubation with a modified O'Dwyer tube and a new graduated air-pump, in its application to medical and surgical practice. Am Med 1902;3:97–103.

[13] Bier A. Experiments regarding the cocainization of the spinal cord. Reprinted in 'Classical File'. Surv Anesthesiol 1962;6:52–9 (orginally from Dtsch Z Chir 1899;51:361–9).

[14] Matas R. Local and regional anesthesia with cocaine and other analgesic drugs, including the subarachanoid method as applied in general surgical practice. Philadelphia Med J 1900;6:820–43.

[15] Hamilton GR, Baskett TF. In the arms of Morpheus: the development of morphine for postoperative pain relief. Can J Anesth 2000;47:367–74.

[16] Shumacker HB. A moment with Matas. Surg Gynecol Obstet 1977;144:93–8.

[17] Keys TE. Historical Vignettes: Dr Rudolph Matas, 1860–1957. Anesth Analg 1975;54:29–30.

[18] Talbott JH. Rodolphe Matas (1869–1957). In: A Biographical History of Medicine. New York: Grune and Stratton, 1970:1030–2.

[19] Scannell JG. Rudolph Matas (1860–1957). J Thorac Cardiovasc Surg 1996;111:1294.

# Alexander Graham Bell and the vacuum jacket for assisted respiration

Thomas F. Baskett

Alexander Graham Bell is, of course, best known for his invention of the telephone which he achieved by the age of 30. However, most of his 50 years of experimentation and innovation were spent in a multitude of other endeavours, many of which never came to fruition. Much of his investigation, most of it carried out in isolation, was aimed at improving the understanding and treatment of the deaf. Among other areas of interest he worked on aviation, air conditioning, distillation of fresh water from seawater, submarines, genetics, eugenics, sheep breeding, x-rays and obstacle-detection devices for the blind [1–3]. This article will highlight some of his medical inventions, particularly as applied to resuscitation.

As a young man Alexander, following in the professional footsteps of his father and grandfather, was interested in teaching speech, phonetics and elocution. As part of his studies on speech therapy he attended anatomy and physiology courses at the University College, London from 1868 to 1870, and became familiar with clinical problems of respiration. He was particularly interested in neonatal asphyxia and respiratory problems of the newborn infant and developed what he called a 'vacuum jacket' or 'infant life-saver' in an attempt to create an apparatus that would allow for assisted respiration in immature or weak infants [1]. Bell's rationale was that a simple mechanism that could produce expansion and contraction of the thoracic cage could help sustain the infant with weak respiratory muscles. He designed a rigid, air-tight jacket of a size that would encompass the chest and abdomen of a cat. This was connected to a piston pump which would mimic respiration by alternately pumping and evacuating the pressure within the jacket. His experiment with a drowned cat failed to revive the cat, but did successfully demonstrate the production of inspiratory and expiratory movements of the chest [1].

When Bell moved from Scotland to Canada in 1870 he left his vacuum jacket in care of a colleague at the Alexandria Hotel in London. It was to be 22 years before he wrote back and found that the jacket was still at the hotel and arranged to have it returned to him in Canada. In late 1881 Bell's wife, Mabel, gave birth prematurely to their first son who died a few hours after birth. As she wrote in her diary: 'He was a strong little fellow and might have pulled through if they could once have established regular breathing' [4]. Bell did not refer to this episode in his notebooks but in the summer of 1882 he presented a paper at the Annual Meeting of the American Association for the Advancement of Sciences: 'Upon a proposed method of producing artificial respiration by means of a vacuum jacket' [1]. Intermittently over the next few years his notebooks contained sketches of a variety of vacuum jackets for assisted respiration. He modified these for adults and in 1892 built an adult-sized vacuum jacket with a piston pump and bellows [5]. This prototype now resides in the Alexander Graham Bell Museum in Baddeck, Nova Scotia (Fig. 1). Bell foresaw one of the potential applications of this jacket to be for victims of drowning. In order to test this he had a sheep intentionally drowned in Baddeck Bay and then used the device to revive the animal. One of his employees was so upset at this 'work of the devil' that he left Bell's employ and would not even accept his final pay cheque [4]. Like many of Bell's inventions the vacuum jacket was not seen through to publication or clinical use. Although, when Alfred Gradwitz described a similar Hungarian invention in 1905 in *Scientific American* [6], Bell noted his priority in a letter to the editor [7].

Bell modified a device known as the induction balance to detect metal in the human body. It was based on the principle that metal introduced into the field of a balanced induced current would break that balance [2]. Bell had used this principle in telephone circuits and thought of applying it in humans to detect metal foreign bodies, such as bullets. His first opportunity came in July 1881 when the United States President, James Garfield, was shot in the back. He survived but his doctors were unable to track the course of the bullet and therefore to locate and remove it [2,8]. Bell modified the induction balance with a needle probe but the attempt

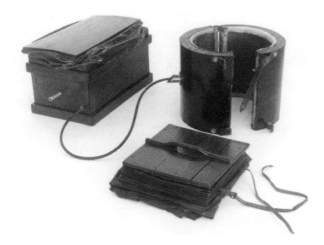

Fig. 1. Alexander Graham Bell's vacuum jacket on display at the Alexander Graham Bell Museum, Baddeck, Nova Scotia (Photo courtesy of Parks Canada/Alexander Graham Bell National Historic Site of Canada).

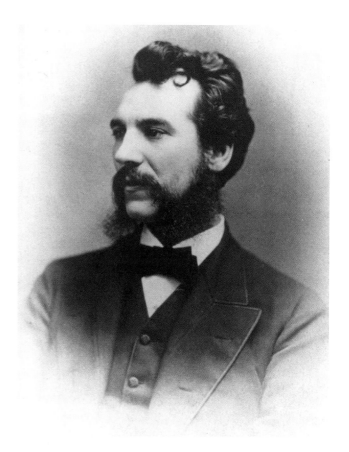

Fig. 2. Alexander Graham Bell, 1847–1922 (Portrait courtesy of Parks Canada/Alexander Graham Bell National Historic Site of Canada).

to locate the bullet in President Garfield was unsuccessful, possibly due to the depth of the bullet and possibly due to the disruption to the balanced current produced by the metal coils in the mattress upon which the President lay [2,9]. Only a few weeks after President Garfield's death, Bell's induction balance technique was used to successfully locate and guide removal of the bullet in a living person [2]. Until the advent of x-rays in 1895 Bell's 'bullet probe' was used successfully in many cases. In recognition of this work he was awarded an honorary doctorate of medicine by Heidelberg University [2,8].

Bell also became interested in the use of radium for the treatment of cancer. He observed the difficulties in treating deep seated cancers with surface application of radium, which also destroyed the tissue between the skin and the underlying cancer. He suggested placing a fragment of radium sealed in a fine glass tube so that it could be inserted into the core of the cancer. He was acknowledged as the first person to suggest this application of radium, although as with many of his inventions, he provided the suggestion and others applied the technique [10,11].

Alexander Bell was born 3 March, 1847 in Edinburgh, the middle of three brothers. His father, Alexander Melville Bell, was a well known teacher of speech, phonetics and elocution and had published more than 20 books on the subject. Alexander was named for his grandfather, Alexander Bell, who had been an actor in his younger years and then taught elocution in London. Alexander's mother, Eliza, was the daughter of a royal navy surgeon. The Bell household in Edinburgh was often full of visitors and relatives. One Canadian visitor was named Alexander Graham and was a former pupil of Alexander's father. Young Alexander liked the name Alexander Graham and, because he was the third consecutive Alexander Bell, he decided, at the age of 10, to change his name to Alexander Graham Bell—a decision which his father endorsed (Fig. 2).

At the age of 13 Alexander went to London and spent a year with his grandfather where he learned elocution and the treatment of speech defects. His initial schooling was at home, but he later attended Edinburgh Royal High School and the University of Edinburgh. Alexander worked with his father in Edinburgh and carried out many experiments on phonetics, seeking instruments that would mimic the sounds of the human voice. After the death of his grandfather in 1865 the family moved to London.

Alexander's two brothers both died from tuberculosis at age 18 and 25 years respectively. His father had traveled to Canada and was impressed with the healthy climate, and in August 1870 Alexander Melville Bell, his wife, and only remaining son emigrated to a 10 acre farm in Brantford, Ontario. Alexander worked from this base but spent much of his time teaching at the Boston School for the Deaf and in similar schools in Massachusetts and Connecticut. In 1877 he married Mabel Hubbard, a deaf pupil at the school, and they took their honeymoon in England, remaining there until their first child, Elsie, was born. They returned to live in Washington, DC, where Alexander Graham Bell eventually became a US citizen. Their second daughter, Marion known as Daisy, was born in 1880.

Bell had become wealthy from his telephone invention and in summer the family would escape the humid, smog-filled cities of the eastern seaboard to holiday in Canada. In

1885 the Bell family visited Nova Scotia and loved the area around the town of Baddeck, Cape Breton which reminded Bell of his home in Scotland. They later bought 70 acres on a peninsula across the bay from the town and named this Beinn Bhreagh—Gaelic for 'beautiful mountain'. They later built a large and impressive home known as Beinn Bhreagh Hall. It was here that Bell found serenity floating on an inner tube smoking cigars while mulling over his ideas. After dark his family could track his whereabouts on the lake from the glowing tip of his cigar. By the late 1890s and early 1900s Bell spent an increasing amount of time in Cape Breton and conducted his experiments with flight and the hydrofoil. In 1919 his hydrofoil, HD4, was to set the world waterspeed record of 70.86 miles per hour which was not broken for 10 years (Fig. 2).

Bell was one of the founders of the National Geographical Society in 1888 and 10 years later was elected President of the Society [12]. In 1920 he returned to Scotland for a 'farewell visit', during which he received the Freedom of the City of Edinburgh. In his later years Bell developed diabetes and pernicious anaemia and, by the summer of 1922, his health deteriorated progressively. He died peacefully at Beinn Bhreagh Hall on 2 August 1922. Two days later he was buried on the highest point of Benin Bhreagh having previously chosen the site of his burial, and later that of his wife, by lying down in various spots at the top of the mountain to find the position with the best view [4]. The site for the grave was blasted out of the rock and on either side one American and one British flag flew at half mast. At the appointed hour of his funeral service all telephones of the American Tele-

phone and Telegraph Company were silent for one minute. Bell's wife died from pancreatic cancer a few months later on 3 January, 1923 and exactly 1 year after Bell's service her ashes were placed in the grave beside him. Bell's home in Beinn Bhreagh remains in the hands of his descendants who still spend their summers overlooking the beautiful bay of the Bras d'or Lake at Baddeck, Nova Scotia.

## References

[1] Henderson AR. Resuscitation experiments and breathing apparatus of Alexander Graham Bell. Chest 1972;62:311–6.

[2] Shephard DAE. Alexander Graham Bell, doctor of medicine. New Engl J Med 1973;288:1166–9.

[3] Langille J. Alexander Graham Bell. Tantallon, Nova Scotia: Four East Publications Limited; 1989.

[4] Grosvenor ES, Wesson M. Alexander Graham Bell: The Life and Times of the Man Who Invented the Telephone. New York: Harry N. Abrams Inc; 1997.

[5] Eisenberg MS. Life in the balance. New York: Oxford University Press; 1997.

[6] Gradwitz A. A novel process of reanimation. Scientific Am 1905;93:276.

[7] Letter to editor. Scientific Am 1905;93:339.

[8] Burden G. Alexander Graham Bell: medical inventor. In: Amazing Medical Stories. Fredericton: Goose Lane Editions; 2003, p. 57–61.

[9] Bliss DW. Report of the case of President Garfield, accompanied with a detailed account of the autopsy. Med Rec 1881;20:393–402.

[10] Sowers ZT. The uses of radium. Am Med 1903;6:261.

[11] Davis KS. The history of radium. Radiology 1924;2:334–42.

[12] Lesage J. Alexander Graham Bell Museum: a tribute to genius. Natl Geogr 1956;110:227–56.

# Jaromir Baron von Mundy—Founder of the Vienna ambulance service

Markus Figl    Linda E. Pelinka

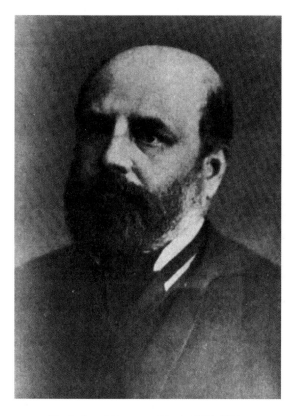

Fig. 1. Jaromir Baron von Mundy (1822–1894).

During a presentation of "The Tales of Hoffmann" by Offenbach on the evening of 8 December, 1881, a terrible fire broke out at the Ring Theater of the City of Vienna (Fig. 1). There was an audience of 1760 people at the theatre on that evening. The fire was caused by a gas lamp hanging over the stage. While the singers were able to escape to safety through the stage exit, the audience was engulfed in deadly chaos. When the theatre lights went out, the chaos grew even worse, and the panic-stricken audience was trapped in the pitch-dark theatre, groping frantically for the exit. The main theatre exit, however, was constructed to open towards the inside only. Therefore, the first ones to reach the entrance could not open the doors against the giant crowd of people pressing forward behind them. Many fell and were trampled to death or suffocated [1].

As a result, those fleeing from the fire were unable to get outside to save themselves and the firemen were unable to overcome the wedge of trampled corpses and get inside the burning theatre. Some of those trapped inside hurried out to the balcony, desperately crying for help, or jumped down in panic to the Vienna Ringstrasse, the street below, to escape. The raging fire, however, had already reached the Ringstrasse. Most of those who jumped were either killed or severely injured. Those who remained in the theatre were soon completely surrounded by flames, without even a slim chance of survival (Fig. 2).

The entire city of Vienna was panic-stricken by that devastating fire, which claimed as many victims as a major battle. Many of those who were injured could have been saved, but ultimately died of their burns and of smoke intoxication because no medical aid was available at the scene of the fire.

The bodies were laid out in the courtyard of the Main Police Station on the Schottenring nearby. Later, municipal workers transported them to the General Hospital in horse-drawn carriages and on stretchers [1].

While the city of Vienna was still in a state of fear and shock, Jaromir Baron Mundy knew it was time for his long-coveted dream of a medical ambulance service to become reality. On 9 December, 1881, 1 day after the fire,

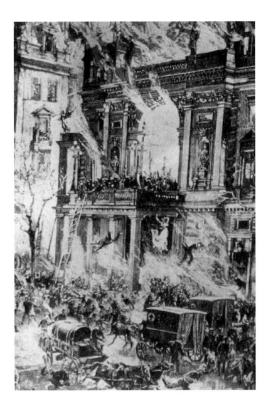

Fig. 2. Fire at the Vienna Ring Theatre.

1848, after 5 years with the military, Mundy became Imperial First Lieutenant in Italy. He spent every minute of his spare time on medical research.

In early 1852 he became Imperial First Captain of the 6th Infantry Regiment. After the Crimean War in 1855 and 12 years with the military, Mundy decided to end his military career. At the age of 33, he fulfilled his greatest wish in life and began studying medicine [1]. He moved to Wuerzburg, where several famous scholars were teaching at that time [4]. One of those scholars was Rudolf Virchow (1821–1902), who discovered the importance of cellular changes for the development of diseases. Mundy was very much impressed by the fact that Virchow was not only a physician and a scientist, but a politician and social reformer as well. Virchow's opinion that physicians should be advocates of the poor corresponded perfectly with Mundy's intent and initiative to help the poorest of the poor, the sick [1].

His talent and diligence as well as his years of experience and research with the military enabled Mundy to graduate from medical school after only four semesters. In those days, to work as a physician was frowned upon in aristocratic circles. Therefore, Mundy always remained an outsider in the eyes of his fellow aristocrats [1].

He left Wuerzburg shortly after his graduation from medical school on 23 March, 1859. After increasing his knowledge in Heidelberg and Leipzig, Mundy moved to Berlin, where he focused his interest on the therapy of mental diseases [5]. Additionally, Mundy repeatedly returned to his former unit as an Imperial Captain. He worked as a physician on several battlefields, including Solferino, where he met the Swiss writer Henri Dunant on 24 June, 1859 [1].

In those days, Solferino on Lake Garda in Italy belonged to Lombardy, which was under Austrian rule. Napoleon III of France had instigated the Lombards against the Austrians. After an ultimatum had expired, the war finally broke out. Approximately 190,000 men on the Austrian side were fighting approximately 180,000 men on the Italian/French side. Slowly but surely, the battle escalated into a massacre. Chaotic mismanagement and conflicting orders worsened matters even more. In the end, 42,000 men had fallen or been severely injured in the terrible Battle of Solferino and were left lying helplessly on the battlefield [1].

Henri Dunant (1828–1910), who was in Solferino of his own accord and as a newspaper correspondent, became an eye witness to the goriest battle of the 19th century and to the greatest failure and lack of care for the injured. He saw how they were left behind on the battlefield, helpless prey to thieves and looters. In his "Recollection of Solferino", published in 1912, Dunant wrote that ". . .lamenting, screams of fear and pain, and heart-rending calls for help rang out in the dead of the night. Who could ever describe the agony of that horrible night". The Solferino experience marked the beginning of Dunant's fight for humanity during wartime. He became the force behind the Geneva Convention, which convened on 22 August, 1864 to improve the situation of injured soldiers and prisoners of war. Moreover, Dunant became the

he founded the "Volunteer Ambulance Service of Vienna" together with Hans Count Wilczek (1837–1922) and Edward Count Lamezan (1835–1903). Mundy had gathered a great deal of experience on various battlefields all over Europe, where he had worked as a care provider for the military, constantly striving to expand the radius and to improve the quality of care. Mundy's immense experience was an enormous advantage for the new civilian ambulance service.

Mundy was born on 3 October, 1822 at Eichhorn Castle in Moravia, a province of today's Czech Republic [2]. He was the youngest son of Johann Baron von Mundy and the Hungarian Isabella Countess Kálnoky von Köröspatak [3]. His mother doted on him, but his relationship with his father, a harsh and tyrannic man, was not close at all. It was Mundy's father who forced him to study theology [1]. Before long, however, Mundy decided to leave boarding school in Brno, where he was supposed to be studying theology and attain priesthood. To Mundy, whose love and interest were devoted to medicine, the idea of spending life as a priest was not attractive at all. His enthusiasm for medicine had become obvious during his boyhood, when he had loved nothing more than accompanying the country doctor and learning from him on his patient rounds. Enraged by that, Mundy's father forbade him to study medicine. Young Jaromir protested vehemently, but in vain—his father enrolled him as a cadet with the 49th Infantry Regiment at the Alser Barracks in Vienna [2].

Not even his father's decision could stop Mundy from devoting his interest to medicine. During his stay in Vienna he paid regular visits to the clinics of the General Hospital. In founder of the International Red Cross. On 10 December, 1901, Henri Dunant was awarded the Nobel Prize for peace.

As an Austrian delegate, Mundy took part in the Paris Conference, held on the occasion of the Paris World Exhibition to discuss the realization of the Geneva Convention [6]. He was a mesmerizing speaker and did everything in his power to support Dunant's cause and to improve social aid for the injured.

While Mundy was on an educational journey through England, the Austro-Prussian War broke out on 7 July, 1866. Mundy immediately contacted the Ministry of War to volunteer as a physician. He treated injured soldiers in the Battle of Koeniggraetz and supervised their transport to Vienna [3]. The injured were bedded on straw and transported back to Vienna from the battlefield in cattle cars without any medical care at all [1]. They were brought to the Prater park grounds, where a casualty clearing station had been set up under Mundy's supervision. Almost as many soldiers died during transport as on the battlefield. Mundy realized that the means of transport were unsatisfactory and racked his brains how to improve this intolerable situation. Thanks to his initiative, freight cars were equipped with shock-proof stretchers and the trains began carrying physicians and nursing personnel as care providers en route for injured soldiers [3].

Moreover, Mundy worked on the constructing of stretchers, ambulances and giant spotlights for the transport of injured soldiers from the battlefield in the dark. Again and again, Mundy criticized the municipal medical aid in Vienna, because he believed that all patients transported from the scene of an accident should be accompanied by medical personnel and because there was no such thing as medical personnel trained to deal with potential disasters. All his warnings had been ignored, however, until the great fire broke out in the Vienna Ring Theatre.

An action committee was founded at a meeting on 10 December, 1881. Wilczek was made President of Honour, Lamezan President and Mundy Secretary and Chief Physician of the Ambulance Society.

On 2 January, 1881, Wilczek and Lamezan submitted their "most humble plea for shelter and protection and for gracious expedition of the official decrees" to Emperor Francis Joseph I. One month later, the Imperial Governorship of Lower Austria certified the statutes and the Volunteer Ambulance Society of Vienna officially took office [1]. Wilczek donated the funds for the Ambulance Society and repeatedly provided financial support in the following years.

The foundation of the "Volunteer Ambulance Society of Vienna" marked the birth of an institution providing first aid by physicians and medically trained personnel anywhere—in the streets, in offices, in homes and in ambulances.

Almost at the same time, Jaromir Mundy, Hans Wilczek and the surgeon Theodore Billroth founded the "Rudolfiner House" under the protectorate of Crown Prince Rudolph [1]. Though at first it was merely a small hospital pavilion with wooden barracks to accommodate the patients, the Rudolfiner

House was soon to become famous. Mundy insisted that Billroth, who was quite reluctant initially, join the Rudolfiner Society. That marked the foundation of the first classic nursing school for the laity in Austria. Nurses were trained directly at the operating table by surgeons. Billroth's supervision and expertise led the institution to international fame. During the First World War (1914–1918) the Rudofiner House became a Red Cross Hospital and thousands of injured soldiers were treated there. After the war, the hospital faced serious problems for many years and more than once it was in danger of being shut down completely. Today, the Rudolfiner House is Vienna's leading private hospital.

The first outpatient service for the patients brought in by ambulance opened its doors in Wilczek's private villa. Since volunteers for the day shifts were difficult to find at first, the Ambulance Society decided to recruit medical students for the work [1].

The citizens of Vienna were encouraged to support the new institution, both financially and personally. Even the Emperor made a donation to the Society. Over the years, several charity balls and other events were organized for the benefit of the new institution for the sick and injured. The famous composer Johann Strauss wrote the "Freiwillige vor" (volunteers forward) march for the Ambulance Service and the "Jakob Lohner Company" built three (electrically powered) ambulance cars according to Mundy's own blue prints [1].

On 1 May, 1883, the first ambulance station was established on the Fleischmarkt in the heart of Vienna. Its car park included four ambulance cars, three horse-drawn carriages, two cars for the mentally ill and two cars for contagious patients. The Ambulance Society was called directly or telegraphically, and later via a direct telephone line to the police. In August of 1889, the Main Ambulance Station moved into a new facility on Stubenring 1. It had its own coach house with stables for the horses and the number of cars increased to 17. In July 1894, 10 more supervising physicians were engaged so that four physicians could be on duty around the clock [7]. In response to every call, one physician and two medically trained assistants, (comparable to today's emergency technicians) drove to the scene of the accident [1].

Mundy, who had been suffering from depression for many years, committed suicide on 23 August, 1894. He walked down to the bank of the Danube Canal under the Sophien Bridge and shot himself in the head with his own pistol. Apparently, Mundy had hoped he would tumble head over heels into the Danube Canal and drift downstream. Instead, he fell backwards into a bush. Shortly thereafter, a woman found him there with his feet dangling down into the water, his face and beard covered in blood from the shot wound behind his right ear. She hastened to call a policeman, but neither he nor any of the onlookers had any idea who the dead man could be. Later, a man who lived nearby was able to identify Mundy for the police. He had seen the Baron several times at accidents and fires and even knew his first

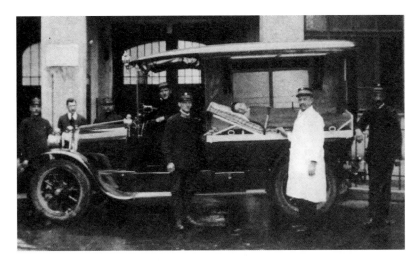

Fig. 3. Automobile ambulance of the Volunteer Ambulance Service of Vienna.

name, Jaromir. The embroidered initials J.M. were found on the dead man's clothing [1]. The City of Vienna provided a grave of honour, and he was buried at the Central Cemetery.

In 1897, the Ambulance Service had to clear its facility on Stubenring to make room for the new subway. Emperor Francis Joseph I designated a piece of land on Radetzkystrasse for the erection of a new Central Ambulance Station, which has remained at that location to this day.

Following the example of the Volunteer Ambulance Society of Vienna, other ambulance societies were founded by several European cities including Prague, Crakow, Trieste, Lemberg and Budapest. The Vienna Ambulance Service also supported similar organizations in Czernowitz, Johannesburg, Kiev, Odessa, Saint Petersburg and Warsaw, as well as volunteer ambulance departments in the Austrian cities Linz, Klagenfurt and Salzburg [1].

The Society also trained its own emergency technicians. The curriculum included eight 2-h lectures on anatomy, physiology, so-called "sudden illnesses", first aid for intoxications, correct handling of hemorrhage, fractures, contusions, sprains and dislocations, transport of accident victims, nursing and hygiene.

On 1 February, 1905, the Vienna Ambulance Service opened a second office at Mariahilfer Guertel 20. On that same day, the first automobile ambulance went into use [1] (Fig. 3).

The Vienna Ambulance Service dispatched well-equipped medical teams to disasters far beyond the city limits of Vienna, such as the earthquake in Ljubljana (1895), the flood in Prague (1897) and the earthquake in Sicily (1908).

During World War I, the Ambulance Service equipped a hospital train with 138 beds and organized transportation from the railway stations to the hospitals, so that injured soldiers could not only be transported directly from the front to the hospitals, but also treated en route the entire way. At the age of 77, Count Wilczek took command over the hospital train, which was under the authority of the Ministry of War [1].

After the Nazis took power over Austria in March 1938, Jewish physicians were forbidden to serve in the Ambulance Society. Because of the Society's financial problems and needs, the Fire Brigade of the City of Vienna took over in September of that same year. Shortly thereafter, the Society was integrated into the Ambulance Service of the City of Vienna under the authority of the Municipal Department of Health. At that time there were five Ambulance Stations and seven ambulances for the entire city of Vienna.

On Christmas Eve, 1944, the ambulance responded to 42 calls to people who had attempted to commit suicide with carburetted hydrogen because of the war [1]. By the end of World War II, most of the ambulance stations and cars had been destroyed. Reconstruction progressed with the help of the Allies and the International Committee of the Red Cross in Geneva, which provided ambulance cars.

Today, the Vienna Ambulance Service has roughly 650 employees, including 70 physicians. Dr. Alfred Kaff has been in charge since 1984.

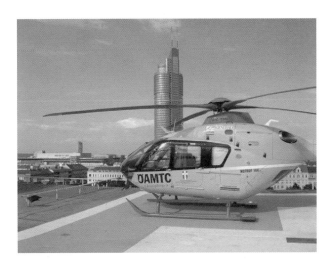

Fig. 4. Emergency helicopter Christophorus 9 of the Austrian Automobile and Touring Club.

The Vienna Ambulance Service responds to more than 170,000 calls annually. The main office relays each call directly to an ambulance in one of its 12 ambulance stations. One physician-staffed helicopter, four physician-staffed ambulance cars, 10 physician-staffed cars and 23 paramedic-staffed ambulance cars are on duty around the clock. Eight additional paramedic-staffed ambulance cars work a 13-hour shift. Special ambulance cars are available for disasters and operate according to the city of Vienna's multi-step disaster plan.

The Vienna Ambulance Service dispatches emergency physicians and technicians for the emergency helicopter Christophorus 9, operated by the Austrian Automobile and Touring Club. Christophorus 9 covers the entire city of Vienna and surroundings, with a radius of approximately 100 km (60 miles) and a range to the northeastern boundaries of Austria (Fig. 4).

Tragic as his life was, Mundy remained a humanitarian and an idealist, and never ceased to fight for the cause he believed in. He spoke up for the poor and was one of the greatest philanthropists of our day. No doubt Mundy deserves a place among the resuscitation greats. His heritage has prevailed to this day and has set a standard in the field of emergency medicine. Every Viennese ambulance car is a memorial to Jaromir Baron von Mundy.

## References

[1] Machala R. 100 Jahre ärztlicher Rettungsdienst in Wien. Wien: Verlag Urania; 1981.

[2] Moller N. Neue Deutsche Biographie. Berlin: Verlag Duncker und Humboldt; 1997.

[3] Höfler I. Jaromir Freiherr von Mundy. Wien: Verlag Helikon; 1994.

[4] Lesky E. Die Wiener Medizinische Schule im 19. Jahrhundert. Graz-Köln: Verlag Hermann Böhlaus; 1965.

[5] Mundy J. Eröffnungs-Vortrag über Psychiatrie. Wiener Medizinische Wochenschrift 1866;101:1615.

[6] Schlesinger W. Die Konferenz in Würzburg und Paris- Porträts aus denselben. Wiener Medizinische Wochenschrift 1868;18:89.

[7] Wyklicky H. Über Jaromir Mundy und die Anfänge eines ärztlichen Rettungsdienstes in Wien, 1881–1894. Wiener Medizinische Wochenschrift 1995;49:1030–1.

# Franz Koenig and Friedrich Maass

Markus Figl   Linda E. Pelinka  , Walter Mauritz

On March 21st, 1892 Dr. Friedrich Maass, resident at the Department of Surgery at the University of Goettingen, Germany, published his paper "Resuscitation technique following cardiac death after inhalation of chloroform" in the Berlin Clinical Weekly [1]. In that publication, Maass described the first successful performance of external cardiac massage.

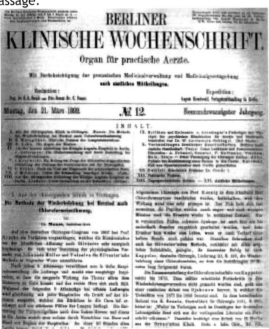

Friedrich Maass was a student of the famous German surgeon Professor Franz Koenig. Koenig was born in Rotenburg, Germany on February 16th 1832. He spent most of his medical school years in Marburg. After graduating, he became a general practitioner and was later appointed Professor of Surgery at the University of Rostock. In 1875, he was summoned to the University of Goettingen as chairman of the Department of Surgery. Koenig's special interest had always been devoted to surgical challenges such as lung injury [2—4]. It was in Goettingen that he developed his resuscitation technique using external cardiac massage.

Prior to 1891, hardly any progress had been made in treating so-called "chloroform syncope". In those days, sudden circulatory arrest during chloroform anaesthesia was usually fatal. In his Textbook of General Surgery [5], Koenig published his resuscitation technique for chloroform syncope, clearly describing how it was performed at the University of Goettingen. Professor Koenig had proposed compression of the "heart region" as an alternative to the ventilatory procedures used in the operating room at the time. Koenig's technique involved manual compression of the xyphoid area and costal margins at the rate of spontaneous respiration and was undoubtedly a form of assisted ventilation. It was generally successful within a few minutes or not at all.

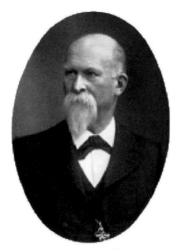

Franz Koenig 1832-1910

Maass discovered his new resuscitation technique in a desperate attempt to save a young life. In his paper published in 1892, Maass presented the case of a 9 year-old boy scheduled for surgery of the palate to correct his hare-lip. Surgery began after the boy had been anaesthetised with chloroform. However, since the patient woke up screaming and bucking the minute a surgical instrument was inserted in his mouth, a gauze swab with a second dose of chloroform was placed over his mask. Suddenly the boy's pupils dilated, his face turned dark blue and soon he stopped breathing altogether. Immediately, the attending physician forced the boy's mouth open, pulled his tongue forward and inserted his finger to lift the boy's epiglottis. Superficial spontaneous breathing now set in, but still no pulse was palpable. At this point the physicians started with Koenig's resuscitation technique, compressing the xyphoid area at a rate of 30—40 compressions per minute. Cyanosis soon disappeared and the boy's pupils contracted again, but still no pulse was palpable. The next step was tracheotomy. Thirty minutes later, the boy's condition had deteriorated to such a point, that his case was considered hopeless according to the medical experience of the day. In order to clear the operating room for the next case, the boy was wheeled into a side room and Friedrich Maass was instructed to continue compressing the xyphoid area until no further effect could be seen upon pupils or breathing.

Maass wrote:

''I kept on working in the same way for 3—4 min and had the impression that less and less air was flowing in and out. The boy's pupils were fully dilated and showed no reaction at all. His eye bulbs were limp, his face was deathly pale. He was not breathing at all and no pulse whatsoever was palpable. At this point I had to believe the boy was dead. Neverthe-less, I immediately started compressing the xyphoid area directly again, now working at a much quicker and forceful rate since I was extremely agitated. Very soon, the boy's pupils contracted a little. I continued compressing at the same rate and not only did the pupils soon grow even smaller than before, but erratic, gasping breathing set in as well during the chest compression interval. For the next half hour, I now continued compressing even more quickly with only a few short intervals. The following changes now took place: the boy's spontaneous breathing during the chest compression intervals appeared to grow stronger at first, and then grew clearly more rapid as well. About 50 min after the beginning of the syncope, I noticed some strange kind of chest movement near the boy's heart. Since I could not hear the heart making any sounds at all, I attributed this strange movement to twitching intercostal muscles. It was over an hour after the beginning of the syncope that I thought I felt something swirling in the boy's carotids. I continued my resuscitation attempts, and the boy's cheeks and lips, which had previously remained pale, became rosy within a very short time. I paused with resuscitation, and the boy continued to breathe very smoothly. A quick, feeble carotid pulse was now well palpable. Having grown quite cold, the boy was now bedded down with hot water bottles. His face grew intensely red. No radial pulse was palpable until approximately 1.5 to 2 h later. The pupils remained much dilated throughout the afternoon, but reacted to light. The boy continued to sleep deeply until the following morning, showing only some warding-off activity when slapped vigorously on the cheek. He did not answer at all. His condition improved very slowly. At first he was fed fluids only, since he was unable to digest solid food. For 8—10 days he remained completely stupid, but gradually regained his former level of intelligence. On December 10, 1891, the boy had recovered completely and was discharged from hospital.''

The second patient Maass described in his paper was a 13 year-old boy suffering from tuberculous coxitis and scheduled for hip joint resection. Surgery was performed under chloroform anaesthesia. After resection of the tuberculous femoral head, the acetabulum was to be cleared of tuberculous debris. When the surgeon pulled his leg to gain better access to the debris, the boy screamed and warded the surgeon off vigorously. More chloroform was then poured over the mask. Suddenly the boy's pupils dilated fully, he stopped breathing, his face turned slightly bluish and his radial pulse was no longer palpable. Again the surgeons began with Koenig's chest compression technique.

Maass wrote:

"Since the initially administered 30—40 chest compressions per minute were obviously showing no effect at all, I increased the compression rate to 120. Soon a carotid pulse wave corresponding to the increased chest compression rate was palpable. As soon as the compressions ceased, that pulse wave ceased as well. The boy's spontaneous breathing grew stronger and stronger during the compressions, so that I could soon feel his chest wall rising and falling with my compressing hand. After this condition had lasted for approximately an hour and 10 min, two weak carotid pulse waves seemed palpable immediately after I stopped compressing. I now continued my resuscitation attempts for three or four more minutes. At this point the boy's lips, which had previously remained very pale, though no longer blue, began to turn rosy. Now a quick feeble carotid pulse wave became clearly palpable during my chest compression intervals. The boy continued to breathe spontaneously and his pupils contracted somewhat. He was taken back to his bed and could then be left to himself."

Fifty-one days later, the boy underwent chloroform anaesthesia again and surgery was completed. This time there were no complications at all.

Maass felt that his main clinical observation was the success encountered with a more rapid rate of chest compression. In his paper, Maass described the technique of external cardiac compression massage as follows:

"One stands to the patient's left, facing his head, and compressing the area of the heart quickly, vigorously and deeply, with one's open right hand placed with the base of the thumb between the apex of the heart and the left sternal margin. The chest compression rate is 120 per minute and more. At such a high compression rate, one usually needs to beware more of carrying out each chest compression with sufficient strength than of compressing too strongly. The technique is somewhat easier to perform if one places one's left hand around the right side of the patient's chest to stabilize the body while compressing with one's right hand. The efficacy of resuscitation is reflected by the chest compression-driven carotid pulse wave and by the contraction of the pupils. Both the strength and rate of chest compressions need to be adapted to the individual patient. In order to check and re-check the effect and simultaneously be sure that the airway is still clear, a helper should be positioned at the head of the patient. As long as the patient's condition has not improved much, intervals between resuscitation attempts should be lim-ited to a minimum, both in number and duration. A certain degree of thoracic elasticity is clearly a prerequisite to chest compression. However, according to my own experience in resuscitating elderly patients, the chest wall rarely lacks the necessary degree of elasticity."

Unfortunately, very little is known about Friedrich Maass and any further efforts to promulgate his resuscitation technique after 1892. He published his two cases in German and French journals. He and Koenig also demonstrated their resuscitation technique at the Congress of Surgery in Berlin [6]. After spending several years in the United States of America (1897—1914), where he practiced surgery in Detroit and New York, Maass returned to Bremen, Germany [7]. Green's review of reported cases of successful internal and external heart massage as of 1906 fails to reference Maass [8]. Apparently, Maass' discovery never caught on outside Germany [9] and was brushed aside completely when attention began to focus upon restoring circulation by open cardiac compression. Sixty-nine years went by before heart massage by external chest compression was rediscovered by William Kouwenhoven, who was completely unaware that Maass had made the original discovery decades earlier. Kouwenhoven's paper [10], published in JAMA 69 years after Maass' paper had been published in the Berlin Clinical Weekly, convinced the world of the efficacy of external chest compression for cardiac arrest [11]. Internationally, Koenig's and Maass' achievement in the field of resuscitation has remained virtually unnoticed to this day. Nevertheless these two true pioneers of resuscitation definitely deserve their place among the resuscitation greats.

## References

1. Maass F. Die Methode der Wiederbelebung bei Herztod nach Chloroformeinathmung. Berliner Klinische Wochenschrift 1892;12:265—8.
2. Müller W. Franz König. Beilage zur Münchener medizinischen Wochenschrift. Blatt 284;1911.
3. Hoffmann K. Der Chirurg Franz König (1832—1910). Archiv des Institutes für Geschichte der Medizin, Wien.
4. Fischer I. Biographisches Lexikon der hervorragenden Ärzte der letzten fünfzig Jahre. Berlin: Urban und Schwarzenberg, 1933.
5. Urban G. Lehrbuch der kleinen Chirurgie. Leipzig: Veit & Comp.; 1896.
6. Boehrer H, Goerig M. Pioneers of cardiac massage. In: Schulte am Esch J, Goerig M, editor. Proceedings of the fourth international symposium of the history of anaesthesia. Dräger, Lübeck, 1998. pp. 389—93.
7. Taw R. Dr. Friedrich Maass: 100th anniversary of "new" cpr. Clin Cardiol 1991;14:1000—2.

8. Green T. Heart massage as a means of restoration in cases of apparent sudden death, with a synopsis of 40 cases. Lancet 1906;2:1708.

9. Overbeck W, Susskind-Schwendi G. Historical considerations on cardiac arrest and resuscitation. Thoraxchir Vask Chir 1969;17(2):177–84.

10. Jude R, Kouwenhoven W, Knickerbocker G. Cardiac arrest—report of application of external cardiac massage in 118 patients. JAMA 1961;178:1063.

11. Safar P. Cardiopulmonary Resuscitation. New York: Churchill Livingstone; 1989.

# Franz Kuhn, his contribution to anaesthesia and emergency medicine.

A. Thierbach

## 1. Medical training

Franz Kuhn (Fig. 1), fifth child of a wealthy landowner, was born on 12. October 1866 in Aschaffenburg, a small town close to Frankfurt.

He began his medical studies in Würzburg and continued in Berlin and Munich. Kuhn obtained the doctorate in Würzburg in 1891 with a dissertation entitled 'Morphologische Beiträge zur Leichenfäulnis' (The Morphology of Cadaveric Decomposition).

His medical training and career began at the Department of Surgery at the University Hospital in Giessen, Germany, in 1895, where he was assistant to Heinrich Bose and Peter Poppert. Bose had been working on various problems associated with tracheostomy, Poppert was known to be an expert in anaesthesia due to his publications on the risks of ether. Presumably, these teachers raised Kuhn's interest in the issue of asphyxia due to anaesthesia [1].

Very early, he was working on techniques of examining the gastro-intestinal tract using flexo-metallic bougies [2].

Slightly resembling the modern flexible non-occlusive endotracheal tube, strengthened by a metal wire in its wall, Kuhn's flexo-metallic tubes consisted of a spiral of thin metal with overlapping edges. Kuhn had proposed and published this principle for different purposes in medicine since 1896 [3]. After experience in examining the gastro-intestinal-tract he started studying its use for intubating the trachea in corpses, presumably influenced by his impressions from the United States.

In 1897, a scholarship enabled Kuhn to undertake an extensive study tour to the United States of America. His journey took him to New York

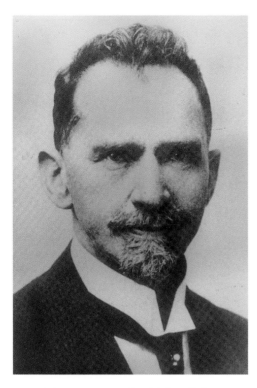

Fig. 1. Franz Kuhn (1866–1929).

City, Philadelphia, and Baltimore. There, he came first into contact with digital intubation techniques of the trachea and the Trendelenburg cone for administering volatile anaesthetics.

## 2. Endotracheal intubation

The newly built Elisabeth Hospital in Kassel, Germany, appointed Kuhn in 1899 director and specialist in surgery.

During the time at Kassel, Kuhn undertook his most important anaesthetic investigations. He published more than 90 papers, one third of which were concerned with orotracheal intubation of the trachea and the technique of positive pressure ventilation.

In 1900, Kuhn was confronted with a patient who died from a sudden haemorrhage in the throat. This incident is thought to have motivated him to develop a technique of securing the airway with his flexo-metallic bougies. In 1900, he had developed a metallic endotracheal tube [4]. The first detailed description of the technique of orotracheal intubation followed in 1901 [5]. He commenced this publication with his intention for his work: "I describe the tubage of the trachea to ensure an uncompromised airway without tracheostomy" (Author's translation).

Kuhn stated that 'the perioral tubage (intubation) keeps the airway open, even without traction of the tongue or protrusion of the mandible'. Another remarkable statement was that 'even the direct ventilation of air into the trachea with a rubber balloon would be workable and is the most appropriate measure in case of asphyxia'. Very early, he had noticed the importance of a secure airway during anaesthesia and surgery and he never stopped promoting this conviction [6]. 'If, during anaesthesia, respiration may become insufficient or even stops, and there is the need for artificial ventilation, what is the first measure to perform? Clear and secure the airway! How could this goal be achieved faster and safer than performing perioral tubage?' [7]

Kuhn's first tubes measured between 12 and 15 cm in length with a cylindrical shoulder close to the distal end, which helped to prevent the tube from being inserted too far into the trachea. At the proximal end of the tube, a shield was fixed to prevent damaging the tube by the teeth. He recommended using tubes with a diameter of 6–7 mm for children, 9 mm for women and up to 10 mm for men.

Although Kuhn mentioned the use of the Kirstein autoscope, a forerunner of the laryngoscope, he usually inserted the tube with a metal introducer by the help of digital palpation of the epiglottis and the arytenoid cartilages. The tube was fixed after insertion into the trachea with a rubber band to a metal hook. The proximal end of the tube could be connected with a Trendelenburg cone filled with gauze to administer chloroform and perform anaesthesia. A stethoscope attached to the cone was used to monitor the patient's breath sounds.

Some years later, Kuhn explained his favour of the flexo-metallic bougie as endotracheal tube in comparison with a rubber tube [8]. He wanted to obtain a drainage of the airway, comparable to surgical principles, to guarantee an open airway from the teeth down to the trachea. Therefore he was looking for a flexible, but non-compressible tube, similar to the natural cartilages of the trachea.

Kuhn performed tracheal intubation using this technique in the awake patient, using local anaesthesia — with cocaine and sometimes added epinephrine — of the upper airways, or under

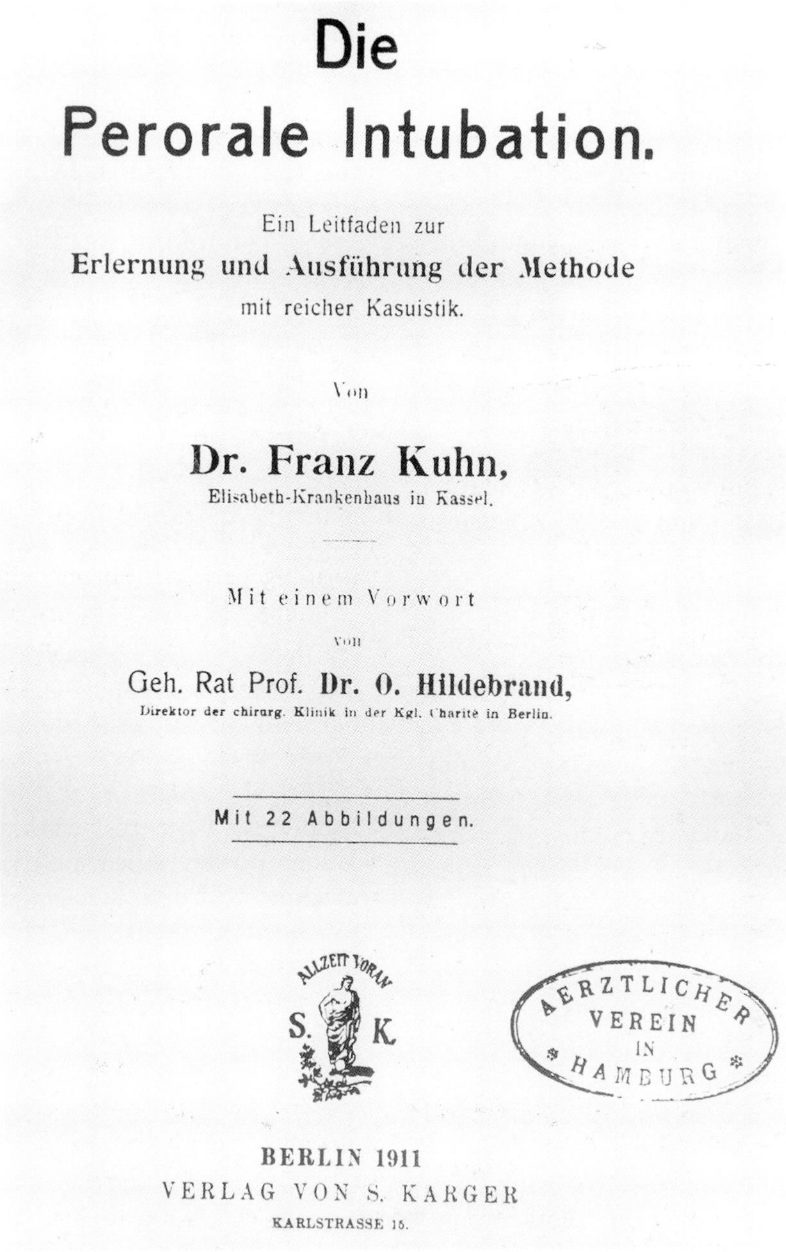

Die

Perorale Intubation.

Ein Leitfaden zur

Erlernung und Ausführung der Methode

mit reicher Kasuistik.

Von

Dr. Franz Kuhn,

Elisabeth-Krankenhaus in Kassel.

Mit einem Vorwort

von

Geh. Rat Prof. Dr. O. Hildebrand,

Direktor der chirurg. Klinik in der Kgl. Charité in Berlin.

Mit 22 Abbildungen.



BERLIN 1911

VERLAG VON S. KARGER

KARLSTRASSE 15.

Fig. 2. First textbook on intubation.

general anaesthesia. For premedication, he used a mixture of atropine and morphine, administered subcutaneously.

He recommended tracheal intubation in patients suffering from asphyxia, to perform resuscitation and, most important of all, during anaesthesia using chloroform. In a wide range of applications, he described the use of this technique in patients undergoing surgery of the gall bladder, resections of tongue and mandible tumors, neurosurgery and others. Kuhn published his findings and studies on intubating the trachea in 1911, presenting the first textbook covering this issue [9] (Fig. 2).

### 3. Emergency medicine

Franz Kuhn also published very modern and, in 1910, revolutionary ideas on resuscitation and airway management in asphyxiated patients by performing endotracheal intubation [10]. According to his findings from animal research, he recommended immediate artificial ventilation after intubation using an air pump, the application of oxygen, the infusion of warmed fluids and cardiac massage performed by rhythmic thoracic compressions in asphxiated patients. These resuscitative efforts should be continued for several hours [11].

Kuhn was also aware of another problem that existed, the individual qualification of doctors to perform emergency measures [12]. He demanded to reform the mechanical–technical part of resuscitation according to scientific knowledge, a very early reference to the now popular 'evidenced based medicine' principle.

In Kassel, Kuhn also worked on the problem of tracheal secretions. Beside premedication with atropine, he used a manually operated suction pump and flexible suction catheters to remove secretions and blood through his tubes.

Beside these anaesthetic studies, he also worked on surgical problems and introduced, to mention just one of the most important, sterile catgut into surgical practice [13].

## 4. The controversy with Sauerbruch

Before Ferdinand Sauerbruch invented the revolutionary concept of a negative pressure operating chamber for thoracic surgery in 1904, surgical interventions on the thoracic organs were extremely uncommon, except for emergency cases. The patient breathed spontaneously while the thorax was placed in a large negative pressure chamber where the surgeons could operate on the thorax avoiding a pneumothorax.

Franz Kuhn, in opposition to the generally accepted opinion, proposed using his endotracheal tube — after tamponade of the hypopharynx — to perform positive pressure directly to the lungs so avoiding a pneumothorax during thoracotomy. He also made experiments with a rubber coating of his metallic tubes to assure its airtightness. Rubber balloons, similar to a tube cuff, were placed in the pharynx, larynx or trachea to seal the airway and enable positive pressure ventilation.

Together with Dräger, an anaesthesia machine manufacturer, he developed the Kuhn–Dräger anaesthesia machine for positive pressure ventilation (Fig. 3) [14].

Unfortunately, Sauerbruch had become such an influential figure, especially in Germany, that Kuhn's novel ideas were met with hostility and — due to Sauerbruch's opposition and Kuhn's intubation difficulties during clinical demonstrations — further development of the routine use of tracheal intubation was considerably delayed [15,16]. Another reason for the very slow spread of this technique of securing the airway was the introduction of local anaesthetics into clinical practice at this time. Some surgeons performed up to 80% of operations under local anaesthesia, because the use of chloroform was thought to be dangerous, even by federal authority and jurisdiction [1].

## 5. Anaesthesia machines

Franz Kuhn also worked on more effective and safe ways of administering volatile anaesthetics, mainly chloroform. Until this time, the liquid chloroform had to be dripped on a Schimmelbusch mask held over the patients face.

Kuhn's very practical and modern solution was an injector system, using the Venturi principle. The Dräger company used this type of injector in many of their anaesthesia machines until the first World War.

The absorption of carbon dioxide in closed anaesthesia systems was also investigated by Kuhn. He developed a closed system anaesthesia machine with two soda lime canisters and valves to direct the gas flow [14]. Due to a large deadspace in the system and the fear of possible

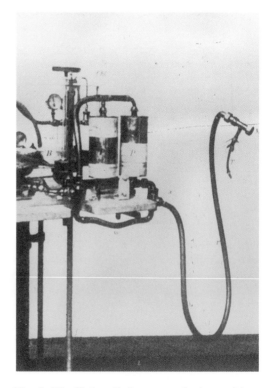

Fig. 3. The Kuhn–Dräger anaesthesia machine.

interaction between the soda lime and the chloroform, he did not finish his investigations on this issue.

## 6. Kuhn's work in Berlin

In 1913, Kuhn became Director of the newly built St. Norbert Hospital in Berlin Schöneberg. During 1912 and 1913, Kuhn developed with the Braun company a dextrose based isotonic infusion, which should be applied to prevent, among other indications, venous thrombosis.

Beside studies on a high pressure applicator for local anaesthetics, Kuhn worked mainly on surgical questions at the St. Norbert Hospital [17].

On 28 March 1929, Franz Kuhn died of lung carcinoma in Berlin.

To modern anaesthesiologists, it seems puzzling that Franz Kuhn with his enormous technical and scientific contribution to anaesthesia was not properly recognised until the second half of the 20th century [18].

In 1974, Zinganell [19] unveiled a plaque at the Elisabeth Hospital in Kassel, where Kuhn performed his major works:

*Here worked from 1899 until 1913*
*Dr Franz Kuhn.*
*His orotracheal intubation was a pioneer work*
*for the anaesthesia today.*
*German Society of Anaesthesia and Resuscitation*
*Society of German Anaesthesiologists.*

## References

[1] Goerig M. Franz Kuhn (1866–1929) on the 125th anniversary of his birthday. Anaesthesiol Intensivrned Notfallmed Schmerzther 26;1991:416–24.

[2] Kuhn F. Die Meta I Isch la uchsonde im Dienste der klinischen Diagnostik, insbesondere des Magen-Darm-Kanals. Münch Med Wochenschr 1896;43:8658.

[3] Kuhn F. Die Bedeutung des Metallschlauchprinzips für die praktische Medizin, Z prakt Ärzte 1896; 21.

[4] Kuhn F. Der Metallschlauch in der Tubage und als Trachealkancile. Wien klin Rdsch 1900;28:554.

[5] Kuhn F. Die perorale Intubation. Zentralbl Chir 1901;28:1281–5.

[6] Kuhn F. Kein Pressen und Erbrechen bei Narkosen. Bin klin Wochenschr 1903;17:402–3.

[7] Kuhn F. Technik der peroralen Tubage. Dtsch med Wochenschr 1902;28:539–41.

[8] Kuhn F. Perorale Tubage mit und ohne Druck. I. Teil: Perorale Tubage und pulmonale Narkose. Dtsch Z Chir 1905;76:148–207.

[9] Kuhn F. Die perorale Intubation; ein Leitfaden zur Erlernung und Ausführung der Methode mit reicher Kasuistik [Oral Intubation; A Guide for Learning and Executing this Method Including a wide Selection of Casuistics], 1911.

[10] Kuhn F. Die Wiederbelebung durch Ventilation der Luftwege per vias naturalis, Münch Med Wochenschr 1910; 57.

[11] Kuhn F. Asphyxie (Scheintod) und Tubage, Therap Gegenwart 1905; 442-54.

[12] Kuhn F. Die erste Hilfe bei Asphyxien mittels direkter Einblasung von Luft, Münch Med Wochenschr 1913; 647-50.

[13] Kuhn F. Katgut vom gesunden Schlachttier. Münch Med Wochenschr 1906;41:2018–20.

[14] Kuhn F. Perorale Tubage mit und ohne Druck. III. Teil: Apparat zur Lieferung des Druckes für die Überdrucknarkose. Dtsch Z Chir 1906;81:63–70.

[15] Sweeney B, Kuhn Franz. His contribution to anaesthesia. Anaesthesia 1985;41:2018–20.

[16] Brandt L. The history of endotracheal anesthesia, with special regard to the development of the endotracheal tube. Anaesthesist 1986;35:523–30.

[17] Klimpel V. Our surgical heritage. On the development of abdominal surgery in the mirror of the controversy between Franz Kuhn and Hans Kehr. Zentralbl Chir 1990;115:919–23.

[18] Luckhaupt H, Brusis T. History of intubation. Laryngol Rhinol Otol 1986;65:506–10.

[19] Zinganell K. Franz Kuhn, pioneer of peroral intubation]. Anaesthesist 1974;23:308–11.

# The 1900s

The 20$^{th}$ century saw an increasing amount of research and discovery in resuscitation, much of it building on the concepts that had been suggested in the previous two centuries. The century opened with discovery of blood groups by **Karl Landsteiner**. Following on the work of **James Blundell** some 80 years earlier, Landsteiner's work brought blood transfusion into clinical reality and probably represents one of the greatest benefits for mankind in this century of war and escalating non-military trauma.

Although **Sir Robert Woods** had demonstrated the efficacy of mouth-to-mouth ventilation in 1906, interest in manual methods of artificial ventilation, based on the earlier work of **Marshall Hall** and **Henry Silvester**, continued during the first half of this century with contributions by **Edward Sharpey Schafer, Holger Nielsen** who understood the protection offered by the prone position, and by **Frank Eve** whose rocking method was surprisingly effective if the equipment was at hand. Airway control remained a difficult problem for many. Simple effective airways were devised by **Arthur Guedel** and **Morris Brook**. The latter offered an opportunity for artificial ventilation as well and was in regular use until the 1960s.

The ravages of the two world wars brought the need for extensive reparative maxillo-facial surgery and this was made possible by **Sir Ivan Magill** whose work on oral and nasal tracheal tubes, laryngoscopes and blind nasal intubation techniques made this surgery feasible. Tracheal intubation remains the gold standard of airway management during resuscitation. **Sir Robert Macintosh** popularised the technique of safe anaesthesia and tracheal intubation throughout the world. Working with Sir Robert the intrepid and courageous **Edgar Pask** demonstrated the success of various methods of resuscitation after immersion, using himself as the subject. **Virginia Apgar** from New York devised a score for resuscitation assessment of the newborn which holds fast today.

With the advent of electricity came accidental electrocution of line workers and the Edison Company sponsored research into the mechanism and potential reversal of electrocution. Early work was carried out in Baltimore by **William Kouwenhoven** who worked on the effects of electricity on animal hearts and developed internal defibrillation. Unknown to the Western world **Naum Gurvich** in Russia was also developing defibrillation at the same time and indeed had made great progress. Once again research and progress was interrupted by another world war but interest in electricity continued soon afterwards and **Claude Beck** was the first to perform internal defibrillation on a patient. **Bernard Lown** and **Paul Zoll** developed the technique of external defibrillation and **Frank Pantridge** made the first portable defibrillator, enabling defibrillation to be used in the pre-hospital situation. **Douglas Chamberlain** was amongst the first to implement a public access defibrillation programme using the new semi-automatic defibrillators.

The second world war had devastated Europe. There was no money for research and many traveled to the United States in search of opportunities. One such person was **Peter Safar** from Vienna who was to make a landmark contribution to resuscitation. When reestablished in Baltimore he met with **James Elam** who was working in an animal laboratory. Together they demonstrated that expired air ventilation was effective and produced normal blood gas values in paralysed human volunteers. Shortly afterwards, also in Baltimore, **William Kouwenhoven** and **Guy Knickerbocker,** working with animals, discovered, almost by accident, that external chest compressions could produce a demonstrable cardiac output. In collaboration with **James Jude,** a clinical colleague, they were able to show that the technique could support the circulation after cardiac arrest in humans. Indeed, the results they achieved using compressions only rival many of the best resuscitation survival figures reported today. Safar was quick to realise the potential for a combination of expired air ventilation and external chest compressions, which he called Cardiopulmonary Resuscitation or CPR. Safar had the energy, drive and persuasiveness to popularise the method and overcome a natural aesthetic resistance to mouth-to-mouth ventilation. At the same time, **Henning Ruben** from Copenhagen had shown the need for head tilt to maintain a patent airway. He also developed the self-inflating bag which probably saved more lives than any other piece of equipment in the early stages of resuscitation. **Brian Sellick** from London demonstrated the value of cricoid pressure in the emergency patient.

CPR was all very well, but how to teach it? This was where **Asmund Laerdal,** a toymaker from Stavanger, came in. He visited **Bjorn Lind** to learn more about the new method of mouth-to-mouth ventilation. They approached Peter Safar to discuss a training manikin: ResusciAnne was born and the problem of training in CPR was largely solved. Since then the company has continued to evolve and thrive under the leadership of Tore Laerdal, Asmund's son, and it is now in the forefront of simulation training and distance learning.

By the early 1970s resuscitation was a well established sub-speciality with the journal *Resuscitation* under the editorship of **Harold Hillman.** Stimulated by the of work of **Frank Pantridge** in Belfast, pre-hospital schemes for resuscitation were developed world wide by **Eugene Nagel** in Miami, by **Cobb** and **Eisenberg** in Seattle, by **Peter Safar** and **Nancy Caroline** in Pittsburgh, by **Rudolf Frey** and **Fritz Ahnefeld** in Germany, by **Stig Holmberg** in Sweden, by **Douglas Chamberlain** and Peter Baskett in Brighton and Bristol in the United Kingdom, and by Pierre Carli in France.

In the paediatric world **Gordon Jackson Rees,** the master of paediatric anaesthesia and critical care was joined by **Leon Chameides** who did so much to promote training in paediatric resuscitation through the Americian Heart Association.

Post resuscitation care was made possible by the introduction of the intensive care unit in the 1950s by **Bjorn Ibsen** and the technique of controlled ventilation using muscle relaxants pioneered by **Cecil Gray** and **Gordon Jackson Rees** in Liverpool. **Vladimir Negovsky** in Moscow had been studying 'reanimatology' since the 1930s and teamed up with Peter Safar in the 'cold war' years to build on the much earlier work of **Temple Fay** on hypothermia at the beginning of the century. It was not until the end of the century that mild hypothermia was introduced into regular clinical practice for comatose survivors of cardiac arrest.

# Karl Landsteiner, the discoverer of blood groups

Markus Figl    Linda E. Pelinka

*"Wherever a blood transfusion is performed in the world today, wherever a worried mother's threatened child is saved, Karl Landsteiner is virtually present".*

Those were the final words of Hermann Chiari's speech at the unveiling of the Landsteiner memorial in the arcades of the University of Vienna in 1961 [1].

One hundred and three years ago, in November 1901, the Viennese Weekly Journal of Medicine published a paper entitled "Agglutination phenomena of normal human blood" by Karl Landsteiner [2]. That paper marked the discovery of blood groups, setting the stage for blood transfusions and further research in various fields of science. In 1930, Landsteiner was awarded the Nobel Prize for this milestone in the field of medicine.

Karl Landsteiner was born in Baden, in the province of Lower Austria, on 14 June 1868 (Fig. 1). His parents, Fanny and Leopold Landsteiner, a Viennese Journalist and newspaper publisher, residents of the Austrian capital of Vienna, were spending their traditional summer vacation in the idyllic nearby spa of Baden [1].

Only 7 years later, Leopold Landsteiner died. Since he had been Mosaic, his son Karl was brought up in the same faith. While Karl Landsteiner was studying at the university, however, he and his mother converted to Catholicism. On 4 December 1890, he was baptised to the name Karl Otto in the Schotten Church in Vienna [1]. Later, he went to great lengths to keep his Jewish background absolutely secret. When his biography appeared in the encyclopaedia entitled "Who's Who in American Jewry", published in the United States in 1937, Landsteiner vehemently protested and sued for $ 100.000. He admitted that his parents had been Jewish, but pointed out that he himself had been living according to the Christian faith since 1890. He lost the lawsuit [3].

Landsteiner, who went to school in Linz, in the province of Upper Austria and in Vienna, the capital of Austria, was a good pupil, particularly gifted in science. He passed his final exams and graduated from the Austrian Imperial High School, Wasagasse, in the 9th district of Vienna in 1885. In autumn of the same year, Landsteiner entered Medical School at the Alma Mater Rudolfina of the University of Vienna. The faculty included famous scientists such as the anatomist Carl Toldt, the internist Otto Kahler, the surgeon Theodore Billroth and the physiologist Siegmund Exner [1].

As a medical student, Landsteiner was fascinated by research, particularly in the field of chemistry. He began performing experiments in the laboratory of his chemistry professor, Ernest Ludwig, where he also published his first papers on chemical topics [1]. These early skills and accomplishments in chemistry formed the basis for Landsteiner's later serological work. He joined the military as a medical student, serving as a volunteer for 1 year with the medical field unit. Landsteiner graduated from Medical School on 18 February 1891. Soon afterwards, in July of the same year, he was awarded the military rank of attending physician of the reserve first class [1].

He began his clinical training at the II. University Department of Internal Medicine under Otto Kahler, the first physician to publish a report on multiple myeloma. Landsteiner's particular interest, however, continued to be devoted to chemistry and he increased his knowledge during numerous visits abroad with Arthur Hantzsch in Zurich, Switzerland, with the 1902 Nobel Prize winner for chemistry Emil Hermann Fischer in Wurzburg, Germany and with Eugene Bamberger in Munich, Germany. After returning to Vienna he began his surgical training at the I. University Department of Surgery under Eduard Albert [1].

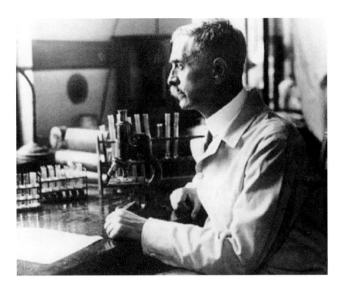

Fig. 1. Karl Landsteiner (1868–1943).

At 27 years of age, Landsteiner completed his clinical training and devoted his entire interest to research. He began at the University Institute for Microbiology and Hygiene under Max von Gruber, who strongly influenced Landsteiner's scientific career. His work in the field of bacteriology and serology began at that institute [1]. He proceeded to the Institute for Pathology under Anthony Weichselbaum, where he remained for the next 10 years. During that time, Landsteiner performed and documented 3639 dissections and wrote several papers dealing with haematology, serology, bacteriology, virology and pathology [1].

His highly interesting experiments, which led to the discovery of blood groups, were performed there. Landsteiner drew samples of venous blood from himself as well as from his colleagues working in the prosectorate and from laboratory assistants [1]. After mixing each one of these samples with each one of the other samples, he observed that in some sample mixtures red blood cells formed clots which were even visible to the naked eye, while other sample mixtures showed no reaction at all. From this observation Landsteiner concluded that red blood cells must be carrying a substance which reacts with corresponding substances carried by some of the samples examined. The reason why agglutination did or did not take place was precisely the reason why previous blood transfusions between humans were not invariably successful and why such medical procedures were even prohibited in some countries. As early as the year 1900, Landsteiner anticipated his later discovery. In a footnote to his publication "Anti-fermentative, lytic and agglutinating effects of blood serum and lymph", he stated that "the serum of healthy humans has an agglutinating effect, not only upon animal blood cells, but frequently upon blood cells from other individuals as well", pointing out that "the question is whether this phenomenon is due to inherent individual differences or to the effect of inflicted damage, e.g. of bacterial nature" [4]. The following year, Landsteiner himself answered this ques-

tion in his publication "Agglutination phenomena of normal human blood" [2] (Fig. 2), attributing this phenomenon to inherent individual differences and describing the human blood groups A, B and O. The setting for safe blood transfusions had finally become reality. The well-known basic immunological rule, the so-called "Landsteiner Rule", which states that the serum of each human contains only iso-haemagglutinins that are *not* directed against the agglutinable substance of that human's erythrocytes, is derived from that publication [2]. The fourth main blood group AB was discovered the following year by Landsteiner's co-workers, Alfred Decastello and Adriano Sturli, at the II. University Department of Internal Medicine [1].

At first, Landsteiner's discovery was only acknowledged to a limited extent by medical circles. Thus, he was forced to continue with research in other fields. In 1903 Landsteiner received his Ph.D. in the field of pathology with the publication entitled "On opaque swelling", a patho-histological study of parenchymatous degeneration [5]. In 1904, Landsteiner and Julius Donath were able to clarify the patho-physiological mechanism of paroxysmal cold-induced haemoglobinuria. By proving that this disease is due to specific antibodies, they provided the first work ever published on auto-antibodies and auto-immune disease [6].

During his years at the Institute of Pathology, Landsteiner was also involved in reasearch on syphilis. Together with Viktor Mucha, an assistant at the Department of Syphilidol-

Aus dem pathologisch-anatomischen Institute in Wien.

## Ueber Agglutinationserscheinungen normalen menschlichen Blutes.

Von Dr. Karl Landsteiner, Assistenten am pathologisch-anatomischen Institute.

Vor einiger Zeit habe ich beobachtet und mitgetheilt[1]), dass öfters Blutserum von normalen Menschen rothe Blutkörperchen anderer gesunder Individuen zu verklumpen im Stande ist. Ich hatte damals den Eindruck, dass in manchen Krankheitsfällen diese verklumpende Eigenschaft des Blutserums fremden Blutkörperchen gegenüber besonders deutlich wäre und meinte, dass sie mit dem von Maragliano[2]) viel früher beobachteten starken Lösungsvermögen pathologischer Sera für normale Körperchen in Zusammenhang sein könne, da ja Agglutinations- und Lösungsvermögen häufig, wenn auch nicht immer, parallel sich ändern. Gegen die Gleichsetzung der Reactionen von Maragliano mit den jetzt so häufig untersuchten hämolytischen Reactionen der Blutsera spricht der Umstand, dass zwar nicht Erwärmen, wohl aber Zusatz von Kochsalz bis zu einem Gehalt, der dem normalen gleichkommt, das Lösungsvermögen der Sera aufhebt. Maragliano selbst unterscheidet seine Beobachtung von der Erscheinung von Landois — der Hämolyse durch artfremdes Serum, dadurch — dass in seinem Fall das Hämoglobin nicht nur gelöst, sondern auch zerstört wird. Ein wesentlicher Unterschied meiner Beobachtung und der von Maragliano besteht darin, dass im Falle von Maragliano das Serum auch auf die Körperchen, die vom selben Individuum stammen, wirkt und dass seine Reaction nur mit krankhaftem Blut gelingt. Meine Beobachtung zeigte aber gerade Unterschiede recht sinnfälliger Art zwischen Blutserum und Körperchen verschiedener anscheinend völlig gesunder Menschen.

ogy and Dermatology, Landsteiner developed a new method of diagnosing spirochetes by microscope, using the darkfield technique [7]. Moreover, Landsteiner and Ernest Finger succeeded in transferring syphilis from humans to monkeys, an important scientific accomplishment which had previously been associated with considerable methodological problems [8,9].

Poliomyelitis was another field to which Landsteiner contributed considerably. By transferring the disease to monkeys, he was able to prove that poliomyelitis is a viral disease [10]. Together with Constantin Levaditi of the Pasteur-Institute in Paris, Landsteiner reported that the poliomyelitis virus can be filtered [11] and is conservable in glycerine [12]. Furthermore and most importantly, they reported that the poliomyelitis virus can be inactivated in vitro by the serum of monkeys that have had poliomyelitis [13].

In 1908 Landsteiner became the Head of the Prosectorate of the Imperial Wilhelminen Hospital in Vienna. His mother, to whom he was extremely devoted, died that same year. Her picture hung in Landsteiner's bedroom for the rest of his life, even after he moved to the United States. On 4 November 1916, he married Helen Wlasto, who bore his only son Ernest Karl [1].

The year 1919 markedly affected Landsteiner's further career. Life in Vienna after World War I was almost unbearable. During the financial and social disaster associated with the collapse of the Austro-Hungarian monarchy, Landsteiner finally decided that he had no choice but to leave his country, since he had no opportunity to continue his scientific work in impoverished post-war Austria. He moved to Holland, where a colleague helped him in find employment as a prosector at the Catholic R. K. Hospital in Den Haag. However, Landsteiner found working conditions there unsatisfactory and was quite disappointed [1].

Thanks to his good reputation, Landsteiner finally received an offer from the board of directors of the Rockefeller Institute for Medical Research in New York. In the spring of 1923 he moved from Scheveningen, Holland to the United States of America. He was provided with a laboratory fully equipped for chemical research. In spite of the good working conditions at the Rockefeller Institute, Landsteiner was only able to do a limited amount of bacteriological and virological research, since the institute was run according to very strict rules and regulations, restricting his work to a closely defined field. During his visits to Vienna, Ludwik Hirszfeld, who discovered the inheritability of blood groups together with Emil von Dungern [14], mentioned that Landsteiner had originally planned to continue his research on poliomyelitis in New York. It turned out that he was unable to do so, however, since another colleague was already assigned to research in that field [1]. Therefore, Landsteiner's work in New York was devoted mainly to immunological, serological and genetic topics. In 1927, Landsteiner and Philipp Levine described three more genetic characteristics of human blood, which they specified as M, N and P [15]. These genetic characteristics are important for the determination of paternity as well as for identification of suspects involved in criminal cases.

The Rhesus factor, another antibody in human blood, was also discovered by Landsteiner [16]. This discovery explained the occasional incompatibility reactions during transfusion of compatible blood groups as they were known at the time, and was essential for understanding the aetiology of haemolytic neonatal disease [17]. While at the Rockefeller Institute, Landsteiner also wrote his book on "The specificity of serological reactions" [18]. This fundamental work in serology and immunology is devoted to the research performed by Landsteiner and co-workers on antigens in general, serological specificity of proteins, cellular antigens and serologic reactions with chemical substances.

Landsteiner became an American citizen in 1929. During his years at the Rockefeller Institute, he received several honours and awards which contributed to his outstanding international reputation. In 1927 the University of Chicago awarded him its honorary doctorate, terming Landsteiner "the world's greatest authority on the mechanism of immunology". In 1929 Landsteiner was President of the American Association of Immunologists [1].

On 10 December 1930 Landsteiner was awarded the Nobel Prize for Medicine in Stockholm. When first informed that he was to receive the prize, Landsteiner took hardly any notice at all. To his co-worker, Philip Levine, he commented later that he would have preferred receiving the Nobel Prize for his contributions to the fundamental chemistry of serological reactions rather than for the discovery of blood groups and their role in blood transfusion [1]. In his lecture at the Nobel Prize ceremony, entitled "On the individual differences of human blood" [19], Landsteiner addressed the school of thought on the development of different structures in flora and fauna. He presented the blood groups he had discovered as proof for the fact that several complex differences exist not only between different species, but between members of the same species as well.

Immediately after being awarded the Nobel Prize, Landsteiner was also honoured by the Republic of Austria, which awarded him the honorary membership of the Society of Physicians in Vienna. Further honours followed, including the honorary doctorates of the Universities of Cambridge and Brussels in 1934. Harvard University awarded Landsteiner an honorary doctorate in 1936, stating that "he founded a school of thought which has penetrated wherever immunologists are at work" [1].

Landsteiner was known as an extremely critical scientist and teacher. His co-workers and assistants were required to repeat all important experiments right before his eyes. All scientific results were checked in detail by Landsteiner himself. He was a private person who shied away from the public and the limelight and detested commotion and quarrelling. According to one story, Landsteiner, a passionate piano player, sold his own piano one day to avoid any further quarrels with his neighbours. The only reason was that his piano music annoyed them while they were listening to the radio [1]. At the laboratory he was a stubborn tyrant, characteristically unsatisfied, sceptical and pessimistic. Levine used to say that Landsteiner's personal relationship with some colleagues at the Rockefeller Institute was not always the best. He frequently heard Landsteiner complain about having been treated unfairly by colleagues and about insufficient financial means. Even Hans Zinsser, Head of the Department of Bacteriology and Immunology at Harvard University, who was very fond of him, once gave Landsteiner a pat on the shoulder when he heard him complaining again and said: "You know, Karl, you are an old crab" [1].

The last years of Landsteiner's life were overshadowed by his concern for his wife, who was suffering from a malignant tumour of the thyroid gland. Day and night he was busy doing research on malignant tumours, hoping to discover some help for his wife. When he realised that he would not be able to do so, he deteriorated physically and mentally. At the age of 75, Landsteiner had a heart attack in the laboratory at the Rockefeller Institute. After resisting stubbornly for some time, he finally agreed to being admitted to a hospital. He died 2 days later on 26 June 1943 [1].

A student of the Vienna Medical School, Landsteiner is among the outstanding scientists of the 20th century. His research and publications in the fields of haematology, bacteriology, virology, and above all in the fields of serology and immunology remain fundamental and indispensable for the world of medicine today. His work on blood groups has made Landsteiner one of the great benefactors of humanity and has saved millions of lives. There is no doubt that Landsteiner deserves his place among the Resuscitation Greats as one of the most accomplished scientists of all time.

# References

[1] Speiser P, Smekal FG. Karl Landsteiner. Wien: Verlag Brüder Hollinek; 1975.
[2] Landsteiner K. Über Agglutinationserscheinungen normalen menschlichen Blutes. Wien Klin Wochenschr 1901;46:1132–4.
[3] Angetter D. Die österr eichischen Medizinnobelpreisträger. In: Österreichisches Biographisches Lexikon- Schriftenreihe 8. Wien: Institut Österreichisches Biographisches Lexikon und biographische Dokumentation; 2003. pp. 44–57.
[4] Landsteiner K. Zur Kenntnis der antifermentativen, lytischen und agglutinierenden Wirkungen des Blutes und der Lymphe. Zbl Bakt 1900;27:357–62.
[5] Landsteiner K. Über trübe Schwellung. Beitr Pathol Anat Allg Pathol 1903;33:237–80.
[6] Donath J, Landsteiner K. Über paroxysmale Hämoglobinurie. Münch Med Wochenschr 1904;51:1590–3.
[7] Landsteiner K, Mucha V. Zur Technik der Spirochätenuntersuchung. Wien Klin Wochenschr 1906;19:1349–50.
[8] Finger E, Landsteiner K. Untersuchung über Syphilis an Affen, Erste Mitteilung. Sitzgsber Akad Wiss Math naturw 1905;114(3):497–503.
[9] Finger E, Landsteiner K. Untersuchung über Syphilis an Affen. Zweite Mitteilung. Sitzgsber Akad Wiss Math naturw 1906;115(3):179–200.
[10] Landsteiner K, Popper E. Übertragung der Poliomyelitis acuta auf Affen. Zeitschr Immun Forsch 1909;2(1):377–90.
[11] Landsteiner K, Levaditi C. La transmission de la paralysie infantile aux singes. Compt Rend Soc Biol (Paris) 1909;67:592–4.
[12] Landsteiner K, Levaditi C. La paralysie infantile experimentale. Compt Rend Soc Biol (Paris) 1909;67:787–9.
[13] Levaditi C, Landsteiner K. La Poliomyelite experimental. Compt Rend Soc Biol (Paris) 1910;68:311–3.
[14] Dungern E, Hirszfeld L. Über Vererbung gruppenspezifischer Strukturen des Blutes. Zeitschr Immun Forsch 1910;6:284–92.
[15] Landsteiner K, Levine P. A new agglutinable factor differentiating individual human bloods. Proc Soc Exp Biol (NY) 1927;24:600–2.
[16] Landsteiner K, Wiener A. An agglutinable factor in human blood recognized by immune sera for rhesus blood. Proc Soc Exp Biol (NY) 1940;43:223.
[17] Levine Ph, Burnham L, Katzin EM, Vogel P. The role of isoimmunization in the pathogenesis of erythroblastosis fetalis. Am J Obstet Gynecol 1941;42:925–37.
[18] Landsteiner K. Die Spezifität der serologischen Reaktionen. Berlin: Springer; 1933.
[19] Landsteiner K. Über individuelle Unterschiede des menschlichen Blutes. Les Prix Nobel en 1930 Imprimerie Royal Stockholm 1931:1–13.

# Cemil Topuzlu Pasha: One of the forgotten pioneers in the history of open chest cardiac massage

Mustafa Karatepe    Erkan Tomatir    Pervin Bozkurt

One of the pioneers of open chest cardiac massage was Cemil Topuzlu Pasha, in Turkey. Although, he had presented his experiences in cardiopulmonary resuscitation in several papers published in Ottoman and French and German, Cemil Pasha does not appear in the context of modern resuscitation literature.[1-3] Other than presenting his experiences he had reviewed the literature and knowledge available at the beginning of the 20th century regarding the open chest cardiac massage. In Cemil Pasha's comments the terminology of ''do not resuscitate'' was introduced.

Cemil Topuzlu was born in 1866 and entered Military Medical School at age of 15. After his graduation from medical school he was sent to Paris to study modern surgery. Between 1887 and 1890 he worked as assistant to the famous French surgeon Jules Pean. After returning to his home country,

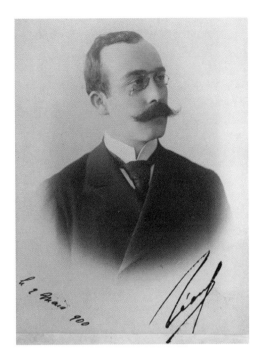

**Figure 1** Portrait of Cemil Topuzlu Pasha.

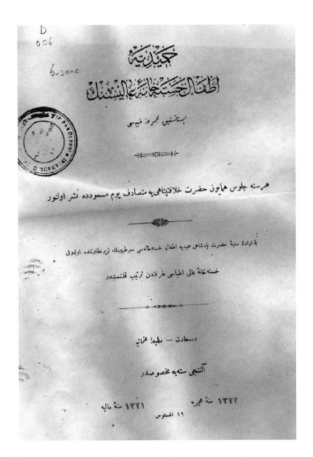

**Figure 2** Cover of the journal from which the translations are presented in this article.[1]

he was assigned to Haydarpasa military hospital as a surgeon and became a member of the teaching staff of the medical school. In 1893, he and his colleagues Pean, Trea, Oluya and a group of surgeons established "Association Française de Chirurgie". He had made great efforts in designing and constructing famous hospitals in Istanbul. At the same time he was the Sultan's personal doctor (Figure 1). After successful work in a short period of time he was made a Pasha by the sultan. He had worked as president of Istanbul municipality (1912–1914, 1919–1920) and introduced major evolutions in the era of public health in Istanbul.[3,4]

On 27 August 1903 in the surgical department of the Medical Faculty, while he was performing an external urethrotomy under chloroform anaesthesia, the patient developed a cardiac arrest and he performed open chest cardiac massage.

He reported this case that same year in the Gazette Medicale d'Orient, a journal published in French in Istanbul.[2] Later the article was translated into Ottoman Turkish and re-published. The extract from Ottoman publication is depicted in Figure 2.[1] He collected all of his submitted papers in a book entitled "Memories et Observations Medicales" in 1905 for the honour of the Sultan as a tradition at that time (Figure 3) and mentioned this case report once again.[5]

Although he had used chloroform anaesthesia in operations on 5000 patients up to that time (Figure 4) Cemil Pasha reported that this was the first case in which he had observed cardiac arrest:

"The chloroform was administered by Junker device. At the time when the cardiac arrest was observed, the chloroform dose was less than 8 grams. Under these conditions although the following known procedures - pulling the tongue out; performing artificial ventilation; giving oxygen and performing electric shock - were followed for more than twenty minutes, it was all in vain and I was bitterly disappointed by my lack of success. Immediately I opened up the left part of the chest, cut open the layer covering the heart and seized the heart in my hand. After rubbing it with my hand for some time, I felt the heart movements and pulse. After a minute, it stopped again. I started to rub it once more. The heart resumed beating. This time the heart movements and the radial pulse were more powerful and the patient started bleeding from the surgical incision and from his tongue. The pale and cyanotic face of the patient started to return to its normal state. After a little artificial respiration, the patient was able to breath by himself. However, a short time later the patient's breathing and radial pulse could no longer be detected. Although we continued rubbing the heart and administering artificial ventilation for

167

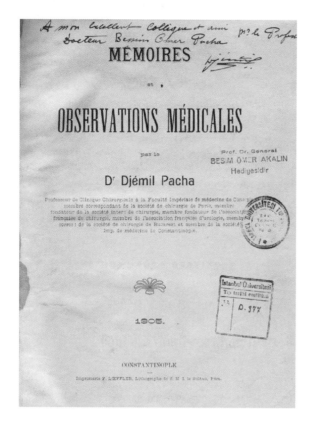

Figure 3 The cover of Cemil Topuzlu Pasha's book published in 1905.[5]

*ten more minutes, the heart did not respond and this meant all our hopes and efforts were in vain.[1]"*

Cemil Topuzlu reported that in the autopsy performed afterwards, no heart and lung pathology was found to explain the cardiac arrest. In the next part of the article it is reported that some other physiologists had met with hopeful results in their experiences with open chest cardiac massage under chloroform anaesthesia. Because of this, open chest cardiac massage was recommended in cases where the desired results were not obtained using classical methods. According to him the real problem was knowing when to start and to stop the cardiac massage when classic methods are not proving successful.

Until Arnaud in 1891 and Hallion in 1903, all previous studies recommended that open chest cardiac massage should not exceed 20 to 25 minutes. In this case, could approximately ten minutes be an acceptable limit? *"If in this period of time the classic methods are not successful, open chest cardiac massage should immediately be initiated... In fact, I was not able to bring this patient back to life. I suppose that I did not start when the conditions were favourable. I am very sad to admit that I was too late in starting open chest cardiac massage.[1]"*

Cemil Pasha also advised that in cases involving serious heart disease and other diseases where life expectancy is very short, open chest cardiac massage should not be performed. It is possible to see one of the first definitions of ''Do Not Resuscitate'' (DNR) principle from this recommendation.

Cemil Pasha also defines the technical details of the procedure he performed: after performing a

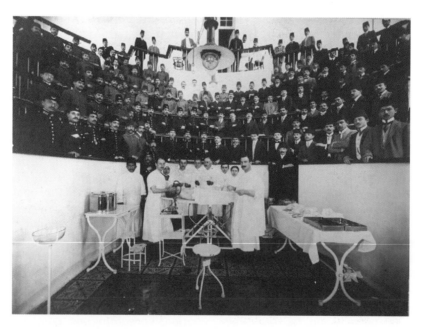

Figure 4 Preoperative stage in the operating room of Cemil Pasha, students observing the operation. The patient had been anaesthetised by chloroform, using Junker apparatus.[4]

left thoracotomy on the fourth and fifth ribs, he broke the other ribs by pulling them with his fingers. He approached the chest cavity and pushed the pleura gently so as not to harm it, cut the pericardium in the shape of a 'T' and thus reached the heart. He then rubbed the heart gently, imitating normal heart movements. He also reported that the pleura should be opened carefully and meticulously.

*"The major objection to opening up the pleura or cutting the pericardium is the risk of deflating the lung due to damage inflicted on the pleura. In my opinion, although Dr Tuffier's case and Monsieur Prus's experiments on animals appeared to show that this was not very dangerous, unfortunately, no proof has been provided to back up this claim.[1]"*

In the article, sixteen cases of cardiac massage reported up to that time were re-evaluated. Amongst these cases; there were Tuffier's case, Lane's and Gray's cases which had been reported by Starling, and Niehans's case by Zesas. Cases where there was no heart movement were considered as unsuccessful and cases where there was some movement for a short period of time were considered partly successful. The first case to survive was reported by Starling and this case was elaborated upon in greater detail. Cemil Pasha reported that in the Starling case, which was performed under chloroform anaesthesia, once all the usual methods had been tried, cardiac massage was carried out through an abdominal incision without having recourse to thoracotomy, while a narrow tube was passed down the trachea and positive pressure air was given.[1]

Although, Cemil Pasha reports Starling's case as the first of its type, we now know that the first case of a patient surviving open chest cardiac massage was performed by Kristian Ingelsrud in 1901, but it was only reported by Keen in 1904.[6] At the time when Cemil Pasha reported his case, therefore, he was not aware of this development.

In the concluding part of his article, Cemil Pasha said that out of thirteen open chest massages seven had been unsuccessful and six partly successful. He thought that it would be wrong to draw the conclusion that this method was not effective just because they had not obtained any success from it.

*"Physiologists have demonstrated to us that cardiac massage performed by opening the chest can be successful in their experiments on animals. There is no reason to doubt that this technique will be unsuccessful on humans. The partial success so far in the clinic gives us reason to hope. We are trying to reach a conclusion from the information we have in hand, but we only have a limited number of cases to discuss. It is therefore impossible to discuss the priority of one technique over another. I believe that performing cardiac massage immediately after the occurrence of cardiac arrest under chloroform anaesthesia can return a patient to life.[1]"*

The history of chloroform anaesthesia in Turkey goes all the way back to 1848. When Sultan Abdulmecit visited the Medical School on 25 July 1848 one of the fifth grade students, Yusuf Efendi, explained the properties of chloroform to him. The Faculty chemistry teacher, Antonie Calleja, showed the effects of chloroform on animals and on Yusuf Efendi.[7] During surgery carried out in the faculty in 1848, chloroform anaesthesia was administered. By the 1880s, chloroform anaesthesia was being performed routinely. Cemil Pasha reported the first open chest cardiac massage during cardiac arrest under chloroform anaesthesia.

The success of open chest massage in animal experiments was reported by physiologist Moritz Schiff in 1874. This technique was first tried by Paul Niehans in 1880 and was published in 1903 by Zesas. Tuffier's report of 1898 stated that the patient's heart movements were observed for some time before they stopped following a second cardiac arrest. The first successful open chest cardiac massage was carried out by the Norwegian, Kristian Ingelsrud in 1901 and reported by Keen in 1904. In 1906, Green reported 40 cases of cardiac arrest of whom nine survived. In 1924 Lee and Downs reported that 25% of 99 cases had been saved thanks to open chest cardiac massage.[6,8–10]

As can be seen from Cemil Pasha's report of 23 August 1903, at that time no successful cases involving open chest massage had been reported. From the above one can understand that Cemil Pasha had made himself aware of all the cases and the experiments of physiologists at that time. In his conclusion, he remarks that this technique is promising and recommends that it should be performed immediately in hopeless cases.

Because of his bravery in performing open chest cardiac massage at a time when it was not yet proven on humans during cardiac arrest due to chloroform Cemil Pasha should be remembered as one of the pioneers in the field of resuscitation.

## Acknowledgement

We are grateful to grandson of Cemil Topuzlu Pasha, our mentor Cemalettin Topuzlu Professor of General Surgery (Istanbul University Oncology Institution) for opening up the private archives of his family generously. The support of Prof. Ayten Altintas (Istanbul University Cerrahpasa Medical Faculty, Department of History of Medicine and Deontology) was invaluable for the authors.

## References

1. Topuzlu C. Kloru nemel ile tenvim esnasında zuhura gelen sekte-i kalbiyede mess-i kalbin fevait ve netayici. Hamidiye Etfal Hastanesi Istatistik Risalesi 1323/1905;6:92—100.
2. Pacha C. Le massage du coeur dans les syncopes chloroformique. Gazette Medicale d'Orient 1903;21:348—54.
3. Batirel HF, Yüksel M. Cemil Topuzlu Pacha and his arterial suture technique. Ann Thorac Surg 1997;64:1201—3.
4. Topuzlu C. In: Topuzlu, C, editor. Istibdat, Meşrutiyet, Cumhuriyet Devirlerinde 80 Yıllık Hatıralarım. 4th ed. Istanbul: Topuzlu Yayınları, 2002.
5. Pacha D. Memoires et Observations Medicales. Constantinople: F. Loeffler; 1905.
6. Vallejo-Manzur F, Varon J, Fromm R, Baskett P. Moritz Schiff and the history of open-chest cardiac massage. Resuscitation 2002;53:3—5.
7. Ulman YI. The early steps of chloroform anaesthesia in Turkey during the Ottoman Empire in 19th century. Ann Françaises d'Anesthesie et de Reanim 2005;24:377—82.
8. Alzaga-Fernandez A, Varon J. Open-chest cardiopulmonary resuscitation; past, present and future. Resuscitation 2005;64:149—56.
9. Hermrec AS. The history of cardiopulmonary resuscitation. Am J Surg 1988;156:430—6.
10. Safar P. Development of cardiopulmonary-cerebral resuscitation in the twentieth century. Int Congress Series 2002;1242:215—27.

# Robert Woods (1865–1938): The rationale for mouth-to-mouth respiration

Thomas F. Baskett

Early records from Egyptian mythology and the Bible suggest that mouth-to-mouth and mouth-to-nose respiration were among the earliest resuscitative efforts using artificial respiration.[1,2] The technique has also been used for many centuries by midwives in attempts to revive apparently still-born infants. One of the first authenticated cases of recovery following artificial respiration using the mouth-to-mouth technique was the resuscitation of a suffocated miner by Tossach in 1744.[3] Indeed, the recommendations of the Humane Societies in Europe and the United States in the latter part of the 18th century advocated mouth-to-mouth respiration for resuscitation of apparently drowned persons.[4] However, the demonstration of carbon dioxide in expired air by Black and the discovery of oxygen by Priestley, along with the germ theory of disease, led to mouth-to-mouth respiration falling into disrepute for almost two centuries. It was replaced by positive pressure ventilation with bellows and a myriad of manual techniques for artificial respiration.[5]

Elam and Safar are largely credited with the restoration of mouth-to-mouth and mouth-to-nose techniques of artificial respiration in the 1950s.[6,7] However, some 50 years earlier a Dublin throat surgeon, Robert Woods, clearly outlined the rationale and technique for mouth-to-mouth respiration and advocated its reinstatement as a technique superior to the manual methods of artificial respiration in vogue at the time. In his paper, read before the Royal Academy of Medicine on 18 May 1906 and published that same year in the *Transactions of the Royal Academy of Medicine in Ireland*, Woods recalled the use of mouth-to-mouth respiration advocated 150 years earlier and how it had come to be replaced by the manual methods of artificial respiration (Figure 1).[8] He made a plea for the restoration of mouth-to-mouth respiration and described the technique as follows[8]:

'The operator first takes a deep breath or two, so as to purify his own lungs, and by a single puff fully inflates the patient. During this act sufficient pressure is applied to the cricoid cartilage to keep the gullet closed, and thus prevent the air from entering the stomach. Then removing his mouth from the patient's mouth or nose, the inflated air is allowed to escape, the last portion of it being expressed by moderate pressure on the chest and abdomen, the process being repeated about every five seconds'.

Woods outlined the rationale for the superiority of the mouth-to-mouth technique compared to manual methods of artificial respiration. He pointed out that the amount of air introduced into the

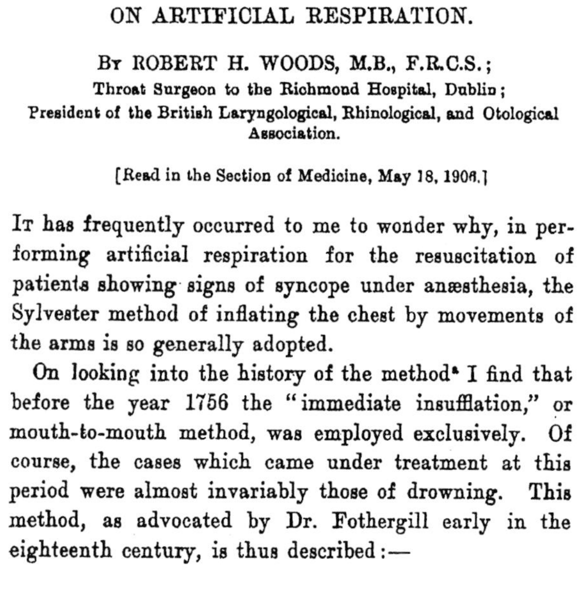

## ON ARTIFICIAL RESPIRATION.

By ROBERT H. WOODS, M.B., F.R.C.S.;
Throat Surgeon to the Richmond Hospital, Dublin;
President of the British Laryngological, Rhinological, and Otological
Association.

[Read in the Section of Medicine, May 18, 1906.]

It has frequently occurred to me to wonder why, in performing artificial respiration for the resuscitation of patients showing signs of syncope under anæsthesia, the Sylvester method of inflating the chest by movements of the arms is so generally adopted.

On looking into the history of the method* I find that before the year 1756 the "immediate insufflation," or mouth-to-mouth method, was employed exclusively. Of course, the cases which came under treatment at this period were almost invariably those of drowning. This method, as advocated by Dr. Fothergill early in the eighteenth century, is thus described:—

Figure 1 Transactions of the Royal Academy of Medicine, Ireland, 1906.

chest by blowing was much greater than that introduced by manual techniques. He then discussed the theoretical aspects of artificial respiration and resuscitation[8]:

'In the resuscitation of the apparently drowned, two effects are sought - first, the starting of the heart mechanism, and, secondly the oxygenation of the blood. In cases of poisoning by volatile drugs, such as chloroform, there is a third effect desired - viz; the elimination of the poison. As far as starting the heart mechanism is concerned anyone can prove on himself that increasing the depth of the respiration increases the force and frequency of the heart beat. It is fair, therefore, to assume that the better the chest is filled the greater will be the stimulus to the heart's action. The method, therefore, by which the largest volume of air is made to ebb and flow will, both from this point of view and that of an elimination of a volatile drug, be the best'.

Woods went on to discredit the 'theorists of the 18th century' who had dismissed mouth-to-mouth respiration because of the 'poisonous gas' exhaled by the lungs[8]:

'They allowed themselves to be frightened from a most excellent practice by the inference drawn from the fact that exhaled air makes lime water turbid. No one doubts that carbonic acid gas is poisonous, but to say that it is present in poisonous quantities is expired air is absurd. Patients breathe and rebreathe the air from the bag of an ether inhaler for a very considerable fraction of an hour

at a time, with no bad effects, though the quantity of carbonic acid gas present must necessarily be very high, and the oxygen minimal'.

Woods' experience was confined to patients in the operating theatre where he noted 'It has fallen to my lot to have seen several cases of syncope under chloroform'. He recounted four cases, two of whom did not recover. In one case of sarcoma of the throat a tracheotomy had been performed and chloroform was administered through the tracheal tube[8]:

'The patient had ceased to breathe, the skin was pallid, the pupils dilated, the cornea anaesthetic, and the pulse absent, or at least impalpable at the wrist. I insufflated the patient through the tracheal tube. In a minute or two his colour returned, and he began again to breathe and bleed'.

He described another case in which a 14-year-old girl under chloroform anaesthesia developed '... a similar condition of profound collapse ... the patient was restored after a moment or two of direct insufflation'.[8] At the conclusion of his paper, Woods outlined the main benefits of the mouth-to-mouth or mouth-to-nose method as follows[8]:

'(1) The quantity of tidal air is greater than by any indirect method, and, therefore, the stimulation of the mechanisms of circulation and respiration, the elimination of the poison, and the oxygenation of the blood are all as great as possible.

(2) The impurities, if present at all, are negligible.

(3) The method can be applied without a moment's loss of time.'

Robert Henry Woods (1865–1938) was born in Tullamore, Ireland on 27 April 1865 (Figure 2). He received his university education at Dublin University graduating BA in 1887 and MB in 1889. The following year he received a travelling scholarship from Trinity College to study in Vienna.[9] Upon his return, he was appointed throat surgeon to the Richmond Hospital, Dublin. He confined his practice to ear, nose and throat surgery—at that time a relative rarity. He was later appointed to Sir Patrick Dun's Hospital in 1906. In his time, he held the offices of President of the Irish Medical Association, President of the British Laryngological Society and, from 1910 to 1912, was President of the Royal College of Surgeons in Ireland. He had an inventive mind which he applied to the development of a number of procedures and instruments in his specialty. In order to reduce glare, he changed the standard white operating drapes to green. He was described in one biographical article as follows:

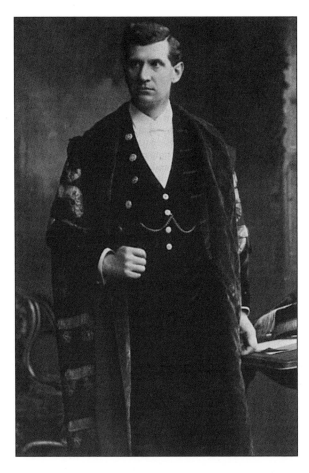

**Figure 2** Sir Robert Henry Woods, 1865—1938.[9] Reproduced courtesy of the Royal College of Surgeons Ireland.

*'His manner was abrupt and unconventional, his presence imposing; he had a bright, eagle glance, an alert mind and a tongue ready with quip and repartee'.*[9]

In 1908, while serving on the Council of the College of Surgeons, Woods unsuccessfully introduced a by-law 'that no one shall be eligible to hold a Professorship of Surgery, Medicine, Midwifery, Forensic Medicine or Public Health in the College after he has passed the age of forty years or any examinership in those subjects after fifty'.[9] At this time, Woods himself was 43 years old and a Professor of Larynogology and Otology. He received a knighthood from King George V in 1913. In 1918, he was elected to Parliament as a representative for Dublin University. He and his wife, Margaret, had five children. Their eldest son was killed in action in Flanders in October 1916. One of his other sons became a Fellow of the Royal College of Surgeons in Ireland and succeeded his father at Sir Patrick Dun's Hospital. Sir Robert Henry Woods died at his home in Dublin on 8 September 1938.[9]

The restoration of mouth-to-mouth respiration as the technique of choice for resuscitation is generally attributed to Elam and Safar in the mid 1950s.[6,7] However, Woods clearly outlined the rationale for and superiority of this method some 50 years earlier. His report probably went unnoticed because of the limited circulation and availability of the journal in which it was published.

## References

1. Baker AB. Artificial respiration, the history of an idea. Med Hist 1971;15:336—46.
2. Fisher JM. Resuscitation greats: the earliest records. Resuscitation 2000;44:79—80.
3. Tossach W. A man, dead in appearance, recovered by distending the lungs with air. Medical Essays and Observations, Edinburgh 1744;5:605.
4. Sternbach GL, Varon J, Fromm R, Baskett PJF. The humane societies. Resuscitation 2000;45:71—5.
5. Karpovich PV. Adventures in Artificial Respiration. New York: Association Press; 1953. p. 26—9.
6. Elam JO, Brown ES, Elder JD. Artificial respiration by mouth-to-mask method: a study of the respiration gas exchange of paralysed patients ventilated by operator's expired air. N Engl J Med 1954;250:749—54.
7. Safar P. Ventilator efficacy of mouth-to-mouth artificial respiration. JAMA 1958;167:335—41.
8. Woods RH. On artificial respiration. Trans R Acad Med, Ireland 1906:136—42.
9. Lyons AB. An Assembly of Irish Surgeons. Dublin: Glendale Press; 1984. p. 34—9.

# Sir Edward Sharpey-Schafer and his simple and efficient method of performing artificial respiration

## Desmond Writer

When Sir Edward Sharpey-Schafer died in 1935, at the age of 84, one obituary referred to him as one of the world's most distinguished physiologists, "whose name is very widely known to the general public, for his method of giving artificial respiration in the prone position has been adopted by all those who have to do with ambulance work and teach the means of saving life" [1]. Schäfer's eponymous method, first described in 1903, was recommended in successive editions of the "American Red Cross: *First Aid Textbook*" until 1959, when the whispers of its detractors rose to a clamour for its abandonment and replacement by mouth-to-mouth respiration [2–5].

Educated at Clewer House School, Windsor, the young Edward Schäfer showed "exceptional promise by the awards of scholarships at London University in zoology, anatomy and physiology" [6]. As a student in University College Hospital, he was impressed by the teachings of William Sharpey, then in his last years as professor of physiology and anatomy. Sharpey's example would influence Schäfer in two ways: first, by defining his career path as histologist and physiologist, and later, in 1918, by causing Schäfer to change his name.

Authors offer different accounts to explain the name change. Talbott writes: "Late in life, Schäfer's surname was extended to Sharpey-Schafer, after dropping the umlaut, a token legally executed for the great esteem and respect held by the pupil for his teacher" [7]. Sharpey-Schafer's 1935 obituarist, referring to him as "the son of James William Henry Schäfer of the free city of Hamburg and of Highgate," offered another explanation: ". . . he came under the influence of William Sharpey, the physiologist, whose name he added to his own in 1918 to emphasize the fact that he was an Englishman by birth and education, at a time when anyone with a German name was regarded with suspicion and hostility by newspaper-inflamed ignorant people" [1]. The writer goes on to state that Schäfer's action was "wholly unnecessary, for both his sons lost their lives in the war. . . " Elaborating on this account, Comroe wrote: "Schäfer was such an admirer of his professor, William

Sharpey, that, when Sharpey died without any known descendants, Schäfer gave the name Sharpey to his own son to perpetuate it. When Schäfer's son was killed in World War I, Schäfer added Sharpey to his own name in 1918 and became Edward Sharpey Schafer" [8]. Comroe further notes that Schäfer's name has caused "much trauma" to medical indexers, since it appears variously as Schäfer, Schafer, Schaefer, Sharpey Schäefer and Sharpey-Schafer.

Although known to generations of first-aid providers for his method of artificial respiration, Schäfer first achieved professional recognition as a histologist. As a student in 1872, he became the first Sharpey scholar, when awarded the studentship founded at University College in Sharpey's honour [6]. Two years later, he was assistant professor of physiology, devoting most of his time to histological research on striated muscle fibres and fat absorption. By 1883 he had succeeded to the post of Jodrell professor of physiology, which he held for 16 years.

Schäfer's textbook, *The Essentials of Histology*, first appeared in 1885 and was revised through 17 successive editions until 1953, Schäfer himself undertaking the revisions over almost 50 years [7]. In his introductory address to the medical students in the year his textbook first appeared, Schäfer "regretted the general assumption of those in charge of medical education. . . that anatomy was the foundation on which the whole surperstructure of medical and surgical science could be reared" [6]. He felt that assumption could only be justified if "the object of medical education were to provide physicians not for the living but for the dead." Dr. W. A. Bain, the last of Schäfer's pupils to have worked with him, said Schäfer "held very strongly to the view that histology should be an integral part of the physiological curriculum, and he never tired of deploring the modern tendency to separate the two subjects and relegate the teaching of histology to the anatomists and the anatomical laboratory" [6].

Elected to the chair of physiology in Edinburgh University in 1899, Schäfer was both admired and feared as a teacher. "Few things could be more dramatic than the sudden transition from the babble of 200 voices to a stillness as of the

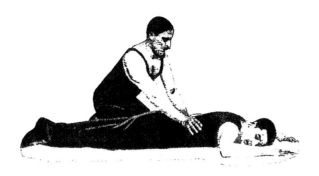

Fig. 1. First position of operator and patient for effecting artificial respiration by the "prone pressure method" described by Professor Schäfer. The operator's hands are over the lowest ribs of the patient. Photograph of E Sharpey-Schafer from Brit Med J 1935;1:741.

grave when Schäfer appeared at the door of his theatre and made his way slowly, and with characteristic step, to the rostrum" [6]. Often the one o'clock gun would go off during his lecture, something which might otherwise have resulted in "pandemonium," but Schäfer was allowed to continue uninterrupted.

Not until his Edinburgh days, did Schäfer describe his "Simple and efficient method of performing artificial respiration in the human subject," in a presentation to *The Royal Medical and Chirurgical Society* [9] (Figs. 1 and 2):

"It consists in laying the subject in the prone posture, preferably on the ground, with a thick folded garment underneath the chest and epigastrium. The operator puts himself in a position athwart or at the side of the subject, facing his head and kneeling upon one or both knees, and places his hands on each side over the lower part of the back (lowest ribs). He then slowly throws the weight of his body forward to bear upon his own arms, and thus presses upon the thorax of the subject and forces air out of the lungs. This being effected, he gradually relaxes the pressure by bringing his own body up again to a more erect position, but without moving the hands: as he does this, air is drawn, by the removal of the pressure from the chest walls and by their elastic reaction, into the lungs. This process is repeated quite regularly and without man-

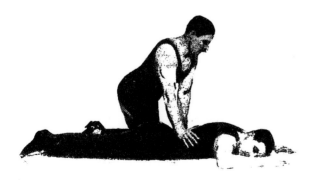

Fig. 2. Second position of operator. Who is throwing his weight vertically on his wrists, thus putting pressure on the thorax and abdomen of the patient. "This pressure is exerted slowly, occupying some three seconds and is then removed for a period of two seconds and again applied from Schafer EA. JAMA 1908;51:802.

ifest intervals between the movements not less often than twelve times a minute: it may be done somewhat more rapidly, but fifteen times a minute would, in any case, be sufficient. By this means it is easily possible in an average man to effect an exchange of fully 6500 cubic centimeters per minute – an amount which is more than enough to maintain complete aëration of the blood."

Schäfer's estimates of minute volume derived from experiments conducted on his laboratory attendant and reported to the *Royal Society of Edinburg* in 1903 [10]. Their description makes fascinating reading. Schäfer first refers to earlier experiments in which he compared his technique to those of Silvester,* Howard,** and Marshall Hall,*** Schäfer writes: "The number of experiments which we were able to make at the time was, however, too limited to enable us to draw any positive conclusion regarding the relative value of the several methods of performing artificial respiration in man..." This limitation did not, however, deter him from continuing: "...although the experiments clearly show the very important part which alternating pressure on the lower part of the chest plays in effecting the emptying and (by resiliency) the consequent filling of the lungs."

In those earlier inconclusive experiments, subjects expired into, or inspired from a counterpoised bell jar, filled with air and inverted over water, which rose and fell with each respiration. These "somewhat rapid movements imparted to it [the jar], a swing of its own which must have affected the record," Schäfer concluded. He therefore discarded the apparatus, replacing it with a "constructed graduated gasometer (spirometer)," and repeated his earlier experiments, comparing the efficacy of his prone pressure method to the other techniques [10]. Schäfer considered the supine position, as recommended by Silvester, "strongly contraindicated on account of the tendency for the tongue to fall back [which] hinders the escape of water" [9].

On the same conscious subject, his 23 year-old male laboratory attendant, who weighed 10 stone, one-and-a-half pounds, and had a chest expansion of 38 inches, Schäfer performed his series of experiments [10]. In each, he recorded minute volumes over five minutes of spontaneous, or artificial respiration. Noting the spirometer had a capacity of only 10 litres, Schäfer stated: "It was necessary to take the amount of air yielded by each minute separately." In the intervening intervals, while the spirometer was emptied and the volume of its contents measured, Schäfer's subject breathed "naturally." Schäfer made one significant assumption, which would not have survived the scrutiny of contemporary research committees: "The air which is pumped out of the chest is alone measured, but *it is clear that an equal amount must afterwards pass in to take its place*" (my italics).

During "natural respiration" Schäfer's attendant, when in the supine position, expired an average minute volume of 6.46 L over five successive minutes. When prone, that figure fell to 5.24 L. With the Silvester method of artificial respiration, the average minute volume was 2.28 L, while, using

Howard's method, Schäfer achieved an average minute volume of 4.02 L. Despite the superior results with Howard's method, Schäfer noted the volume exchange was "not up to the tidal air standard" [10]. With Marshall Hall's method, the average minute volume proved similarly inadequate at 3.3 L. Perhaps unsurprisingly, given the strength of Schäfer's conviction in the superiority of his prone pressure method, the minute volumes achieved by that method exceeded those of the other techniques, averaging an impressive 6.76 L. In his extensive review, Comroe, in cynical vein, suggests that Schäfer's laboratory attendant "may well have wanted to please his professor" [8].

In his communication to the *Royal Society of Edinburgh*, Schäfer stated: "Results similar in character to the above have been yielded by many experiments, both upon the same and different individuals" [10]. However, he offered no other data than those achieved on his attendant. Comroe writes: "The editor of today's *Sunday Supplement* would have published Schäfer's single case as gospel, but the editor of today's *American Review* would have returned the manuscript and asked for a peek at Schäfer's additional data" [8].

When his paper was read before *The Royal Medical and Chirurgical Society*, Schäfer "was unable to be present either at the reading of his paper or at the subsequent discussion" [9]. The president of the society introduced Schäfer's paper, noting that it was the outcome of an earlier paper presented to the society by Schäfer, on behalf of its "Committee on Suspended Animation." The president left no doubt that the paper "represented Professor Schäfer's own individual views." The subsequent discussion was lively and unsympathetic to the absent Schäfer. Acknowledging that Schäfer's method was simple, Dr. Bowles said "it was exactly and no more than the first movement in [his] own method" [9,11]. Bowles also pointed out that pressure on the back alone with the patient prone could not be expected to "effect sufficient gaseous exchange... under the conditions existing in the drowned," and he advocated rolling the patient from the prone position on to his right side, "to introduce more air and relieve the heart and circulation." Others also supported Bowles. Dr. M.S. Pembrey, "speaking from the physiological side," felt the important thing was to start circulation "so as to get oxygen to the medulla." In his view, Bowles's method established negative pressure and inspiratory movement, to achieve this end. Dr. Henry Silvester, no doubt resentful of Schäfer's dismissive treatment of his method, said the method advocated by Schäfer "had the merit of being extremely ancient." Having damned Schäfer with such faint praise, Silvester humiliated him further by stating: "the instructions given by Professor Schäfer would be generally admitted to be faulty in principle, for it was sought... to make expiration precede inspiration, whereas in natural breathing expiration was always second in order..." Silvester also objected to the posture of the operator "athwart the patient" as being "undesirable... in respect of female patients."

Undeterred by these criticisms, Schäfer responded to them in writing, and with comparable vitriol. Concerning Silvester, he wrote: "... as was perhaps natural, [he] continues to hold the view that the only suitable means for effecting artificial respiration is that introduced by him and known by his name." Further skewering his detractors, Schäfer continued: "So far as I am aware, no one of these gentlemen who have expressed their opinion on this matter has made any measurements or comparative experiments as to the relative efficiency of the several methods which have been advocated..." Later, he added: "The experimental evidence (which I have given at length in 'The Proceedings of the Royal Society of Edinburgh,' and which is also stated briefly in an appendix to the report of the Committee on Suspended Animation) leaves no room for uncertainty as to the relative efficiency of the several methods under discussion. The special advantages of the prone-pressure method as against other methods hitherto in use are summarised in this paper, and no single one of the statements there made has been seriously traversed in the above discussion" [9].

The story of the successive committees that investigated "suspended animation" and resuscitation of the apparently drowned is equally charged with intrigue and speculation [8]. Between 1861 and 1889, *The Royal Medical and Chirurgical Society* constituted four such committees [8,12]. Each reported promptly. After Bowles read his paper "On the resuscitation of the apparently drowned" before the society in 1889, another committee was convened [11,12]. Schäfer joined the committee, as one of its five members. It took them almost 11 years to produce an interim report, signed by Schäfer and three other members, only one of whom remained from the original committee. The committee's final report came three years later in the form of Schäfer's paper to *The Royal Medical and Chirurgical Society* [9]. One of Schäfer's contemporaries, Arthur Keith, later stated: "He (Schäfer) ultimately became the committee" [8].

Another five years would elapse before the Royal Society of Medicine made its recommendation to the Metropolitan Police concerning "the subject of suspended animation and the best methods of restoration from it" [12]. With commendable equanimity, but obvious hesitation, the committee wrote: "... whilst we consider the Schäfer method the best for what may be called first aid in cases of drowning, there may be circumstances which may render other and additional means desirable."

Within a year, although Schäfer's method had been widely adopted, Keith, delivering his Hunterian lectures, criticised Schäfer's choice of a healthy volunteer, who had suspended respiration during the test, as being the greatest weakness in his method [8,13]. Other criticisms followed [2,3]. Writing eight years after Schäfer's death, Eve, author of the rocking method used by the Royal Navy, praised Schäfer's "splendid [1908] Harvey lecture," but took issue with Schäfer's comment: "Of course, on relaxing the pressure [on the chest] the same volume of air must pass in again as the chest resumes its former shape and size" [3,14]. "Unfortunately,"

Eve wrote, "this perfectly natural assumption, justified by his experiments on normal people, does not hold good in the nearly drowned..."

Comroe and Dripps compared the Schäfer and Eve methods in two apneic unconscious subjects, suffering from terminal neurological complications [4]. The Schäfer method produced a maximum minute volume of 1.4 L in one patient and 2 L in the other, in contrast to Eve's method (6 L and 5 L respectively). The authors concluded that their data "cast grave doubt on the efficacy of the Schäfer prone pressure method" [4]. In studies performed on curarized, anaesthetized subjects, Gordon et al. compared six manual techniques [15]. They concluded: "... of the methods... investigated, the Schafer prone pressure method is the least effective." Further evidence of the inadequacy of Schäfer's method followed, but it was not until 1958 that a Commission of the U.S. National Research Council found mouth-to-mouth respiration superior. In 1959, the American Red Cross began teaching the technique [8].

In his long and distinguished academic career, Schäfer garnered many honours. He became a Fellow of the Royal Society at the age of 28, and in 1924 received the society's Copley Medal, its highest honour. He was knighted in 1913. The recipient of honorary doctorates from many universities, Schäfer also lectured in Johns Hopkins University and Stanford. With George Oliver he discovered "the remarkable action on blood pressure which followed an injection of an extract of the suprarenal gland," and continued his physiological researches until his retirement in 1933 [1]. Schäfer enjoyed "long years of vigour ... due in part to the excellent golf which he played on the famous links at North Berwick, where his charming house was situated," until he died in 1935, from pneumonia following surgery [1].

Was Schäfer one of *The Resuscitation Greats*? Set against his many scientific achievements, Schäfer's method of artificial respiration seems an anachronism, and it is somewhat ironic that the eponymous technique, by which he was widely known, should have generated so much contemporary and subsequent criticism. Writing in appreciation of Schäfer, his teacher and mentor, Sir Leonard Hill, another Sharpey scholar, said: "A superb intolerance of intellectual dishonesty was combined in him with a kindly generous tolerance of the inevitable slips and errors of his assistants and students" [1]. Bain noted that Schäfer's "uncanny genius for assessing the significance of a result... sometimes led him to make prophetic utterances, the wisdom of which was demonstrated years later..." [6]. At best, Schäfer's work and views on artificial respiration might be forgiven as *ex cathedra* utterances from the lofty heights of Edinburgh's professorial chair, the wisdom of which was *not* subsequently demonstrated. At worst, if not examples of intellectual dishonesty, we might see them, with the surety of hindsight, as "inevitable slips and errors," more characteristic of his students. History, nonetheless, should accord them "kindly generous tolerance."

Schäfer did not live to see the demise of his method, which continued to be taught for more than 20 years after his death. That it should have been supplanted by mouth-to-mouth respiration, an ancient technique performed in the supine position, is, perhaps, the ultimate ignominy [16].

\* Silvester's method advocated forcible arm traction, to augment inspiration, followed by return of the arms to the side of the chest, and pressure on the chest to facilitate expiration. The patient remained supine, with the attendant risk of airway obstruction and further aspiration.

\*\* Howard's technique called for intermittent pressure on the lower ribs with the patient prone.

\*\*\* In the Marshall Hall method, the patient lies prone, and is then rolled alternately to one side and the other, each time returning to the prone position. When the subject is prone, pressure is exerted on the chest to induce expiration.

## References

[1] Anonymous. Obituary, Sir Edward Sharpey-Schafer: Brit Med J 1935;1:741–742

[2] Drinker P, Shaw LA. The prolonged administration of artificial ventilation. J Franklin Inst 1932;213:355–372.

[3] Eve FC. Complacency in resuscitation of the drowned. Brit Med J 1943;1:535–537.

[4] Comroe JH, Dripps RD. Artificial respiration. JAMA 1946;130:381–383.

[5] Heimlich HJ. Subdiaphragmatic pressure to expel water from the lungs of drowning persons. Ann Emerg Med 1981;10:476–480.

[6] Anonymous. Obituary, Sir Edward Sharpey-Schafer. Lancet 1935;1:843–845.

[7] Talbott JH. Sir E. A. Sharpey-Schafer (1850–1935). In: A Biographical History of Medicine. New York: Grune and Stratton, 1970:953–956.

[8] Comroe Jr JH. "... In comes the good air." Pt.I. Rise and fall of the Schäfer method. Am Rev Resp Dis 1979;119:803–809.

[9] Schäfer EA. Description of a simple and efficient method of performing artificial respiration in the human subject, to which is appended instructions for the treatment of the apparently drowned. Med Chir Trans 1904;87:609–614 (discussion pp. 615–623).

[10] Schäfer EA. The relative efficiency of certain methods of performing artificial respiration in man. Proc Roy Soc Edin 1903;25:39–50.

[11] Bowles RL. Resuscitation of the apparently drowned. Med Chir Trans 1889;72:407–431.

[12] Church WS, Champneys FH, Haward JW, et al. Resuscitation of the apparently drowned. Report of the committee appointed by the Council of the Royal Society of Medicine to consider the request of the Chief Surgeon to the Metropolitan Police that the society should pronounce as to the best method to be adopted. Proc Roy Soc Med 1908;2:1–8.

[13] Keith A. Three Hunterian lectures on the mechanism underlying the various methods of artificial respiration practised since the foundation of The Royal Humane Society in 1774. Lancet 1909;1:745–749, 825–828, 895–899.

[14] Schäfer EA. Artificial respiration in man. In: Harvey Lectures. Philadelphia: J.B. Lippincott, 1907–8;223–243. Philadelphia.

[15] Gordon AS, Sadove MS, Raymon F, et al. Critical survey of manual artificial respiration. JAMA 1951;147:1444–1453.

[16] Comroe Jr JH. "... In comes the good air." Pt.II. Mouth-to-mouth method. Am Rev Resp Dis 1979;119:1025–1031.

# Sir Ivan Whiteside Magill

## Peter Baskett

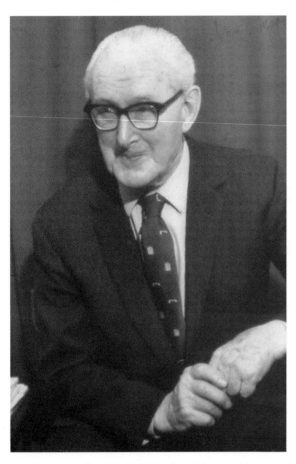

Fig. 1. Sir Ivan Magill on his 90th birthday. This portrait hangs at the home of the Association of Anaesthetists of Great Britain and Ireland at 21 Portland Place, London. (Reproduced with permission).

There is little doubt that optimal control of the airway and ventilation is achieved by tracheal intubation in competent and experienced hands. Sir Ivan Magill perfected the technique like no other. He invented and designed the equipment, including the tubes for both tracheal and bronchial intubation and their connectors, the modified laryngoscope, the breathing circuits and the intubating offset forceps—all a godsend in the resuscitation process, and all originating from his good practice of anaesthesia (Fig. 1).

Ivan Whiteside Magill was born in Larne, County Antrim, Northern Ireland in 1888 [1]. His parents, Samuel Magill and Sara (nee Whiteside) had five children. His father, Samuel, was a prominent business-man in the clothing trade and a local politician. The family had no medical background, but after education at Larne Grammar School, Ivan studied medicine at Queens University Belfast, graduating in 1913.

As a medical student he played rugby football and boxed at heavyweight for the university.

It is recorded that at medical school he gave about 60 anaesthetics (without any formal training) and qualified (like the author of this article, some 40 years later) with a certificate indicating that he had "received practical instruction in the administration of anaesthetics and had personally administered an anaesthetic" [2]. His degree awarded by the Queens University, Belfast was entitled not only MB, BCh (Batchelor of Medicine and Surgery) but with an additional BAO (Batchelor in the Art of Obstetrics—which was peculiar to the Irish Universities).

After qualification he came to England and took up resident posts (principally in surgery) at the Walton Hospital, Liverpool [3]. A year later the Great War of 1914–1918 loomed, and soon after the outbreak of conflict Magill was commissioned as a Captain in the Royal Army Medical Corps (RAMC). He served with the Irish Guards at the Battle of Loos and with a field hospital in Rouen in France. The casualty rate in that war was quite horrendous on both sides both from trauma and intercurrent illness in the diabolical conditions of trench warfare.

During a short period of leave in 1916 he returned to the United Kingdom to marry Edith Robinson from Banbridge in County Down in Northern Ireland. She was then a school doctor with the London County Council. They did not have any children.

Upon his return to Britain at the end of the war he was posted to Barnet War Hospital (now Barnet General Hospital). Soon he moved to take up an appointment at the 600 bed Queen's Hospital for Facial and Jaw Injuries (now Queen Mary's Hospital) in Sidcup in Kent.

There, significantly, he met up again with Stanley Rowbotham, another ex RAMC officer. Together they decided to opt for anaesthesia as their chosen interest and they were to make fundamental and pioneering advances to what was then, a fledgling specialty. The work at Sidcup was extremely challenging for the anaesthetist because, in many cases, it involved sharing the airway with the surgeon. The surgeon was Major, later Sir Harold, Gillies, who was embarking on the new field of facial plastic surgery in the aftermath of horrendous war injuries and burns.

Magill was a master of invention that was based on a sound knowledge of gas physics, practical engineering ingenuity and clinical need based on extensive experience. Many of these inventions are essential to resuscitation practice today. He was a master of the airway. The rather primitive anaesthetic technique of the time consisted of insufflation of ether through a Phillips oropharyngeal airway with a side piece, made from a 303 rifle cartridge case, and was standard practice when he and Rowbotham arrived at Sidcup. The patients were frequently prone to airway obstruction and pulmonary aspiration.

"We worked out that the whole essence of success in these cases was control of the larynx" [4]. And so they developed insufflation of ether directly into the trachea through a catheter using an air pump with a flow rate which was sufficient to blow away any blood or debris lurking in the pharynx above. To convince sceptical spectators, Magill, a true Irish showman, would demonstrate the safety of the method.

"I took a jug of water at the end of the operation and poured it into the patient's mouth to show that respiration was completely under control" [5].

Is it worth pondering that tracheal insufflation of oxygen is a possible way forward in the ventilation aspect of CPR in the present day debate concerning the primacy of chest compressions?

There were short comings of the method used by Magill. The surgeon was covered with a spray of blood and obliged to inhale ether fumes. Gillies remarked "Maggi – you seem to get the anaesthetic into the patient alright, don't you think you could devise some method of getting it out, so that I am not anaesthetised as well" [6].

Together with Rowbotham, Magill devised the "two tube method of anaesthesia" supplementing the insufflation catheter with a wide bore tracheal tube as a conduit for the expiratory gases. A pack could now be placed in the pharynx to protect the surgeon from blood and ether fumes.

The expiration tube was generally passed through the nose and Magill designed his unique offset forceps to lift the tip of the tube into, and through, the laryngeal

isthmus [7]. From this concept Magill developed the wide bore tracheal tube for to and fro respiration using a breathing circuit of his own design, incorporating a rebreathing bag and expiratory valve [8,9].

There was difficulty in obtaining rubber tubing of the correct consistency. Wound drainage tubing used in hospital was too thin walled and was subject to kinking. Eventually Magill found a source of suitable material from a rubber shop in Tottenham Court Road in London which sold footballs and coils of rubber tubing. It is said that Magill would leave the tubing coiled inside his top hat which imparted precisely the correct curvature! He cut the bevel to face the left side of the patient as the right nostril was generally preferred for introduction of the tube. Later the renowned manufacturer and supplier of anaesthetic equipment, Charles King, started to stock and supply tracheal tubes to Magill's specification.

Magill would pass his tracheal tubes through either the mouth or nose, according to the operation to be performed. He preferred the nasal route because generally this did not involve using a laryngoscope. He was a master at blind nasal intubation. Success hinged on the correct alignment of the head and neck. Magill described this as the "sniffing the morning air" position, with some flexion of the cervical spine achieved by a pillow placed under the occiput and the head extended at the atlanto-occipital joint. Listening carefully to the breath sounds when the tube entered the pharynx he would slip it through the larynx during inspiration. Not as easy as he made it appear!

When working with some reactionary practitioners, who did not approve of any alternative anaesthetic techniques except open drop chloroform or ether using a mask, he would divert their attention for a few seconds by a remark such as: " Could you please look at the clock and tell me the exact time?". During the time that the practitioner was turned away Magill would have intubated the patient blindly through the nose and had replaced the mask over it without the practitioner knowing that it had been done [10].

Magill designed his own laryngoscope (which took several forms), tracheal tube connectors that gave access for tracheal aspiration, reinforced unkinkable tracheal tubes ("surgeon proof" as he called them!) and endobronchial tubes and blockers for use in thoracic anaesthesia—much in demand at the time for the ravages of tuberculosis and bronchiectasis.

Magill worked on a part time basis at Sidcup, and also held appointments at the Brompton and Westminster Hospitals in central London. The anaesthetic department at the Westminster (now the Chelsea and Westminster Hospital) bears his name. He was in great demand in private practice and would give an anaesthetic virtually anywhere – in private houses, nursing homes, and even in a bathroom at the Ritz Hotel! He would bring his anaesthetic apparatus with him carrying the cylinders of nitrous oxide and oxygen in a shoulder yoke hidden under his greatcoat [11]. He was not a huge man but was immensely wiry and strong – a legacy from his rugby and boxing days at university.

He anaesthetised many foreign dignitaries and several members of the Royal Family including the Dowager Duchess of Gloucester in 1937, Princess Margaret in 1955, the Duke of Windsor, Prince Charles, and Princess Anne [12]. In a personal interview, I once asked him what it was like to anaesthetise members of the Royal Family. He told me, in his Ulster brogue; "It is really very demanding. It can interrupt your holidays. And they don't pay, ye know!" [13] But the Royal Family did show their appreciation, for King George VIth invested him with the honour of Commander of the Royal Victorian Order in 1946 and he was knighted KCVO in 1960 by the present Queen. The Royal Victorian Order is a special honour bestowed by the Royal Family for personal services to them.

Magill was keen to establish anaesthesia as a specialty in its own right. He realised that this would involve setting standards and examinations and as Honorary Secretary of the Section of Anaesthetics of the Royal Society of Medicine he proposed the creation of a Diploma of Anaesthetics [14]. As this innovation could not be achieved by the Royal Society of Medicine under its charter, the Association of Anaesthetists of Great Britain and Ireland was established in 1932 under the Presidency of Harry Featherstone from Birmingham. This body was responsible for the introduction of the first diploma in anaesthetics of the Conjoint Board of the Royal College of Surgeons of England in November 1935.

Magill received many honours during his lifetime, probably more than any other anaesthetist. He was elected President of the Section of Anaesthetics of the Royal Society of Medicine in 1937 and was awarded the Hickman Medal of the Society in 1938 and the Medal of the Ulster Medical Society in 1939. The Association of Anaesthetists of Great Britain and Ireland awarded him Honorary Membership and their John Snow Silver Medal in 1958 and later named their most prestigious award—the Magill Gold Medal in his honour. He was also made an Honorary Fellow of the Royal Society of Medicine and of the Faculty of Anaesthetists in both England and Ireland and the Royal College of Surgeons. From abroad, he received awards from the Canadian Society of Anaesthetists and the American Association of Plastic Surgeons.

His alma mater, Queens University, Belfast, treated him strangely. In 1920 he submitted a thesis for an MD on endotracheal anaesthesia. This was rejected by a professor of medicine, of very little perspicacity, on the grounds that it was unlikely to be of much value! [15]. A bit like rejecting Elvis Presley or the Beatles for a

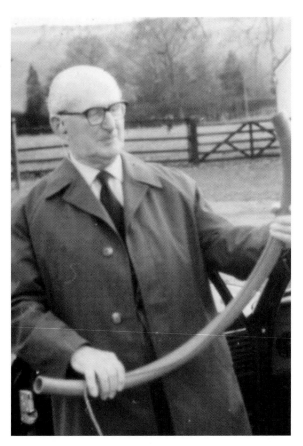

Fig. 2. Sir Ivan Magill at the University of Bristol School of Veterinary Medicine at Langford. Photo by John Zorab. (Reproduced with permission).

recording contract! In 1945, the University attempted to make amends for their monumental error of judgement a quarter of a century earlier, and awarded him an Honorary Doctorate of Science. "Paddy" Magill liked to dine out on that one!

He was also made an Honorary Member of the Society of Anaesthetists of the South Western Region of England during a meeting of the Society held at Bristol University Veterinary School at Langford. On that occasion he was presented with a cuffed tracheal tube about one metre long—used at Langford for intubation of horses (Fig. 2)!

Trout fishing was his beloved pastime. He was a master of this sport in the rivers of Ireland and on the River Test at Stockbridge in Hampshire where he was a member of the exclusive fishing club, The Houghtons. He caught a 5 pound (2.5 kg) trout on his 97th birthday! [16].

He remained in London during the 1939–1945 war. His house was bombed but "it was not a problem because I was out at the time" [17]. He gave his last anaesthetic at the age of 84.

In his latter years he was dysarthric, which seemed to accentuate his Ulster accent. Coming from that part of the world, I was one of the few who could understand him. He loved food, "strong" drink, Burma cheroots and practical jokes. There was an impudent sparkle in his eyes right up to the time of his death in November 1986 in his 99th year. He spent his last days under the care of his nephew in Leigh Woods in Bristol. I was privileged to visit him several times there and talk about old times.

Sir Ivan Magill was a household name and a legend in his own lifetime. This modest, sane, practical man, of great humour gave us wonderful tools and techniques that are key elements of resuscitation today. We thank and honour him for that.....

## Acknowledgements

I am grateful to the Association of Anaesthetists of Breat Britain and Ireland for permission to reproduce the photograph in Fig. 1, and to my colleague and friend, John Zorab, for permission to reproduce Fig. 2 and for giving me the digital images of both figures.

## References

[1] Page R. The Barnhill lad who became a consultant to Royalty. Larne Times1987, January 22nd.

[2] Magill IW. Anaesthesia: The Magill story. In: Gillies H, Millard DR (Eds) The Principles and Art of Plastic Surgery, vol 1, Little, Brown, Boston and Toronto.

[3] Rowbotham S. Ivan Magill. Brit J Anaesth 1951;23:49–55.

[4] Pallister WK. Sir Ivan Whiteside Magill (1888–1986) and tracheal intubation. In: Atkinson RS, Boulton TB, editors. The History of Anaesthesia. London and New York: Royal Society of Medicine Services, 1889:606.

[5] Pallister WK. Sir Ivan Whiteside Magill (1888–1986) and tracheal intubation. In: Atkinson RS, Boulton TB, editors. The History of Anaesthesia. London and New York: Royal Society of Medicine Services, 1889:607.

[6] Pallister WK. Sir Ivan Whiteside Magill (1888–1986) and tracheal intubation. In: Atkinson RS, Boulton TB, editors. The History of Anaesthesia. London and New York: Royal Society of Medicine Services, 1889:607.

[7] Magill IW. Forceps for intratracheal anaesthesia. Brit Med J 1920;2:670.

[8] Magill IW. Endotracheal anaesthesia Proc Roy Soc Med 1929;22:83–7 (also reproduced in Anaesthesia 1978; 33: 580-586).

[9] Magill IW. Techniques in endotracheal anaesthesia. Brit Med J 1930;1:818–9.

[10] Pallister WK. Sir Ivan Whiteside Magill (1888–1986) and tracheal intubation. In: Atkinson RS, Boulton TB, editors. The History of Anaesthesia. London and New York: Royal Society of Medicine Services, 1889:606.

[11] Maltby JR. Magill Forceps. Sir Ivan Whiteside Magill (1888–1986). In: Maltby JR, editor. Notable Names in Anaesthesia. London: Royal Society of Medicine Press, 2002:124.

[12] Lee KG. The life and work of Sir Ivan Magill KCVO. In: Atkinson RS, Boulton TB, editors. The History of Anaesthesia. London and New York: Royal Society of medicine Services, 1989:603–4.

[13] Magill IW. Personal Communication, 1976.

[14] Minutes of a meeting of the Council of the Section of the Royal Society of Medicine held on Friday November 6th 1931;300–301.

[15] Lee KG. The life and work of Sir Ivan Magill KCVO. In: Atkinson RS, Boulton TB, editors. The History of Anaesthesia. London and New York: Royal Society of medicine Services, 1989:603–4.

[16] Maltby JR. Magill Forceps. Sir Ivan Whiteside Magill (1888–1986). In: Maltby JR, editor. Notable Names in Anaesthesia. London: Royal Society of Medicine Press, 2002:125.

[17] Magill IW. Personal Communication, 1976.

# Eve's rocking method of artificial respiration

Thomas F. Baskett

In the quest for effective artificial respiration a variety of methods using thoracic compression were introduced in the 19th and early 20th centuries. These included the techniques devised by Marshall Hall, Henry Silvester, Edward Schafer and Holger Neilsen [1]. All of these methods relied, to some extent, upon the elastic recoil of the muscles of the thorax to provide the inspiratory phase following the expiratory compression. Frank Eve, a consulting physician in internal medicine and paediatrics, took a different approach. In his 1932 publication in the *Lancet* he outlined his rationale [2] (Fig. 1):

---

## ACTUATION OF THE INERT DIAPHRAGM
### BY A GRAVITY METHOD

By Frank C. Eve, M.D. Camb., F.R.C.P. Lond.
CONSULTING PHYSICIAN, ROYAL INFIRMARY, HULL

---

Formerly I regarded the breathing thorax as a concertina-bellows ; my present work suggests that it resembles rather a cylinder and piston. In older men the cylinder wall is often rigid and is scarcely used in respiration at rest. Hence in artificial respiration it seems much better to exploit the piston action of the diaphragm rather than to try to compress the rigid walls of the cylinder—leaving the piston flapping passively up or down and thus frustrating much of one's efforts to squeeze air in and out of the trachea.

The efficacy of the following method—simple but apparently novel—is illustrated by my first two cases : (1) post-diphtheritic paralysis of the diaphragm (successful) ; (2) Landry's paralysis, dying of failure of the heart, not of respiration.

Essentially the method consists of laying the patient on a stretcher, which is pivoted about its

Fig. 1. Lancet 1932;1:95 [2].

"Formerly, I regarded the breathing thorax as a concertina-bellows; my present works suggest that it resembles a cylinder and piston. In older men, the cylinder wall is often rigid and scarcely used in respiration at rest. Hence, in artificial respiration it seems much better to exploit the piston action of the diaphragm rather than try to compress the rigid walls of the cylinder . . . . Essentially, the method consists of laying the patient on a stretcher, which is pivoted about its middle on a trestle and rocking up and down rhythmically so that the weight of the viscera pushes the flaccid diaphragm alternately up and down. Anyone can convince himself that this method of artificial respiration is adequate by lying on the apparatus in action. He will find that he need not breathe; it is done for him. Oxygen is not required—only air."

Eve provided two illustrative case reports to support his contentions. The first was a 2-year-old girl with post-diphtheritic diaphragmatic paralysis. The child's respiratory distress was partially relieved by placing her in the lateral head-down position. Eve was worried that the weight of the abdominal contents would push up the diaphragm and cause collapse of the lungs, which would increase the risk of pneumonia [2]. He therefore modified a rocking-chair into a bed with several blankets. He taught the parents to tilt the rocking-chair through 30° on each side of the horizontal about 10 times a minutes; this they did for the next two days other than during feeding. This apparently reduced the child's respiratory distress and she slept intermittently. A portable X-ray apparently showed the desired excursion of the diaphragm in the head-up and head-down position [2]. By the third day, the child was greatly improved and eventually recovered completely. In the other case, a 24-year-old man with Landry's paralysis, Eve initiated his rocking method by using a stretcher pivoted over a trestle. Although the man later died from cardiac failure the rocking movement was seen to relieve his cyanosis and Eve felt, "the apparatus did what it was asked to do" [2].

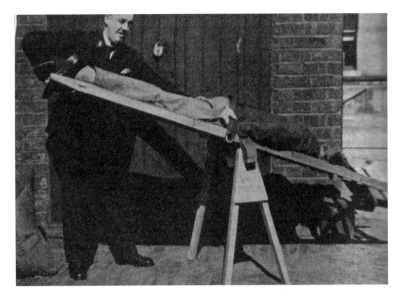

Fig. 2. Illustration of Eve's rocking method of artificial respiration [2].

In experiments on himself and his 18-year-old son, Eve had chest X-rays taken, which showed that the diaphragmatic movement was 5 cm. Using their chest measurements he calculated that this 5 cm excursion of the diaphragm amounted to 1800 cc of air movement. In contrast, he said that, "Schafer's method produced only 1000 cc air movement." In addition to this efficient movement of air in and out of the lungs, Eve felt the main benefit of his technique was the fact that it could be performed by the rescuer for many hours without exhaustion—in contrast to the other manual methods of artificial respiration. He acknowledged that there would often be a delay while the stretcher and trestle were gathered or improvised and advised that Schafer's method be used in the interim, and his own technique employed if long-term artificial respiration was necessary (Fig. 2).

In a subsequent publication, one year later, Eve and a colleague, Esther Killick from the Department of Physiology in the University of Leeds, reported the results of their physiological experiments on the rocking and other methods of artificial respiration [3]. They compared the tidal air during artificial respiration in healthy subjects and found that with Silvester's method the tidal air was about 200 cc, with the Schafer technique it was 350–550 cc and with the rocking method 450–600 cc. They also found that carbon dioxide elimination was increased when the rocking rate exceeded 15 min$^{-1}$ and that the percentage of oxygen absorbed declined as the rocking rate increased. They concluded that an excessive rocking rate would eliminate too much carbon dioxide, removing this stimulus to the respiratory centre and potentially delaying the onset of spontaneous breathing. For this reason, and the fact that the oxygen absorption diminished at high rates of rocking, they concluded, "Since measurements of the lung ventilation show that rocking the stretcher 10 times or more a minute induced adequate ventilation, we may conclude that for most subjects the optimum rate rocking the

stretcher lies between 10 and 15 per minute—i.e., the normal rate of breathing" [3]. In contrast, Gordon et al. [4] studying the measurement of pulmonary air exchange in "recently deceased warm corpses, prior to the onset of rigor mortis and ... within one hour of cessation of the heart beat" found that the rocking technique averaged 225 cc, the Schafer method 185 cc and the Silvester technique 520 cc. In a subsequent publication, Gordon, after further evaluation, recommended the Holger Nielson (arm-lift, back-pressure) method of artificial respiration [5].

During the Second World War, Eve made a plea for an improved approach to resuscitation of the drowned, "now so urgent a problem ... especially in these days of U-boats [6]". While Eve advocated the use of the Schafer method in the first instance he felt that it had considerable limitations in the management of the nearly drowned, "in whom the elastic tone of the respiratory muscles failed progressively" [6]. He found that the inspiratory phase required elastic recoil of the muscles in the Schafer technique and this elasticity was diminished in the nearly drowned. Working with colleagues in the Royal Navy, Eve helped them install the equipment and establish resuscitation drills. One of the practical difficulties was providing resuscitation in the small boats sent out from the larger ships to pick up the nearly drowned from the water. In these small boats, it was virtually impossible to provide any of the normal techniques of manual resuscitation. With his naval colleagues they worked out a method whereby two sailors opposite each other would grasp each other's forearms and use them as the pivot across which the body could be rocked until they reached the ship when a stretcher could be provided and rocked over "a trestle or rope from hammock hooks placed under the middle of the stretcher" [6]. Eve also pointed out that warmth was an essential component of resuscitation. His technique was officially adopted and endorsed by the Royal Navy during the Second World

War. In general, however, Eve's method was limited by the need to set up or improvise a rocking stretcher. Like all other methods of manual artificial respiration, it was supplanted by mouth-to-mouth respiration.

Frank Cecil Eve was born in 1871 at Silsoe, Bedfordshire. From Bedford school he obtained a scholarship in 1890 to Emmanuel College, Cambridge, where he took first class honours in the Natural Sciences Tripos. He worked as a demonstrator of Physiology at Yorkshire College, Leeds, and then completed his clinical work at St. Thomas's Hospital, London, where he was a university scholar [7]. He graduated MB in 1900 and followed this with the MRCP in 1901 and MD in 1903. He held posts as a house officer at St. Thomas's Hospital and the Hull Royal Infirmary. He was then appointed honorary physician and later consulting physician to the Hull Royal Infirmary and Victoria Hospital for Sick Children. He carried on a busy consulting practice in Hull but maintained his interest in physiology and made a number of practical contributions to the diagnosis and management of diabetes and pernicious anaemia. As a young man he was a considerable golfer, figure-skater, skier and fisherman. After retirement, he lived in the town of Beverley, Yorkshire where he died on 7 December 1952. His wife and only son were both physicians [7,8].

## References

[1] Thangam S, Weil MH, Rackow EC. Cardiopulmonary resuscitation: a historical review. Acute Care 1986;12:63–94.
[2] Eve FC. Actuation of the inert diaphragm by a gravity method. Lancet 1932;1:995–7.
[3] Killick EM, Eve FC. Physiological investigation of the rocking method of artificial respiration. Lancet 1933;2:740–2.
[4] Gordon AS, Fainer DC, Ivy AC. Artificial respiration: a new method and comparative study of different methods in adults. JAMA 1950;144:1455–64.
[5] Gordon AS, Sadove MS, Rayman F, Ivy AC. Critical survey of manual artificial respiration. JAMA 1951;147:1444–53.
[6] Eve FC. Complacency in resuscitation of the drowned. BMJ 1943;1:535–7.
[7] Eve FC. BMJ 1952;2:1362 [obituary].
[8] Eve FC. Lancet 1952;2:1276 [obituary].

# Arthur Guedel and the oropharyngeal airway

## Thomas F. Baskett

The oropharynx is the primary site of airway obstruction in the unconscious or anaesthetised patient. The obstruction is usually caused by relaxation of the tongue and musculature of the mandible, allowing posterior movement of the tongue and epiglottis to obstruct the airway. Oropharyngeal airways are used to establish a patent unobstructed airway and to act as a bite block. The original airways were made of metal but this was liable to cause trauma to the teeth and soft tissues of the lips and tongue. Arthur Guedel designed an oropharyngeal airway made of rubber with a metal insert to reinforce the proximal portion and prevent obstruction, if the patient bit down on the tube. There was a phalange at the oral end to keep it in front of the patient's teeth and lips and prevent over insertion. The curved portion of the tube conforms to the contours of the oropharynx, while a central channel allows exchange of respiratory and anaesthetic gases and the passage of a suction catheter. Guedel's original paper describing this enduring piece of anaesthetic equipment was 14 lines of a half column in the *Journal of the American Medical Association* in 1933 [1] (Fig. 1). Subsequent modifications have been made of plastic, but Guedel's principles remain and the eponymous Guedel airway has endured.

When discussing pharyngeal spasm, Guedel emphasized prevention and the use of the oropharyngeal airway to maintain oxygenation. If such an airway was not in place pharyngeal spasm could be difficult to manage: "The mouth is held rigidly shut so that the introduction of an oral-pharyngeal airway is difficult or impossible, and the posterior pharynx is so constricted that a soft rubber nasal airway will be of little or no help. By holding the gas mask tightly to the face a small amount of oxygen may be forced past the obstruction" [2]. Having discussed the condition and its management Guedel finished with a typical whimsical summation: "This accident although it is rarely of serious consequence, does, because of the ugly appearance of the patient, worry the gallery and embarrass the anesthetist considerably" [2]. He also emphasised the use of the oropharyngeal airway during anaesthesia when "there is sufficient muscular relaxation to permit the lower jaw to fall backward allowing the base of the tongue to lie against the posterior wall of the pharynx. Depending upon the anatomical structure of the pharynx, this may partially or completely obstruct inspiration. It is usually remedied at once by the insertion of a pharyngeal airway which will hold the tongue forward from the pharyngeal wall" [2].

One of Guedel's other major contributions was to standardise the clinical observations to estimate the depth of anaesthesia. These principles formed the core of his later text *Inhalation Anesthesia: A Fundamental Guide* first published in 1937 [2] with a second edition in 1951. The opening sentence of his book set the practical tone: "This subject is treated concisely, avoiding confusing details, in order that the student may have a helpful picture to aid him in his early work" [2]. The genesis of his observations was one of necessity during his service with the American Expeditionary Force in France during the latter part of the First World War. The paucity of trained medical and nursing staff to administer anaesthesia was highlighted by the overwhelming numbers of soldiers requiring this service. As he wrote in the forward to his book [2]:

"Due to the deplorable lack of knowledge of anesthesia in the medical corps of the American Army during the World War, the author of this little book found himself in the embarrassing position of providing pain relief for our wounded soldiers in several base hospitals of the war zones. The only available personnel was made up of nurses and enlisted men of the army medical corps, with little or no medical training or background. By means of a motorcycle, he was able to visit once daily, a number of base hospitals and there to instruct and supervise untrained and inexperienced men in the art of anesthesia. The necessity was obvious for a simple and rapid

# Clinical Notes, Suggestions and New Instruments

## A NONTRAUMATIC PHARYNGEAL AIRWAY

ARTHUR E. GUEDEL, M.D., BEVERLY HILLS, CALIF.

The pharyngeal airway has become an indispensable part of the anesthetist's equipment. Heretofore, various forms have been made of metal; but metal airways are all more or less traumatizing, even when carefully used, frequently producing cut or bruised lips, chipped or broken teeth, or lacerations of the pharyngeal mucosa.

The airway herewith depicted is made of rubber and is sufficiently soft and flexible not to traumatize yet amply rigid

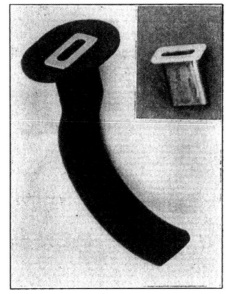

Pharyngeal airway made of rubber, with metal insert for mouthpiece.

to maintain an open oropharyngeal air passage under all conditions. Its flexibility permits it to conform to the varied oropharyngeal curves in different individuals.

The metal insert extends into the airway for about 2 cm. from the oral opening and prevents collapse of the rubber between the teeth.

520 North Bedford Drive.

Fig. 1. Journal of the American Medical Association 1933;100: 1862.

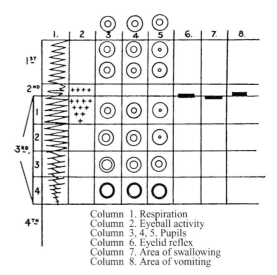

Column 1. Respiration
Column 2. Eyeball activity
Column 3, 4, 5. Pupils
Column 6. Eyelid reflex
Column 7. Area of swallowing
Column 8. Area of vomiting

Fig. 2. From: Guedel AE. Inhalation Analgesia: A Fundamental Guide. New York: The MacMillan Company, 1937. p. 25.

sia at the Indianapolis General, St. Vincent's and Protestant Deaconess Hospitals [4].

Even before his stint in the army Guedel showed his initiative and practical nature in his first paper published on the administration of nitrous oxide in obstetrics [6]. Although this had first been proposed by Klikovich in 1881 [7] ether and chloroform were almost exclusively used for pain relief in labour if, indeed, any analgesia was provided at all. Guedel devised a technique with a mixture of nitrous oxide and air analgesia, which could be self-administered by the patient [6]. He emphasized the advantage of the woman controlling the analgesia herself: "She soon learns that her relief depends

means of teaching physical signs and danger signals which could be readily grasped by the uninitiated. Evidence was needed which could tell him at a glance, on his short daily inspection visits, whether the man was applying instruction which he had previously received."

Guedel created a wall chart with a grid of physical signs, with emphasis on the eyes, that allowed the untrained personnel to assess the depth of anaesthesia (Fig. 2). This battleground experience was to form the basis of Guedel's subsequent publications and teaching on the assessment of the depth of anaesthesia [3,4].

Arthur Ernest Guedel was born in Cambridge City, Indiana on 13 June 1883. He graduated from the Medical College of the University of Indiana in 1908. While an intern at the City Hospital in Indianapolis part of his duties was to administer ether and chloroform anaesthesia [5]. He started in general practice, but increasingly confined his practice to anaesthe-

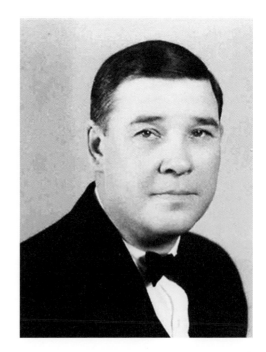

Fig. 3. Arthur Ernest Guedel (1883–1956). Reproduced with permission from the Wood Library-Museum of Anesthesiology, Park Ridge, IL, USA.

upon the results of a race between the actions of the gas and the pain, with the gas winning always if given an even start" [6].

Another of Guedel contributions was in the development of safe endotracheal intubation. In his home laboratory, and using the fingers of rubber gloves, he designed inflatable cuffs for endotracheal tubes [5]. In conjunction with an anaesthetic colleague, Ralph Waters from Madison, Wisconsin, he developed a new endotracheal tube with the inflation bag situated in the trachea just beneath the larynx [8,9]. Guedel dramatically displayed the integrity of the system by anaesthetizing his own dog, named "Airway", followed by intubation and total emersion of the dog in an aquarium. The dog remained anaesthetized in this position for one hour during the lecture demonstration. Anaesthesia was then stopped and the dog was removed from the water tank, revived, shook himself vigorously and, after a short nap, left the stage—presumably to sustained applause [5,8]. Among other innovations Guedel devised a straight blade for the laryngoscope [10].

After service in the first World War Guedel returned to Indianapolis and the private practice of anaesthesia with an appointment in the School of Medicine at Indiana University. In 1928 he moved to Pasadena, California as Clinical Professor of Anaesthesia at the University of Southern California and worked at the Cedars of Lebanon Hospital in Los Angeles [5,11]. It was here that he developed the oropharyngeal airway. Guedel worked hard, long and fast with a personal motto, 'maintain flying speed' [11]. Suffering from insomnia he took barbiturates to sleep and then found he needed amphetamines to counteract the effect in the mornings. Recognizing his addiction he had the courage and conviction to stop both drugs. In his student days he was a considerable athlete but his later years were marred by arthritis and ischaemic heart disease, such that he retired from clinical practice in 1941 [5]. He continued to stimulate and investigate with his large cadre of anaesthetic friends and colleagues. His contribution to anaesthesia was recognized by award of the Henry Hickman Medal in 1941 and, in 1950, the Distinguished Service Award of the American Society of Anesthesiologists [12].

Arthur Guedel was from the era of anaesthetists who, to some extent, made it up as they went along. However, his innovations were marked by careful observation, exhaustive testing and pragmatic common sense. Although his oropharyngeal airway was one of his simplest inventions it remains an essential piece of anaesthetic and resuscitation equipment more than 70 years after he introduced it with a succinct 14 line report.

## References

[1] Guedel AE. A nontraumatic pharyngeal airway. J Am Med Assoc 1933;100:1862.

[2] Guedel AE. Inhalation Anesthesia: A Fundamental Guide. New York: The MacMillan Company; 1937. pp. 25, 102-5.

[3] Guedel AE. Third stage ether anaesthesia: a sub-classification regarding the significance of the position and movements of the eyeball. Am J Surg (Anesth Suppl) 1920;34:53–7.

[4] Faulconer A, Keys TE. Foundations of Anesthesiology. Springfield: Charles C. Thomas; 1965, vol. 2, p. 1216.

[5] Maltby JR, Arthur E. Guedel (1883–1956). In: Maltby JR, editor. Notable Names in Anaesthesia. London: RSM Press, 2002. p. 84–6.

[6] Guedel AE. Nitrous oxide air anesthesia self-administered in obstetrics—a preliminary report. Indianapolis Med J 1911;14:476–9.

[7] Klikovich S. Uber das Stickstoffoxydul als Anaesttheticum bei Geburten. Arch Gynak 1881;18:81–108.

[8] Guedel AE, Waters RM. A new intra-tracheal catheter. Anesth Analg 1928;7:238–9.

[9] Waters RM, Rovenstine EA, Guedel AE. Endotracheal anesthesia and its historical development. Anesth Analg 1933;12:196–203.

[10] Dorsch JA, Dorsch SE. Understanding Anesthesia Equipment. 4th ed. Baltimore: Williams & Wilkins; 1999. p. 516.

[11] Waters R. Emminent anaesthetists, No. 7: Arthur E. Guedel. Br J Anaesth 1952; 24: 292–9.

[12] Keys TE. The History of Surgical Anesthesia. Park Ridge (Illinois): Wood Library-Museum of Anesthesiology, 1996. p. 76–8.

# Martin Kirschner: 1879—1942—A surgeon in prehospital care

## W. Dick

The Martin Kirschner AWARD (5.000 €) for scientific research in pre-hospital emergency medicine is awarded each year by the South West German Association of Emergency Physicians (Figure 1).

Who was the man behind this award?

In 1942, Rudolf Zenker, chairman of the Surgical University Hospital Heidelberg, opened his obituary on Martin Kirschner by quoting Johann Wolfgang von Goethe:

"The surgeon dedicates himself to the most divine of all occupations, to cure without miracles and to work miracles without words".[17]

Martin Kirschner is looked upon as the "father of pre-hospital emergency care" by emergency physicians in German-speaking countries.

In 1938 he stated that "it is not the emergency patient who should be taken to the hospital to be seen by the doctor, but the hospital doctor should go out to see and treat the emergency patient at the scene of an accident" (a postulate later extended to any life-threatening situation) (Figure 2).

Kirschner also called for the use of aircraft for the monitored transfer of critically ill patients from one hospital to the other.[4] Surprisingly, his surgical colleagues, who were appreciative of the merits of Martin Kirschner's other innovative ideas, failed to recognise the value of this concept, whose time was to come later.

Many of his articles on topics of emergency medicine document Kirschner's extensive experience gained as one of the leading military surgeons on the battlefields of World War I (and World War II).

Let us take a look at his life and his invaluable contributions to emergency medicine in a chronological manner for a complete portrayal of the man and his work:[2,4,13,15,16,18]

Martin Kirschner was born on October 28th, 1879 in Breslau (today: Wroclaw, in Poland). He studied medicine at the Universities of Freiburg and Straßbourg, where he earned his doctoral degree in 1904, before going on to study and train first in Zürich and later in München to obtain his licence to practice medicine.

As was customary at that time, he spent a few years in internal medicine in Berlin (von Renvers) before going to Greifswald in 1908 to study with the surgeon E. Payr. He followed Payr to Koenigsberg 1910, and soon thereafter began to embark on his academic career with the publication of his first scientific articles, and by regular participation

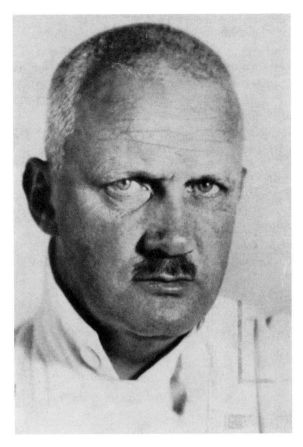

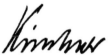

Figure 1 Martin Kirschner: Galerie hervorragender Ärzte und Naturforscher. From ref. 17. Beilage zur Münchn. Med. Wschr. Blatt 567, 1942. With kind permission of Urban und VOGEL 30.5.2005.

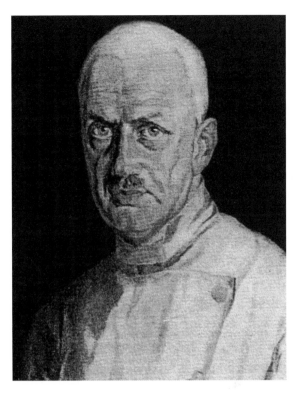

Figure 3 Martin Kirschner on the occasion of his birthday. From ref. 15. Georg Thieme Verlag KG. With kind permission of Georg Thieme Verlag 1.6.05.

in the annual congresses of the German Society of Surgery.

He completed his postdoctoral dissertation (Habilitation) successfully in 1911. At the age of 37 years, Kirschner was appointed professor of surgery at the University of Koenigsberg in 1916. Not long thereafter he was offered the chair of surgery at the University of Tuebingen, a position he filled from

1927 to 1934. In 1934 he was appointed chairman of the University Hospital of Surgery in Heidelberg, where he remained until the end of his academic career (Figure 3).

The following achievements emphasise Kirschner's importance as a pioneer of modern emergency medicine:

1. First pulmonary embolectomy[7]

    This operation was first described by Kirschner's colleague Trendelenburg and became famous under the latter's name as a life-saving surgical intervention. However, Martin Kirschner was the first surgeon to carry out this procedure successfully in a patient in 1927.[3]

2. Kirschner—wire extension and splints[8,14]

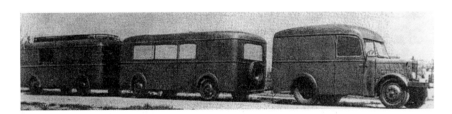

Figure 2 Mobile Life Support Unit (Notarztwagen). From ref. 4. Georg Thieme Verlag. With kind permission of Georg Thieme Verlag 1.6.05.

This well-known procedure, which is still widely used today, was developed during World War I, and facilitated the initial care of wounded patients considerably.

3. Kirschner's bloodlessness
4. Kirschner's operations I and II
5. Kirschner—Perthes cuff
6. Treatment of pain[5,6,12,18]

Motivated by his experience as a military surgeon, Kirschner made the improvement of the treatment of pain a focus of his scientific research, which led to the development of

- high pressure local anaesthesia;
- target controlled spinal anaesthesia;
- rectal anaesthesia with Avertin.

The use of Avertin did, however, not gain wide acceptance and was soon replaced by short-acting barbiturates.[11]

- The development of SEE (scopolamine-Eucodal (oxycodon-HCL)-ephedrine) analgo-sedation in trauma victims. This combination was used extensively over many years, but was later replaced by more advanced agents.
- Electrocoagulation of the trigeminal nerve (Gasserian ganglion), a procedure applied in chronic pain management.

On the occasion of a symposium held in Heidelberg in 1980 to commemorate the 100th anniversary of Kirschner's birthday, Rudolf Frey underlined that M. Kirschner's scientific endeavours had created the basis for the future development of pain clinics.[18]

The statement, ''... even in visceral surgery and traumatology, this man left his foot prints.'', taken from the Newsletter of Vascular Surgeons documents that the importance of the name Martin Kirschner is by no means limited to vascular surgery. This also holds true for the fame of Kirschner's surgical clinic teaching institution:[1] In the 1930s DeBakey, who subsequently became surgical chief of the Texas Heart Institute and introduced coronary bypass procedures into cardiac surgery, underwent part of his postgraduate surgical training with Martin Kirschner at the Heidelberg institution. DeBakey was later honoured with the title Alumnus of the University of Heidelberg.[1]

In addition to his varied medical activities, Martin Kirschner was one of the few surgeons at that time who engaged themselves intensively on planning and designing university surgical hospitals (Tübingen, Heidelberg, Koenigsberg). One of his contributions to hospital design consisted of the separation of wards from functional complexes by establishing independent diagnostic and therapeutic areas, facilities for teaching and training, as well as for emergency care.[9,10]

Considering all of his activities and commitments, Kirschner's scientific publication activity was astonishing, comprising 200 papers in respected scientific journals, eight book chapters, and more than three comprehensive, or sets of, books.

Kirschner is not only justly considered the 'father' of pre-hospital emergency medicine in Germany, but also, as Goerig and Schulte am Esch emphasised in 1994, as one of the pioneer anaesthetists, intensivists and pain therapists, in parallel to his lifelong commitment to surgery.[4]

# References

1. Kirschner M. Heidelberg Alumni International-Service: Alumni Review—September 2001. Alumni Spotlight University of Heidelberg.
2. Kirschner M. Badische Landesbibliothek.
3. Birks W. History of cardiac surgery in Germany— in consideration of her relation to the German Cardiac Society. Z Kardiol 2002;91(Suppl. 4):81—5.
4. Goerig M, Schulte am Esch J. Martin Kirschner: Anaesthesiologist, Intensive Care Physician-Pain Therapist (German) Anästh. Intensivmed., Notfallmed, Schmerzth. 1994;29:343—53.
5. Kirschner M. Berichte über die erste Hilfsexpedition nach Bulgarien. Beiträge zur Kriegsheilkunde: Central Komitee der Deutschen Vereine vom Roten Kreuz: Berlin; 1914.
6. Kirschner M. Kriegschirurgische Erfahrungen vom Balkankriegsschauplatz Dtsch Med. Wschr. 1914;2:99.
7. Kirschner M. Ein durch die Trendelenburg Operation geheilter Fall von Embolie der Art. Pulmonalis, Arch Klin Chir 1924;133:312—27.
8. Kirschner M. Verbesserung der Drahtextension. Arch Klin Chir 1927;148:650—8.
9. Kirschner M. Zum Neubau der Chirurgischen Universitätsklinik Tübingen II Der Krankenbau Chirurg 1930;2: 54—61.
10. Kirschner M. Zum Neubau der Chirurgischen Universitätsklinik Tübingen III Der Behandlungbau Chirurg 1930;2: 202—15.
11. Kirschner M. Intravenöse Kurz.-und Rauschnarkose mit Evipan. Arch Klin Chir 1933;177:48—51.
12. Kirschner M. Die Schmerzbekämpfung im Felde. Chirurg 1936;8:269—76.
13. Rheder K, Shampo MA, Kyle RA, Kirschner M. JAMA 1982; 247:1302.
14. Rieger A, Ebel H, Laun A. Modified Kirschner wire insertion for direct ventral screw fixation of dens fracture (German). Zbl Neurochir 1995;56:97—101.
15. Schmitt W. Martin Kirschner on the occasion of his 100th birthday (German). Zbl Chirurgie 1979;104:1434—7.
16. Kirschner M. www.whonamedics.com.
17. Zenker R, Kirschner M. Münchner Medizinische Wochenschrift 1942:41;876—7.
18. Zenker R. Die Chirurgie Martin Kirschners in unserer Zeit. Münch. Med. Wschr, 1980;122:318—9.

# Breaking the thermal barrier: Dr. Temple Fay

Ana G. Alzaga , Gloria A. Salazar , Joseph Varon

Dr. Temple Fay (1895–1963), one of the most talented and skilled neurosurgeons of his time, is also considered a pioneer in therapeutic hypothermia. He was an inquisitive thinker who encountered multiple difficulties experimenting in such an unknown field. Fay believed that body temperature was an important physiopathological factor in certain diseases such as cancer. He conducted several clinical trials and broke ''the thermal barrier''. The vast majority of Fay's patients with terminal diseases experienced beneficial outcomes after ''refrigeration'' and the mortality rates were low. The cooling methods he implemented form the basis of the methods we use today to induce hypothermia. Dr. Fay's discoveries led to today's indications and techniques for therapeutic hypothermia.

Dr. Temple Fay, since the age of 12, knew where he was heading, followed his mentors and became one of the most talented and skilled neurosurgeons of his time.[1,2] His endless questions and thirst for knowledge led him to breakthroughs in several areas in neurosurgery and science, seeking for new and innovating ways for treatment through his research.[1] Like many geniuses in history, he was ahead of his time and was not fully recognized by his peers, sometimes confronting harsh criticism and isolation.

Temple Fay is remembered for several achievements but one of them makes him standout.[3] He was a pioneer of what we now know as therapeutic hypothermia, a recognized medical procedure nowadays, but an unexplored field in Dr. Fay's time. He, nevertheless, was an unconventional man, breaking barriers of time, prejudice, thought and most of all, temperature.[3]

## His beginnings

Temple Fay was born on January 9, 1895 in the city of Seattle. His parents both came from families of great scientists and naturalists. As a child, Fay was brought up in an environment of academic achievement and high expectations.[2,3]

Fay was pressurised by his family to go into the clergy but he was set on becoming a doctor.[2] He attended the Medical School of the University of Pennsylvannia.[3] Fay spent all his free time on the wards with Dr. William G. Spiller and Dr. Charles H. Frazier, who were well known as a neurologist and a surgeon respectively.[2,3] He began as Dr. Spiller's assistant and later he assisted Dr. Frazier in surgeries to become assistant in neurological surgery and instructor in neurology.[3] He learned everything he could from his mentors and became a neurologist and neurosurgeon of outstanding skill. He always demanded perfection from the people around him as well as loyalty and honesty.[2]

In 1929, he became a professor of neurosurgery and head of the department at the Temple University.[2] In 1931, he founded the Harvey Cushing Society with doctors Van Wagenen, Glen Spurling and Eustace Semmes, which, years later, became the American Association of Neurological Surgeons.[2] Dr. Fay was the Society's sixth president (see Figure 1).

## His early work

Dr. Fay's interests, in the 1920s, were mainly focused on water balance and metabolism, particularly applied to reducing intracranial pressure.[1-3] In patients with intracranial hypertension, he would use hypertonic solutions, especially magnesium sulphate which could be given orally or rectally. Then remove by lumbar puncture as much spinal fluid as possible and restrict fluid intake.[2-4] These dehydrating measures were also applied to patients with migraine and epilepsy.[1-3] The same principle was applied in eclampsia, with a therapeutic modality named Arnold-Fay in 1930.[2,5]

He considered his research on biochemical and biophysical balances at the cellular level of the central nervous system to be the most important contribution of his life.[3]

He invented and modified several surgical instruments and ventured into new surgical procedures.[3]

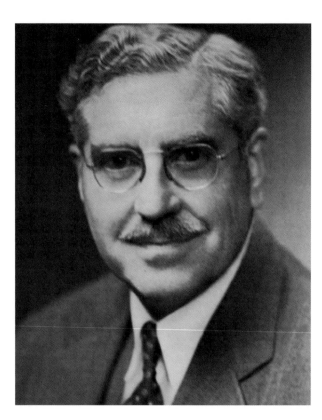

**Figure 1** Dr. Temple Fay.

In 1923, he developed, with Dr. Francis C. Grant, a ventriculoscope which could be adapted for intraventricular photography.[1,2,3,6] He elaborated on an instrument which combined suction and irrigation for intracranial surgeries.[3,7] He was one of the first surgeons to approach neuralgia of the glossopharyngeal nerve with an intracranial approach.[1,2,3,8]

## Breaking the thermal barrier

While Dr. Fay was still in medical school, he participated in a knowledge quiz. Directing the quiz was Dr. Allen Smith who asked Fay if he knew why metastatic cancer rarely appears in the limbs.[3] He answered that he did not know and his professor acknowledged he did not know either; this question would leave a great impression in Fay's mind.[3]

In the late 1930s, he finally decided to pursue the answer to this question and started his research on the matter. He hypothesized that the differences in the location for cancer growth had to do with temperature and soon started collecting data of temperatures at different body sites.[2] He used a thermocouple device and a galvanometer determining variations of segmental or dermatomal temperature elaborated by George C. Henny of the Department of Biophysics at Temple University.[3,9] He found a decrease in temperature of 12–22 °F below knees and elbows compared to the rest of the body.[3,10] In contrast, he observed that common cancerous sites, were mostly located in areas with higher temperatures.[3,10]

Fay also investigated the effects of different temperatures in chicken embryos at his farm in Maryland.[3] With the assistance of Dr. Lawrence W. Smith from the Department of Pathology at Temple University, he found a marked retardation and inhibition of embryonic growth with the use of low temperatures as he discovered that cellular differentiation seemed to cease almost entirely at 90 °F.[10] Dr. Fay determined that cellular temperature levels were a factor in the evolution of cancer cells.[2,10] He found through tissue culture methods that the growth of tumor cells was affected by temperature.[2,10]

The next step was to apply this in the clinical setting.[10] He was the first physician ever to perform "cooling" trials on humans. Patients with terminal, inoperable cancers were treated with local "refrigeration", as he would call it.[10,11] Local refrigeration was reached with the application of ice water and ice at first.[10] The first attempts included a water cooler, rubber tubing and a discarded $CO_2$ gas capsule with two small metal tubes soldered into its neck.[12–14] Later on, Fay implemented cooling devices designed individually using coils, hollow metal capsules or appropriately fitted rubber bags to fit the structures in which the tumors were located and to secure the maximum distribution of cooling process (see Figure 2).[10,12,13]

The first reported patient of Dr. Fay to undergo hypothermia (July 1936) was suffering from intractable pain from massive pelvic extension of a cervical carcinoma.[10] The capsule, connected to a continuous circulation of ice water, was inserted deep in the vaginal mass and continuous refrigeration of the local area was maintained by constant circulation of water through an enclosed system at approximately 36 °F.[10] At the end of 48 h, the patient was pain free. Within 5 days, the carcinomatous area had definite devascularization and shrinkage of the gross mass.[10]

In cases in which Dr. Fay wanted to implement hypothermia into deep areas of the body, mainly the brain, he used local implants of subfreezing metal capsules or "bombs".[14] These capsules with connecting tubing were sterilized and introduced into the brain through a trephine or craniotomy adjacent to the lesion.[14] The results in patients with cerebritis, osteomyelitis, skull fractures or after neurosurgical removal of the necrotic core

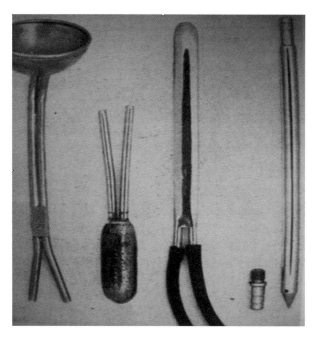

**Figure 2** Instruments used by Dr. Fay for "local refrigeration".

of gliomata were very encouraging.[14] Fay noticed a reduction in pain and swelling in the area of trauma or infection, as well as a bacteriostatic effect. This approach was used before antibiotics were available.[14]

Dr. Fay continued to perform local refrigeration and serial biopsies at varying intervals in several patients with carcinomatous lesions near body surfaces. It became obvious that local hypothermia, when applied to involved areas, promptly controlled pain, retarded malignant cellular metabolism and growth, was bacteriostatic, reduced inflammation and was well tolerated by the brain.[14] Dr. Machteld Sano from the Department of Neuropathology established the critical level of temperature for division of malignant cells in vitro.[14] This critical level was reached at 67.5 °F.[14]

The following question naturally arose as to the possibility of reducing the entire body temperature below the "normal level", in hopes of retarding the growth of deep metastatic tumors inaccessible by local hypothermia methods.[14] It was also intriguing to know how far it would be safe to carry the body temperature below the standards of "normal" and for how long.

The first attempt of general "refrigeration" was made on November 28, 1938.[14] It was a cool crisp day and Fay opened the window in the patient's room and shut off the heat. One hundred and fifty pounds of ice chips were placed over the patient as he lay in bed.[14] Soon after the patient received sedation and her body temperature dropped to the low 30's °C.[14] Clinical hypothermia was experimentally achieved that afternoon.[14] The patient's blood pressure and pulse virtually disappeared, and although the patient continued to breathe, the fear of cerebral hypoxia persisted.[14] The patient was rewarmed to normal temperature values again with heat applied to body surfaces and a hot coffee enema.[14] Within a few hours, the patient had returned to conscious levels and was not aware of the experience.[14]

The majority of Dr. Fay's early hypothermia patients were physicians or nurses who understood the inevitable outcome of metastatic malignancies.[14] Each patient was prepared differently before inducing hypothermia.[14] Each individual's personality and emotional state were evaluated closely at least 18–24 h before the induction of "refrigeration".[14] Most patients received chloral hydrate and sodium bromide by mouth or rectum the night or the morning before the induction.[14] Moments before the period of actual "refrigeration", paraldehyde was given.

Fay believed that the fact that the patients knew the truth about their terminal condition gave them a new found self-confidence.[14] He believed every patient had to be ready before initiating hypothermia rather than rushing them to fit into the schedule of the hospital.[14] When the patient's body temperature began dropping beyond 33 °C, pulse pressure, hemoglobin, pH and $CO_2$ determinations, urine and blood analysis were monitored regularly.[14]

The nursing staff at first was quite concerned about working in the "Refrigeration Service".[14] The nurses had difficulties getting the patient's temperature with the long-stemmed laboratory thermometers, difficulty getting the readings for the blood pressure, and water and ice were everywhere in the room.[14] The programme was almost shutdown when some nurses started getting "colds" and other illnesses.[14] Fortunately, special blankets made of rubber tubes devised to carry a cold solution from a special "beer cooler" machine pumps were commercially available and were found to be useful in this technique (see Figure 3).[14] Electric thermocouples for 24-h charting of rectal temperatures were also designed. The need for cold rooms disappeared with the use of this apparatus and no further complaints were received from the nursing staff.[14]

The preliminary results of Dr. Fay's program were presented at the Scientific Session and Exhibit of the American Medical Association in St. Louis in 1939.[14] Even though the potential of "refrigeration" was evident in many aspects, his work received a "cold reception".

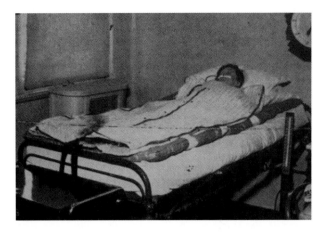

**Figure 3** Patient in "general refrigeration" with the help of a special blanket containing rubber tubing, continuous circulation of chilled solution and automatic temperature control. Picture also shows rectal thermocouple.

During World War II, the Germans apparently captured one of his manuscripts, 'Observations on Prolonged Human Refrigeration', sent to Belgium for publication and became familiar with the technique. Refrigeration was used experimentally in concentration camps and became an infamous procedure.[14] This was thought to delay the progress of hypothermia for about 10 years.

From July 9th, 1936 to October 1st, 1940, Fay conducted 169 episodes of "refrigeration" treating a total of 126 patients, mostly with terminal cancer (112 patients), five patients with brain tumors, four with leukemia, three with Hodgkin's disease, one patient with filariasis and another one with syphilis.[12] In 83 instances, the patients were treated with local "refrigeration" maintained at 7 °C.[12] In 66 patients, general "refrigeration" was induced from 12 to 24 h to 8 days, ranging rectal temperatures from 33 to 25 °C.[12]

The most remarkable effect of hypothermia in these patients was the relief of pain that the vast majority of the patients experienced.[11,14] The basal metabolism was reduced on average by 20–25%.[11] Acute anemia was noted in some patients who underwent several periods of generalized refrigeration. In the first 24–48 h, a number of patients experienced a rise in the leukocyte count of 15–20,000 with a normal differential count. A drop in the urea levels and blood sugar was also seen in some patients. Kidney function was noted to be maintained if intravenous fluids were provided.[11]

Repeated neurological examinations were also performed in 42 of the patients subjected in all to 83 episodes of refrigeration with the assistance of Dr. Gerald W. Smith.[13,14] Each period varied in duration from 24h to 5 days and a total of 400 examinations were performed.[13] Increase in deep tendon reflexes was seen at a temperature range of 36—30 °C which corresponded to the shivering stage. Abolition of deep tendon, abdominal and gag reflexes occurred at 25 °C. The pupils remained equal, regular and normal in size but the response to light became progressively sluggish until it was abolished at 25 °C. Dysarthria began at 35 °C and retrograde amnesia remained below 35 °C. Cerebration was delayed and mental faculties were preserved until the temperature reached 35 °C. The relief of pain was seen in 95.3% of the patients.[13]

As happens to most innovators, Dr. Fay was roughly criticised by his peers since at that time the general understanding was that survival below 35 °C was impossible.[3,14] All the clinical thermometers were calibrated down to only 35 °C, the lowest temperature compatible with human life.[14]

Dr. Fay always acknowledged the use of refrigeration as an ancient art.[14] In the clinical setting, scientists such as Thomas Bell (Bell's palsy) (1829), John Hughes Bennett (1849), James Arnott (1851), Thomas Weedon Cooke (1865), J.W. Bright (1871), and S. Weir Mitchell (1872), reported favorable results in a variety of clinical conditions.[14]

The last article Fay published, in 1959, looked back to his earlier studies in hypothermia and acknowledged the group of courageous young people who worked with him.[14] He felt ''fortunate, because when one strays from the conventional paths of medicine, there is a great comfort and encouragement in the assurance and confidence of the younger minds to offset the disapproval and outright condemnation from the older and more conventional members of the profession''.[3,14] It was then, and not 20 years before, that he could now talk about human refrigeration to most of his colleagues without the criticism and antagonism of the past.[14]

## His last days

Dr. Fay's last years of clinical research were focused on studying mental paralysis and rehabilitation.[1] In 1960, after developing hypertensive encephalopathy, he spent his last few years at his home close to a small nucleus of family and friends, continuing to study and write, still looking ahead.[2,3]

Therapeutic hypothermia has become part of the armamentarium for clinicians over the past 5 years.[15—17] Use of this technique has clearly shown significant neurological improvement in a variety of settings.[18,19] This improvement is mainly due to Dr.

Fay's efforts at breaking the thermal barrier and many others that worked in this field.[20]

## References

1. Wolf JM. Temple Fay, M.D.—Inquisitive scientist, prolific scrivener. Pathol Med J 1965;68:47—51.
2. Murtagh F. Temple Fay, M.D. 1895—1963. Surg Neurol 1991;36:167—9.
3. Henderson AR. Temple Fay, M.D., unconformable crusader and harbinger of human refrigeration. J Neurosurg 1963;20:627—34.
4. Fay T. The administration of hypertonic salt solutions for the relief of intracranial pressure. JAMA 1923;80:1445—8.
5. Arnold JD, Fay T. Eclampsia; its prevention and control by means of fluid limitation and dehydration. Surg Gyn Obs Internat Abst Surg 1932;55:129—50.
6. Fay T, Grant FC. Ventriculoscopy and intraventricular photography in internal hydrocephalus. JAMA 1923;80:461—3.
7. Fay T. New instrument combining suction and irrigation for intracranial surgery. JAMA 1927;89:25—6.
8. Fay T. Intracranial division of glossopharyngeal nerve combined with cervical rhizotomy for pain in inoperable carcinoma of the throat. Ann Surg 1926;84:456—9.
9. Fay T, Henny GC. Correlation of body segmental temperature and its relation to the location of carcinomatous metastasis. Clinical observations and response to methods of refrigeration. Surg Gyn Obs Internat Abst Surg 1938;66:512—24.
10. Smith LW, Fay T. Temperature factors in cancer and embryonal cell growth. JAMA 1939;113:653—60.
11. Smith LW, Fay T. Observations on human beings with cancer, maintained at reduced temperatures of 75—90 °F. Am J Clin Pathol 1940;10:1—11.
12. Fay T. Clinical report and evaluation of low temperature in treatment of cancer. Proceed Inter-state Post Grad Med Ass N Am 1940:292—7.
13. Fay T, Smith GW. Observations on reflex responses during prolonged periods of human refrigeration. Arch Neurol Psychol 1941;45:215—22.
14. Fay T. Early experiences with local and generalized refrigeration of the human brain. J Neurosurg 1959;16:239—59.
15. Holzer M, Cerchiari E, Martens P, et al. The hypothermia after cardiac arrest study group: mild therapeutic hypothermia to improve the neurologic outcome after cardiac arrest. N Engl J Med 2002;346:549—56.
16. Bernard SA. Therapeutic hypothermia after cardiac arrest. MJA 2004;181:468—9.
17. Bernard S, Buist M. Induced hypothermia in critical care medicine: a review. Crit Care Med 2003;31:2041—51.

18. Nolan JP, Hazinski MF, Steen PA, Becker LB. Controversial topics from the 2005 International Consensus Conference on cardiopulmonary resuscitation and emergency cardiovascular care science with treatment recommendations. Resuscitation 2005;67:175—9.

19. Safar PJ, Kochanek PM. Therapeutic hypothermic after cardiac arrest. N Engl J Med 2002;346:612—3.

20. Safar P. Mild hypothermia in resuscitation: a historical perspective. Ann Emerg Med 2003;41:887—8.

# The Holger Nielsen method of artificial respiration

## Thomas F. Baskett

Widespread teaching and application of manual techniques of artificial respiration for both lay people and medical personnel developed in the last half of the 19th century and into the early 20th century. One of the first methods to achieve acceptance was that of Hall,[1] followed by the techniques of Silvester,[2] Howard,[3] and Shafer.[4] Until the early 20th century the two most commonly used methods were those of Hall and Silvester. Both the Hall and Silvester techniques suffered from the fact that the tongue was likely to fall back and obstruct the airway and similar criticism was levelled against the Howard technique. In 1904, the prone pressure method developed by Shafer was increasingly accepted, although it was shown subsequently to be the least effective of all the techniques.[5]

In Copenhagen, Colonel Holger Louis Nielsen (1866–1955), who was a physical fitness instructor in the Danish Army and an experienced teacher of life saving methods, began to work on an improved technique of artificial respiration[6] (Figure 1). Nielsen had taught both the Silvester and Shafer methods to his students. However, he felt that neither of these techniques was ideal: the supine position of the Silvester method with its potential for airway obstruction by the tongue, and the prone pressure method of Shafer which lacked an active inspiratory phase component. He thus developed his method in which the victim was placed prone with the elbows bent and the hands placed under forehead. The expiratory action was the same as Shafer's with prone pressure on the posterior part of the chest and the inspiratory phase was accomplished by lifting the elbows.[7,8] Initially Nielsen proposed two operators, one each for the inspiratory and expiratory phases, respectively. He presented this proposal to the Danish Red Cross in 1930 but they rejected it on the grounds that it was impractical to expect two operators to be present.[6] The answer to the one-man approach came to Nielsen fortuitously when he attended a masseur seeking relief from muscular pain in his shoulders. During the massage, while Nielson lay on his stomach he noted that when the masseur, who was positioned at the head of the table, pressed down on his shoulder blades it caused a forced expiration.[6,9] Nielsen had the answer: he placed one rescuer at the head of the victim with instructions to press down on the shoulder blades then pull up on the bent elbows (Figure 2). The method, which became known as the 'push–pull' technique, was described as follows[8]:

'The victim's arms are folded and his face turned sideways and placed on his hands. The operator kneels about 6 inches from the head...he places the

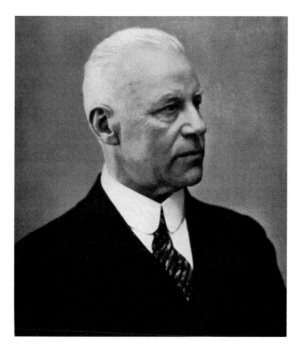

**Figure 1** Holger Nielsen (1866—1955).

heels of his hands on the upper edge of the shoulder blades with the fingers spread out obliquely. He slowly rocks forward on straight elbows until his arms are nearly vertical, exerting steady pressure on the chest; then rocks back slowly, sliding his hands to the victims arms, just above the elbow, grasps the arms and continues to rock backward, raising the arms until tension is felt, and then draws them slightly towards himself; finally, he lowers the arms, completing the cycle. The whole cycle should take about six seconds, so that it is carried out at a rate of about 10 times a minutes. Two seconds should be allowed for pressure on the back and two seconds for traction on the arms, allowing one second for every change of the hand position.'

As Nielsen developed his technique he sought assistance from senior physiologists in Denmark who assured him that the amount of pulmonary ventilation with his manoeuvre was equal to or superior to other techniques.[10] He then published his method in the Danish literature[11] (Figure 3).

In 1933 the Danish Red Cross accepted and endorsed Nielsen's one-man method. The Holger

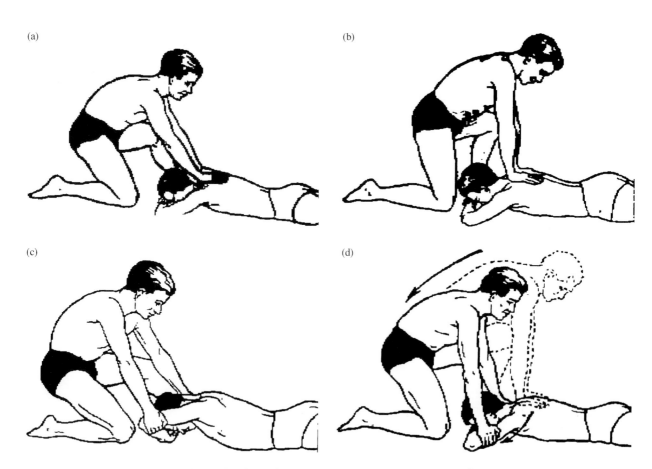

**Figure 2** The Holger Nielsen method of resuscitation.[8]

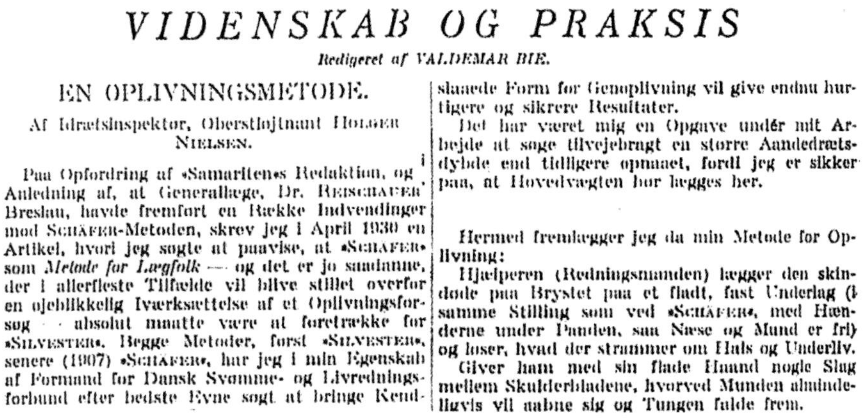

VIDENSKAB OG PRAKSIS

Redigeret af VALDEMAR BIE.

EN OPLIVNINGSMETODE.

Af Idrætsinspektør, Oberstløjtnant HOLGER
NIELSEN.

Paa Opfordring af »Samariten«s Redaktion, og
Anledning af, at Generallæge, Dr. REISCHAUER,
Breslau, havde fremført en Række Indvendinger
mod SCHÄFER-Metoden, skrev jeg i April 1930 en
Artikel, hvori jeg søgte at paavise, at »SCHÄFER«
som Metode for Lægfolk — og det er jo saadanne,
der i allerfleste Tilfælde vil blive stillet overfor
en øjeblikkelig Iværksættelse af et Oplivningsfor-
søg — absolut maatte være at foretrække for
»SILVESTER«. Begge Metoder, først »SILVESTER«,
senere (1907) »SCHÄFER«, har jeg i min Egenskab
af Formand for Dansk Svømme- og Livrednings-
forbund efter bedste Evne søgt at bringe Kend-

skabede Form for Genoplivning vil give endnu hur-
tigere og sikrere Resultater.
    Det har været mig en Opgave under mit Ar-
bejde at søge tilvejebragt en større Aandedræts-
dybde end tidligere opnaaet, fordi jeg er sikker
paa, at Hovedvægten bør lægges her.

    Hermed fremlægger jeg da min Metode for Op-
livning:
    Hjælperen (Redningsmanden) lægger den skin-
døde paa Brystet paa et fladt, fast Underlag (i
samme Stilling som ved »SCHÄFER«, med Hæn-
derne under Panden, saa Næse og Mund er fri)
og løser, hvad der strammer om Hals og Underliv.
    Giver ham med sin flade Haand nogle Slag
mellem Skulderbladene, hvorved Munden alminde-
ligvis vil aabne sig og Tungen falde frem.

**Figure 3** Nielsen's original paper.[11]

Nielsen method of artificial respiration was rapidly accepted in Scandinavian countries and in Europe by the late 1930s. In 1935 Nielsen introduced his technique at the 4th International Congress for Live-saving and First Aid in London. Acceptance of his method spread throughout Europe and North America and by 1953, at the International Red Cross Conference in Toronto, Nielsen's technique was officially adopted as the method of choice for first-aid teaching.[12] However, by the late 1950s the evolution of cardio-pulmonary resuscitation with mouth-to-mouth respiration rendered obsolete Nielsen's and the other techniques of manual artificial respiration that had been developed over the previous 100 years.

# References

1. Hall M. On a new mode of effecting artificial respiration. Lancet 1856;1:229.
2. Silvester HR. A new method of resuscitating still-born children, and of restoring the persons apparently drowned or dead. BMJ 1858;2:576—9.
3. Howard B. The more usual methods of artificial respiration. With demonstrations of the ''direct method'' of the author. Lancet 1877;2:194—6.
4. Shafer EA. Description of a simple and efficient method of performing artificial respiration in the human subject especially in drowning to which is appended instructions for the treatment of the apparently drowned. Med Chir Trans 1904;87:609—15.
5. Gordon AS, Fainer DC, Ivy AC. Artificial respiration: a new method and comparative study of different methods in adults. JAMA 1950;144:1455—64.
6. Karpovich PV. Adventures in Artificial Respiration. New York: Association Press; 1953. p. 63—6.
7. Garland TO. Artificial respiration: with special emphasis on the Holger Nielsen method. London: Faber and Faber Ltd.; 1955.
8. Resuscitation drill—the Holger Neilson method. The Royal Life Saving Society's handbook of instruction. 22nd ed.; 1958.
9. Eisenberg MS. Life in the Balance. New York: Oxford University Press; 1997. p. 82.
10. Asmussen E, Nielsen M. Efficacy of artificial respiration. J Appl Physiol 1950;3:95—102.
11. Nielsen H. En oplivningsmetode (method of resuscitation). Ugesk f Laeger 1932;94:1201—3.
12. Gentle HW. A new method of artificial respiration. Natl Safety News 1935;32:34.

# Naum L Gurvich: A pioneer of defibrillation

Ludmila V. Ussenko, Alexander V. Tsarev , Yaroslav A. Leschenko

It is difficult to imagine modern cardiopulmonary resuscitation (CPR) without using electric defibrillation as its principal component. Our knowledge of the ventricular fibrillation (VF) mechanism and possibilities of practical application electric defibrillation today is expanding from the introduction of automated external defibrillators (AED) and automated implantable cardiovertor defibrillators (AICD) to the fundamental investigation of chaotic properties of VF as complex nonlinear systems. But such outstanding investigators as PC Abilgaard, JL McWilliam, JL Prevost, F Batelli, CJ Wiggers, CS Beck, P Zoll, WB Kouwenhoven, AN Diack, A Winfree, VI Krinsky and B Lown were the first to study VF and create electric defibrillation methods. Among them a special place belongs to the Russian scientist Naum Lasarevich Gurvich (Figure 1).

Naum L Gurvich was born 15 April 1905 in Timkovich (Byelorussia) in a teacher's family. In 1923 he entered the medical faculty of the State Crimean University. A year later, in connection with the breakup of the University, he moved to Saratov and continued his study in the Medical Institute from which he graduated in 1928. After graduating from the institute, Gurvich worked as an ordinary doctor in the Moscow region for 4 years. In 1932—1935 he was a postgraduate student at the Physiology Institute of Narcompross. Then he worked as an assistant Professor at the physiology department of Veterinary Institute and Second Moscow State Medical Institute.

In 1937 he was promoted to be a scientific worker in the Physiology Institute. His leader was the director of the institute Professor LS Shtern. Shtern had graduated from Geneva University and for many years she worked under the leadership of Professor JL Prevost.[1] In 1899 Prevost and Batelli published their first work on possibility of treating VF by electrical defibrillation, and in 1900 they described the use of an electrical discharge from a capacitor.

In the Physiology Institute Shtern organized a group of investigators to undertake research into the mechanism of arrhythmia and the influence electrical shock. Naum Gurvich was a participant in this group. In 1939, Gurvich along with GS Yuniew published his classical work ''Restoration of regular rhythm in the mammalian fibrillating heart'' in which they proposed using a single discharge from a capacitor for converting VF.[2] That year Gurvich graduated with a doctorate in medicine with a thesis entitled ''About stimulation of intramural system by sinusoidal low frequency current.'' In these works he concluded that electrical influence on the heart within definite current parameters caused a stimulant effect and could lead to two contrary results. On one hand, alternating current with a fre-

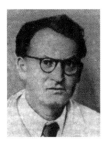

**Figure 1** Naum L Gurvich.

quency of 50—500 Hz could not be tolerated by the hearts conducting mechanism and, as a result, VF occurs. On the other hand a single discharge from a capacitor through inductance caused synchronization of excitation process and stops VF.[3-5]

In 1939 Gurvich together with GS Yuniev resuscitated a dog, which had been subjected to induced ventricular fibrillation, with combined transthoracic electrical defibrillation and closed chest cardiac massage. In 1947 Naum Gurvich published his next work which showed that heart massage can be done in a dog by frontal compression of the thorax. However, when the thorax is wide, compression through the open thorax is a more effective way. Using this method he succeeded in supporting the circulation for 15 min and through transthoracic defibrillation the normal work of heart recovered.[6,7] Though these facts were ahead of their time they were not picked up in the classical works of Kouwenhoven et al.

In 1948 after the closure of the Physiology Institute, Gurvich began to work with Professor Vladimir Negovsky on resuscitation of the organism in the experimental physiology laboratory of the USSR Academy of Medical Sciences. Negovsky wrote about their first meeting: *On the question about the principal direction of his research Gurvich answered: ''Electric physiology of heart and defibrillation in particular.'' ''We are interested in brain, — was my answer, — could you help us in research into electrical physiology in the dying man and reviving the brain?'' His answer: ''I could. Only for that I'll have to study this scientific direction. Aren't you interested in working out heart defibrillation methods?'' I answered: ''We cope anyhow with fibrillation but research into the brain, dying and resuscitation is still for us ''tabula rasa'''''. Gurvich remarked: ''But if we together continue to work out defibrillation methods we'll be able to defibrillate heart not ''anyhow'' but safely and steadily''. In conclusion I said: ''I take you on our staff. Go on working on heart electrical physiology and later we will determine the direction of your scientific work''.*[8]

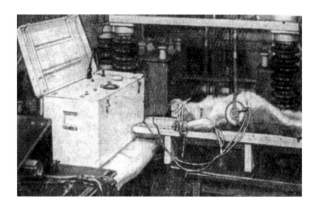

**Figure 2** The impulse defibrillator ID-I-UEI 1952.

The first impulse defibrillator ID-1-UEI (the First USSR Electro-engineering Institution) was made and produced in 1952 (Figure 2). It was based on a new method of heart transthoracic defibrillation. Synchronisation of excitation was achieved by a strong current of 8—10 ms on the heart.

In 1957 Gurvich summed up the results of his researches and his accumulated experience in one of the first monographs on this subject ''Fibrillation and defibrillation of heart'' (Figure 3).[9] The next

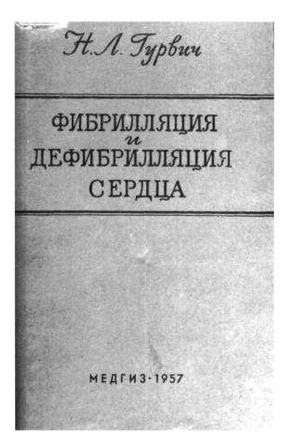

**Figure 3** Cover of the monograph ''Fibrillation and defibrillation'' published in 1957.

important discovery was Gurvich's proposal about using biphasic waveforms. A hypothesis suggesting the effectiveness of a symmetric biphasic waveform was suggested by Gurvich and Makaraechev,[10] independently of the earlier work of Kouwenhoven and Knickerbocker published in 1963 in an engineering journal. They described the first "diphasic" — now called biphasic defibrillator — but this did not attract any attention from medical public.[11,12] Gurvich's biphasic defibrillators were manufactured and used in the USSR in the 1970s but the biphasic waveform in defibrillators in the West was not realized until the 1990s.

In 1968 engineers Venin et al. suggested a scheme for a biphasic quasi-sinusoidal impulse with a given pattern of half-waves. Experimental research on animals demonstrated that an impulse with equal half-waves (called symmetric biphasic quasi-sinusoidal impulse) was less effective than a monophasic impulse. A group of research doctors from Institute of General Reanimatology of USSR (since 1991 Russia) Academy of Medical Sciences — Gurvich, Tabak, Bogushevich (Moscow, Russia) together with engineers from USSR Institute of Radio Electronic Medical Apparatus (REMA) — Venin, Pasechnik, Baluashvilli (Lviv, Ukraine) worked out the concept of a biphasic asymmetric quasi-sinusoidal defibrillating impulse. Effectiveness increased almost twice as a result of summing, the highest aspect of both half-waves and it was named the Gurvich—Venin impulse.[13,14] In 1970 the USSR began the industrial production of defibrillators ID-03 and DKI-01, generating a biphasic waveform 25 years before the West. In 1975 Gurvich published his second monograph "The main principles of cardiac defibrillation"[15] in which he summed up his experience of more than 30 years of experimental and clinical research.

Naum L Gurvich died on February 25, 1981.

We must thank him for being one of the first, ahead of his time, who could shoot an arrow of knowledge into the research of ventricular fibrillation and electrical defibrillation of heart.

## References

1. Negovsky VA, Bogushevich MS, Gurvich NL. Founder of theory of fibrillation and defibrillation of the heart. In: Moroz V, editor. Fundamental problems of reanimatology, vol. 2. Moscow; 2001. p. 3—16 [book in Russian].
2. Gurvich NL, Yuniev G. Restoration of regular rhythm in the mammalian fibrillating heart. Bull Exp Biol Med 1939;8:55—8; Gurvich NL, Yuniev G. Am Rev Sov Med 1946;3:236—9 [translated].
3. Gurvich NL, Yuniev GS. About restoration of normal rhythm in the fibrillating heart by a capacitor discharge. Bull Exp Biol Med 1939;8(1):54—8 [in Russian].
4. Gurvich NL. Dependence of threshold size of tension and capacity of capacitor discharges on halting fibrillation of heart. Bull Exp Biol Med 1943;16(12):66—9 [in Russian].
5. Gurvich NL. Stopping fibrillation by the repeated capacitor discharge of threshold force. Bull Exp Biol Med 1945;20:55—6 [in Russian].
6. Gurvich NL. Restoration of regular rhythm in heart with prolonged fibrillation. Bull Exp Biol Med 1947;23(1):28—32 [in Russian].
7. Gurvich NL, Yuniev G. Restoration of heart rhythm during fibrillation by a condenser discharge. Am Rev Sov Med 1947;4:252—6.
8. Negovsky VA. Old and always new problems of reanimatology. Anesthesiol Reanimatol 1996;5:4—9 [in Russian].
9. Gurvich NL. Fibrillation and defibrillation of heart. Moscow: Medgis; 1957 [book in Russian].
10. Gurvich NL, Makaraechev VA. Optimum electric impulses at defibrillation. In: Negovsky VA, editor. Actual questions of reanimatology and hypothermia. Moscow: Medicina; 1964. p. 14—5 [book in Russian].
11. Chamberlain D. Never quite there: a tale of resuscitation medicine. Resuscitation 2004;60:3—11.
12. Acosta P, Varon J, Sternbach GL, Baskett PJF. Kouwenhoven, Jude and Knickerbocker the introduction of defibrillation and external chest compressions into modern resuscitation. Resuscitation 2005;64:139—43.
13. Gurvich NL, Makaraechev VA. Defibrillation of heart by the biphasic waveform. Cardiology 1967;7:109—12 [in Russian].
14. Gurvich NL, Tabak VY, Bogushevich MS, Venin IV. Defibrillation of heart by the biphasic waveform in experiment and clinics. Cardiology 1971;8:126—30 [in Russian].
15. Gurvich NL. The main principles of cardiac defibrillation. Moscow: Medicina; 1975 [book in Russian].

# Claude Beck and ventricular defibrillation

George L. Sternbach    Joseph Varon    Robert E. Fromm Jr

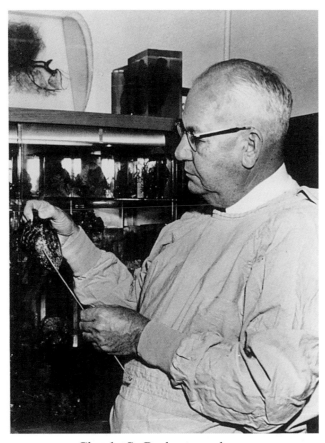

Claude S. Beck at work.

The first case of successful resuscitation of a patient from ventricular fibrillation was reported by Claude S. Beck in 1947 [1]. Beck, the innovative surgeon at Western Reserve School of Medicine in Cleveland, described the course of cardiac arrest occurring during surgery for sternal resection of severe pectus excavatum. The patient, R.H., a 14 year-old boy tolerated the surgery well but sustained cardiac arrest during closure. The electrocardiogram confirmed ventricular fibrillation. The incision was reopened, internal cardiac massage initiated, and the patient given intravenous epinephrine and digitalis.

For 45 min he failed to respond to these measures. An electric shock was then applied directly to the heart, but ventricular fibrillation persisted. A second series of shocks produced ventricular standstill, but this was followed almost immediately by the appearance of regular, though feeble myocardial contractions. Heart massage was continued for 5 min, until it was apparent that cardiac activity was adequate.

Although the systolic blood pressure was only 50 mmHg at this point, the patient's pupils had remained constricted and no cyanosis had appeared throughout the course of the resuscitation. The thorax was closed after a perfusing rhythm had been present for 20 min. The patient proceeded to make a full recovery, exhibiting no subsequent signs of cardiac or neurological impairment.

Although it is now recognized that the rhythm responsible for the vast majority of cardiac arrests is ventricular fibrillation, this mechanism remained obscure for many centuries. Throughout most of the nineteenth century, it was commonly assumed that sudden cardiac death was caused by the abrupt cessation of the heart's activity in diastole. Hoffa and Ludwig, two German physiologists, first described canine ventricular fibrillation in 1850 [2]. They considered this to be merely a laboratory phenomenon, irrelevant to clinical medicine.

Nearly 40 years later, John McWilliam, of the University of Aberdeen, Scotland, published a radical hypothesis in the British Medical Journal [3]. Extensive animal experimentation had convinced him that cardiac arrest was usually due to ventricular fibrillation rather than diastolic ventricular standstill. Though McWilliam had not actually witnessed this arrhythmia to occur in humans, it seemed to him "in the highest degree probable that a similar phenomenon occurs in the human heart" [3]. He proceeded to describe the terminal cardiac activity in poetic terms. Ventricular fibrillation constituted a "violent, though irregular and uncoordinated manifestation of ventricular energy. Instead of quiescence, there is tumultuous activity, irregular in its character and wholly ineffective as regards its results. The cardiac pump is thrown out of gear, and the last of its vital energy is dissipated in a violent and prolonged turmoil of fruitless activity in the ventricular walls" [3].

No successful treatment for this calamity was attained to be for the next decade. In 1899, the French physiologists Prevost and Battelli terminated ventricular fibrillation in dogs by passing high-voltage current between scalp and rectal electrodes [4]. Achieving a more conventional electrode placement took somewhat longer. Hooker et al. successfully demonstrated transthoracic defibrillation in dogs in 1933 [5]. By this time, Claude Beck was already well known, most notably for his descriptions of the cardiac compression trials with which his name is associated [6].

Beck was born in Pennsylvania in 1894. He trained at Johns Hopkins University and Harvard University before going to Cleveland in 1924. Although predominantly a thoracic surgeon, he made numerous contributions to vascular and neurological surgery. During thoracic operations, he developed an interest in open chest massage and defibrillation. For a number of years, Beck made efforts to defibrillate patients who developed ventricular fibrillation intraoperatively. By 1941 he had restored stable rhythms in several such patients, but all died without ever regaining consciousness [7].

When he finally succeeded in the case of R.H., he used his standard method for intra-operative defibrillation. The heart was "placed between two large electrodes and ordinary 110 volt alternating current with 1.5 amperes is momentarily impressed through the heart between the electrodes. Usually a series of shocks is necessary to accomplish defibrillation" [1]. Beck attributed success in this case to the combination of electric shock and continuous cardiac massage. It was his stated hope that the case would induce operating rooms to "be equipped to handle cases of sudden ventricular fibrillation and that personnel will be trained in the method" [1].

## References

[1] Beck CS, Pritchard WH, Feil HS. Ventricular fibrillation of long duration abolished by electric shock. J Am Med Assoc 1947;135:985–6.

[2] Hoffa M, Ludwig C. Einige neue versuche uber herzbewegung. Z Ration Med 1850;9:107–44.

[3] McWilliam JA. Cardiac failure and sudden death. Br Med J 1889;1:6–8.

[4] Prevost JL, Battelli F. Sur quelques effets des decharges

electriques sur le coeur des mammiferes. C R Seances Acad Sci 1899;129:1267–8.

[5] Hooker DR, Kouwenhoven WB, Langworthy OR. The effect of alternating electrical currents on the heart. Am J Physiol 1933;103:444–54.

[6] Sternbach G, Beck C. Cardiac compression triads. J Emerg Med 1988;6:417–9.

[7] Beck CS. Resuscitation for cardiac standstill and ventricular fibrillation occurring during operation. Am J Surg 1941;54:273–9.

# Vladimir A. Negovsky the father of 'reanimatology'

## Peter Safar

Vladimir A. Negovsky of Moscow (Figs. 1 and 2) created the science of resuscitation medicine [1,2]. This he calls 'reanimatology' [3], which includes the prevention and treatment of critical terminal states and post-resuscitation disease. This term makes more sense than our terms 'resuscitation' and 'intensive care' for two reasons: First, it focuses on 'anima' the mind or spirit, indicating that resuscitation efforts must aim for survival without brain damage. Secondly it focuses on science ('--ology') while our terms mean methods. Americans, however, may think of 'anima' as animation for Disney movies. A compromise would be to equate 'critical care medicine' (CCM) with 'resuscitology' [4] and to identify CPR as methods of basic, advanced, and prolonged life support, i.e. *'cardiopulmonary–cerebral resuscitation'* (CPCR) [5].

Negovsky was a pathophysiologist when he initiated scientific work for what later became resuscitation medicine. Throughout the latter half of the 20th century, he and his associates have researched acute terminal states and clinical death and their reversibility, considering a global view of the whole organism. His work has influenced many around the world.

In 1936, Negovsky founded the first resuscitation research laboratory in the world [6]. In 1986 his 'laboratory' was renamed Institute of Reanimatology of the USSR (since 1991 of the Russian) Academy of Medical Sciences. His countrymen in the 1940s and 1950s, and his colleagues around the world since the 1960s, have been inspired by his concepts and the terminologies. He introduced the terms 'terminal state', 'agonal state', 'clinical death' (i.e. the period of no blood flow that is potentially reversible to complete recovery), 'biological death' (cardiac arrest with brain death which is irreversible) and the 'post-resuscitation disease' of multiple organ systems [7], particularly of the most vulnerable organ, the brain [7–9].

Already in 1951, he had published in Russian his observations on cerebral changes during dying and resuscitation. One can only speculate on whether resuscitation research would have flourished more rapidly had Negovsky's findings and spirit been accessible to the outside world between 1936 and 1962, when World War II and the Iron Curtain isolated our colleagues in communist countries.

## 1. Negovsky the scientist

Negovsky was born on March 19, 1909, in Kozelts, the Chernygov region of the Ukraine (a part of the Russian Empire at that time). He grew up in a family of teachers, with many brothers and sisters. In 1933, he graduated from the Second Medical Institute in Moscow and started working as a physician and later as a scientific worker in the Institute of Experimental Physiology and Therapy. In 1936, he initiated the first laboratory in the world that focused on restoring vital processes during acutely life-threatening conditions, especially on dying and resuscitation, starting with systematic studies in animal models. He developed an exsanguination cardiac arrest model in dogs, reversing the arrest with centripetal arterial pressure infusion of oxygenated, warm blood with epinephrine, accompanied by artificial ventilation with bellows; the heart stopped in electro–mechanical dissociation and resumed beating under arterial infusion, without requiring cardiac massage [10]. During the second World War, in the spring of 1943, Negovsky formed front-line resuscitation teams and achieved effective resuscitation of more than 40 wounded men with clinical death,

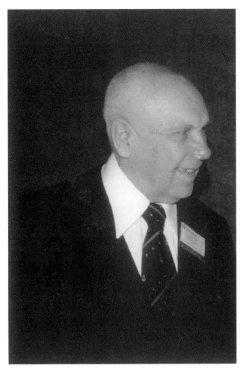

Fig. 1. Portrait of Vladimir Negovsky in the 1980s.

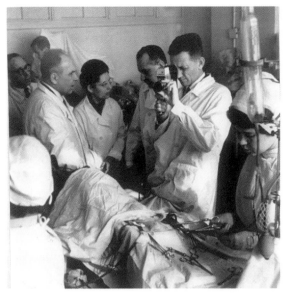

Fig. 2. The Pittsburgh–Moscow Connection as it began in 1962. Vladimir Negovsky (left), with Peter Safar, Chairman of Anesthesiology and Critical Care Medicine, University of Pittsburgh (right), and Hugh Rosomoff, Professor of Neurosurgery, University of Pittsburgh (center), visiting in 1963 at the reanimatology laboratory of the USSR Academy of Medical Sciences on 25th October St., Moscow. This picture was taken during one of Negovsky's exsanguination cardiac arrest-arterial resuscitation dog experiments. Guy Knickerbocker of Baltimore was also present, then working on defibrillation with Naum Gurvich in Negovsky's laboratory.

using the above method [11]. Later his team also used other models of dying, including electrically induced ventricular fibrillation and asphyxia.

In Europe, a 'doctorate' requires a thesis. In 1943, Negovsky presented his thesis on the 'pathophysiology and reversal of death' [12], in which he stated the main principles of the pathophysiology of terminal states and of complex resuscitation methods. His thesis became his first book, which was translated later into English in eight issues of the American Review of Soviet Medicine [12]. In 1945, his war resuscitation experience became his second book [11]. In the 1950s, his first book was updated in Russian and translated into Dutch, Romanian, Polish, and German. Soon after the war, in 1947, he was promoted to professor.

In Negovsky's laboratory, since the 1940s, external chest compression to provide heart massage was used on animals [6–12]. This was more than 10 years before the re-discovery and clinical introduction of this method of emergency artificial circulation without thoracotomy in Baltimore [13]. In the 1880s, German surgeons had successfully used external chest compression in patients, but did not pursue it [14]. Some laboratory researchers around the world, however, continued using chest compressions at a rapid rate on animals, for both artificial ventilation *and* circulation, mostly for anaesthesia induced apnea and pulselessness [6,7,15–17]. Negovsky's associates studied issues of pathophysiology and therapy of terminal states caused by different mechanisms, including trauma, blood loss, myocardial infarction,

drowning, electric trauma, and asphyxia of the newborn.

Since the 1940s, Negovsky's associate Naum L. Gurvich [15] had studied the aetiology and pathogenesis of ventricular fibrillation and issues of electric defibrillation. Gurvich demonstrated for the first time the feasibility of reversing ventricular fibrillation in dogs with an 'external impulse charge' using direct current (DC) countershock, which made it possible to create the first battery-powered portable defibrillators. This was about 10 years before the first successful use of external defibrillation with alternating current (AC) in patients by Zoll in Boston [18], with DC in patients by Peleska in Prague [19] and Lown in Boston, and with AC and DC in animals by Kouwenhoven in Baltimore [20]. Later, in the 1960s, Negovsky and his students improved the Gurvich defibrillator by applying a bipolar-shaped impulse which later received the name 'Gurvich's impulse'. A number of defibrillators were created which generated an impulse which was safer and more effective than other defibrillators.

Negovsky also employed and inspired neuroscientist Alexander Gurvitch [21], who had joined him in 1953. Alexander Gurvitch was among the first to study, in animals and patients, the general principles of decreasing and restoring cortical and subcortical activity in various regions of the brain, during different patterns of dying and resuscitation. He showed that the electroencephalogram was a reliable diagnostic tool for following post-insult restoration of brain activity.

Fundamental studies and clinical experience allowed Negovsky, at the International Conference of Traumatologists in Budapest in 1961, to declare the appearance of a new medical science of *reanimatology*, which had as its goal the prevention and therapy of terminal states and clinical death [22]. Negovsky was mentor to several generations of 'reanimatologists' in communist countries, for some of whom anaesthesiology, out-of-hospital emergency care, and other acute clinical practices, had become subspecialties of reanimatology.

Alexander Gurvitch and biochemist Zolotokrylina were co-authors with Negovsky for his pioneering book (in English) on the post-resuscitation disease [7]. The authors' descriptions of post-cardiac arrest derangements, pursued systematically in animal models and patients, concern all vital organs. This was a 'first'. They raised the possibility of post-insult self-poisoning by 'toxic' blood. I had the privilege of recommending and chaperoning this book for publication in the West. The post-insult derangements described include what was later labeled in the West, 'reoxygenation injury'. Negovsky's post-resuscitation disease, however, includes more than free radical reactions, which until the 1980s could only be suspected, not proven. Other areas where Negovsky made major contributions since the 1960s concern the understanding of lethal accidents in pregnant women, resuscitation of the newborn, determination of brain death, and issues related to organ donation [23].

Negovsky's laboratory team responded to hospitals and maternity homes for resuscitation attempts. Since 1946 the laboratory's associates rendered resuscitation aid to patients in the Institute of Chest Surgery led by the cardiac surgeon A. Bakulev. In 1955, physicians from his laboratory were assigned for permanent work in the Department of Emergency Surgery in the S.P. Botkin Hospital to help patients with massive blood loss and severe trauma. In 1959, Negovsky created the first Moscow Center for the treatment of shock and terminal states, and later, in 1962, the first resuscitation unit. E. Zolotokrylina, V. Kassil and other members of his laboratory took an active part in the organization and work. In 1964, a centre for advanced intensive care ambulances was set up in Moscow.

The first hospital Intensive Care Unit (ICU) in the USSR was set up at the Botkin Hospital in 1962, by Negovsky's associate Kassil and others [2]. The hospital ICU developments in the 1950s in Scandinavia [24] and Baltimore [25] may have stimulated the development of similar units in the USSR. While Negovsky's base specialty was pathophysiology, he leaned heavily on clinical disciplines, particularly anaesthesiology, the base specialty of his successors as Institute directors, Professor Victor Semenov (1987–95) and Professor Victor Moroz (since 1995). They all have shared my view that every modern anesthesiologist is (should be)

also a reanimatologist, an expert in basic, advanced, and prolonged life support.

Negovsky became an 'academician of the USSR' in 1975. He is the author or co-author of more than 300 scientific publications and 14 monographs, some of which, since the 1960s, have been translated into several Western languages. He was twice awarded the state prize of the USSR, with gold medals from the Soviet Peace Fund. Negovsky is also a corresponding (honorary) member of the Academy of Medicine in Toulouse (France), the Slovenian Academy of Science and Arts, and other scientific and medical societies abroad. At the time of his 85th birthday, he was in good health. Until then he had maintained throughout a reputation of tenaciously pursuing unanswered questions. I visited him last in 1999, for his 90th birthday celebration, hosted by his successor, Professor Victor Moroz.

## 2. The Moscow–Pittsburgh connection

I have been privileged to share a friendship with Vladimir Negovsky since 1962. Although we had the opportunity to honour him before [1–3,26,27], I wish to pay tribute to him again through this article. The sentiments also come from the University of Pittsburgh, its International Resuscitation Research Center (IRRC) [28] (renamed in 1994 by its current director Patrick Kochanek, 'The Safar Center for Resuscitation Research'), and its alumni, peers and colleagues worldwide.

Though I began resuscitation research in Baltimore in 1956 I did not know about Negovsky's work until the early 1960s when I read his earlier work through the English translation of his book, 'Resuscitation and Artificial Hypothermia' [23]. We first met in September 1962, at the first European Congress of Anesthesiology in Vienna, organized by Vienna's anesthesiology chairman, Professor Otto Mayrhofer [29]. Karl Steinbereithner and I had invited Negovsky to be a member of a panel on 'Controversial Aspects of Resuscitation'. We were thrilled that the iron curtain had been pierced with scientific communication and collegiality. Although Negovsky came to Vienna 'chaperoned', he and I established a form of openness for clinician–scientists then and there, long before Gorbachev initiated 'glasnost' for the entire USSR. In the same year, presidents Kennedy and Kruschev had met in Vienna in a futile attempt to de-fuse the nuclear war confrontation. In Vienna [29], our stimulating panel ranged from the steps of CPCR [5] to Negovsky's concept of post-resuscitation disease [7]. As this was 4 years after the launching of Sputnik, Negovsky was also asked about space capsule technology, such as its oxygen environment. When questions and disagreements arose on resuscitation topics, including those from participating colleagues of other Eastern countries, Professors Jiri Pokorny and Hugo Keszler from Prague, Negovsky handled them with collegiality. Our panel discussion of 1962 was published as the first monograph of the 'Anesthesiology and Resuscitation' series by Springer-Verlag [29].

At that meeting of 1962 in Vienna, Negovsky invited me to Moscow. Keszler and Pokorny of Prague also invited me to Prague. For this trip in September 1963, I invited my friend and hypothermia pioneer neurosurgeon Hubert Rosomoff (then of Pittsburgh) [30] (Fig. 2). Our study tour was supported by the US Army. In both cities collegial military physicians rolled out the 'red carpet', probably because they had seen our US Army-made documentary film on mouth-to-mouth ventilation and CPR research made in Baltimore. In Moscow we met Guy Knickerbocker, PhD research fellow of the Johns Hopkins University [13], who then spent several months with Naum Gurvich in defibrillation research [15]. Knickerbocker spoke Russian. In those days we were 'chaperoned' by 'administrators' and attractive Intourist translators in Negovsky's laboratory, at our hotel, and at official events. Otherwise, we were left alone to roam the streets unchaperoned. This kindled warm feelings toward the Russian people.

In the spartan environment of the Negovsky laboratory, in an old building on 25 October Street, near Red Square, Negovsky was the obvious father of the team. During this and subsequent visits, his imaginative ideas and writings, and his personality, made us add to our resuscitation research a greater interest in pathophysiology-orientated research. When, in 1979, we consolidated our resuscitation research projects as the IRRC in Pittsburgh, we did so in an old brick building on Pittsburgh's Fifth Avenue [28], which resembles Negovsky's laboratory [6]. His historic building is gone now and his Institute has moved to a new building at 25 Petrovka Street. Our IRRC building (in the distant past used for a casket factory near the hospital) has remained our home. It was honored when Negovsky and his successors visited us.

Soon after our historic visit to Moscow in 1963, President John F. Kennedy was murdered; we received warm condolences from Vladimir. I then learned that US Senator Hubert Humphrey, later vice-president of the US, had visited the Negovsky laboratory in 1959. Humphrey reported to the US Congress on the outstanding achievements of the Russian scientists. I urged the US Congress to support resuscitation research centers in the U.S. The National Institute of Health had other priorities.

Persistence ensured that there was continuous communication and scientific cross-fertilization between resuscitation researchers in Moscow and those in Pittsburgh, fueled by regular meetings at medical congresses, and reciprocal visits to Moscow and Pittsburgh between 1963 and 1999 (Fig. 3). In 1987, we were keynote speakers at the Clinical Death Researchers'

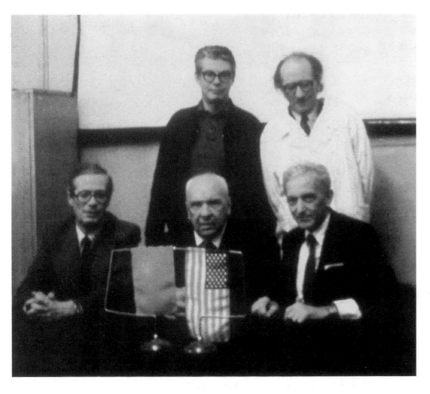

Fig. 3. Practicing 'glasnost' while promoting friendships between East and West during the cold war, at Negovsky's laboratory in 1973. Standing (left to right) Drs A Gurvitch, and Tabak. Seated Drs, Kassil, Negovsky and Safar.

Symposium in Pittsburgh, at the centennial of the University of Pittsburgh [31,32] and we published side-by-side in the proceedings of several congresses [31–34]. The University of Pittsburgh awarded Negovsky a certificate of recognition (comparable to an honorary doctorate in other universities) for 'visionary and pioneering research for more than 40 years'. In the early 1990s, the USSR Academy of Medical Sciences, Scandinavian anaesthesiology professors, and the University of Pittsburgh honoured us for our introduction of modern resuscitation medicine, with prestigious nominations. In 1994, the European Resuscitation Research Council made us both Honorary Members [1,35].

Scientific disagreements between us were resolved by mutual collegial review of publications. We have been special advisors to the journal, 'Resuscitation', since we helped its initiator, physiologist Hillman, in the 1970s. Our research has been complementary. Negovsky has focused more on pathophysiology and on protective and preservative hypothermia (before and during the insult) [23,36]. I have focused more on CPCR methods and on resuscitative hypothermia (after the insult).

Communication between Pittsburgh and Moscow was facilitated by Miroslav Klain, M.D., Ph.D., Professor of Anesthesiology and CCM in Pittsburgh, who through his roots in Prague also speaks Russian. There has been much ongoing communication, but no joint laboratory work between the two groups, probably because of the language barrier and different styles of conducting and reporting research. There was however, thanks to Klain's leadership, full collaboration in disaster medicine. Negovsky was installed as a founding member of the Club of Mainz [World Association for Disaster and Emergency Medicine (WADEM)], created by Rudolph Frey of Mainz in 1977 and at the second WADEM congress, in Pittsburgh in 1981 [33,34], Negovsky, his successor Semenov, and others from communist countries, contributed significantly. Following the earthquake in Armenia in 1987, my colleagues from Pittsburgh joined with Negovsky and colleagues from the USSR and Armenia to apply semi-quantitative methods to determine the resuscitability of earthquake victims who are not instantaneously crushed to death, but who die within minutes or hours. Immediate life-supporting first aid by uninjured co-victims would have made the greatest impact [37–39].

Our collaboration was also active in what I call 'peace medicine' [40]. In 1981 Negovsky and colleagues from Israel, Canada, Britain and the US agreed that medical planning for nuclear war was senseless, and the only effective approach was prevention. In 1983, Negovsky and I met with the 'Soviet Peace Committee' in Moscow, which had tried to dispel the feeling in the West that there could be aggressive military intentions against Western Europe on the part of the USSR. In 1990, when some of us visited Moscow for a disaster medicine congress, it was evident that glasnost and peace medicine efforts had succeeded.

The first English language publication of Negovsky's work appeared in the West in the early 1960s [23]. Since then he has also had to overcome nonpolitical hurdles; the practice of Soviet scientists to publish their often imaginative new ideas only in the Russian language, and using a format of reporting that is not customary in the West. All of this created a barrier to collaboration. In the 1980s he had overcome some of these hurdles with more frequent participation in international medical meetings and with publications in English [12]. Since the end of the cold war, however, his successors as leaders of his Institute, Semenov and Moroz, both leading anaesthesiologists, have had new hurdles to overcome. In the 1990s, further developments of reanimatology in Russia have been stymied by fiscal anarchy in spite of open communication and travel.

Negovsky is featured prominently in a forthcoming article on the Pittsburgh-Moscow connection by Klain, Semenov and Moroz [26], and my own autobiography [41].

## 3. Negovsky the man

Negovsky has been visionary, determined, kind and collegial, and at times tough. Even now, at age 92, he regularly visits his office and laboratory. In the 1960s and 70s, his staff perceived him as a benevolent dictator. His physical appearance has not changed much during the 40 years we have known him [Figs. 1–3]. In the 1970s, although already then perceived as being a 'senior citizen', this perception was quickly proven wrong. His eyes lit up in the company of charming females. When he broke his leg on a joint trip from Moscow to a Congress in Riga, he bandaged his leg and kept on walking, ignoring pain. Upon his return he resumed cross-country skiing. His hospitality warmed his team and his guests. In the early years, translators often were chaperones. He could not speak English at first, but he understood it quite well. Over the years, his communication skills in English improved and he did not hesitate to debate and even lecture in English.

He was persona grata in the upper circles of Soviet politics. To be effective he had to be. Nevertheless, he retained openness for free speech with the West. He used every opportunity possible to travel to the West. Under Gorbachev he succeeded in also obtaining such permission for some of his associates to go as well. His daughter was, and is, very close to him and always likes to accompany and pamper him. His grandson Vladimir Godsunov, a good pianist and a cardiologist, has been the apple of his eye.

Vladimir A. Negovsky will go into the history of medicine in general and resuscitation medicine in particular as 'the father of reanimatology', the science of resuscitation medicine. During and after World War II, he inspired scientists and clinicians in many countries to understand the pathophysiological changes that occur when the whole organism undergoes clinical death, and the disease process that can follow emergency resuscitation. From the start he focused on restoration of our humanity, namely survival without brain damage. His and my goal has been restoring a socially active person.

Personally, I thank Vladimir for a lasting friendship which cross-fertilized resuscitation research programs in Pittsburgh, Moscow, and beyond and may even have helped sustain peaceful co-existence of people of both East and West while their governments were waging a cold war. Professor Robert White of Cleveland, Ohio, neurosurgeon and pioneer in therapeutic hypothermia, and Distinguished Professor Hugh E. Stephenson of Columbia, Missouri, a famous resuscitation historian, both also longstanding friends of Vladimir Negovsky, have contributed to the cross-fertilization in resuscitation medicine between East and West with frequent joint visits to Moscow. Since 1991, Negovsky, an eminent product of the USSR, has had to watch his resuscitation research center go through difficult economic times. Our most recent visits, by Klain, Zelman, White, Shoemaker and I to Moscow for Negovsky's 90th birthday in 1999, and by Negovsky's successor, Victor Moroz, to Pittsburgh in 2000, signal the start of further communications and cross-fertilization in resuscitation medicine, and perhaps even some collaborations by the next generation.

## Acknowledgements

Drs Victor Moroz, Vladimir Kassil, and Miroslav Klain made valuable suggestions.

## References

[1] Safar P. Citation for Vladimir Negovsky for Honorary Membership of the European Resuscitation Council. Resuscitation 1994;28:175–6.

[2] Kassil VL. Remarks on P. Safar Citation for Vladimir Negovsky for Honorary Membership of the European Resuscitation Council. Resuscitation 1994;28:176–7.

[3] Negovsky VA. Reanimatology today: some scientific and philosophic considerations. Crit Care Med 1982;10:130–3 (editorial).

[4] Safar P. Reanimatology — the science of resuscitation. Crit Care Med 1982;10:134–6 (editorial).

[5] Safar P, Bircher NG. Cardiopulmonary–Cerebral Resuscitation. An Introduction to Resuscitation Medicine. World Federation of Societies of Anaesthesiologists, A Laerdal, Stavanger, 3rd edn. London: WB Saunders, 1988.

[6] Negovsky VA. Fifty years of the Institute of General Reanimatology of the USSR Academy of Medical Sciences. Crit Care Med 1988;16:287.

[7] Negovsky VA, Gurvitch AM, Zolotokrylina ES. Postresuscitation Disease. Amsterdam: Elsevier, 1983.

[8] Negovsky VA. Reanimatology as a neurological science. Minerva Anestesiol 1994;60(10):479–82.

[9] Negovsky VA. Neurologic stage in reanimatology. Resuscitation 1995;29:169–76.

[10] Negovsky VA. Resuscitation after lethal blood loss. Bull Exp Biol Med 1938;6(3):35–6 (in Russian).

[11] Negovsky VA. Therapy of Agonal States and Clinical Death in an Army Region. Moscow: Medgiz, 1945 (book in Russian).

[12] Negovsky VA. Resuscitation of the Organism: Agonal States and Clinical Death. Moscow: Unknown, 1943 (book in Russian). Published also in English in Amer. Rev. of Soviet Med., 1945, vol .2; and 1946, vol. 3.

[13] Kouwenhoven WB, Jude JR, Knickerbocker GG. Closed-chest cardiac massage. J Am Med Assoc 1960;173:1064–7.

[14] Maass: Die Methode der Wiederbelebung bei Herztod nach Chloroformeinathmung. Berlin Klin Wochschr 1892;29:265–8.

[15] Gurvich N, Yuniev SG. Restoration of a regular rhythm in the mammalian fibrillating heart. Amer Review of Soviet Medicine 1946;3:236–9.

[16] Safar P. History of cardiopulmonary–cerebral resuscitation. In: Kaye W, Bircher N, editors. Cardiopulmonary Resuscitation. New York: Churchill Livingstone, 1989:1–53 Chapter 1.

[17] Safar P. On the history of modern resuscitation. Crit Care Med 1996;24/S:S3–11.

[18] Zoll PM, Linenthal AJ, Gibson W, Paul MH, Norman LR. Termination of ventricular fibrillation in man by externally applied electric countershock. New Engl J Med 1956;254:727–32.

[19] Peleska B. Transthoracic and direct defibrillation. Rozhl Chir (CSSR) 1957;26:731.

[20] Kouwenhoven WB, Milner WR. Treatment of ventricular fibrillation using a capacitor discharge. J Appl Physiol 1954;7:253–7.

[21] Gurvitch AM. Determination of the depth and reversibility of postanoxic coma in animals. Resuscitation 1974;3:1–26.

[22] Negovsky VA. International Traumatology Conference, Budapest. Traumatology and Orthopedics 1961;3-4:259.

[23] Negovsky VA. Resuscitation and Artificial Hypothermia (USSR). New York: Consultants Bureau, 1962 (in English).

[24] Ibsen B. The anesthetist's viewpoint on treatment of respiratory complications in poliomyelitis during the epidemic in Copenhagen, 1952. Proc R Soc Med 1954;47:72–4.

[25] Safar P, DeKornfeld TJ, Pearson JW, Redding JS. Intensive care unit. A three year experience at Baltimore City Hospitals. Anaesthesia 1961;16:275–84.

[26] Klain M., Semenov V., Moroz V., Reanimatology developments by the Pittsburgh–Moscow connection, 1962–2000. In preparation.

[27] Safar P. The mechanisms of dying and their reversal. In: Schwartz GR, Safar P, Stone JH, Storey JH, Wagner DK, editors. Principles and Practice of Emergency Medicine. Philadelphia: WB Saunders, 1978:17–50 Chapter 2.

[28] Safar P. Resuscitation Research Center, University of Pittsburgh. Resuscitation 1979;7:69–70.

[29] Safar P. Resuscitation: controversial aspects. International Symposium, Vienna 1962. In: Anesthesiology and Resuscitation Series, vol. 1. Berlin: Springer-Verlag, 1963.

[30] Safar P, Rosomoff H. Study tour to Prague and Moscow. Der Anaesthesist 1964;13:317–9 Also, more detailed intramural publication by the authors.

[31] Safar P. Resuscitation from clinical death: Pathophysiologic limits and therapeutic potentials. Crit Care Med 1988;16:923–41.

[32] Negovsky VA. Postresuscitation disease. Crit Care Med 1988;16:942–6.

[33] Safar P. Resuscitation research programs in three spheres. Prehospital Disaster Med 1985;1(1):4–6.

[34] Negovsky V. Reanimatology: The Science of Resuscitation. Prehospital Disaster Med 1985;1(1):1–3.

[35] Baskett PJF. Citation for Peter Safar, MD (Vienna), Dr.h.c. (Mainz), FCCM, FACCP for Honorary Membership of the European Resuscitation Council. Resuscitation 1994;28:173–4.

[36] Negovsky VA. Reanimatology — the science of resuscitation. In: Stephenson H, editor. Cardiac Arrest and Resuscitation. St Louis: CV Mosby, 1974.

[37] Klain M, Ricci E, Safar P, Semenov V, Pretto E, Tisherman S, Abrams J, Comfort L, and other members of the Disaster Reanimatology Study Group, Disaster reanimatology potentials: a structured interview study in Armenia I. Methodology and preliminary results, Prehospital Disaster Med, 1989;4(2):135-154.

[38] Ricci EM, Pretto EA, Safar P, Klain M, Angus D, Tisherman SA, Abrams J, Crippen D, Comfort L, Semenov V, and other members of the Disaster Reanimatology Study Group, Disaster reanimatology potentials: a structured interview study in Armenia II. Methods, Prehospital Disaster Med, 1991;6:159-166.

[39] Pretto EA, Ricci E, Klain M, Safar P, Semenov V, Abrams J, Tisherman S, Crippen D, Comfort L, and other members of the Disaster Reanimatology Study Group, Disaster reanimatology potentials: A structured interview study in Armenia III. Results, conclusions, and recommendation, Prehospital Disaster Med, 1992;7:327-337.

[40] Safar P, Baskett PJF, WADEM, Resolutions concerning disaster medicine and nuclear war, Prehospital Disaster Med, 1985;1:15.

[41] Safar PJ. An autobiographical memoir. In: Fink BR, McGoldrick KE, editors. Careers in Anesthesiology, vol. V. Chicago: Wood Library-Museum of Anesthesiology, 2000.

# The Brook airway

## Thomas F. Baskett

The various methods of artificial respiration using manual chest compression, with or without associated arm movements, were introduced in the 19th and early 20th centuries. By the late 1950s the improved effectiveness of mouth-to-mouth respiration was established.[1] In 1954, Elam et al. showed that mouth-to-mask ventilation produced adequate gas exchange in apnoeic adults,[2] and subsequently, Safar demonstrated superior gas exchange using mouth-to-mouth ventilation compared to manual methods of artificial resuscitation.[3–5] In 1958, Safar and McMahon described an S-shaped oropharangeal airway which consisted of two Guedel-type airways soldered together and provided 'a new and aesthetic modification of mouth-to-mouth artificial respiration'.[6] A smaller version was made for infants and children. In addition to the aesthetic improvement the airway kept the tongue forward when the patient was in the supine position; Safar having shown previously how the tongue fell backwards to obstruct the airway in the unconscious patient.[5] This airway had the advantage of portability and was apparently carried by personnel of the Baltimore Ambulance Service at that time.

The existence of this portable airway was unknown to the general practitioner Morris Brook when, in July, 1957, he was called to the Potash Company of America mine near Saskatoon in Canada. There had been a cave-in at the mine and, while most of the personnel involved were extracted alive and recovered, one man was unconscious and not breathing. Brook performed mouth-to-mouth respiration and the victim was resuscitated successfully. However, Morris Brook was put off by the amount of dirt, blood and vomit that he encountered during the resuscitation. He thought that there must be a better way and went on to develop what came to be known as the Brook airway. Like Safar he started with a Guedel airway to which he attached a mouth guard flap to fit snugly over the patient's lips. To this was attached a flexible rubber neck leading to a straight plastic tube containing a built-in spring one-way valve so that air could be blown into the tube but the expired air from the victim would escape via the valve through a side exit (Figure 1).

Although mouth-to-mouth respiration had become established as the technique of choice for first aid resuscitation of the unconscious non-breathing patient, many people, including medical and nursing personnel, were put off by the need for oral contact with mucous, blood and sometimes vomit. Indeed, the Canadian Red Cross in 1959 gave up teaching mouth-to-mouth respiration because most people would not do it, as they stated: 'the difficulty is to persuade a layman to place his lips against the lips of a presumed corpse'.[7] The

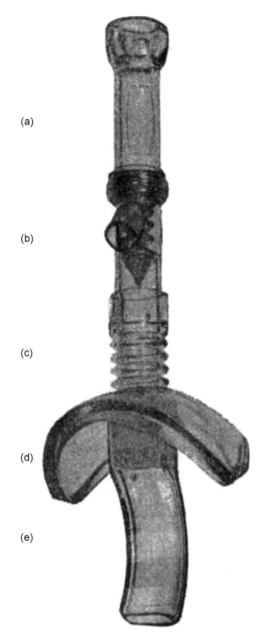

**Figure 1** Brook airway (a) blow-tube (b) non-return valve (c) flexible neck (d) mouthguard (e) oral airway (from literature,[11] p. 1565).

NY, Dr. P. Safar of Baltimore and Dr. H. Ruben of Copenhagen for their invaluable assistance in keeping us abreast with their progress in this field through personal communications'.[9] Brook also offered 'special thanks to Dr. Safar for his assistance in development of an improved airway: a result of the critical tests to which he exposed earlier Brook airway prototypes; and for imparting some of his great enthusiasm'.[9] In some of the later models the airway had a suction channel with an attached suction-bulb to aspirate mucous. Brook first demonstrated his airway at the Refresher Course in Obstetrics, Gynaecology and Paediatrics at the University of Saskatoon in February 1959. The airway was evaluated by the Department of Anaesthesia in St. Paul's Hospital in Saskatoon and in a trial of over 200 anaesthetised patients was found 'to work beautifully and be the best thing out'.[7] The first models were made locally in Saskatoon and distributed to all the Potash Company of America miners and clipped into a band on their helmets.[7] The airway was produced by Woodbridge Moulded Plastics of Toronto and later manufactured in England. It was made available to the public under patent in ten countries. Soon after his prototype airway was produced Brook outlined the advantages of his flexible airway in two publications in Britain and Canada.[10,11] The advantages of the airway included the simplicity of the method, the flexibility of the tube, allowing its use when patients were trapped in an awkward position and the fact that a single operator could perform both artificial respiration and external cardiac compression without changing position (Figure 2).

In December 1959 Morris Brook took part in a symposium with the United Services Section of the Royal Society of Medicine in London.[12] In this meeting Brook emphasised the need for 'safe and practical methods of teaching and group training in the direct method of artificial resuscitation'.[12] He demonstrated the training aids he had developed, including the 'air passage demonstrator'--a wooden model showing the airway and how obstruction occurred when the neck was flexed and the importance of placing the head in the hyperextended position. Other aids included a plastic manikin developed to teach mouth-to-mouth respiration and a documentary film ''That They May Live''. Dr. Brook lectured widely on emergency resuscitation with the Saskatchewan Safety Council, the Nursing Training Programme at the University of Saskatchewan and with the Department of Education Grade 7 school compulsory resuscitation training classes. Twenty years after the development of the Brook Airway, in August 1977, the Coun-

advantage of Brook's airway was the flexible neck so that the tube could be angled if necessary to provide access when victims were trapped in an awkward position. His other main incentive was to obviate the aesthetic difficulties mentioned above. Brook was undoubtedly influenced and guided by the work of Elam and Safar, as well as by the Danish anaesthetist Henning Ruben, the latter having developed the self-inflating, 'AMBU Bag' with its combined non-rebreathing and air inlet valves.[8] Indeed, in their 1960 article on artificial respiration the Brook brothers thank 'Dr. J.O. Elam of Buffalo,

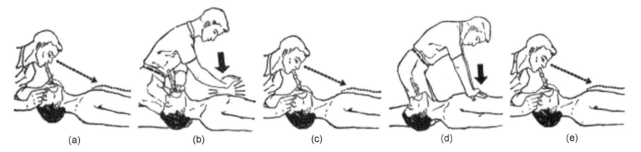

(a)                 (b)                (c)                (d)                (e)

**Figure 2** Illustration of emergency resuscitation. Mouth-to-mouth resuscitation (using the Brook airway when available) plus external cardiac resuscitation. (a) Begin artificial respiration at once. Place victim on back, tilt head fully back, insert airway over tongue. Raise the chin and pinch nostrils closed. Blow every 3—4 s. Watch for chest raise, and listen for sound of air returning from victim. (b) If there is no response after 1—2 min, as evidenced by no improvement in colour, no spontaneous respiration, no detectable pulse, dilated pupils, in the absence of any chest injury, thump lower third of breast-bone sharply with butt of hand three times. (c) Resume direct artificial respiration. (d) If there is still no response after 1 min, begin external cardiac resuscitation. Place heel of hand on lower third of breast-bone. Place other hand over first as illustrated, keep arms straight, press sharply 60—80 times per minute. (e) After 1 min, resume direct artificial respiration. If required, alternate 15 chest compressions and 2 airway breaths until assistance arrives or victim is rescued. (From literature,[11] p. 1564).

cil of the Canadian Medical Association passed a resolution advising commercial airlines to carry the airway as part of the emergency kit on all aircraft.[13]

Morris Harry Brook was born in Winnipeg, Manitoba on 25 May 1911 (Figure 3). He received his medical degree from the Manitoba Medical College in 1935. In 1937 he moved to Kindersley, Saskatchewan, and carried out general practice there until 1943. He served with the R.C.A.M.C. from 1943 to 1946.[14] In 1946 he established a practice in Saskatoon accompanied by his younger brother Joseph, who had qualified in medicine from the Manitoba Medical College in 1941. His other brother Max Brook practised dentistry in Saskatoon. His brother Joseph, who was co-author on some of his articles, helped during the early experiments with the airway and it was he who suggested the valve to separate the patient's expired air.

Morris Brook died on Thursday, 5 October 1967 in Saskatoon, at the age of 56. His experience of resuscitation of a miner following a 'cave-in' had led him to develop a logical and practical airway so that artificial respiration could be performed without direct mouth-to-mouth or mouth-to-nose contact. His aim was always to have this available to the general public as well as health workers. He achieved this aim and the airway was made available in many countries and sold to the public in the 1960s and 1970s. However, the simplicity, success and widespread availability of Ruben's AMBU Bag and other technical advances meant that Brook's airway fell from common use.[15]

## Acknowledgement

Thanks to Jo-Anne Wolan, Director of Communications/Education, College of Physicians and Surgeons of Saskatchewan, for the photograph and information on Morris Brook.

## References

1. Thangam S, Weil MH, Rackow EC. Cardiopulmonary resuscitation: a historical review. Acute Care 1986;12:63—94.
2. Elam JO, Brown ES, Elder JD. Artificial respiration by mouth-to-mask method: study of respiratory gas exchange of paralysed patients ventilated by operator's expired air. N Engl J Med 1954;250:749—54.
3. Safar P. Ventilator efficacy of mouth-to-mouth artificial respiration. Airway obstruction during manual and mouth-to-mouth artificial respiration. JAMA 1958;167:335—41.

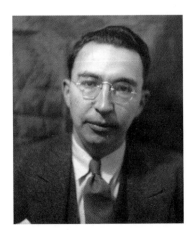

**Figure 3**   Morris Brook (1911—1967).

4. Safar P, Escarraga L, Elam JO. Comparison of mouth-to-mouth and mouth-to-airway methods of artificial respiration with the chest pressure arm lift methods. N Engl J Med 1958;258:671–7.
5. Safar P. Failure of manual respiration. J Appl Physiol 1959:1484–8.
6. Safar P, McMahon M. Mouth-to-airway emergency artificial respiration. JAMA 1958;166:1459–60.
7. Saskatoon star-phoenix; 7 February 1959.
8. Ruben H. Combination resuscitator and aspirator. Anaesthesiology 1958;19:408–9.
9. Brook MH, Brook J. Direct artificial respiration (D.A.R.): present-day teaching and group training requirements. Can Med Assoc J 1960;82:245–8.
10. Dobkin AB, Brook MH, Brook J. Emergency (on the spot) resuscitation of collapse using direct artificial respiration (D.A.R.) and external cardiac compression (E.C.C.). Can Med Assoc J 1961;84:889–92.
11. Brook MH, Brook J, Wyant GM. Emergency resuscitation. BMJ 1962;2:1564–6.
12. Brook MH. Discussion on artificial respiration. Proc Roy Soc Med 1960;53:311–5.
13. Saskatoon star-phoenix; 3 August 1977.
14. Saskatoon star-phoenix; 6 October 1967.
15. Baskett PJF, Zorab J, Henning Ruben MD, FFARCS(I), FFARCS. The Ruben valve and the AMBU bag. Resuscitation 2003;56:123–7.

# Professor Sir Robert Macintosh

## T.M. Craft

Robert Reynolds Macintosh was born in New Zealand on the 17th October 1897. The son of an All Blacks rugby player, he spent his early childhood in Timaru. His father developed overseas business interests that took his family all over the world but in particular to Argentina and it was here that Robert learnt to speak fluent Spanish. His teenage years, however, were spent at school back in New Zealand in the town Oamaru.

With the outbreak of war in Europe in 1914, Macintosh travelled to England and enlisted in the Royal Scots Fusiliers even though he was still under age. Later he transferred to the Royal Flying Corps and became a successful fighter pilot. Before the end of the war, however, he was shot down behind enemy lines in France and made a prisoner of war in Germany. Whilst in captivity Mac learned to speak fluent German and, together with two fellow detainees, escaped captivity on several occasions only to be recaptured before he could make it back to Britain.

After demobilisation, Macintosh decided to stay in the United Kingdom and commenced medical training at Guy's Hospital Medical School. He qualified in 1924 and intended to pursue a career in surgery. He passed the examination for Fellowship of the Royal College of Surgeons in 1927 but, in order to earn money whilst looking to develop his surgical career, he began to give anaesthetics in London. His interest in anaesthesia developed rapidly and he founded a successful private anaesthetic practice administering anaesthesia in the dental and surgical clinics of the West End of London in the late 1920s. Techniques in practice at this time included inhalational induction with nitrous oxide, but Macintosh developed an early interest in the intravenous administration of barbiturates. Criticism of such new-fangled techniques was rife and Mac soon found himself defending the practice at the Royal Society of Medicine in London and in many articles in print.

Macintosh became friendly with the car manufacturer, Sir William Morris, who later became Lord Nuffield. They played golf together and during the walks from green to green Nuffield recounted the numerous experiences he had had with anaesthesia as a young man, consequent upon the need for a number of dental and general surgical operations. Nuffield complained about the discomfort and unpleasantness of nitrous oxide induction. He described in particular the feeling of prolonged suffocation he remembered after one anaesthetic given so that some of his teeth could be pulled together with the subsequent nightmares. Nuffield was impressed by the smooth transition to unconsciousness that Mac described following the administration of intravenous barbiturates and questioned him further about it. When, in the early 1930s, Nuffield needed to have a small operation in London he asked Macintosh to anaesthetise him and was astonished at the difference in his experience.

In the summer of 1936 the annual meeting of the British Medical Association was held in Oxford. Sir Farquhar Buzzard, the University Profession of Medicine in Oxford, gave the presidential address. In it he stressed how fitting it would be for Oxford to develop as a postgraduate medical centre of learning and appealed to Lord Nuffield, who by then was very wealthy, to support such a development by funding three new clinical chairs, in Medicine, Surgery, and Obstetrics. When Nuffield told Mac of this at Huntercombe, the golf club to which they both belonged, Macintosh joked that once again anaesthetics had been forgotten. The comment was ignored but clearly not forgotten as some weeks later Lord Nuffield insisted on the endowment of a Chair of Anaesthesia at Oxford as a condition of supporting the other medical professorships at the University. Buzzard tried to decline the offer of the fourth chair, claiming that it would lead to ridicule of both the University and of Nuffield, but Nuffield simply withdrew the offer to support any of the chairs without one being created in Anaesthesia. Even more surprising for the University establishment in Oxford, Nuffield also insisted that, despite his youth, Robert Macintosh be appointed the first Chair. There had never been a University Department of Anaesthesia in Britain before this date and indeed Macintosh became the first Professor of Anaesthetics in Europe just a few years after the establishment of the first Chair in the United States occupied by Ralph Waters at the University of Wisconsin at Madison.

Macintosh used his continued friendship with Lord Nuffield to good effect: collaboration between the Department of Anaesthetics and his Morris Motor Works at Cowley in Oxford led to the development and manufacture of negative pressure respirators (iron lungs) for use in treating patients with polio and other paralytic diseases. Nuffield ensured that these were made available to any hospital in the British Empire that asked to have one.

The Second World War saw promotion for Macintosh and he was awarded the rank of Air Commodore as well as becoming an adviser in anaesthetics to both the Royal Air Force and the Royal Navy. Despite these responsibilities he continued to administer his Department at Oxford. Here an important role in training doctors in anaesthesia for the British and Allied Services soon developed. At the same time new equipment was required and Macintosh developed the Oxford vaporisers for ether and chloroform that were used in many field-hospitals during the Second World War. These were the fore-runners of the EMO (Epstein, Macintosh, Oxford) vaporiser and the OMV (Oxford Miniature Vaporiser) that continued to play an important role in the development of anaesthesia in the immediate post-war period. Squadron Leader Edgar Pask, who later became a Professor of Anaesthesia himself, collaborated with Macintosh at the RAF Research Institute at Farnborough. In a now-celebrated piece of work, Macintosh would repeatedly anaesthetise Pask and then throw him, unconscious, into a swimming pool while wearing a variety of life jackets designed to keep the head of the victim above water. The motivation for this came from the fact that pilots who crashed into the sea would invariably die of drowning if they were not fully conscious at the moment of immersion. This was because the life jackets of the day almost always resulted in the victim floating face down. Macintosh redesigned the life jacket so that, when inflated, it would indeed keep the head above water and just, as importantly, maintain a clear airway. Mac repeatedly tested and modified his designs in the swimming pool with the fully anaesthetised Pask, anaesthesia being maintained via a long anaesthetic breathing circuit. These experiments are testimony both to Pask's bravery and to the depth of friendship that developed between the two men. The resulting life vest design undoubtedly saved hundreds of British airmen forced down in the English Channel during the Second World War. This work in particular led to Robert Macintosh being honoured by the Queen with a widely acclaimed and popular knighthood in 1955.

Unlike some medical professors, Robert Macintosh was first and foremost a clinician. Despite the onerous responsibility of organising and directing a large and growing Department in Oxford, throughout his time there Macintosh was most often to be found in the operating theatres. Because of his close association with clinical anaesthesia, he was readily able to identify opportunities to improve clinical practice and the equipment employed in it. He built around him a team of experts most of whom were not primarily anaesthetists. Epstein for instance was a physicist whilst Richard Salt, Macintosh's chief technician, worked on developing mechanical devices to improve the practice of anaesthesia.

After the war, Robert Macintosh developed a keen interest in regional anaesthesia, promoting the use of lumbar puncture and spinal anaesthesia as well as local analgesia techniques for the head and neck, and brachial plexus analgesia. He was an early advocate of sub-arachnoid anaesthesia for Caesarean section rather than general anaesthesia, despite a large body of opinion that disagreed with him at the time. Macintosh and Salt developed a range of spinal and epidural needles with various adaptations including one designed to indicate the successful location of epidural space (the Macintosh balloon).

The polio outbreak in Copenhagen in 1952 led to the successful use of manually controlled ventilation and alerted Macintosh to the need for improved techniques of respiratory intensive care and the ultimate development of the positive pressure Radcliffe ventilator, designed to replace the negative pressure tank respirators. Mac's most famous and widely used piece of equipment, however is, of course, the eponymous laryngoscope blade. This has been adopted as a standard for adult intubation throughout the world. Macintosh had noticed that the Boyle-Davies gag used at tonsillectomy provided an excellent view of the glottis. It was this observation then that led to the development of the now very familiar curved Mac blades.

Macintosh's most productive years were undoubtedly at a time of great development in anaesthesia. Perhaps his greatest contribution, however, came not from the large number of pieces of equipment that he helped to develop but from his contributions as a teacher. Macintosh was a quiet and well-mannered man for whom public speaking at large meetings did not come easily. What he excelled at, however, was teaching a small group of people in the anaesthetic room or operating theatre. His love of clinical anaesthesia and a drive for clear simple thinking made such learning opportunities both a delight and a privilege. Macintosh was both modest and disarming, with a sparkling sense of humour. He was always generous and supportive to the trainees and associates that worked in his Department, whilst at the same time playing down the importance of his own role.

Macintosh retired in 1965 but continued to have a close relationship with the Nuffield Department of Anaesthetics and the Royal Society of Medicine. Twenty-two years after his retirement, the Nuffield Department of Anaesthetics celebrated its 50th anniversary and Mac his 90th birthday. Even at this advanced stage of his life, Mac would attend academic meetings in Oxford.

As a trainee in the Nuffield Department of Anaesthetics I remember the anxiety of presenting my own research findings for the first time to a large and august audience. Macintosh sat quietly at the back of the lecture theatre, making occasional entries in his notebook. Later, when most of the discussion had finished, this small, bald, bespectacled man quietly raised his hand and gently asked the most insightful questions of all.

Sir Robert died at the age of 91; he tripped whilst walking his dog, sustaining a head injury from which he never recovered. He was admitted to the Radcliffe Infirmary, the Hospital that housed his own academic Department. The fact that he died a few days later would have pleased Mac as he had made no secret of the fact that an active life ending with sudden death was far preferable to him than an existence in a geriatric facility.

Professor Sir Robert Macintosh was not just an inventor of anaesthetic and resuscitation equipment but also a master in the art of anaesthesia and the skills it requires. He was a resuscitation great, but was also a great and generous man.

## Further reading

Beinart J. A History of the Nuffield Department of Anaesthetics: 1937–1987. Oxford, University Press. 1987.

Boulton TB. Professor Sir Robert Macintosh, 1987–1989: Personal Reflections on a Remarkable Man and His Career. Regional Anaesthesia 1993:18:145–154.

Macintosh R. Modern Anaesthesia, with Special Reference to the Chair of Anaesthetics at Oxford. In Rupreht J et al, eds. Anaesthesia - Essays on its History. Berlin: Springer-Verlag, 1985.

Mushin WW. Professor Emeritus Sir Robert Reynolds Macintosh, MA, DM, FRCSE, DA DSc(Hon)Wales, FFARCS(Hon), FFARCSI(Hon), FRCOG(Hon), 17 October 1897–28 August 1989. Anaesthesia 1989:44:951–952.

Sykes MK. Obituary. Robert Reynolds Macintosh, MA, DMOxon, FFARCS. Lancet 1989:2:816.

# Paul M. Zoll, —The father of "modern" electrotherapy and innovator of pharmacotherapy for life-threatening cardiac arrhythmias

Stafford I. Cohen

Paul Zoll (Figure 1) has a prominent permanent place in history because of his discoveries while developing a broad management plan for life-threatening cardiac arrhythmias.

In 1948, Zoll became the attending physician to a 60-year-old woman with Stokes-Adams attacks. Syncopal attacks increased in frequency as her idioventricular rhythm slowed or temporarily stopped. Death occurred after several weeks of intensive comprehensive medical care. The postmortem examination demonstrated a healthy heart with a clinically flawed conduction system. She had, in Claude Beck's oft quoted phrase, "*A heart too good to die.*"[1] Zoll was dismayed at the outcome. This was his private patient. He had the burden of responsibility to stabilize the rhythm. Zoll was deeply troubled, so much so that he later acted with resolve to prevent others who were similarly afflicted from suffering the same fate. The quest had a slow start and a complex course. The ultimate goal was achieved 12 years later with the implantation of the Zoll—Belgard version of a fully contained permanent implantable pacemaker.[2]

There were several groundbreaking discoveries along the way. Zoll, an astute clinician, had insight not readily apparent to others regarding the subtle relationships among the hazardous heart rhythms. The deadly ones are absence of electrical activity, pulseless electrical activity and chaotic fibrillatory electrical activity. Zoll had a broad vision of the problems and of their solutions. He developed short-term, bridging and long-term approaches with electrical devices and pharmacology.

Paul Zoll was a premier clinical investigator who shuttled back and forth between his patients and his laboratory bench. It was the patients that energized his achievements, always the patients. His most important discoveries are summarized in Table 1.

Paul Zoll's achievements will not be forgotten by future generations of physicians. However, they should be reminded of the personal characteristics and strengths that helped him to succeed. His defining personal traits were as follows:

- Demanding much of himself and expecting no less from others.[14]

220

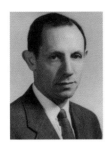

**Figure 1** Paul M. Zoll (1911–1999).

- A man on an important mission and in a hurry to get there.[15]
- A good listener.[16]
- Honesty in academic issues and in personal relationships.[14]
- Exceptionally shy, quiet and modest.[14]
- A man of few words.[16] (Being laconic gave him credibility in pronouncing that, ''people died from eating too much, smoking too much, drinking too much and talking too much.'')
- Being close to family and a few friends.[16] Paul married Janet Jones in 1939. They had two children; Mary, a medical editor with a doctorate in biochemistry, and Ross, a physicist and anesthetist who collaborated with his father in the development of the later model transcutaneous pacer. After Janet's death, Paul married Ann Blumgart Gurewich.
- Perhaps his greatest strengths were an extraordinary confidence that he could solve most any problem coupled with an extraordinary perseverance while completing the task. He was not discouraged by ''the devil in the details'' or by his critics.[17]

Paul solved important problems that benefited humanity. He was acclaimed in the scientific community for his discoveries. His crowning recognition

was likely to be the Albert Lasker Award in 1973 for clinical medical research, which is the highest national award for scientific achievement.[18] Yet Paul Zoll remained humble throughout his career, attributing his success to able co-workers.

Paul Maurice Zoll was born and raised in Boston, MA. He was the second child of Latvian immigrants. Paul attended Boston Latin School, a public school with entry only to those with high achievements on competitive testing. There is an anecdote[19] told about young Paul by a hospitalized patient who was moving towards a needed permanent pacemaker. He had been Paul's boyhood friend and next door neighbor. The patient referred to Dr. Zoll by his boyhood nickname, Pauly, or by his adulthood synonym—the inventor of the pacemaker. They had played football together in the street or a nearby field. If they forgot the time or the need to do their homework, the light in Paul's room might be on all night. The patient closed with, ''He was a good student you know.''

Indeed, Paul was a good student. He went on to graduate summa cum laude from Harvard College. Apparently, academic excellence was easier to achieve than the mandatory swimming requirement. There are two versions of Paul's tribulations in passing the swimming test. One is that Paul passed, but nearly drowned as he dog-paddled across the pool.[20] The other version is that he failed, but was given a ''pass'' by a sympathetic instructor after a promise to improve.[14] In later years, Paul kept his promise, if one had been made, by becoming an excellent swimmer and expert water skier.

Paul Zoll entered Harvard Medical School and worked with Soma Weiss during his last year (1936). Internship was at Boston's Beth Israel Hospital. Residency was at New York's Bellevue Hospital. Paul returned to Beth Israel Hospital in 1939 with an

**Table 1**  Noteworthy achievements

| Year | Achievement |
| --- | --- |
| 1952 | Transcutaneous cardiac pacer in man.[3] A first in world competition (gold medal) |
| 1955–1956 | Continuous cardiac rate monitor with adjustable alarmed limits. A first in world competition (gold medal). Continuous cardiac rate monitor with adjustable alarmed limits and a visual rhythm display.[4] A first in world competition (gold medal) |
| 1956 | Transcutaneous cardiac defibrillator in man.[5] A first in world competition (gold medal) |
| 1956 | Automatic standby pacing on demand. An optional operational mode on the Electrodyne PM-65 for transcutaneous or internal pacing. Refer Appendix A for details |
| 1958–1963 | Pharmacological methods of managing symptomatic slow heart rates[6] and overdriving hazardous or potentially rapid foci[7] |
| 1960 | Implantable fully self-contained permanent pacemaker. A second in world competition (silver medal)[2] |
| 1963–1971 | Algorithms for reviving patients with cardiac arrest[8–12] |
| 1981 | Non-invasive transcutaneous cardiac pacer.[13] Improved version of that introduced in 1952 |

appointment as a Josia Macy Foundation Research Fellow investigating the clinical pathological relationships of coronary artery disease. The work was interrupted by World War II (WWII) after which Zoll returned to further explore the manifestations and outcomes of coronary artery disease while working with Monroe Schlesinger and Herman Blumgart in injecting and then dissecting the coronary arteries.

During WWII, Paul Zoll was Chief of Medicine at an Army Hospital in England where Dwight Harken, a Harvard Medical School classmate and thoracic surgeon, was extracting bullets and foreign bodies from in and around the heart. Paul's intraoperative responsibility was heart rhythm management. He observed that the heart had contractile sensitivity to the mere touch of a finger or instrument.[21] That observation remained embedded in memory to be recalled years later when Paul searched for an approach to prevent death from Stokes-Adams Disease. After the war, Dwight Harken and Paul Zoll each returned to neighboring Harvard Teaching Hospitals.

Throughout his career, Paul spent half time in clinical practice and half time in research. Not long after becoming established at the hospital, Zoll sought support for his own cardiac arrhythmia projects. His Chief, Herman Blumgart, and the Associate Chief of Research, A.S. Freedberg, were supportive and provided Paul with a laboratory and funding. Soon he was performing experiments on pigs with heart block surgically produced by Dr. Leona Norman Zarsky. She was a surgeon who had previously worked with Dwight Harken at Boston City Hospital during the momentous development of closed mitral valve commissurotomy. Dr. Zoll was also joined by Dr. Arthur Linenthal, who had a background in electrophysiology and knowledge of the complex properties of anti-arrhythmic drugs. Arthur added critical analytical interpretation of the miles of ECG rhythm strips generated in the animal lab and on the hospital wards. He also developed novel pharmacological approaches to controlling arrhythmias.

Paul's initial approach at managing heart block was electrical. He recalled how readily the heart contracted to varied stimuli while collaborating with Dwight Harken in England. Dr. Zoll was familiar with historic investigations relating to direct electrical stimulation of the heart. The accepted approach to resuscitating an arrested heart had been proposed by Carl Wiggers and later implemented by Claude Beck, a thoracic surgeon from Cleveland, who had succeeded in resuscitating pulseless cardiac arrest by rapidly performing a left-sided thoracotomy and compressing the heart by hand. He also invented a defibrillator with James

Rand to be applied to the exposed fibrillating heart. Beck is credited with the first such success in man. Although the setting was in an operating room,[22] Claude Beck was evangelistic in training physicians, nurses and dental personnel to respond in any circumstance. Those disciples drawn to heroic acts carried a penknife on their person at all times.

Paul Zoll sought a non-invasive alterative to open-chest resuscitation. He was intrigued by a paper delivered at a meeting of the Boston Surgical Society by John Callaghan and Wilfred Gordon Bigelow on transvenous sinus node pacing in hypothermic animals. After the meeting, Zoll questioned Callaghan about the nature of their stimulator and was told that a commercially available Grass stimulator should suffice. Paul borrowed a Grass Thyratron stimulator from Otto Krayer's physiology laboratory at Harvard Medical School. The stimulator was used to pace the ventricles of an animal using an esophageal-anterior chest lead configuration. The recording was on a modified Sanborn photographic videoscope or cardioscope machine with a fluorescent rotating screen.[23]

Paul described the moment when he noted ventricular contractions in response to the electrical stimuli, *"It seemed to me that the whole problem of cardiac arrest was solved, at least in theory."*[24] Zoll abandoned the esophageal lead after he proved that a transcutaneous anterior chest configuration worked well and could be applied rapidly. When Zoll published the first three cases of transcutaneous pacing in humans, he speculated that transcutaneous electrical stimulation might also be applicable to correcting ventricular fibrillation.[3] The paper created a tectonic shift. Barriers collapsed. New approaches were formulated. *"In 1952, Paul Zoll in Boston had invented a transcutaneous pacemaker to be used during asystole... The achievement motivated all of the later development in cardiac pacing."*[25]

The early transcutaneous paced patients with bradycardia were managed with a Grass stimulator, which Zoll found to be too cumbersome, too complicated and somewhat underpowered. In an anecdote, Paul relates that he approached Mr. Grass with details of the project and generic specifications for a new stimulator design. Mr. Grass declined to help. Zoll's project was a gamble. Even if it succeeded the outcome would be undesirable because of a need to work harder and the company's need to pay more taxes![26]

Zoll then formed an alliance with Alan Belgard, an engineer and co-owner of the small medical device firm, Electrodyne. Using Paul's input on research and specifications; Electrodyne produced commercially the Zoll version of the transthoracic pacemaker, the alarmed visual cardiac rhythm monitor, the transcutaneous alternating current (A/C) defibrillator and the implantable permanent self-contained, self-sustaining battery powered pacemaker. The implanted permanent pacer was to maintain an adequate heart rate while preventing a bradycardic or asystolic crisis. The transcutaneous pacer and defibrillator were machines to be used in a crisis. They had a specific lifesaving short-term purpose. Solving the problem of potential recurrence required a transitional bridging therapy from restarting an asystolic heart to a permanent pacemaker and from defibrillating the ventricle of a heart to implanting an internal defibrillator.

Paul Zoll worked with Arthur Linenthal to stabilize pharmacologically the asystolic heart, which was excessively slow or irritable. More than a decade later, Zoll was both aware of and approved of Michael Mirowski's internally placed defibrillator device.[27]

Paul Zoll and Arthur Linenthal used dilute solutions of epinephrine (adrenaline) or isoproterenol to increase the heart rate in the presence of hazardous bradycardia[6] or to elevate a lowly natural pacemaker to a dominant position in the hierarchy of pacemakers which could stabilize rhythm and rate by suppressing unstable competing foci.[8] Although the solutions of epinephrine or isoproterenol required frequent titration, constant attention and unusual commitment, Dr. Zoll believed that his approach to temporary stabilization of rhythm and rate was superior to that of Seymour Furman's advocacy for temporary transvenous intracardiac pacing.[28] In spite of Furman's success in stabilizing Stokes-Adams patients for long periods of time with transvenous pacing, Zoll raised objections which included possibilities of creating portals for infection, provoking a hazardous arrhythmia, perforating the heart, electrode displacement and encouraging an atmosphere of complacency.

To Paul Zoll's credit, he developed nearly all of the essential instruments that are required in response to a cardiac arrest. Zoll recalls a meeting with Hughes Day in Boston during which they discussed the best approach to reducing mortality in victims of acute myocardial infarction. The concept was raised of concentrating necessary services in a specialized coronary care unit. Day asked Zoll why he had not established such a unit. Paul answered that the administrators of his hospital turned him down because they had more important priorities.[29]

Hughes Day went on to establish the nation's first coronary care unit in Bethany Kansas.[30] Paul Zoll and Alan Belgard likely took a measure of pride in the fact that nearly all of the critical resuscitative apparatus in that unit was developed by Paul and manufactured by Electrodyne. The equipment included transcutaneous pacers and alarmed cardiac oscilloscopic rhythm monitors, which were combined in the model PM-65 cardiac monitor automatic pacemaker, and the A/C transcutaneous defibrillator. The only exception was a battery operated external−internal transistorized stimulator (Medtronic) to couple with transvenous or epicardial temporary electrodes.

Paul Zoll was a pioneer in the art and science of cardiac resuscitation. "*The science of resuscitation stems from the demonstration by Zoll and others that the human heart can be defibrillated by a shock administered across a closed chest.*"[31] Paul developed programs to approach ventricular asystole and fibrillation (Figure 2).[7,9] Hazardous arrhythmias were Paul Zoll's clinical and research interest. He identified three phases of resuscitation which were restoration of circulation, restoration of intrinsic cardiac rhythm, and prevention of recurrent episodes.[9] Zoll later added the prevention of primary cardiac arrest.[11,12] He was a member of his hospital's resuscitation committee, early response team and was Chairman of the Massachusetts Heart Association's Committee on Cardiac Arrest. He was among the "first generation" of experts to gather at the initial Wolf Creek Conferences on cardiopulmonary resuscitation which was a think tank for those who were at the forefront of new knowledge in the field.[32] Paul Zoll's early works provided a large portion of the platform for advanced cardiac life support (ACLS). Some elements have been retained in the current ACLS Guidelines such as transcutaneous thoracic pacing for a heart rate too slow to sustain an adequate cardiac output, infusions of dilute solutions of epinephrine to support blood pressure and heart rate and most importantly, rapid transcutaneous defibrillation—a prioritized intervention for the majority of victims of cardiac arrest. Zoll also emphasized preparedness. "*Once the arrest has been recognized, a prearranged and well rehearsed program of action must be instituted promptly.*"[33] (Figure 3)

Paul's electrotherapy research started in response to ventricular bradycardia or asystolic cardiac arrest during Stokes-Adams attacks. Those patients presented in relatively small numbers whereas the majority of cardiac arrests resulted from ventricular fibrillation. At times, asystole and ventricular fibrillation were two sides of the same coin—each occurring in the same patient. Zoll began work on transcutaneous defibrillation as soon as he succeeded with transcutaneous pacing.

| | |
|---|---|
| **FOR A MAJOR ATTACK: EMERGENCY RESUSCITATION** | Slap Precordium<br>Cardiac Puncture<br>Intracardiac Epinephrine<br>Cardiac Pacemaker |
| **FOR PERSISTENT VERTRICULAR STANDSTILL** | Cardiac Pacemaker<br>Sympathomimetic Drugs<br>To arouse idioventricular rhythm:epinephrine<br>To maintain blood pressure: Norepinephrine |
| **FOR FREQUENT ATTACKS** | Drugs to maintain adequate idioventricular rate: ephedrine, epinephrine<br>To prevent variations in conduction: atropine<br>To prevent ventricular irritability: Cardiac pacemaker |

**1955 [7]**

*The Three Problems of Stokes-Adams Disease and Cardiac Arrest. Program for Their Management*

1. *Restoration of Circulation.*
   Precordial blow
   External electrical stimulation or countershock
   External cardiac compression
   Cardiac puncture and intracardiac epinephrine
   Thoracotomy and massage
      If other methods fail
      If adequate help is available
      If prognosis is favorable:
         No irreversible cerebral damage
         General condition good
   Artificial Respiration
2. *Restoration of intrinsic cardiac rhythm*
   Electrocardiograph or monitor
   Electric stimulation or countershock
   Drugs: Epinephrine, isoproterenol, procainamide
      calcium salts, norepinephrine, sodium bicarbonate
3. *Prevention of recurrent episodes*
   Intravenous epinephrine, isoproterenol, atropine
   Oral ephedrine and isoproterenol
   Internal electrical pacemaker

**1963 [9]**

**Figure 2** Programs for the treatment of Stokes-Adams disease. 1955 program emphasizes electro and pharmacotherapy. 1963 program adds chest compression[43] and a permanent internal electrical pacemaker.

He was familiar with the large body of animal experimentation relating to open-chest defibrillation and Claude Beck's success in open-chest termination of ventricular fibrillation in a young man who was still in the operating room at the conclusion of a pectus excavatum repair.

When Paul Zoll started to grapple with the issue of transthoracic defibrillation, he was unaware of Naum Gurvich's success with transthoracic defibrillation in animals. Gurvich was associated with the Scientific Research Institute of Physiology and the

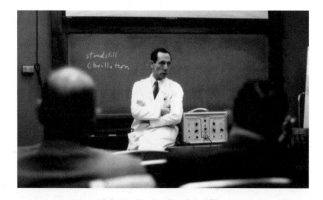

**Figure 3** Dr. Zoll teaching his favorite subject; the approach to cardiac arrest. The instrument is an Electrodyne PM-65, which combined a cardiac monitor with a transcutaneous or internal pacemaker. It could automatically pace when asystole was detected. Courtesy of Archives Beth Israel Deaconess Medical Center.

Academy of Sciences in the USSR. His works spanned decades. During his long experience, defibrillation was achieved in small and large animals with both A/C and direct current (D/C) defibrillators.[34] Gurvich favored D/C and speculated that success should be achievable in man.[35] These important experiments were either unknown to or were overlooked by workers who were rooted in the West.

In 1956, Zoll used Belgard's early version transcutaneous defibrillator to terminate ventricular fibrillation in man[5] and by doing so fulfilled both his own and Gurvich's prediction. The Electrodyne A/C defibrillator also succeeded in terminating every type of rapid arrhythmia in animals and ventricular tachycardia in man.[36,37] Six years later, Bernard Lown electively converted ventricular tachycardia with an A/C[38] and then with a D/C defibrillator that had a synchronizing circuit.[39] Lown coined the term "cardioversion" whereas Zoll preferred the term "countershock" in deference to Carl Wigger's classic animal experiments during which ventricular fibrillation was induced with an electrical shock and then terminated with a second so called "countershock."

Alternating current defibrillators served the medical community well between 1956 and 1962. However, the introduction of the D/C defibrillator with a synchronizing circuit capable of discharging during the absolute refractory period of the cardiac cycle provided a theoretically safer alternative for a large population of patients with troublesome, but not life-threatening arrhythmias. Although Zoll defended A/C, he ultimately accepted the medical community's preference for D/C defibrillation and countershock/cardioversion.

Within 4 years, Zoll developed electrotherapy for the two major causes of cardiac arrest, which are asystole and ventricular fibrillation. He knew that the long-term solution to asystole or severe bradycardia was a reliable permanent implantable pacemaker. He and his co-workers hoped to be the first to achieve that goal. In 1958, the first permanent pacemaker was placed in Sweden.[40] It promptly failed. The unit's power source required recharging from an external source. A number of centers and individuals were competing to develop a reliable permanent pacemaker. In 1960, William Chardack and Wilson Greatbatch were the first to succeed in placing a reliable fully implanted self-contained pacemaker powered by a self-sustaining battery.[41] Paul Zoll and Alan Belgard's version was implanted by Howard Frank about 3 months later.[2]

These early workers encountered multiple technical problems. The most troublesome was developing a reliable lead. There were early unacceptable elevations in the stimulation threshold and frequent electrode fractures. In 1963, Zoll relates being referred by some engineers from the Massachusetts Institute of Technology to the Simplex Wire Company in nearby Cambridge, Massachusetts. Zoll told their representative that he needed a wire that could flex 36,792,000 times a year for 50 years. He cited a young patient in her 20s with a recently placed pacemaker. He needed electrodes that would serve this patient for another 42–50 years. The company's representative conceded that their best wire would fracture after a few thousand flexions.[26] Drs. Zoll and Frank along with Belgard developed their own electrode[42] and implantation techniques, which minimized threshold and electrical fracture problems. At this writing, the young woman that Zoll referred to at the Simplex Wire Company remains fully functional with continuous pacemaker dependence.

In another of Paul's recollections of the seminal discovery that he could stimulate the ventricle in an animal with a closed chest externally, he wrote, *"I think I recognized at that time that a new field of electric cardiac stimulation had begun. I think I foresaw almost all of the implications of what has followed in the next 25 years."*[10] What followed was his developing transcutaneous pacing in man; increasingly complex arrhythmia detection systems some of which had an option for standby automatic pacing on demand; a transcutaneous defibrillator; a permanent implantable pacemaker; and resuscitation programs which combined electro and pharmacotherapy to confront cardiac arrest. He lived to see others extend his work with the introduction of the implantable internal and the automatic external defibrillator.

When historians reflect on Paul Zoll's achievements, they should recall that each was developed in response to the needs of his cardiac patients. When Paul Zoll retired, he was asked, *"Do you have any regrets?"* He answered, *"I did so little...there is so much more I should have done."*[20]

## Acknowledgement

This work was supported in part by a gift from the Simons Foundation.

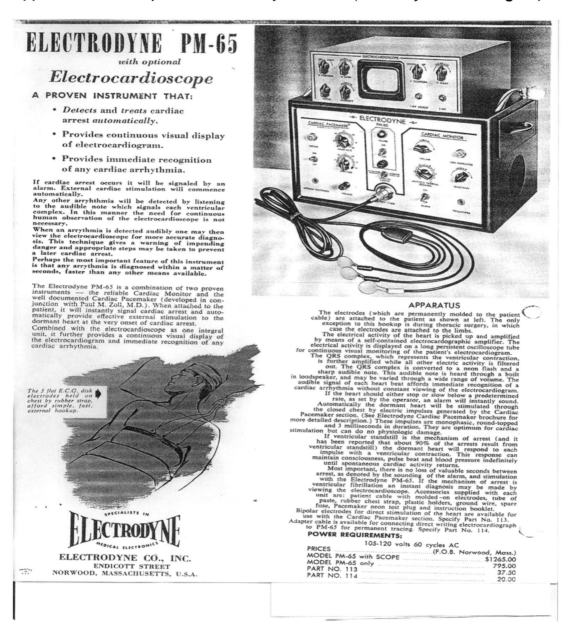

*Legend*: The PM-65 could automatically stimulate the heart after an adjustable predetermined asystolic interval.[44] Dr. Seymour Furman's famous case #2[28], identified as MH78921,P.S. (or in other publications as Pincus Shapiro), had frequent Stokes-Adams attacks. Mr. Shapiro experienced intolerable pain during transcutaneous pacing. So, a dedicated nurse was at the bedside continuously to manually activate the pacemaker only when absolutely necessary.

During the second half of the hospitalization, a temporary transvenous pacemaker electrode was placed from the arm and the automatic internal pacing mode of the Electrodyne PM-65 substituted for the nurse operated manual transcutaneous external pacing mode. The pacer was programmed to activate after 5 s of asystole. Thereafter, there was reliable automatic painless cardiac pacing on demand via the PM-65 accessory bipolar electrode for direct cardiac stimulation, which Dr. Furman adapted to his transvenous endocardial catheter. Pincus Shapiro was the first to receive what is now known as transvenous endocardial VVI mode pacing. A fascinating brief film about a patient with Stokes-Adams attacks, which co-features the Electrodyne PM-65 is available on the internet.[45]

# References

1. Beck CS, Leighniger DS. Death after a clean bill of health. JAMA 1960;174:133—5.
2. Zoll PM, Frank HA, Zarsky LR, et al. Long-term electrical stimulation of the heart for Stokes-Adams Disease. Ann Surg 1961;154:330—46.
3. Zoll PM. Resuscitation of the heart in ventricular stand-still by external electrical simulation. New Engl J Med 1952;247:768—71.
4. Zoll PM, Linenthal AJ, Norman LR, et al. Treatment of unexpected cardiac arrest by external electric stimulation of the heart. New Engl J Med 1956;254:541—6.
5. Zoll PM, Linenthal AJ, Norman LR, et al. Termination of ventricular fibrillation in man by externally applied countershock. New Engl J Med 1956;254:727—32.
6. Zoll PM, Linenthal AJ, Gibson W, et al. Intravenous drug therapy of Strokes-Adams disease. Effects of sympathomimetic amines on ventricular rhythmicity and atrioventricular conduction. Circulation 1958;17:325—39.
7. Zoll PM, Linenthal AS, Norman LR, et al. External electrical stimulation of the heart in cardiac arrest. Arch Int Med 1955;96:639—53.
8. Linenthal AJ, Zoll PM. Prevention of ventricular irritability in Stokes-Adams disease by intravenous sympathomimetic amines. Circulation 1963;27:5—11.
9. Zoll PM, Linenthal AJ. Program for Stokes-Adams disease and cardiac arrest. Circulation 1963;27:1—4.
10. Zoll PM, Linenthal AJ. External and internal electric cardiac pacemakers. Circulation 1963;28:455—66.
11. Zoll PM. Prevention and treatment of ventricular fibrillation and ventricular asystole. In: Surawicz G, Pellegrino ED, editors. Sudden cardiac death. NY: Gruen & Stratton Inc.; 1964. p. 145—58.
12. Zoll PM. Rational use of drugs for cardiac arrest and after cardiac resuscitation. Am J Cardiol 1971;27:645—9.
13. Zoll PM, Zoll RH, Belgard AH. External noninvasive electrical stimulation of the heart. Crit Care Med 1981;9:393—4.
14. Freedberg AS. In memoriam. Harvard Med Alumni Bull 1999;72:56—7.
15. Freedberg AS. Interview with Stafford I. Cohen, 8 March 2006.
16. Abelmann WH, Axelrod P, Cohen SI, et al. Faculty of medicine—memorial minute. Harvard University Gazette April 19, 2001; p. 12.
17. Personal observations of the author, Stafford I. Cohen.
18. Albert & Mary Lasker Foundation. Citations. JAMA 1973;19:876.
19. Personal experience of the author, Stafford I. Cohen.
20. Mahler EJ. Memorial Service for Paul Maurice Zoll M.D., Beth Israel Hospital, 23 February 1999.
21. Zoll PM. Development of electrical control of cardiac rhythm. JAMA 1973;226:881—6.
22. Beck CS, Pritchard WH, Feil HS. Ventricular fibrillation of long duration abolished by electrical shock. JAMA 1947;135:985—6.
23. Zoll PM. The intermediate history of cardiac pacing. In: Harthorn JW, Thalen HJT, editors. Boston colloquium on cardiac pacing. The Hague, Holland: Martinus Nijhoff's Boekhandel en Unitgeuersmaatshappij BV; 1977. p. 27—32.
24. Schechter DH. Electrical cardiac stimulation. In: Modern era of artificial pacemakers. Medtronic Inc.; 1983 [Chapter 9, p. 112].
25. Furman S. Forward. In: Greatbatch W, editor. The making of the pacemaker. Amherst, NY: Prometheus Books; 2000. p. 13.
26. Harken DE. History of pacemaker development. Biomed Instrum Technol 1991;25:319.
27. Mirowski M, Reid PR, Mower MM, et al. Termination of malignant ventricular arrhythmias with an implanted automatic defibrillator in human beings. New Engl J Med 1980;303:322—4.
28. Furman S, Schwedel JB. An intracardiac pacemaker for Stokes-Adams seizures. New Engl J Med 1959;261:943—8.
29. Weisse AB. Heart to heart, the twentieth-century battle against cardiac disease. An oral history. Chapter on Paul Zoll, M.D. New Brunswick, New Jersey & London: Rutgers University Press; 2002.
30. Day H. A cardiac resuscitative program. Lancet 1962;82:153—6.
31. Kravitz AE, Killip T. Cardiopulmonary resuscitation. Status report. Editorial. New Engl J Med 1972;286:1000—1.
32. Advances in cardiopulmonary resuscitation.Safar P, editor. Preface. Proceedings of the 1975 Wolf-Creek conference. Springer Verlag; 1977.
33. Zoll PM, Linenthal AJ. External electrical simulation of the heart. Ann NY Acad Sci 1969;165:932—7.
34. Gurvich NL, Yuniev GS. Restoration of regular rhythm in the mammalian fibrillating heart. Am Rev Sov Med 1945—1946;3:55—8.
35. Gurvich NL, Yuniev GS. Restoration of heart rhythm during fibrillation by a condenser discharge. Am Rev Sov Med 1946—1947;4:252—6.
36. Zoll PM. Effects of external electrical currents on the heart; control of cardiac rhythm and induction and termination of cardiac arrhythmias. Circulation 1956;14:745—6.
37. Zoll PM, Linenthal AJ, Zarsky LR. Ventricular fibrillation; treatment and prevention by electrical currents. New Engl J Med 1960;264:105—12.
38. Alexander S, Kleiger R, Lown B. Use of an electric countershock in the treatment of ventricular tachycardia. JAMA 1961;77:916—8.
39. Lown B, Amarasingham R, Newman J. New method for terminating cardiac arrhythmias; use of synchronized capacitor discharge. JAMA 1962;182:548—55.
40. Jeffrey K. Machines in our hearts. Baltimore & London: The Johns Hopkins University Press; 2001. p. 90—2.
41. Chardack WM, Gage AA, Greatbatch W. A transistorized, self-contained, implantable pacemaker for long-term correction of complete heart block. Surgery 1960;48:643—54.
42. Zoll PM. Historical development of cardiac pacemakers. Prog Cardiovasc Dis 1972;14:421—9.
43. Kouwenhoven WB, Jude JR, Knickerbocker GG. Closed chest cardiac massage. JAMA 1960;73:94—7.
44. Nicholson MJ, Eversole UH, Orr R, et al. A cardiac monitor--pacemaker: use during and after anesthesia. Anesth Analg 1959;38:335—47.
45. Heart Rhythm Society. Electricity and the heart. Tony's cardiac pacemaker. http://www.hrsonline.org/ep-history/.

# Bernard Lown and defibrillation

## Mickey Eisenberg

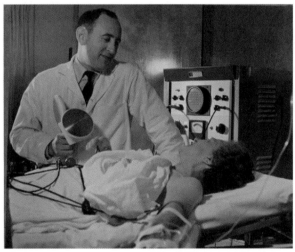

I suspect Bernard Lown is most proud of his achievements as a clinician[1] and Nobel Peace Prize winner. But to those of us in resuscitation science, he is known for his contributions to defibrillation.

Bernard Lown was born in Utena, Lithuania on June 7, 1921. Driven by anti-semitic persecution, his father emigrated and later brought him to the United States in 1935, when Lown was 13 years old. Lown graduated summa cum laude from the University of Maine in 1942, receiving his B.A. in the classics. Lown was accepted at Johns Hopkins Medical School and received his M.D. in 1945. After serving in the Army Lown interned in medicine at the Jewish Hospital in New York City and later worked at Montefiore Hospital in New York City. In 1950 he took a position as a researcher in cardiology at Peter Bent Brigham Hospital in Boston, and he has had successive positions at the Brigham since then, including director of the Levine Coronary Care Unit. He has also had prestigious positions at Harvard University and at various hospitals in Boston and other cities, working as a consultant to the World Health Organization, the National Institutes of Health, and other national and international organizations. He is currently cardiology professor emeritus at the Harvard School of Public Health.

In the late 1950s, Lown's interest in defibrillation was catalyzed by the frustration of attempting to treat patients with ventricular tachycardia. In 1959 Lown had such a patient. Pharmacological therapy with procainamide offered little to the patient and in fact, worsened the condition. Lown recalled an article by Zoll et al.[2] describing alternating current electric therapy for ventricular fibrillation. Lown was in uncharted territory and decided electrical cardioversion offered the only hope for his patient. He recalled, ''I didn't know the first thing about how to use AC on a patient, what type of current settings, amperage, and what not." Nevertheless, the patient responded well to the shock. As Lown describes what happened next in his 1996 book, *The Lost Art of Healing*, "I heard ... a slow, regular lub-dub. These heart sounds gave me a ... thrill, recalling my first hearing, as a youngster, the opening bars of Beethoven's Fifth Symphony."

The patient's tachycardia stopped at once, his blood pressure returned to normal, and he was quickly discharged from the hospital. Within two weeks, though, he was back with a severe tachycardia. Again Lown used the AC defibrillator to cardiovert the man's heart back to normal but this time the AC current caused the heart to go into ventricular fibrillation. Nothing worked at that point, even open heart defibrillation, and the patient died. Lown was devastated by this episode and set out to discover just what alternating current did to the heart. In a series of experiments with dogs he found that alternating current induced fibrillations in a normal heart about 25% of the time. "Obviously, we had a technology that was very hazardous," recalled Lown.[1]

He decided to study safe and effective ways of delivering a lifesaving shock to the heart. Direct current was the logical current to study, but little was known about its effect on the heart. A series of animal experiments on dogs in 1960 and 1961 established that DC shocks were extremely effective in shocking the heart. An article in 1962 in the *American Journal of Cardiology*, confirmed his early findings that AC current was dangerous to the heart.[3] Lown noted that the incidence of ventricular fibrillation was 10 times more frequent after AC than DC cardioversion. Lown also discovered one short period of time during the procedure when a DC shock could induce ventricular fibrillation, the so called "vulnerable period" shortly after the T wave in the heart's cycle of depolarization.

Lown and his colleagues also studied the different type of DC waveforms to determine the most effective type. An electrical engineer at the American Optical Company in Buffalo hand-built several different types of DC machines for Lown to test. Eventually, they hit upon the right combination of voltages and waveform. The first clinical opportunity to use the DC cardioverter came in 1961 at the Peter Bent Brigham Hospital in Boston. An elderly woman with an acute myocardial infarction developed a serious ventricular tachycardia. Drug treatment slowed the ventricular tachycardia but sent her into shock.39 The resident treating the woman contacted Lown, who was then doing some work at the Harvard School of Public Health, across the street from the Brigham. It was about 2:00 a.m.,

but Lown and another doctor "carried the device to the Brigham and set it up," Lown recalled. The patient was muttering that she was dying—"with adequate reason," Lown would later write. Lown gave her a single jolt from his new DC cardioverter. "She came right out of the tachycardia rhythm," said Lown. "It was so remarkable." The woman's heart failure improved at once, and her blood pressure went back to normal. "The funny story about her," recalled Lown, "was that she felt so good that she thought she'd died and we were angels! It took me about an hour to persuade her that I wasn't the angel Gabriel." Lown's report of this case and several others like it was published in the November 3, 1962 issue of *JAMA*.[4] It was reprinted in the same journal 24 years later and honored as a Landmark Article, a distinction given to only a handful of scientific reports. Although others were also working on direct current defibrillators at the same time, Lown's machine was the first to be actually built and successfully used on humans.

The initial studies in the late 1950s and early 1960s focused exclusively on how to treat tachycardic rhythms effectively.[5,6] Defibrillation for the treatment of ventricular fibrillation was not on the early agenda. Lown appreciated, however, that a shock for a racing ventricle would likely to be equally effective for a fibrillating ventricle. Thus, Lown worked with engineers from AO Optical to develop a DC machine that could do both cardioversion and defibrillation. He later said he saw his DC defibrillator as something best used in a hospital setting, easily accessible to a large population. In fact, it was his breakthrough to DC that eventually made the portable defibrillator practical. The development of small but powerful DC batteries and small capacitors would be the next technologic link. At that point, the need to carry a 50-lb step-up transformer to the patient and the need to find an electrical outlet in which to plug an AC-based defibrillator vanished. Lown's work to perfect a DC defibrillator takes on greater significance because its development coincided with that of modern mouth-to-mouth ventilation and chest compression. Prior to CPR, the opportunity to defibrillate was a rare event. It had to happen in a hospital with a defibrillator immediately at hand. Lown, in an era without CPR, would have invented a better mousetrap but there would be few mice to catch. The ability to prolong the dying process with CPR suddenly gave an urgency to find the best type of defibrillatory shock. Now it was possible to rush the machine to the patient because CPR bought a few precious minutes of time. The real significance of DC defibrillation is that small and portable defibrillators were now possible to build. Lown envisioned his machines being used primarily in hospitals, but in moments of unbridled imagination he hoped his machines would be used to attack sudden death directly in the community. With the development of DC defibrillation, Lown made a considerable contribution to resuscitation.

Though this biographical sketch stresses Lown's contribution to management of cardiac arrest, I believe he is equally, if not more, proud of his work to reduce the likelihood of nuclear catastrophe culminating in his Nobel Peace Prize in 1985. He received this honor for founding, with Soviet cardiac researcher Yevgeny Chasov, the society that became known as the International Physicians for the Prevention of Nuclear War. Not surprisingly, the two Nobelists first met while working on ways to prevent sudden cardiac death. The official announcement of the Nobel Committee on October 11, 1985 commended him for ''a considerable service to mankind by spreading authoritative information and by creating an awareness of the catastrophic consequences of atomic warfare.'' Lown spoke with passion about the role of medicine and the dangers of nuclear weapons. In his Nobel acceptance speech he said, ''We physicians protest the outrage of holding the entire world hostage. We protest the moral obscenity that each of us is being continually targeted for extinction. We protest the ongoing increase in overkill. We protest the expansion of the arms race to space. We protest the diversion of scarce resources from aching human needs. Dialogue without deeds brings the calamity ever closer, as snail-paced diplomacy is out-distanced by missile-propelled technology. We physicians demand deeds which will lead to the abolition of all nuclear weaponry.''

Lown's achievements are impressive—a lifelong impassioned commitment to limit, reduce, and eliminate nuclear weapons and a lifelong commitment to find better treatment for ventricular tachycardia and sudden cardiac arrest. There is a common theme here: reducing the risk of death, from external horror from the sky and internal chaos from the heart.

Portions of this article are based on biographical material on Bernard Lown contained in Eisenberg MS, *Life in the Balance: Emergency Medicine and the Quest to Reverse Sudden Death.* Oxford University Press, New York, 1997, pp. 196—199.

Unattributed quotes are from an interview I conducted with Bernard Lown on June 2, 1992.

# References

1. Lown B. The lost art of healing. New York: Houghton Mifflin; 1996.
2. Zoll PM, Linenthal AJ, Gibson W, Paul MH, Norman LR. Termination of ventricular fibrillation in man by externally applied electric countershocks. New Engl J Med 1956;254:727—32.
3. Lown B, Neuman J, Amarasingham B, Berkovits BV. Comparison of alternating current with direct current electroshock across the closed chest. Am J Cardiol 1962;10:223—33.
4. Lown B, Amarasingham R, Neuman J. New method for terminating cardiac arrhythmias. Use of synchronized capacitor discharge. JAMA 1962;182(November):548—55.
5. Lown B. Cardioversion of arrhythmias (I). Modern Concepts Cardiovasc Dis 1964;33:863—8.
6. Lown B. New method of terminating cardiac arrhythmias. Modern Concepts Cardiovasc Dis 1964;33:548—55.

# Edgar Alexander Pask—a hero of resuscitation

Gary Enever

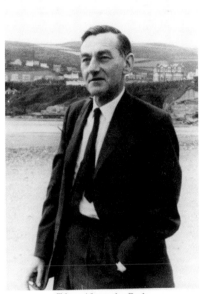

Edgar Alexander Pask

Some older anaesthetists have heard the name "Pask", but few know who he was or what he did. The Association of Anaesthetists of Great Britain and Ireland has an award named after him, for anaesthetic acts over and above the call of duty, but few know why. The man was a legend in his lifetime and set an example that was to have tremendous influence on future generations.

## 1. The early years

Edgar Alexander Pask, later often known as "Gar", was born on the 4th of September, 1912. His father, Percy Pask, had started out as a barrow boy in Liverpool, United Kingdom, but soon progressed to be an important fruit importer.

Percy married Mary Speedie, a Manxwoman (as natives of the Isle of Man are known) and a staunch Methodist, and they had three sons. Alfred was the eldest, and became a Methodist minister. Edgar was next, born when the family had moved out of Liverpool to West Kirby in Cheshire. Their youngest son, Gordon, was born much later, in 1928, eventually becoming famous as a professor of cybernetics.

Edgar was educated at Rydal School in Colwyn Bay, and won a scholarship to Downing College, Cambridge to read natural sciences [1]. Following a double first class honours in his Tripos examinations in 1933, he progressed to The London Hospital to complete his undergraduate education, and qualified MBBCh. in 1937.

Pask spent 2 years at The London in junior hospital posts, and then in 1939 took up the appointment that was to change his life. With his impressive academic record, his scientific credentials and his experience of anaesthesia, the Nuffield Department in Oxford was the place for Pask. Professor Macintosh had been head of Britain's only academic anaesthetic department since it's inception in 1937 when Pask joined as the first assistant. He became one of a small but growing band of anaesthesia's elite, and had only just settled in when war was declared [2].

In September 1939, the Nuffield Department was a hive of activity. It was not only providing anaesthetic services for the Oxford hospitals and generating a wide variety of research, but was also drawn into supporting the war effort. Macintosh, a First World War fighter pilot, was made a Group Captain to advise the RAF on anaesthesia. The Department began running short training courses for military service anaesthetists, which were very popular. They were particularly enjoyed when Macintosh packed them into his Bentley for picnics by the Thames. Staff joined and left, moving into the forces or on secondments. Pask was made the Mayo Fellow, and sent south to the Royal Sussex Hospital to help deal with casualties evacuated from Dunkirk. He was then finally drawn into a blue uniform, and followed his professor in the RAF.

## 2. The RAF years

Edgar Pask was a remarkable physiologist. Probably with Macintosh's encouragement, he was posted to the Physiological Laboratory in the RAF Research Station at Farnborough, where he was presented with a number of urgent questions to solve. RAF aircrew were exposed to terrible dangers, not only directly from their enemies, but also from the hostile environments they inhabited. Farnborough hosted a number of remarkable human experiments, many devised by Pask and his colleagues and using themselves as experimental subjects. He stated in the introduction to his MD thesis, submitted after the war, that he "had certain experience in the clinical and experimental practice of anaesthesia and believed that the methods used in such practice could usefully be employed in the solution of the problems under consideration" [3].

Four of the important problems considered were high altitude parachute descent, artificial ventilation, effectiveness of lifejackets and survival in cold water.

### 2.1. Parachute descent from aircraft flying at high altitude

In 1941, lease-lend from the United States presented the RAF with a number of B17 bombers, the legendary "flying fortresses". They were supposedly designed for accurate high altitude daylight bombing, but imposed incredible risks on the aircrew. They flew higher than Everest in a thin, unpressurised aluminium tube, exposed to bitter cold and severe hypoxia. Pask's job was to see what would happen to aircrew if they bailed out at such altitudes.

The first series of experiments, simulated parachute descent, was undertaken by the five young doctors posted to the laboratory at Farnborough. They were aged from 28 to 32 years, and described themselves as "in good health but not in good training". They were all heavy smokers, with Pask well known as a 60-a-day man. Sixteen experiments were undertaken, with Pask as the subject for seven of them. They were exposed to hypoxic gas mixtures in a decompression chamber, with the mixtures designed to simulate the inspired oxygen concentrations encountered while descending. The experimental notes make fascinating, as well as disturbing, reading. They describe young men being asphyxiated, and then slowly recovering. The experiments on Pask undertaken with him hanging in a parachute harness were particularly hazardous (Fig. 1).

It is interesting to note that the volunteers varied markedly in their ability to cope with hypoxia, and in their rates of recovery. It is not known whether they suffered sufficiently to have permanent damage, but the assessment of the risks resulted in portable oxygen cylinders being made available for high altitude crew, should they have needed to bail out over 20,000 feet.

The subsequent experiments involved Pask both as experimenter and subject. He used himself, as it was convenient to do so, in a number of hazardous situations. He was anaesthetised to the point of apnoea then was the subject used to test the available methods of artificial ventilation. Finally, he was anaesthetised wearing a variety of lifejackets and placed into a swimming pool to test their efficiency. Anaesthesia was directed, and often given, by Macintosh himself. The professor commented that Pask did most of the important work for his MD thesis whilst asleep.

### 2.2. The efficiency of the methods of artificial respiration

Many aircrews were forced to ditch into the sea, where cold and injuries would eventually end in drowning. Even when rescued by the RAF's high speed launches, they were often in a poor state, and many collapsed. Artificial respiration, if required, was extremely difficult. The Schafer method [4,5] was used universally at the outbreak of war, but was almost impossible to apply below the cramped, jolting decks of a rescue vessel at full tilt. Medical staff were empowered to call for the launch to slow to allow resuscitation, but this exposed to whole crew to enemy action, and was not popular.

Faced with these problems in 1943, Pask went back to the original papers on artificial respiration, to find a method that was likely to be applicable. It had to be easy to apply in difficult conditions. As the majority of studies had either used conscious subjects or corpses, the efficacy of any particular method was uncertain. So, he allowed himself to be anaesthetised to the point of apnoea, was intubated and his minute volume was recorded on a smoked drum using a range of methods of artificial respiration in vogue at the time.

The following table gives the results:

| Method | Position | Inspired minute volume (L) |
|---|---|---|
| Schafer's | Prone | 3.44 |
| Sylvester's | Supine | 4.12 |
| Eve's 45/45 smooth | Prone | 5.82 |
| Eve's 45/45 jerky | Prone | 5.91 |
| Eve's 30/30 smooth | Prone | 3.54 |
| Eve's 30/30 jerky | Prone | 3.65 |
| Eve's 45/45 smooth | Supine | 3.80 |
| Eve's 45/45 jerky | Supine | 4.09 |
| Eve's 30/30 smooth | Supine | 2.17 |
| Eve's 30/30 jerky | Supine | 3.03 |
| Oxford inflating bellows | Supine | 4.12 (estimated) |
| Mouth to mouth | Supine | 6.16 (estimated) |
| Oxford inflating bellows | Prone | 5.50 (estimated) |

At the time of the study, Pask was 31 years old, 10 stone (65 kg) in weight and a heavy smoker. Following review of the results, once awake, Pask decided that the Eve's Rocking Board method could be most easily and safely applied, and this was duly adopted by the RAF and then the Navy [6,7].

As a point of interest, Pask obtained some early curare from his friend Harold Griffith in 1945. He then persuaded Macintosh to repeat the experiments on him, and was fully paralysed for 2 h, to compare results with his earlier experiment.

**Descent No. 14.** Subject - E.A.P. Gas mixture - Nitrogen/Oxygen
Posture - suspended in parachute harness.
Simulated altitude - 35,000 ft.

This and the next descent caused certain anxiety and necessitated close attention to the subject. As a result, the clinical notes were compiled after the experiment, not during it.

**Clinical Record.**

The period of anxiety was more prolonged than in the "descent" from 35,000 ft., with the subject sitting, and not until the 6th minute was it certain that the "descent" could be completed.

The subject made two attempts to raise himself in the harness by pulling on the parachute risers during 1¼-1½ mins. These attempts he could not remember afterwards. At 1½ mins., the subject became limp and relaxed, the head falling forward, but although it must have been merely a matter of chance, it was not thought that laryngeal or pharyngeal obstruction actually developed, though vigorous inspiratory efforts were made.

Sweating was very profuse and liquid sweat fell from the forehead and formed a noticeable pool on the floor.

Muscular twitching of the left arm was seen between 5th and 9th minutes.

The pulse was not rapid - indeed a good deal slower than in previous "descents" with this subject, but between 2nd and 6th minutes it was recorded as very feeble.

Fig. 1. The experimental record of one of Pask's "descents".

## 2.3. *The efficiency of lifejackets*

It was thought to be a good idea to prevent unconscious aircrew from drowning, should they parachute into the sea, but the lifejackets available that were used had never been investigated. It was a fact that many crew were found dead, face down, floating in their lifejackets. So again, Pask and Macintosh set to it. Anaesthetised and set adrift in a pool, a number of different jackets and suits were tested on Pask, breathing ether through a cuffed Magill tracheal tube via an extremely long co-axial circuit (Fig. 2). The experiments were both traumatic and dramatic. They were filmed, so that they could be shown to aircrew to boost morale and to show that something was being done. After each experiment, Pask was admitted to hospital to recover, and anecdotally he was not very well after each episode, which is hardly surprising. Often he sank completely, greatly increasing the risks of aspirating pool water (Fig. 3).

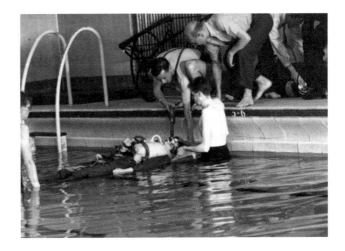

Fig. 2. Pask being placed into the pool by professor Macintosh and his team.

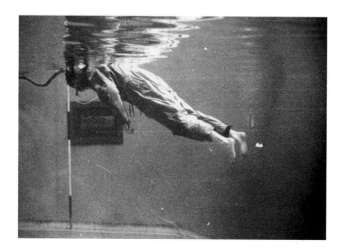

Fig. 3. Pask sinking face down below the surface of the pool.

### 2.4. Temperature maintenance in cold water

Aircrew ditching into the seas around Britain were likely to suffer hypothermia, and so an effective immersion suit was required. Pask experimented with a number of materials and thermal linings, to try and design a suit that was comfortable, warm and water-proof. Once created, these immersion suits were tested in typical Pask fashion. He was parachuted into the sea in winter. Pask's suits became standard issue for the RAF and Fleet Air Arm.

These extreme experiments became Pask's MD thesis, "Anaesthetic Techniques in Research", and his MD was duly awarded by the University of Cambridge in 1947. Little was known of the work, because of wartime security restrictions, and few knew that Pask had used himself as the subject. It was many years before some of the lifejacket work was published [8].

### 3. After the Second World War

As a non-combatant, Pask was not eligible for military medals to recognise his bravery, and was therefore presented with the OBE by King George 6th in 1944, as well as being presented with one of the first John Snow Medals by the Association of Anaesthetists. He left the RAF as a Squadron Leader, and went back to Oxford. Following the lead set by the Nuffield departments there, other universities began to establish academic departments of anaesthesia, and Pask was offered the post of Reader in Anaesthesia at King's College, Newcastle-upon Tyne (part of the University of Durham at the time). However, before taking up the post he went to Madison, Wisconsin, in the United States to learn from the "master", Ralph Waters. At the time, Pask was considering physiology as a career, but Waters persuaded him to return to the Royal Victoria Infirmary at Newcastle.

In 1947, he entered the department that was to be his home until his death in 1966. It had many similarities with Oxford, with laboratories, workshops and its own anaesthetic nurses.

Side by side with his technician, Norman Burn, he built some of the earliest British ventilators, many of which still remain in the historical collection in Newcastle [9]. Not surprisingly, after his wartime experiments, Pask was fascinated with the problems of artificial respiration. He gave many lectures on ventilation and resuscitation, in both Britain and the USA, and it is interesting to note that he emphasised the importance of blood flow and cardiac output, the use of high inspired oxygen concentrations, and the maintenance of a clear airway. He also developed some of the earliest electronic monitoring equipment used in anaesthesia.

Pask also continued his interest in lifejackets. Having become a professor (the second professor of Anaesthesia in Britain), it was not deemed appropriate for his self-experimentation to continue. A chance reading of "Popular Mechanics" magazine in 1954 informed him of the existence of the very first "test dummies", being used by the American airforce. He set off for California, and a year later "Seaworthy Sierra Sam" joined the Newcastle Department. This was the first, and possibly only, manikin designed to be water-proof, and was used extensively in a new series of experiments, which continued even after Pask's death [10].

### 4. Pask the man

It is clear that Pask was a quite remarkable man of phenomenal courage. Norman Burn, his technician, worshipped him. He describes a man of incredible intellect, able to understand and solve complex problems, while still able to work a lathe with great skill. Macintosh, on hearing of his death, wrote "In my opinion he was the best brain in our speciality—and I have yet to meet anyone more reliable and considerate". He was a leading figure both regionally and nationally. He lectured extensively, although it was said that he rarely spoke for more than 30 min, as by then he would need another cigarette. He was not perfect. He would shuffle past colleagues in the hospital corridor, and not acknowledge their greetings. He expected nothing but total dedication from his juniors, because his commitment was also total. They were expected to smoke, so that they would always have cigarettes and a box of matches in their pocket should the professor come by, as he persisted with his 60-a-day until his early death. Pask often appeared in theatre in the middle of the night, at the shoulder of a junior with a difficult case. His advice was invaluable, although his anaesthetic skills were not polished—he did not like "slick" anaesthetists. It is said that the juniors feared the need for surgery, in case they had to have one of the Professor's anaesthetics. But deep down they knew that the professor was driven by compassion for his fellow man.

Pask married late in life. It may have been that the huge risks he took in the Second World War prevented him from marrying, only to leave a widow. It may also have been out of respect for his staunchly Methodist mother, because his wife to be, Muriel, was a Catholic. They did not marry until after

234

the death of his mother. They bought a cottage on the Isle of Man as a retreat, and family trips there to 2 Queen Street, Castletown took place whenever they could, especially after their daughter Susan was born. Pask also travelled to America and Canada many times. At one point, he was considering moving to McGill University in Montreal, but his ill health precluded the move. He suffered from Crohn's disease, and had a number of not wholly successful operations that left him increasingly unwell. He died suddenly, on the 30th May 1966, at the age of only 53. He left many shocked and saddened friends, and the letters of condolence came from the worlds leading anaesthetists. He left relatively few published papers and no textbooks to remember him by, but he had set the direction for many who were to be anaesthesia's future leaders. Sadly, today, he is virtually forgotten, even in Newcastle.

## Acknowledgements

The author would like to acknowledge the University of Cambridge for extracts from Pask's Thesis, and Dr. Joe Stoddart for his photograph of Pask on the beach.

## References

[1] Taylor A. Professor Edgar Alexander Pask. Curr Anaesth Crit Care 1998;9:156–60.

[2] The Nuffield Department of Anaesthetics 1937–1962, Oxford University Press, 1963.

[3] Pask EA. Applications of Anaesthetic Techniques in Physiological Research, M.D. Thesis, University of Cambridge, 1946.

[4] Schafer EA. Description of a simple and efficient method of performing artificial respirationin the human subject, to which is appended instructions for the treatment of the apparently drowned. Med Chir Trans 1904:609–14 (Discussion 615–623).

[5] Sir Edward Sharpey Schafer and his simple and efficient method of performimg artificial respiration, Resuscitation, 2004;61: 113–6.

[6] Eve FC. Activation of the inert diaphragm by a gravity method. Lancet 1932;1:995–7.

[7] Baskett TF. Eve's Rocking method of artificial respiration. Resuscitation 2005;65:245–7.

[8] Macintosh RR, Pask EA. Testing of lifejackets. Br J Ind Med 1957;14:168.

[9] Enever GR. The early Newcastle respirators. CPD Anaesth 2001;33:120–1.

[10] Pask EA. The design of lifejackets. Br Med J 1961:1140–2.

# Virginia Apgar and the newborn Apgar Score

## Thomas F. Baskett

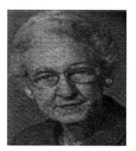

It has been said that "every baby born is first seen through the eyes of Dr. Virginia Apgar" [1]. It is now almost 50 years since Virginia Apgar first described her new method for evaluation of the newborn infant at the joint meeting of the International Anesthesia Research Society and the International College of Anesthetists at Virginia Beach in September 1952. This work was published the following year in *Current Researches in Anesthesia and Analgesia* [2] (Fig. 1). She began her paper with the following observation on the resuscitation of infants at birth: "Seldom have there been such imaginative ideas, such enthusiasms, and dislikes, and such unscientific observations and study about one clinical picture......but the poor quality and lack of precise data of the majority of papers concerned with infant resuscitation are interesting." She went on to review "the objective signs which pertained in any way to the condition of the

Current Researches in Anesthesia and Analgesia—July-August, 1953

### A Proposal for a New Method of Evaluation of the Newborn Infant.*

**Virginia Apgar, M.D., New York, N. Y.**
*Department of Anesthesiology, Columbia University, College of Physicians and Surgeons and the Anesthesia Service, The Presbyterian Hospital*

 ESUSCITATION OF INFANTS at birth has been the subject of many articles. Seldom have there been such imaginative ideas, such enthusiasms, and dislikes, and such unscientific observations and study about one clinical picture. There are outstanding exceptions to these statements, but the poor quality and lack of precise data of the majority of papers concerned with infant resuscitation are interesting.

There are several excellent review articles[1][2] but the main emphasis in the past has been on treatment of the asphyxiated or apneic newborn infant. The purpose of this paper is the reestablishment of simple, clear classification or "grading" of newborn infants which can be used as a basis for discussion and comparison of the results of obstetric practices, types of maternal pain relief and the effects of resuscitation.

The principle of giving a "score" to a patient as a sum total of several objective findings is not new and has been used recently in judging the treatment of drug addiction.[3] The endpoints which have been used previously in the field of resuscitation are "breathing time" defined as the time from delivery of the head to the first respiration, and "crying time" the time until the establishment of a satisfactory cry.[4] Other workers have used the terms mild, moderate and severe depression[5] to signify the state of the infant. There are valid objections to these systems. When mothers receive an excessive amount of depressant drugs in the antepartum period, it is a common occurence that the infants breathe once, then become apneic for many minutes. Evaluation of the breathing time is difficult. A satisfactory cry is sometimes not established even when the infant leaves the delivery room, and in some patients with cerebral injury, the baby dies without ever having uttered a satisfactory cry. Mild, moderate and severe depression of the infant leaves a fair margin for individual interpretation.

A list was made of all the objective signs which pertained in any way to the condition of the infant at birth. Of these, five signs which could be determined easily and without interfering with the care of the infant were considered useful. A rating of zero, one or two was given to each sign depending on whether it was absent or present. A score of ten indicated a baby in the best possible condition. The time for judging the five objective signs was varied until the most practi-

*Presented before the Twenty-Seventh Annual Congress of Anesthetists, Joint Meeting of the International Anesthesia Research Society and the International College of Anesthetists, Virginia Beach, Va., September 22-25, 1952.

Fig. 1.

Table 1
The Apgar Score

| | Sign | 0 | 1 | 2 |
|---|---|---|---|---|
| **A**ppearance | Colour | Pale or blue | Body pink: extremities blue | Completely pink |
| **P**ulse | Heart rate | Absent | $<100$ | $>100$ |
| **G**rimace | Reflex irritability | No response | Grimace/some motion | Cry |
| **A**ctivity | Muscle tone | Limp | Some flexion | Well flexed, active motion |
| **R**espiration | Respiration | Absent | Slow, irregular | Vigorous cry |

infant at birth." She came up with "five signs which could be determined easily and without interfering with the care of the infant....." These were: heart rate, respiratory effort, reflex irritability, muscle tone and colour. Depending on the presence, absence and degree of each of these signs they were rated as 0, 1 or 2 (Table 1). Following study, Apgar felt that 60 s after the complete birth of the baby was the most practical time to assign the score. Apgar acknowledged that colour was "by far the most unsatisfactory sign". She noted that all infants were cyanotic at birth and that peripheral cyanosis had rarely disappeared by 1 min, even in the normal infant. Her original report was on 1021 infants and showed an inverse relationship between the score and neonatal death. Those with a poor score (0–2), a fair score (3–7), and those in good condition (8–10) had a neonatal mortality of 9–14, 1.1–2 and 0.13–1% respectively. Apgar said, "the purpose of this paper is the re-establishment of simple, clear classification or 'grading' of newborn infants which can be used as a basis for discussion and comparison of the results of obstetric practices, types of maternal pain relief and the effects of resuscitation".

A subsequent report, *Further observations on the newborn scoring system*, was published by Apgar and her colleague Stanley James 10 years later [3]. This paper summarised the experience of 8 years between 1952 and 1960 with newborn scoring in 27 715 live births. It confirmed the correlation of a poor score with neonatal mortality as well as the acid-base status of the newborn. They felt the main benefit of the scoring system was in the selection of infants for resuscitation: "The method has been found to be a valuable guide both in teaching and clinical practice in deciding which infants to resuscitate. By its use, delivery room personnel learn to observe several physical signs at once, evaluating them rapidly, and act accordingly." They also hoped that "the newborn scoring

system of infants should afford a basis of comparison for future mental and musculo-skeletal development". Subsequent work has shown that the correlation between the Apgar score and neonatal acidosis is much less precise than anticipated [4]. The hoped for correlation with future neurological development has also not been fulfilled. Even a low (0–3) Apgar score at 5 min is poorly predictive of future neurological outcome. While it does correlate with an increased risk of cerebral palsy in term infants, this increase is only from 0.3 to 1% [5–7].

Dr Virginia Apgar was born in Westfield, New Jersey on 7 June, 1909. Twenty years later, she graduated BA from Mount Holyoke College in Massachusetts. Four years later she completed her MD from Columbia University College of Physicians and Surgeons in New York. The first 4 years of her medical career were spent as a surgical intern and resident at the Presbyterian Hospital in New York. She then switched to anaesthesia and served her residency at the Presbyterian Hospital, in the Wisconsin General Hospital in Madison, and at the Bellevue Hospital in New York. In 1939, she was the second woman to take the Diploma of the American Board of Anesthesiology. She was appointed to the Columbia-Presbyterian Medical Center and, in 1949, was the first woman to receive a full professorship at Columbia Univeristy. During her 21 years as an anaesthetist, she was said to have given 20 000 anaesthetics, and have provided analgesia for a similar number of women during delivery [8]. It was at the Sloane Women's Hospital that she developed and applied the Apgar Score.

In 1959, on her 50th birthday, she received the degree of Master of Public Health from Johns Hopkins University. At this point, she joined the staff at the National Foundation-March of Dimes where she became Head of the Division of Congenital Malformations. By 1967, she was appointed Director of the Basic Research Department within the Foundation and the following year became Vice-President for Medical Affairs. At the same time, she held an appointment as Clinical Professor of Pediatrics in Teratology at Cornell University Medical College. Her stature and energetic speaking schedule ensured that recognition and funding for research in birth defects increased considerably during her tenure at the Foundation.

The tributes paid to Virginia Apgar during her life and after her death provide a picture of a single, very energetic woman with a broad range of interests and talents. She was apparently a fast talker, fast walker and fast driver — claiming that her car tyres never wore out as they rarely touched the ground. She started flying lessons when she was 59 years old. Apgar was a considerable musician and played viola and cello in a string quartet in her home town of Teaneck, New Jersey and, occasionally, with the Teaneck Symphony. She was one of the founders of the Amateur Chamber Music Players and the Catgut Acoustical Society. Under the influence and tutelage of a former patient, Apgar became a skilled instrument maker. This began when the patient was convalescing in hospital and noticed that a shelf in the public phone booth was made of "a fine, well-seasoned piece of curly maple", which apparently had a good resonance to the drumming fingers. She felt it would make an ideal back of a viola and asked Apgar if she could arrange to have the shelf removed and replaced with another. In keeping with the standard mentality of hospital administration they refused. Thus, late one night Apgar and the patient, suitably equipped with carpentry tools, liberated the shelf and replaced it with a piece of identically stained plywood. It was with this piece of wood that Apgar crafted her first viola under the guidance of her former patient. Over the years, she made three other string instruments — the last of which was finished by her tutor just after Apgar's death. Ultimately, the instruments — a cello, violin, viola, and mezzo violin — were purchased by a group of paediatricians and donated to Columbia University College of Physicians and Surgeons [1].

In 1994, a twenty-cent stamp with Virginia Apgar's portrait was issued in the US Postal Service's Great Americans Series. Ironically, Apgar herself had a considerable stamp collection and was a member of the American Philatelic Society. That same year, at the American Academy of Pediatrics Annual Clinical Meeting in Dallas, Texas, a quartet of paediatrician musicians played some of Apgar's favourite chamber music on the instruments she had crafted.

Virginia Apgar's newborn score is used almost universally. She claimed that her main reason for developing this method of early appraisal of the neonate was to redirect some of the attention from the mother to the newborn infant at a very critical stage when, if required, resuscitation efforts would yield great benefit. As she later said, "I wanted to find a way to get doctors to pay attention to the baby" [1]. As her scoring system became widely used the wording and sequence of the five cardinal signs were altered to provide the acronym APGAR: Appearance, Pulse, Grimace, Activity and Respiration [9].

Virginia Apgar died in her sleep on 7 August, 1974. The memorial service held in her local church was attended by a mix of prominent medical and local people, including the local traffic policeman with whom she had so many encounters during her fast driving days.

# References

[1] Skolnick AA. Apgar quartet plays perinatologist's instruments. JAMA 1996;276:1939–40.
[2] Apgar V. A proposal for a new method of evaluation of newborn infant. Curr Res Anesth Analg 1953;32:260–7.
[3] Apgar V, James LS. Further observations of the newborn scoring system. Am J Dis Child 1962;104:419–28.
[4] Sykes GS, Johnson J, Ashworth F, Molloy PM, Gu W, Stirrat GM. Do Apgar scores indicate asphyxia? Lancet 1982;1:494–6.
[5] Nelson KB, Ellenberg JH. Apgar scores as predictors of chronic neurologic disability. Pediatrics 1981;68:36–44.
[6] Stanley FJ. Cerebral palsy trends: implications for perinatal care. Acta Obstet Gynecol Scand 1994;73:5–9.
[7] American College of Obstetricians and Gynecologists. Committee Opinion: Use and abuse of the Apgar score. Washington, DC: ACOG, 1996.
[8] Little DM. Classical file. Surv Anesthesiol 1975;19:399–401.
[9] Butterfield LJ, Covey MJ. Practical epigram of the Apgar score [letter]. JAMA 1962;181:353.

# James O. Elam

## Peter Safar

James Otis Elam MD, was a pioneering anesthesiologist during the adolescence of this specialty in the 1950s [1–3]. He was a clinician and respiratory physiologist who made important original measurements on humans. Many colleagues remember him as an imaginative inventor and developer of devices that have helped those in anaesthesia. Health professionals and lay persons who are interested in first aid should remember Elam primarily for the fact that he was the first person to prove that exhaled air can be an adequate resuscitative gas [4].

I have a personal reason to thank him for having motivated me, through a chance encounter, not only to teach and practice, but also to research resuscitation, which became my lifelong pursuit [3,5]. I will remember him as a catalyst for research and development in resuscitation in the latter half of the 20th century, who influenced several colleagues. This laudatio of Elam as a 'resuscitation great' has input from Mark Lema, MD, Ph.D., present professor and chairman of Anesthesiology, University at Buffalo [2] and from Jim's widow, Marjorie Elam, CRNA.

Jim Elam was born on May 31, 1918 in Austin, TX. Sands and Bacon [1] remind us that he was born prematurely and needed external stimuli to start breathing. He had a creative and dynamic professional life and a family life that included five children with his first wife Elinor. In the 1990s, he suffered from a prolonged illness and died on July 10, 1995, in Valparaiso, Indiana, cared for by his wife Marjorie.

Elam's professional career took him from a bachelor of arts degree at the University of Texas in 1942, to an MD at the Johns Hopkins University School of Medicine in Baltimore in 1945, and via a rotating internship at the US Navy Hospital in Washington (Bethesda, MD) in 1945/1946, physiology training at the University of Minnesota in 1946/1947, internship and fellowship in surgery at Barnes Hospital of Washington University in St. Louis, Missouri, in 1947–1949, to an anesthesiology residency at the Massachusetts General Hospital in Boston and the University of Iowa in 1949–1951. In 1951–1953, he served as a research assistant professor at the Barnes Hospital. From there he went to Buffalo, NY, where he became chief anesthesiologist ('Chief Cancer Research Clinician') of the Roswell Park Memorial Institute, now called Roswell Park Cancer Institute (and hospital), from 1953 to 1964 [2]. During his 11 years at Roswell Park, he rose to the rank of major in the US Army while finishing his Army obligations in 1954–1956 at the Army Chemical Corps Medical Laboratories (Research and Engineering Command) at Edgewood, MD (near Baltimore). His earlier military obligation had been interrupted by his residency training. The combination of US Army-funded research from 1951 to 1970 ($\approx$ \$30,000 per year, present value over ten times this amount) and the opportunity to study anaesthetized patients at Roswell Park, created the environment for his contributions to anesthesiology and resuscitation in general, and to exhaled-air ventilation in particular. That research took place before the advent of institutional review boards, which now have to give approval for patient research. Before the 1970s, Elam and I and other resuscitation researchers studied patients and human volunteers by assuming personal responsibility and seeking approval only from our local peers.

The decade in Buffalo came to an end when Elam became increasingly disappointed that the lack of medical students and anaesthesia residents at the Cancer Institute would prevent his innovations being disseminated and continued. Therefore, in 1964, he left Buffalo to become professor and chairman of the Department of Anesthesiology at the University of Missouri at the

Kansas City General Hospital. He again experienced disappointments and, in 1966, went on to become a professor of anesthesiology at the University of Chicago, working mainly in obstetric anaesthesia, from 1966 until his retirement in the mid-1980s. Retirement gave him the freedom to innovate and further develop his devices privately. The frequent change in locations reflects the restlessness of a creative individual.

## 1. Respiratory physiology and anesthesiology

Before his anesthesiology residency, while in Minnesota under the influence of physiologist Maurice Visscher, he used one of the first oximeters, an ear oximeter [6]. Designed by Glen Millikan, this device was then used by the US Air Force. He also used the Liston-Becker (Model 16) infrared $CO_2$ analyzer for research [7,8]. Elam was probably the first to use it in anaesthesia and resuscitation research. Excited by research in general, Elam continued some studies part-time during his residency in anesthesiology. Present-day anesthesiology board requirements preclude such a mixed experience of patient care, clinical research and laboratory research, although for workaholic, pioneering, young anesthesiology trainees like Elam, that experience was not uncommon in the 1940s–1960s. Moreover, it was not unusual at that time to seek out colleagues of other specialties who had something new to offer.

After his residency, when at Barnes Hospital, he was committed, under US Army funding, to study humans. The chairman of Surgery (anesthesiology was a division of the Department of Surgery) first accepted human studies, but later demanded that they be replaced by work on animals. Since this would be unrealistic and would have jeopardized his Army contract, Elam and collaborators Elwyn Brown, John Elder and Raymond Ten Pas, went to Roswell Park [2]. There, anesthesiology received departmental status. Elam's team established a school for nurse anesthetists, which enabled him to continue focusing on his experiments in respiratory physiology. Physicians directed all of the anaesthesias administered by the nurses. His group then explored, for the Army, new valves designs, a flashlight laryngoscope and, most important, exhaled-air ventilation devices for nerve-gas-poisoned casualties (see later). They also acquired some patents. During his Army duty at Edgewood, he re-visited Roswell Park every week or two to study the data his associates had produced there. An effective synergy developed between Elam, who 'dreamed and schemed' and Brown, the practical engineer [2].

Elam himself was ahead of others in drawing attention to the elimination and monitoring of carbon dioxide [9]. Using the infrared $CO_2$ analyzer, he described the 'alveolar plateau'. Soon after his anesthesiology

training, based on closed-circle anaesthesia systems introduced by Sword, Waters, Adriani and others, Elam questioned the efficacy of the $CO_2$ absorbers in use at the time. He designed a better system for $CO_2$ absorption in anaesthesia circuits [10–17]. Elam and Brown greatly improved the $CO_2$ absorber by making it larger, packing the granules better, using baffles, doubling the canisters and determining that the absorbers' interstitial space should at least equal tidal volume [16]. His successors at Roswell Park wrote [2]: "Every anaesthesia machine over the last 30 years has used a carbon dioxide absorbence system essentially designed by these two physicians."

Elam and his collaborators also constructed a human respiration simulator, for various long-term ventilation experiments. That lung model was further developed into the Roswell Park ventilator, a bellows-in-box ventilator, powered by intermittent compression of the bellows by gas pressure in the box. This machine became the Air Shields Venti-meter Ventilator, which was in use throughout the 1950s, 1960s and 1970s [18]. They first used a windshield-wiper type power source obtained from the TRICO plant adjacent to the Cancer Institute. The ventilator could function by pressure or volume-cycling, with intermittent positive or positive–negative pressure patterns. The novel idea was that this bellows-in-box device was also useful for spontaneous breathing. The anesthetist, when squeezing the bag connected to the box, could monitor and control tidal volumes by watching excursions of the bellows connected to the anaesthesia circuit.

## 2. Exhaled-air ventilation

Before Elam became an anesthesiologist, his interest in respiratory resuscitation was aroused by having been given responsibility for the care of paralyzed polio patients in 1946 in Minneapolis [4]. While assigned to the polio floor, when he temporarily ran out of tank respirators (the Iron Lung), Elam instinctively performed mouth-to-mouth or mouth-to-nose ventilation, sometimes for hours, he said. During his residency in Iowa City, under the direction of Stuart Cullen, when moving patients from induction areas to operating rooms, he again instinctively used mouth-to-tracheal tube ventilation, as I and other anesthesiologists had done quite routinely.

Around 1952, when Elam was assistant professor of anesthesiology at Barnes Hospital, he found in the literature descriptions of over 100 manual (push–pull) methods of artificial respiration, but only brief mention of the mouth-to-mouth method for use in the newborn. He noted that no one had investigated the physiology of exhaled-air ventilation [4]. He and Brown embarked on studies of patients experiencing residual muscle paralysis in the post-anaesthesia recovery room, under renewed succinylcholine paralysis. Elam demonstrated that mouth-to-mask or mouth-to-tracheal tube ventilation could maintain normal arterial blood-gas values, as recorded by the $CO_2$ analyzer and tedious blood-gas analyses by the VanSlyke system. These first data on exhaled-air ventilation were published as a landmark paper in the 'New England Journal of Medicine' soon after his arrival in Buffalo [19] (Fig. 1).

Elam documented that it requires "doubling the tidal volumes, because you are breathing for two". After Elam and I had met (in 1956), he published these blood-gas data in greater detail, in the 'JAMA' of 1958 [20], simultaneously with my data on airway control and the controlled comparison of direct mouth-to-mouth with manual methods [21] and the data by Gordon on mouth-to-mouth versus manual methods in children [22].

Between 1953 and 1956, Elam's breakthrough data [19] seemed to have been dormant, with no one in anesthesiology or first-aid circles paying much attention to them. Gordon [23] had earlier found in curarized adult human volunteers, that the prone back-pressure

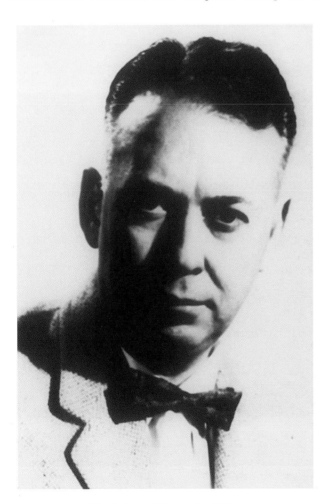

Fig. 1. James Elam in the 1960s.

arm-lift (Holger–Nielsen) method moved more air than the then widely taught prone back-pressure-only method (Schafer)—both techniques were studied *with* a tracheal tube. The views of my mentors of 1950, Comroe and Dripps [24] and similar data obtained using tracheal tubes by Nims et al. [25] in Dripps' department, also questioned the efficacy of the Schafer method. Only the US Army took Elam's work seriously. When Elam worked for the Army Chemical Corps, he found the chest- or back-pressure methods too weak to ventilate nerve-gas-poisoned animals. These animals developed bronchoconstriction, massive bronchial secretions, bradycardia and paralysis. At Edgewood, Elam worked side-by-side with John Clements, a brilliant civilian researcher at the Army Chemical Center (who pioneered pulmonary surfactant). Elam and Clements developed prototypes of valved mask-to-mask devices for intended resuscitation of nerve-gas-poisoned humans [27–29]. A gas filter could be put on the air intake for the rescuer. Clements recently recalled: "Adam Muir and I [26] found that the Holger–Nielsen method did not move any air in rhesus monkeys (with nerve-gas poisoning), and I designed a flow-valved, non-rebreathing mask-to-mask device that was effective enough to overcome severe bronchoconstriction and led to long-term survival [26]."

The research and development of modern emergency resuscitation exploded after Elam and I met, by coincidence, in 1956. I described this event roughly as follows [3,5]: The spark that started my lifelong commitment to resuscitation research, including interest in pre-hospital first aid, was a chance contact with James Elam. It happened at the American Society of Anesthesiologists (ASA) meeting in October 1956 in Kansas City. For the previous 100 years, various chest-pressure arm-lift methods had been used; since the early 1950s, the back-pressure arm-lift method was favored, because of data obtained by Archer Gordon (then in Chicago) who used *intubated* curarized human volunteers [23]. Until that ASA meeting of 1956, I had not been aware of the 1954 publication by Elam [19] that documented normal blood-gas values in apnoeic patients during IPPV with mouth-to-mask or mouth-to-tracheal tube ventilation. On October 12, 1956, Eva (Safar) and I had supper with James Elam. This was the first time I talked with him. Elam asked to hitch a ride back to Baltimore with us. During that ride on October 13 and 14, 1956 from Kansas City via Chicago to Baltimore, I was inspired by his first published proof that exhaled air is an adequate resuscitative gas [19], and by his imaginative personality. Elam revealed to me that his results were not widely known. He gave me the impression during that trip that neither he nor others had challenged the current doctrine, and that first-aid agencies continued to adhere to teaching the back-pressure arm-lift method.

Elam recalled later [4] that he did try to persuade Army physiologist Bruce Dill (research director at Edgewood), Army generals, and the Red Cross "to recognize the method of Elisha. I even told them that Elam was a biblical name and that I (Elam) might be a prophet disguised as a major." I do not know whether this happened before or after we met. Dill, who recognized that the Schafer method would be ineffective for nerve-gas casualties, created the US Army contract for Elam on artificial respiration. Dill promoted the first Army conferences of investigators for artificial respiration and originated the first National Academy of Sciences (NAS) conferences on this subject. Dill, Elam and Dripps probably recommended funding of my first research proposal to the Army in 1956.

I further recalled [3] that when Elam, in October 1956, told me about his results [19], it occurred to me that anesthesiologists' know-how in handling upper-airway obstruction had not penetrated beyond the operating room. On that fateful car trip, I proposed that we conduct the following needed studies and documentations: (1) A study of upper-airway soft-tissue obstruction on curarized adults. (Elam had used a mask, a pharyngeal tube and a tracheal tube in his landmark study [19], but had not explored backward tilt of the head, which I considered crucial.) (2) A controlled study in which ventilation volumes and oxygenation produced by the 'push–pull methods' would be compared with those produced by direct mouth-to-mouth inflations, using both methods on the same apnoeic adult curarized volunteers and on patients, *without* the use of a tracheal tube, pharyngeal tube, or mask, with each subject serving as his own control and mouth-to-mouth ventilation performed by lay persons. Elam agreed that this should be done. I suggested that we do it together at the Baltimore City Hospital where I was chief anesthesiologist. He attended the first two or three experiments in December 1956 [30,31] and then moved to Buffalo and continued on his own. Elam and I maintained some communication thereafter until his death. When Elam left the Army to return to Roswell Park, Brown took his research position in the Army. I thank Jim also for having brought me in touch with John Clements, who gave valuable advice for our human volunteer experiments [31]; John the pianist and his wife Margot, a superb professional singer, made classical music with the Safars and other medical amateur musicians in Baltimore.

Our preliminary [30] and definitive data [31] from the human volunteer experiments in 1957 and my first documentation of the failure of manual methods of artificial ventilation [32]; the mechanisms of upper-airway soft-tissue obstruction in coma and need for backward tilt of the head, jaw thrust, and open mouth [21,33–35]; and the efficacy and techniques of exhaled-air ventilation without adjuncts [20–22], were received as a bombshell in the US and Europe.

On March 8, 1957, the NAS held a meeting in Washington DC, chaired by Julius Comroe, concerning artificial respiration for children. Elam and I presented the data of our first experiments on adult volunteers. Mouth-to-mouth ventilation was recommended for children but not yet for adults. At that meeting, Archer Gordon learned about our preliminary results on adults [30] and gathered similar data on anaesthetized children and adults [22]. On May 10, 1957, Dill gathered Army researchers in Denver; Elam's and my data were hot topics. On November 3, 1958, after our definitive data had been published [20–22], the NAS held its second meeting on artificial respiration, chaired by visionary surgeon Sam Seeley. Backward tilt of the head with direct mouth-to-mouth ventilation was decided upon as the preferred method of artificial respiration. The recommendation applied to adults as well as children. Within 1 year, medical associations, the Armed Forces and the American and International Red Cross organizations changed from the manual methods to the exhaled-air methods of artificial ventilation.

In 1960, Elam was honored by the US Army Chemical Center with an Award of Achievement and by the New York Medical Society with its highest honor, the Albion O. Bernstein Award of Distinction for Contributions to Medicine. He was honored by the American Heart Association as one of the pioneers of CPR.

As was to be expected, there were controversies. Elam had recommended mouth-to-mask ventilation and had produced a green plastic pocket mask. To my knowledge, this never came to market. I introduced blowing through an S-shaped Guedel-type oro-pharyngeal tube. We agreed that use of devices should be restricted to health care professionals. After Elam had returned from Baltimore to Buffalo, he enticed Henning Ruben of Denmark into collaborating with him. Ruben had earlier introduced the self-refilling bag-valve-mask unit, a breakthrough in resuscitation devices [36]. Gordon and I recommended to try blowing into the mouth first [21,22] because of frequent nasal obstruction [33–35], while Elam and Ruben recommended to blow into the nose first [37]. 'Mouth first and nose second' became the national [38] and international guidelines [39]. Elam popularized exhaled-air ventilation in the state of New York and beyond by writing manuals and making teaching films. After the first volunteer experiments at Baltimore City Hospital, Elam produced a film that included a medical student paralyzed with succinylcholine on whom he demonstrated the various ventilation methods, accompanied by ear oximetry. Elam was also sought after in the early years as a lecturer because of his message and impressive speaking style.

Airway control became step A of CPR. Ruben and Elam [40–42] confirmed my head-tilt data [21,33–35]. Elam tried to minimize gastric insufflation and regurgitation by blowing into the narrower nasal passage, which reduced pharyngeal pressure [37]. I found gastric distension to be self-limiting [21] and documented expiratory nasal obstruction as a greater obstacle [33–35]. Exhaled-air ventilation [20–22] became step B of CPR. I combined steps A and B with step C, external cardiac massage, re-discovered by Kouwenhoven et al. [43], into basic life support (BLS) [44,45] and added advanced and prolonged life support for the cardiopulmonary-cerebral resuscitation (CPCR) system [39,45]. Elam continued to promote exhaled-air ventilation together with me [46,47] and reported on actual cases of successful resuscitation [48]. He became co-initiator (with Gordon, Jude and Safar) of the first American Heart Association CPR-Emergency Cardiac Care Committee [49]. Elam joined me in advising Laerdal in the creation of the Resusci-Anne manikin [50]. He also advised the Ambu Company of Denmark concerning resuscitation devices. Elam served on the first American Society of Anesthesiologists acute medicine committee that I had initiated [51]. Later, Elam co-initiated, with Jude and me, the first Wolf Creek Conference of CPR Researchers [52]. At that conference in 1975, Elam contributed imaginative ideas on bag-valve-mask $O_2$ ventilation [53], intrapulmonary administration of CPR drugs [54], the esophageal–pharyngeal airway [55], esophageal electrocardiography [56] and esophageal defibrillation [56].

## 3. Chicago and semi-retirement

With rescue breathing as the climax of his professional career, one can consider Jim Elam's years at the University of Chicago (from 1966 to 1980), a professorship at the University of Texas Southwestern Medical School in Dallas (in 1981–1983) and his semi-retirement in Valparaiso, Indiana (from the mid-1980s to the 1990s) as a continuum (Fig. 2).

Starting in the 1970s, he had turned his attention to new airway-control devices. His conception, design and promotion of devices spanned many years. Most of the recently invented devices have so far not become commercially available. One reason was the bureaucratic demands and delays posed by institutional review boards against human trials, which since the 1980s have been essential to bring devices to fruition. Another reason for some of his inventions having remained dormant may have been a lack of publications.

Since the 1960s he had tried the use of soft rubber nasopharyngeal tubes in both nasal passages as an alternative to tracheal intubation [57,58]. Reportedly, more than 1000 patients at the Lying-In Hospital in Chicago received this airway in operating rooms between 1966 and 1970. Connecting one nasopharyngeal tube directly to an anaesthesia or resuscitation system

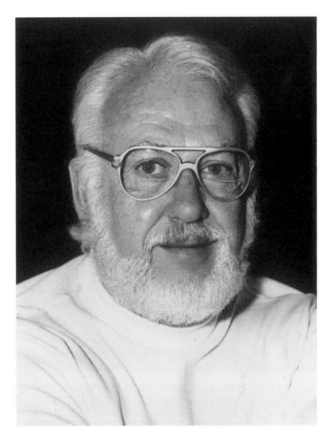

Fig. 2. James Elam in the 1980s.

was not new. Reducing airway resistance by doubling the tube was new. The nasopharyngeal tube connected directly to the anaesthesia circuit did not become a widely accepted method for prolonged general anesthesias, since anesthesiologists and nurse anesthetists felt that patients were safer with a cuffed endotracheal tube. When in Chicago, Elam also made contributions to anaesthesia method [59–61].

He promoted sound principles when he sought new approaches and devices: (1) As alternative to tracheal intubation, he developed a pharyngeal airway with a pharynx-occluding balloon [62], which actually became a forerunner for the laryngeal mask airway (LMA) designed and published by Brain. (2) He designed a double-barreled plastic tube to be inserted into the mouth without a laryngoscope, with one barrel as a conduit for a tracheal tube and the other for a nasogastric tube. The idea was that people without medical knowledge could safely intubate blindly and decompress the stomach at the same time. This was a forerunner of the 'Combitube'. (3) He wanted to develop a non-distensible manual bellows ventilator for use in nerve-gas-poisoned stiff lungs, as he initiated it in the 1950s with the Army. (4) His further work with the Air-Shields ventilator focused on an assist/control mechanism that would allow patients to regulate their own spontaneous breathing volume and rate [63].

Elam's US patents and developments between 1952 and 1983 included $CO_2$ absorbers, ventilators, valves, masks, airways, sensors, a tracheal tube double-cuff, and a cuff monitor. Between 1947 and 1984, he published about 120 works, including peer-reviewed papers, reports, books and abstracts.

During Elam's retirement, we honored him as visiting professor at the opening of the International Resuscitation Research Center facility at the University of Pittsburgh in 1980. After that, we met occasionally at resuscitation conferences sponsored by the American Heart Association. In January 1994, I invited Jim to the May 1994 International Conference of Resuscitation Researchers in Pittsburgh. Elam had to decline because of health reasons: "too many diagnoses including cardiac myopathy and diabetes ... When you asked me why I was still working on gadgets, the answer is that in retirement, with no access to patients, developing better equipment was about all I could do. For example, regurgitation during resuscitation ... we should be concerned about it ... if I could attend your symposium, I would report on my recent project which utilizes (combines) a conventional endotracheal tube, an Ewald (esophago-gastric) tube, and the method of rapidly establishing (inserting) both before aspiration occurs. I have arranged for clinical testing of the method by others. I shall send you the results when the project is done." Sadly there was no follow-up because, according to his wife Marjorie, he became increasingly ill.

At Roswell Park, he had a godfather for his research and development in surgeon and Institute Director George Moore [2]. Thereafter, he lacked such support. In the early 1990s, feeling that time was running out, Jim re-visited Roswell Park in attempts to obtain patients for trials of his novel devices. I believe that airway and ventilation methods and devices would have been further improved had Elam succeeded during the 1970s and 1980s in translating his ideas into prototypes, testing in patients, publishing results and bringing some of the devices to the open market. Helping inventors like Elam should be among the important roles of academic medical centers. Industry and academia may have (incorrectly) perceived him more as a gadgeteer than as a visionary, which I believe he was.

Jim's wife, Marjorie Elam of Valparaiso, Indiana, wrote to me after his death: "Jim died around 10:00 pm on July 10 (1995). He had suffered what seemed to be a small stroke, in addition to kidney failure, chest pain, and diabetes. ... He died very peacefully. Life had become a struggle. His son Michael lives in Los Angeles, son Peter in Minnesota, son David in San Francisco, daughter Joann in Chicago, and daughter Susan in Boston."

## 4. Conclusion

James Elam started as a patient-focused respiratory physiologist and became a visionary inventor of devices that improved the safety of general anaesthesia and contributed to more effective resuscitation methods. He has been called charismatic, determined, innovative and ingenious [2]. His most important contribution was to the noble endeavour of emergency respiratory resuscitation: the documentation that exhaled air can be adequate for artificial ventilation. This sparked the development by others of modern external CPR and beyond. Elam's influence on me and on others, and our subsequent influences on resuscitation researchers who followed, with cross-fertilization between them, which will continue for decades to come, reminds us that each one of us represents one or more links in the chains of human evolution. Elam was a strong link from which modern CPR, cerebral resuscitation (CPCR), trauma resuscitation, emergency medical services and critical care medicine developed during the latter half of the 20th century.

Jim Elam helped put the Roswell Cancer Institute in Buffalo on the map [2]. His legacy has been summarized in several documents on the history of modern resuscitation. I would like to conclude this laudatio by quoting Sands and Bacon [1]: "James Elam, from his early work on $CO_2$ homeostasis, leading to the first human capnograhic tracing, leading to the modifications of the soda lime canister, to his recent work on an airway that laymen can use to intubate victims of cardiac arrest outside the hospital, Elam has always strived to improve the quality of life of his fellow humans. Battling through hardships of his own ... including debilitating osteoarthritis necessitating multiple hip replacements and ultimately confinement to a wheelchair, Elam persevered."

## References

[1] Sands RP, Bacon DR. An inventive mind. The career of James O. Elam, M.D. (1918–1995). Anesthesiology 1998;88:1107–12.

[2] Peppriell JE, Bacon DR, Lema MJ, Ament R, Yearley CK. The development of academic anesthesiology at the Roswell Park Memorial Institute: James O. Elam, MD, and Elwyn S. Brown, MD. Anesth Analg 1991;72:538–45.

[3] Safar P. From Vienna to Pittsburgh for anesthesiology and acute medicine. Careers in Anesthesiology. Autobiographical Memoirs. Vol. V, American Society of Anesthesiologists, Wood Library-Museum, 2000. (Wood Library Museum, 515 Busse Highway, Park Ridge, IL 60068).

[4] Elam JO. Rediscovery of expired air methods for emergency ventilation. In: Safar P, Elam JO, editors. Advances in Cardiopulmonary Resuscitation. New York: Springer-Verlag, 1977:263–5 Chapter 39.

[5] Safar P. From back-pressure arm-lift to mouth-to-mouth, control of airway and beyond. In: Safar P, Elam JO, editors. Advances in Cardiopulmonary Resuscitation. New York: Springer-Verlag, 1977:266–75 Chapter 40.

[6] Sleator W Jr, Elam JO, Elam WN Jr, White HL. Oximetric determinations of cardiac output responses to light exercise. J Appl Physiol 1951;3:649–64.

[7] Luft K. Methode der Registrieren gas Analyse mit Hilfe der Absorption ultraroten Strahlen ohne spectrale Zerlegung. Z Tech Phys 1943;244:97.

[8] White JU, Liston MD. Performance of double beam recording infrared spectrophotometer. J Soc Am 1950;40:93–101.

[9] Brown EB, Miller F. Ventricular fibrillation following a rapid fall in alveolar carbon dioxide concentration. Am J Phys 1952;169:56–60.

[10] Elam JO, Brown ES, Ten Pas RH. Carbon dioxide homeostasis during anaesthesia. I. Instrumentation. Anesthesiology 1955;16:876–85.

[11] Elam JO, Brown ES. Carbon dioxide homeostasis during anaesthesia. II. Total sampling for determination of dead space, alveolar ventilation, and carbon dioxide output. Anesthesiology 1955;16:886–902.

[12] Elam JO, Brown ES. Carbon dioxide homeostasis during anaesthesia. III. Ventilation and carbon dioxide elimination. Anesthesiology 1956;17:116–27.

[13] Elam JO, Brown ES. Carbon dioxide homeostasis during anaesthesia. IV. An evaluation of the partial rebreathing system. Anesthesiology 1956;17:128–34.

[14] Elam JO. Channeling and over packing in carbon dioxide absorbers. Anesthesiology 1958;19:403–4.

[15] Elam JO. The design of circle absorbers. Anesthesiology 1958;19:111–2.

[16] Brown ES. Factors affecting the performance of absorbents. Anesthesiology 1959;20:198–203.

[17] Brown ES, Senniff AM, Elam JO. Carbon dioxide elimination in semiclosed systems. Anesthesiology 1964;25:31–6.

[18] Elam JO, Brown ES, Janney CS. A fixed volume respirator for controlled ventilation during anaesthesia. Anesthesiology 1956;17:504–10.

[19] Elam JO, Brown ES, Elder JD Jr. Artificial respiration by mouth-to-mask method. A study of the respiratory gas exchange of paralyzed patients ventilated by operator's exhaled air. New Engl J Med 1954;250:749–54.

[20] Elam JO, Greene DG, Brown ES, Clements JA. Oxygen and carbon dioxide exchange and energy costs of expired air resuscitation. J Am Med Assoc 1958;167:328–34.

[21] Safar P. Ventilatory efficacy of mouth-to-mouth artificial respiration. Airway obstruction during manual and mouth-to-mouth artificial respiration. J Am Med Assoc 1958;167:335–41.

[22] Gordon AS, Frye CW, Gittelson L, Sadove MS, Beattie EJ. Mouth-to-mouth versus manual artificial respiration for children and adults. J Am Med Assoc 1958;167:320–8.

[23] Gordon AS, Sadove MS, Raymon F, Ivy AC. Critical survey of manual artificial respiration for children and adults. J Am Med Assoc 1951;147:1444–53.

[24] Comroe JH Jr, Dripps RB. Artificial respiration. J Am Med Assoc 1946;130:381–3.

[25] Nims RG, Conner EH, Botelho SY, Comroe JH Jr. Comparison of methods for performing manual artificial respiration on apneic patients. J Appl Physiol 1951;4:486–95.

[26] Muir A, Clements JA. Studies in therapy of G-poisoning. Porton Technical Paper No. 273, 1953.

[27] Clements JA, Elam JO, Johnson RP, Beaton RE. Respiratory effects of an anticholinesterase agent, DFP. Chemical Corps Medical Laboratories Special Report, 1954.

[28] Elam JO, Clements JA, Brown ES, Elton NW. Artificial respiration for the G-agent casualty. Armed Forces Med J 1956;7:797–810.

[29] Elam JO, Brown ES, Clements JA, Greene DG, Janney CD. Mask-to-mask studies in paralyzed human subjects. Chemical Warfare Laboratories Technical Report No. 2082, 1956, p. 43.

[30] Safar P, Elam J. Manual versus mouth-to-mouth methods of artificial respiration. Anesthesiology 1958;19:111–2.

[31] Safar P, Escarraga LA, Elam JO. A comparison of the mouth-to-mouth and mouth-to-airway methods of artificial respiration with the chest-pressure arm-lift methods. New Engl J Med 1958;258:671–7.

[32] Safar P. Failure of manual respiration. J Appl Physiol 1959;14:84–8.

[33] Safar P, Aguto-Escarraga L, Chang F. Upper airway obstruction in the unconscious patient. J Appl Physiol 1959;14:760–4.

[34] Morikawa S, Safar P, DeCarlo J. Influence of head–jaw position upon upper airway patency. Anesthesiology 1961;22:265–70.

[35] Safar P, Redding J. The 'tight jaw' in resuscitation. Anesthesiology 1959;20:701–2.

[36] Ruben H. Combination resuscitator and aspirator. Anesthesiology 1958;19:408–9.

[37] Elam JO, Ruben AM, Greene DG, Bittner TJ. Mouth-to-nose resuscitation during convulsive seizures. J Am Med Assoc 1961;176:565–9.

[38] American Heart Association (AHA) and National Academy of Sciences-National Research Council (NAS-NRC). Standards for Cardiopulmonary Resuscitation (CPR) and Emergency Cardiac Care (ECC). J Am Med Assoc 1966;198:372–9 1974;277:S833–868. 1980;244:S453–478. 1986;255:S2841.

[39] Safar P, Bircher NG. Cardiopulmonary-cerebral resuscitation. In: Laerdal A, Stavanger A, editors. An Introduction to Resuscitation Medicine. World Federation of Societies of Anaesthesiologists, 3rd ed. London: Saunders, 1988 1st ed. 1968; 2nd ed. 1981.

[40] Elam JO, Greene DG, Schneider MA, Ruben HM, Gordon AS, Husted RF, Benson DW, Clements JA, Ruben AM. Head-tilt method of oral resuscitation. J Am Med Assoc 1960;172:812–5.

[41] Greene DC, Elam JO, Dobkin AL, Studley CL. Cinefluorographic study of hyperextension of the neck and upper airway patency. J Am Med Assoc 1961;176:570–3.

[42] Ruben H, Elam JO, Ruben AM, Greene DG. Investigation of upper airway problems in resuscitation. Anesthesiology 1961;22:271–9.

[43] Kouwenhoven WB, Jude JR, Knickerbocker GG. Closed-chest cardiac massage. J Am Med Assoc 1960;173:1064–7.

[44] Safar P, Brown TC, Holtey WH, et al. Ventilation and circulation with closed chest cardiac massage in man. J Am Med Assoc 1961;176:574–6.

[45] Safar P. Community-wide cardiopulmonary resuscitation, J Iowa Med Soc, 1964;629–635.

[46] Safar P, Escarraga L, Elam JO, Greene D. Respiratory Resuscitation. Scientific exhibit produced by Army Institute of Pathology, AMA Convention, 1958.

[47] Safar P, Elam JO, Jude JR, Wilder RJ, Zoll PM. Resuscitative principles for sudden cardiopulmonary collapse. Dis Chest 1963;43:34–49.

[48] Elam JO, Greene DG. Mission accomplished: successful mouth-to-mouth resuscitation. Anesth Analg 1961;40:440–2 also pp. 578–580; 672–676.

[49] Cole WH, Birch LH, Elam JO, Gordon AS, Jude JR, Safar P, Scherlis L, Flynn RL, Vandam LD, Seeley SF. Ad hoc Committee on Cardiopulmonary Resuscitation: cardiopulmonary resuscitation. J Am Med Assoc 1966;198:372–9.

[50] Tjomsland N. From Stavanger with care. In: Laerdals First 50 years. Stavanger, Norway: Laerdal Medical, 1991.

[51] Smith A. American Society of Anesthesiologists Committee on Acute Medicine, Safar P (Chairman), Cheney FW Jr, Elam JO, Hamilton WK, Nagel L: Community-wide emergency medical services. J Am Med Assoc 1968;204:595–602.

[52] Safar P, Elam J, editors. Advances in Cardiopulmonary Resuscitation. Proceedings of the Wolf Creek Conference of October 1975. New York: Springer-Verlag, 1977.

[53] Elam JO. Bag-valve mask $O_2$ ventilation. Efficiency versus convenience; $O_2$ versus valve lock. In: Safar P, Elam JO, editors. Advances in Cardiopulmonary Resuscitation. New York: Springer-Verlag, 1977:65–71.

[54] Elam JO. The intrapulmonary route for CPR drugs. In: Safar P, Elam JO, editors. Advances in Cardiopulmonary Resuscitation. New York: Springer-Verlag, 1977:132–40.

[55] Elam JO, Lim-Tan P, Shfieha M, Robert M. Airway management with oesophageal pharyngeal airway. In: Safar P, Elam JO, editors. Advances in Cardiopulmonary Resuscitation. New York: Springer-Verlag, 1977:132–7.

[56] Elam JO, ViaReque E, Rattenborg CC. Oesophageal electrocardiography and low energy ventricular defibrillation. In: Safar P, Elam JO, editors. Advances in Cardiopulmonary Resuscitation. New York: Springer–Verlag, 1977:167–74 Chapter 26.

[57] Weisman H, Weis TW, Elam JO, Bethune RM, Bauer RO. Use of double nasopharyngeal airways in anaesthesia. Anesth Analg 1969;48:356–61.

[58] Weisman H, Bauer RO, Huddy RA, Elam JO. An improved binasopharyngeal airway system for anaesthesia. Anesth Analg 1972;51:11–3.

[59] Huffman JP, Elam JO. Prisms and fiber optics for laryngoscopy. Anesth Analg 1971;50:64–7.

[60] Titel JH, Lowe HJ, Elam JO, Grasholz JR. Quantitative closed-circuit halothane anaesthesia. A clinical study on pressurized temperature-compensated vaporizer. Anesth Analg 1968;47:560–9.

[61] Elam JO. Catheter subarachnoid block for labor and delivery: A differential segmental technique employing hyperbaric lidocaine. Anesth Analg 1970;49:1007–15.

[62] Elam JO, Sterling R. Airway management I. M-A-S: a mouth-mask-airway-sump system airway control. II. Elastomeric cuffs for long-dwelling endotracheal tubes. Crit Care Med 1981;9:425.

[63] Elam JO. A volumetric system for monitoring minimal respiration in man. Anesth Analg 1975;54:232–7.

# Rudolf Frey

## Wolfgang F. Dick

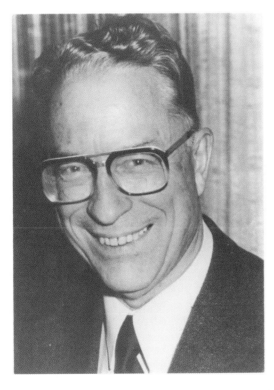

In 1972, Rudolf Frey, John Bonica, Francis Foldes, Torsten Gordt, Harold Griffith, Karl Hutschenreuther, Hans Kilian, Jean Lassner, Sir Robert Macintosh, Otto Mayrhofer, K.T. Ritzema van Eck and Helmut Schmidt edited and published the results of a scientific session titled 'Experienced History of Anaesthesiology' arranged in honour of the 80th birthday of Hans Kilian [2]. On page 16 of this publication, Rudolf Frey added his name to a scientific family tree showing himself as a direct line 'descendant' of Hans Kilian, Henry Beecher, Sir Robert Macintosh and Epstein, as well as of Kern, Lassner and Allgöwer, the "sons of a marriage of surgery and anaesthesiology".

In a personal letter of 1952 to Sir Robert Macintosh, Professor Dr. K.-H. Bauer, Chairman of the German Society of Surgery and Director of the Clinic of Surgery in Heidelberg, wrote, "I would be particularly delighted if you were kind enough to critically examine the advances in anaesthesia in Heidelberg..., we have many anaesthetists visit us, and the Chairman of my anaesthesia department, Dr. R. Frey, himself frequently visits foreign clinics and institutes. He spent, for instance, 6 months each at a Swiss institute and at the Mayo Clinic in the United States, where he participated in the daily work. He will soon become a Private Docent for anaesthesia and thus the first academic teacher of anaesthesia in Germany". In August 1952 Professor Bauer wrote to Sir Robert (translation), "I must reveal to you quite openly that the speciality of anaesthesia, which here in Germany is still so young, is passing through a crisis. You know yourself that I have worked with all my influence on its development in every respect, not only in the clinic under my direction, but also particularly before the various German surgical congresses. Already years ago I had the opportunity to discuss with you the very steeply rising percentage of severe postoperative atony of stomach and intestines. Furthermore, other complications are much more frequent than we think happen in your country...". Professor Bauer wrote to Sir Robert in December 1951: "As President of the next Surgical Congress at Munich, I have for the first time in the history of the Surgical Society arranged for a session on modern anaesthesia. While I am presiding over the whole congress, Professor Frey will preside over this section. As a chief surgeon he is particularly interested in anaesthesia".

This exchange of letters between K.-H. Bauer and Sir Robert Macintosh clearly emphasises the most important role played by Rudolf Frey in German anaesthesia at a time when he was still involved in the clinical work of the surgical department in Heidelberg.

It was in the late 1950s when the former administrative director of the Mainz University Hospital, became the father of an infant suffering from what later became known as a diaphragmatic hernia. At that time, treatment of this disease represented a complicated and rather dangerous procedure particularly because of the anaesthetic problems involved. The surgeon—Professor Brandt—obtained information on a hospital where these procedures were frequently performed and learned that an anaesthetist by the name of Docent Rudolf Frey, a staff member of the surgical department, worked as a specialist in this area at the Heidelberg University Hospital. Dr. Frey was invited to come to Mainz to examine the infant and to decide whether he was prepared to anaesthetise the infant for the operative procedure to be carried out by Professor Brandt. The surgical intervention was successful and from that time on the later Chief Administrator of the hospital, who was still working at the Ministry of Culture of Rhineland–Palatinat at that time, tried everything in his power to convince Administrators, the medical faculty and clinicians that the Mainz University Hospital urgently needed a department of anaesthesia, or at least an anaesthetist. After an apparently brief administrative process (the minister took an open post of the protestant faculty), Professor Rudolf Frey, who was still the Head of the Anaesthesia Division of the Surgical Clinic of the Heidelberg University Hospital, gave his first lectures in Mainz in 1959. In 1960 he was appointed Head of the Department of Anaesthesia at the Mainz University Hospital and was soon named extraordinary professor of anaesthesia, i.e. holder of the first professorship of its kind in Germany. The department became an independent institution in 1962, and the extraordinary professorship was changed into a full professorship in 1967. Rudolf Frey was already interested in emergency medicine when he was still at the Heidelberg University Hospital, an institution with a longstanding tradition in emergency medicine. As early as 1938, for example, the Chief Surgeon, Professor Martin Kirchner, stated that not the patient should go to the doctor, but the doctor should go to see a patient in a life-threatening situation. In 1958 K.-H. Bauer brought the first mobile hospital advance life support unit into operation. This was a large truck outfitted with operating room equipment. The concept of this mobile unit was developed by Martin Kirchner, and taken a step further, allowing surgical interventions to be performed immediately in the mobile operating theatre in trauma victims and other emergency patients. Thus a logical step in the development of anaesthesia in Mainz was the introduction in 1964 of a mobile life support unit by Rudolf Frey together with Fritz Ahnefeld, who later developed the 'chain of survival concept'. This mobile life support unit was staffed by an anaesthetist, an anaesthesia nurse and an emergency medical technician, who also served as the driver. This concept has undergone continuous development, and today the emergency section of the Department of Anaesthesia operates two mobile life support units, one of which is integrated into a rendezvous system, in addition to an emergency and intensive care helicopter.

While the mobile life support unit performed only one prehospital operation in 1964, the number continually increased to over 50 in 1965, 100 in 1966, 150 in 1967, and to more than 200 in 1968. Already at that time patients with ventricular fibrillation were defibrillated outside hospital with a manual defibrillator, making the Mainz mobile life support units as well as those used in Cologne and other German centres comparable to the mobile coronary care units described by Frank Pantridge in a paper referred to recently in this journal. In contrast to today, 30% of the patients were treated outside the hospital for intoxication, and acute myocardial or pulmonary insufficiency. Between 16 and 28% were surgical or neurosurgical cases, mostly victims of trauma, while the remaining cases had psychiatric, obstetric, paediatric and ENT diseases. Today only 10% of interventions are related to major trauma, whereas 90% deal with various complex conditions, such as acute myocardial infarction, cardiac arrest of various origins, TIA and stroke, drug intoxications, paediatric and obstetric cases, etc.

In the late 1960s an army helicopter was in operation at the emergency centre of the Department of Anaesthesiology in Mainz. In view of the fact that its cost effectiveness could not be demonstrated at that time, it was relocated and operated from a centrally located German army base.

Today the emergency physicians of the department serve two Mobile Life Support Units on 4074 missions and one helicopter on nearly 1000 missions in 2000, 2/3 of which were dedicated to emergency procedures and 1/3 to interhospital transport of ICU patients to major intensive care centres.

The man who initiated all this many years ago together with others—Rudolf Frey—was born on August 22nd 1917 in Heidelberg, where he qualified in medicine in 1943 and submitted his dissertation (Promotion) in the following year. After becoming a specialist in surgery in1949 and undergoing training in anaesthesia at various centres inside and outside Europe, he achieved specialist status in this field in 1952. He earned his PhD for a scientific project on mechanism of action of different muscle relaxants [7,8].

Frey was appointed professor of anaesthesia at the University of Heidelberg in 1956 and, as already mentioned, lecturer in anaesthesia at the University of Mainz in 1959. Only 1 year later he became Head of the Division of Anaesthesia and the first extraordinary professor of anaesthesiology in Germany. The Institute of Anaesthesiology gained official recognition in 1962 and Rudolf Frey was appointed its director. In 1967 he became full and ordinary professor of anaesthesiology in Mainz. Although for a long time the Department of Anaesthesiology of the University of Hamburg and the respective institution in Mainz both claimed to have been the first in Germany to appoint an ordinary and a full professor of anaesthesiology, it is now agreed that Rudolf Frey was the first extraordinary full professor of anaesthesiology while Professor Karl Horaz in Hamburg was the first and Rudolf Frey the second ordinary full professor of anaesthesiology.

Rudolf Frey was actively involved in the foundation of the German Society of Anaesthesiology in 1952, he was elected vice president of the WFSA in 1955. He served as co-editor of the journal, Der Anästhesist, the first book on anaesthesiology published in Germany, and the series 'Anaesthesiology and Reanimation', all of which were published by Springer, Heidelberg.

The work of Rudolf Frey has been honoured by nearly all societies and organisations involved in anaesthesiology, intensive care medicine, and, in particular, in emergency medicine. Treatment of intensive care patients by anaesthesiologists was initiated in 1961, and performed with the most modern intensive care methods available at that time. Intensive care measures focused especially on neurosurgical and surgical patients with tetanus, polytrauma and postoperative care being the major areas of research. Medical students underwent training in emergency measures already at that time, and this training was later extended to nurses and doctors from almost all medical disciplines.

From 1971 onwards the institution in Mainz was intensively involved in training courses in intensive care and anaesthesiology for nurses. The training programme developed in Mainz later became recognised as the official training programme nationwide.

Innumerable publications in national and international journals feature Rudolf Frey as the leading or senior author. From the very beginning his lectures on emergency medicine, pain treatment, etc. were orientated toward the future. For instance, when he gave his inaugural lecture in 1959 in Mainz [1], it was dedicated to the principles and future orientation of treatment in chronic pain patients. At that time only a few researchers, e.g. John Bonica, were doing work in this area [3]. A great number of Rudolf Frey's clinical and academic trainees were later appointed chairmen of university departments, large community and other hospitals, and not a few of them dedicated their life to practical and theoretical work in emergency medicine.

At a meeting in February 1972 in Mainz, Rudolf Frey asked Peter Safar if the foundation of the Club of Mainz on disaster medicine might be a reasonable idea. This conception was re-discussed in 1973, and in December 1976 Rudolf Frey invited ten internationally recognised specialists in the field of disaster medicine to a meeting in Geneva. After further deliberations Peter Safar and Rudolf Frey founded the Club of Mainz, today's World Association of Disaster and Emergency Medicine (WADEM) [5]. Frey initiated and chaired the first World Congress of the Club of Mainz, which was followed by other meetings in Pittsburgh, Rome, Brighton, etc. [4]. The goals and objectives of the Club of Mainz were similar to those of the Club of Rome and were primarily focused on improving the medical treatment and organisational procedures in mass disasters. At the time of the foundation of the Club of Mainz in 1976, there was a great reluctance to become involved in disaster medicine because especially the young generation in Europe as well as in the USA equated disaster medicine with war medicine. The term war medicine was still used as much as 30 years after the end of the Second World War. More than another 10 years were needed to change these views, and to make physicians of the younger generation aware that civil disasters like earthquakes, train and plane crashes, floods, nuclear accidents, etc. make disaster medicine an indispensable part of today's medicine.

The future orientated ideas of Rudolf Frey, Peter Safar and others were advanced by the Club of Mainz and attracted a great many respected and distinguished individuals worldwide [6]. In 1983 the journal 'Disaster Medicine' was initiated and is published today under the title 'Prehospital and Disaster Medicine". WADEM celebrated its 25th anniversary in May 2001 with more than 500 members at the World Congress on Disaster and Emergency Medicine in Lyon.

Although Rudolf Frey was actively involved in a great variety of other activities, those outlined above characterise most distinctly his personality and the range of his initiatives, ideas and activities. Many young physicians from different parts of the world sought the opportunity of working with him, and being taught and trained by him. Those who were his guests at the many congresses and other meetings that he organized enjoyed his extraordinary hospitality and friendship. Even at the time of the Cold War, Rudolf Frey was among those who continued to visit the countries and major emergency and disaster institutions behind the Iron Curtain. He was always prepared to offer assistance and support to anyone in need thereof. For many years he unfortunately suffered from a disease, which lead to his untimely death in December 1981.

He will be remembered as a tireless catalyst who developed resuscitation systems and inspired all those who had the privilege to work with him.

# References

[1] Frey R. New methods of pain treatment. Inaugural lecture. Mainz; 1961.

[2] Frey R, Bonica JJ, Foldes FF, Gordh T, Griffith HR, Hutschenreuther K, Killian H, Lassner J, Macintosh R, Mayrhofer O, van Eck R, Schmidt H. Erlebte Geschichte der Anästhesie (experienced history of anaesthesia). Mainz University Press; April 1972.

[3] Gerbershagen HU, Frey R, Magin F, Scholl W, Müller-Suur N. The Pain Clinic—an interdisciplinary approach to the problem of pain. Br J Anaesthesia 1975;47:526–9.

[4] Frey R, Nagel E, Safar P, editors. Mobile intensive care units. Advanced emergency care delivery systems: Anaesthesiology and resuscitation 95. Springer Heidelberg; 1976.

[5] Frey R. The Club of Mainz for improved worldwide emergency and critical care medicine systems and disaster preparedness. Crit Care Med 1978;6:389.

[6] Frey R, Dürner P, von Baumgarten R. First aid and resuscitation on board of space shuttles (German). Münch Med Wschr 1980;122:145–6.

[7] Mayrhofer O. Rudolf Frey—60 years (German). Anaesthesist 1977;26:373–4.

[8] Editors. We salute Rudolf Frey, MD., FFARCS. Anesth Analg 1961;40:52–4.

# Peter J. Safar, the early years 1924–1961, the birth of CPR

## Peter J.F. Baskett

Peter Safar is a truly remarkable man. His contribution to resuscitation, in the widest sense of the word, is so extensive that it cannot be summarised in any justice in one short paper in this series. I have chosen therefore, to write about him in two articles.

This, the first article, concerns his early years in Austria and the US and extends to the end of his time in Baltimore in 1961 (Fig. 1). His work during this period brought about the development of CPR as we know it today and upon that he built his enormous contribution to prehospital and critical care medicine. The sequel will deal with his career in Pittsburgh, his passion for emergency and disaster medicine, his building of international bridges and relationships, his remarkable devotion to his young researchers in training and his unique International Resuscitation Research Centre, where he still follows his quest for improved cerebral resuscitation after cardiac arrest. I have acquired many of the facts for this article from Peter Safar's autobiographical memoir published in the series 'Careers in Anesthesiology' [1] and from letters and conversations with Peter himself.

Peter Safar was born in Vienna in 1924. His grandfather, Josef, originated from Lukavice, a small village near Josefstadt in the Adler Mountains, now in the Czech Republic. As a poor teenager, Josef had sought to earn a living in nearby Vienna. He became a successful medical publisher—'Der Medizinische Buchverlag Josef Safar'. In 1925, this company was taken over by Springer-Verlag and became 'Minerva', their branch in Vienna.

Peter's father, Karl, was an eminent and successful ophthalmic surgeon. His mother Vinca, who had studied the ancient Greek classics in her teens, was a paediatrician. She was one of the first women medical students in Vienna and met Karl as they were studying together. Both had a profound effect on their son Peter and imbued him with a dedication to achievement married to a sense of fairness, honesty and generosity and an almost naïve belief in the virtues of his fellow man. These qualities have been the hallmark of his professional and private life and have stood him in very good stead.

Peter grew up in a relatively well-to-do household but his teenage years were clouded by the disastrous

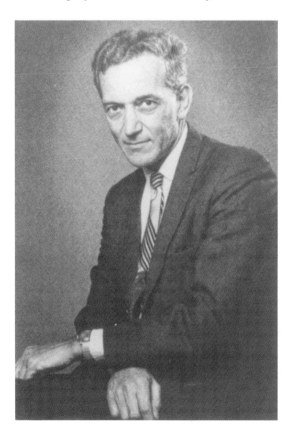

Fig. 1. Peter Safar in 1961.

financial and political events of the time. The economic slump of the 1930s had a profound effect on middle Europe, culminating in the sinister rise of the Nazi movement that apparently took many innocent people by surprise. When they realised what a force for evil it was, it was too late and Austria was occupied by Germany without significant resistance in 1938. Karl and Vinca Safar were dismissed from their university posts because they refused to join the Nazi party and because Vinca was a 'Mischling' and therefore, partly 'non-Aryan'. Karl was allowed to continue in private ophthalmic practice and when war broke out the following year, was assigned to work in the government hospitals where his clinical expertise was sorely needed.

Peter, at the age of 18 (1942), on leaving school had set his heart on being a doctor but was conscripted into a labour camp in Bavaria. He did not know that it was very close indeed to the infamous concentration camp at Dachau, scene of some of the most outrageous medical experimentation in history. After 6 months in this labour camp, where he was abused mentally and physically by sadistic officers, he was drafted into the German Army. There was apparently no way out—"Our generation was trapped. Active resistance was suicidal…but I was determined not to go to the Front to kill and be killed" [1].

Ironically, he was saved from this fate partly by his eczema and partly by his initiative. His eczema was aggravated by the rough army woollen shirt to such a degree that he was admitted to the army field hospital as a 'patient/soldier'—that is, he was expected to work as an orderly during his hospital stay. This suited him well and he began to study medicine on his own, reading day and night when the opportunity arose. His eczema gradually receded and he was due to be sent to the Front, probably to Stalingrad, where the slaughter on both sides was almost unimaginable. His nocturnal studies had given him some medical knowledge and, on the night before the final medical examination to determine his fitness for active service, he smeared his body with tuberculin test ointment. His eczema once again became fulminant overnight. The SS inspectors were confused but decided that his was not fit and so he escaped the Front.

Thanks to the courageous and benign director of the army hospital (who was Austrian), Peter was able to continue his work as a 'paramedic' in the hospital and began his studies as a medical student in 1943. During the final years of the war (1944 and 1945) he saw at first hand the ravages of starvation, infection including typhus, typhoid, tuberculosis, dysentery and pneumonia and the trauma of the final stages of the battle of Vienna. "Soap was scarce—gloves were only used for aseptic surgery. With one hand I would eat a sandwich, hastily prepared by the always caring nurses, while with the other I was helping a dying infectious patient" [1].

The immediate post war period was saddening because many of his school friends did not survive the combat at the Front. Many others came back horribly mutilated. His pacifist beliefs became even more deeply rooted by this experience.

There was one bright spot. He met Eva, a 16-year-old Viennese girl, in 1947 at a house ball and immediately they fell in love. They shared similar values and aspirations and a love of music. They were to be married in 1950 and remain so to this day.

Peter qualified in 1948 and studied pathology as a postgraduate for 9 months before becoming a surgical intern in the university hospital in Vienna in 1949. During his time as an intern, he developed an interest in anaesthesia and perioperative care. A significant feature, later to become very highly significant, was his appreciation of the backward tilt of the head to maintain an open airway practised instinctively by anaesthetists.

In 1949, he applied for and won a Fellowship in Surgery at Yale in New Haven, Connecticut. He wanted to go to the US because of the opportunities there, because the Cold War was on, ("I was a disappointed European, sick of the still present 'isms'"—Naziism, Communism etc" [1]) and because of the dictatorial roles played by professors in medicine in central Europe (the Geheimrat system). Many bright young people from continental Europe and the UK at that time followed the path to the US—the land of opportunity—for their own personal benefit. This was surpassed only by the benefit that they brought to a far sighted host nation. The 'brain drain' was in full flow.

In New Haven, his monthly scholarship stipend of $30 a month was insufficient, even in those days, to feed him. He made a few extra dollars by fitting TV aerials on the steep rooftops of New England and made friends with a nice Greek lady who gave him his meals near the hospital at less than half price. He slept in a corner of a room in the university library and read and read and read.

Peter was amazed that professors invited student opinion and ate lunch with them. There seemed to be no seniority barriers. Patients were told of their ailments and their prognosis quite openly. This was a major contrast with the system he had been brought up with in Austria, where there was a rigid hierarchy and little patient autonomy.

During his time in New Haven, he undertook some surgical research but also reinforced his interest in anaesthesia. The speciality there was much more advanced and sophisticated than it was in Austria at the time. He became convinced that surgery could not advance without improvements in anaesthesia and perioperative care.

By the end of his year in New Haven he had decided that the US was where he wanted to settle. He had secured a place in the residency training programme at the Hospital of the University of Pennsylvania, Philadelphia. This was arguably the finest centre for the speciality in the US at the time. The department was lead by Robert Dripps, a doyen of anaesthesia, who had come from Wisconsin where he had worked with the famous Ralph Waters. In the department at Philadelphia were household names, such as Leroy Vandam, James Eckenhoff and in the pulmonary physiology laboratory, Julius Comroe. This was the place to be.

He had to return to Vienna to satisfy US immigration regulations. During the summer of 1950, he married Eva who agreed to return with him to the US to make their future there. They left Austria in September. The flight from Luxembourg in a converted bomber via Iceland and Newfoundland to Philadelphia took over 20 h. They arrived with $5 and four suitcases.

In Philadelphia, Safar was given a secure grounding in anaesthesia by the outstanding faculty of the time, who led by example and befriended all of the residents personally. This was also to be the hallmark of Safar's character throughout his career. After 2 years, he was offered leadership positions in the US and Austria, but chose (partly because of visa restrictions in the US) to go to Lima, Peru for a year. He was to give support, leadership and teaching to the rudimentary anaesthesiology department there, while Peruvian doctors were trained up for the position. In Peru he learned what could be done with very basic equipment. He taught the local residents in his newly acquired but very basic Spanish. He led from the front in the clinical duties, as he had been shown by Dripps and his colleagues in Philadelphia.

Peter and Eva grew to love Peru and its people. They travelled widely outside the capital. Their local knowledge of the country and understanding of the people was to stand Peter in good stead some 18 years later when he returned there in the aftermath of the devastating earthquake that was to kill 80,000. By then, Peter had become a renowned expert in what he labelled 'disaster reanimatology' (the term reanimatology had been coined to mean the science of resuscitation by his friend and colleague in Moscow, Vladimir Negovski [2]). After studying the pattern of injury, he concluded that there were lives to be saved by the uninjured providing lay person life supporting first aid [3,4].

Upon his return to Philadelphia in 1954, Peter learned that he could not be granted a licence to practice medicine in the state of Pennsylvania without first going back to medical school as a student for 5 years. However, the state of Maryland had no such restrictions and so it was, that on Dripps's recommendation, he was appointed instructor in anaesthesiology at Johns Hopkins Hospital in Baltimore. Dripps had warned him that there were medico-political difficulties

at Hopkins and so it turned out to be. Surgeons and their residents were sometimes competent but always arrogant and were determined to dominate other specialities, especially anaesthesia. This was in direct contrast to the friendly collaboration that had been established at Philadelphia. The surgeons, led by Blalock, did not like to have physician anaesthesiologists in the operating room. They preferred nurse anaesthetists that they could overbear and override. Eventually, things came to a head after confrontations in the operating room and the committee room and the courageous leader of the anaesthesiology department, Don Proctor, resigned. The other anaesthesiologists resigned en mass in his support. The negative attitude by the surgeons was to keep academic anaesthesia, and thus surgery, at Johns Hopkins in the doldrums for 30 years more [1].

Safar moved across town to the smaller Baltimore City Hospital to become the first full time academic chief of the anaesthesiology department. Here was a totally different atmosphere—"the six happiest years of my professional life" [1]. He saw to it that anaesthesia was entirely physician based and there was a very productive academic environment. He retained faculty appointments at Johns Hopkins University and the University of Maryland. Safar had a good chief of surgery to work with, Mark Ravitch. Peter set up a residency programme and worked all hours to see that his young colleagues had supervision throughout the days, nights and weekends. In such a way is experience achieved and respect gained.

Peter had started some research in his new department concentrating initially on lung compliance studies [5,6] and suitable anaesthetic techniques for primitive conditions [7,8]. A chance meeting with James Elam in October 1956 at the American Society of Anaesthesiologists meeting in Kansas City was to change the face of resuscitation. Elam hitched a lift from Safar back from Kansas to Baltimore. It was a long journey and during the trip Elam revealed that he had found that expired air delivered by the mouth to mask or mouth to tracheal tube was capable of maintaining normal blood gases [9]. Elam was interested in this because the manual methods of artificial ventilation of Schafer, Silvester and Holger Nielsen did not work in animals which he used in his research work in the US Army Chemical Warfare Centre. Like all anaesthetists of the time, he had applied mouth to tube ventilation for short periods in paralysed patients when anaesthetic circuit failures had occurred. This was in the days before universal 15–22 mm fittings were introduced and a wide variety of fittings were available that did not fit together. Safar wished to apply the principles of expired air ventilation in life saving resuscitation.

To look into this further, he set about studying methods of overcoming the airway obstruction by the

VENTILATORY EFFICACY OF MOUTH-TO-MOUTH ARTIFICIAL
RESPIRATION

AIRWAY OBSTRUCTION DURING MANUAL AND MOUTH-TO-MOUTH ARTIFICIAL RESPIRATION

Peter Safar, M.D., Baltimore

JOURNAL OF THE AMERICAN MEDICAL ASSOCIATION 167:335-341, 1958

*Conclusions.* In coma without a tracheal tube, direct MMV is effective
because of the ability of the rescuer to support head and jaw for upper airway
patency and because of controllable high inflation pressures and volumes,
whereas manual methods frequently fail to ventilate, mainly because of upper
airway obstruction. We recommend that backward tilt of the head plus exhaled
air inflation methods be taught for general use on adults and children.

Anesthesiology 2001, paper #1 of "classic papers revisited section"

Fig. 2. A landmark paper in mouth-to-mouth ventilation.

tongue and soft tissues that usually occurs in unconscious humans. He also wished to compare the tidal
volumes achieved in paralysed volunteers by mouth to
mouth ventilation with the manual methods used at the
time. Finally, he planned a study of the feasibility of
mouth to mouth ventilation performed by lay persons.

He showed that soft tissue airway obstruction could
be overcome by the head tilt and chin lift method in
most cases [10,11] (the technique that he had seen used
by anaesthetists in the early days in Austria). In the
refractory cases jaw thrust (described first in Germany
in the 1800s as the Esmarch–Heiberg manoeuvre [12])
relieved the problem [13,14]. The majority of this work
was performed on anaesthetised patients.

The next phase of the work must go down as one of
the most courageous pieces of experimental work performed in medicine [15–17] (Fig. 2). Safar's standing
was so good in the Baltimore City Hospital that 31
physicians, medical students and one nurse volunteered
for 49 experiments, while the efficacy of the various
forms of ventilation techniques were evaluated (Fig. 3).
The experiments were carried out on the floors of the
operating rooms on Saturdays when there was little
operating. The first was carried out on December 8,
1956. Tidal volumes were monitored by a pneumograph
applied to the chest and abdomen for volunteers receiving mouth to mouth ventilation and a bell spirometer
taped to a face mask was used for manual methods. An
ear oximeter and an infra red carbon dioxide analyser
were available. Manual methods were applied by professional rescuers from the Baltimore City Fire Department and mouth to mouth by 167 volunteer lay persons
aged 10–70, including Eva and a number of Boy
Scouts. The volunteers received just one live demonstration on a subject by Safar himself as their training.

The subjects were monitored and the results recorded
by resident anaesthesiologist Lourdes Aguto (also
known as Lourdes Aguto Escarraga and Lourdes
Africa), medical students and a number of fellow
anaesthesiologists.

For the study, each volunteer was sedated and
paralysed. For sedation, Safar used large doses of
scopolamine (0.5 mg increments up to 2 mg) and

pethidine [meperidine] (50 mg increments up to 600
mg). For paralysis, succinyl choline was given from an
intravenous infusion totalling 1–3 G. This was titrated
to produce 2–3 h of paralysis at a time while the
experiments were conducted. Safar himself ventilated
each subject between experiments with 50% nitrous
oxide and oxygen. Volunteers were preoxygenated for
1–2 min before each experiment was started. At the
end of the day, they were intubated to obtain control
measurements and to ensure that there had been no
tracheal soiling. All volunteers ate supper at the end of
the day—few were nauseated and Safar noted that
recovery was much more rapid and complete than in
comparable patients who had undergone surgery—not
really a surprise!

It is a tribute to the esteem in which Safar was held
by his colleagues that they willingly submitted themselves to this experiment. It is a measure of Safar's
expertise that no one came to any serious harm.

Such experiments would not receive ethical approval
today and it is fitting to note that if Safar had been
undertaking this work 40 years later, we might not have
resuscitation as we know it. Rather we might be continuing with the ineffective manual methods. Safar's relationship with his volunteers was based on trust—a
sentiment that has largely been discredited by our legal
colleagues.

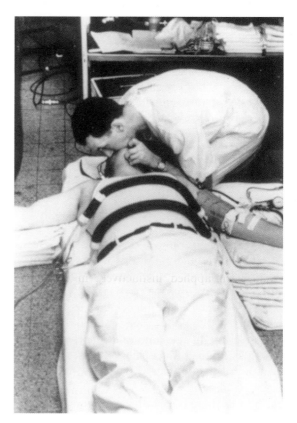

Fig. 3. The early evaluation of mouth-to-mouth ventilation by Peter
Safar in 1957.

The experiments were filmed and financial support came from the US Army Walter Reed Research Institute [18]. The Army supported Safar's research for a further decade. James Elam and Henning Ruben completed further work on airway patency [19]. Elam and Ruben studied mouth to nose ventilation. Archer Gordon had described mouth to mouth ventilation in children [20].

Safar reported his findings in Washington to the National Research Council and to the American Society of Anaesthesiologists in Los Angeles in 1957 [16]. The results were received as a 'bombshell'. In 1958, Safar spoke at the Scandinavian Society of Anaesthetists meeting in Norway. Bjorn Lind of Stavanger was present. This was one of the most fortuitous meetings in resuscitation history.

The US Army, generous though it was, had not seen fit to support the development of a resuscitation training manikin. Bjorn Lind knew Asmund Laerdal, a toy maker in Stavanger who felt he could help. Laerdal immediately flew to the US to meet Safar. Thus, it was that Resusci Anne was developed in 1959–1960. Resuscitation training would never have got off the ground without her.

In 1957, while Safar was conducting his volunteer experiments at Baltimore City Hospital, across town at Johns Hopkins, William Kouwenhoven, professor of electrical engineering, was studying electrical defibrillation in animals. Defibrillation had first been reported in humans by Zoll in 1956 [21,22]. The technique worked if applied within a few minutes of ventricular fibrillation, but soon after that the hypoxic ischaemic myocardium would not respond. Safar and Kouwenhoven met to discuss the problem. The head and neck could be aligned to provide a clear airway, mouth to mouth provided ventilation and oxygenation and defibrillation, when available, appeared to restore an effective circulation after ventricular fibrillation. But there was still no way of producing an artificial circulation to tide the patient over until they were brought to a defibrillator, other than open chest cardiac massage.

External chest compressions had been sporadically reported over the previous 50 years starting with Koenig and Maass in Germany. Mostly the compressions had been applied instinctively in experimental animals and patients with cardiac arrest due to chloroform.

Almost by chance, Kouwenhoven and his colleague Guy Knickerbocker made the rediscovery of external chest compressions in animals when they noticed that the forcible placement of the defibrillator paddles on the chest produced a pulse on the arterial trace. They performed external chest compressions in dogs in cardiac arrest that produced a passable circulation. Soon after, with James Jude, they conducted human clinical trials with remarkably successful results [23,24].

Safar, realising that external chest compressions alone did not produce significant tidal volumes in man due to airway obstruction [25], decided to combine airway alignment, expired air ventilation and external chest compressions to produce the ABC of basic life support—or CPR as it came to be known [25–27]. With his colleague Harris working on dogs, he hit upon the ratio of 1:5 (two rescuer) and 2:15 (one rescuer) [28]. Safar, in his recent autobiography [1] admits that other ratios gave similar results.

In Australia, the technique of mouth to mouth ventilation was accepted rapidly by the water life saving societies and in Norway, Bjorn Lind had started to teach schoolchildren the technique [29,30]. In Baltimore, CPR was practised by the fire department ambulance rescuers but defibrillation (alternating current) was only available in the hospital emergency department. In Eastern European countries, portable defibrillators had been designed by Gurvich in Moscow [31] and Peleska in Prague. However, the information was not disseminated to the West because they published in Russian. It was left to Bernard Lown at Harvard to introduce a direct current defibrillator to the West [32] and Frank Pantridge from Belfast to put defibrillators into the community [33,34].

It was now apparent to Safar that immediate CPR with defibrillation and drugs was not enough for many patients. Long term therapy and support was required for a wide variety of critically ill and injured patients. Following the example of Bjorn Ibsen in Copenhagen, who had introduced a 24-h respiratory intensive care unit to combat the polio outbreak [35], Safar introduced the first physician staffed medical and surgical Intensive Care Unit in the US in Baltimore in 1958 [36]. This unit was designed to cater for all patients with failure of any vital organ system. Inevitably, they came across patients with what was later to be termed adult respiratory distress syndrome (ARDS). He employed positive end expiratory pressure (PEEP) for the condition, but thought it such an obvious remedy as not to be worthy of publication.

Experience in the Intensive Care Unit at Baltimore stimulated Safar's interest in long term life support and the need to support brain function as a primary objective. This was to dominate the second half of his career. In 1961, Peter was appointed as the first Chairman of the department of anaesthesiology at the University of Pittsburgh. The 40 plus years that he worked there will be described in a sequel to this article.

This episode seeks to give just a brief resume of the early career and a mere insight into the drive, sensitivity and gentleness of spirit of this outstanding physician.

# References

[1] Safar PJ. Careers in Anesthesiology, vol. 5. Illinois: The Wood Library Museum of Anesthesiology, 2000.

[2] Safar P. Vladimir Negovski, The Father of Reanimatology Resuscitation, 2001 (in press).

[3] Safar P. Resuscitation potential in mass disasters. In: Manni C, Magalini SJ, editors. Emergency and Disaster Medicine. New York: Springer-Verlag, 1985:28 (First R. Frey memorial lecture).

[4] Safar P, Ramos V, Mosquera J, Ames A. Anecdotes on resuscitation potentials following the earthquake of 1970 in Peru. Prehosp Disas Med 1987;3:124.

[5] Safar P, Bachman L. Compliance of the lungs and thorax in dogs under the influence of muscle relaxants. Anesthesiology 1956;17:334–46.

[6] Safar P, Aguto-Escarraga L. Compliance in apneic anesthetized adults. Anesthesiology 1959;20(3):283–9.

[7] Safar P, Gedang I. Inexpensive system for administration of ether. Anesthesiology 1961;22:323–4.

[8] Pearson JW, Safar P. General anesthesia with minimal equipment. Anesth Analg 1961;40:664–71.

[9] Elam JO, Brown ES, Elder JD Jr. Artificial respiration by the mouth-to-mouth method. A study of the respiratory gas exchange of paralysed patients ventilated by the operators expired air. New Engl J Med 1954;250:749–54.

[10] Safar P, Aguto-Escarraga L, Chang F. Upper airway obstruction in the unconscious patient. J Appl Physiol 1959;14:760–4.

[11] Safar P. Mouth to mouth airway. Anesthesiology 1957;18:904–6.

[12] Esmarch JF. The Surgeons Handbook on the Treatment of Wounded in War. New York: Schmidt, 1878:113.

[13] Safar P, Redding J. The tight jaw in resuscitation. Anesthesiology 1959;20:701–2.

[14] Morikawa S, Safar P, De Carlo J. Influence of the head jaw position upon upper airway patency. Anesthesiology 1961;22:265–70.

[15] Safar P, Escarraga L, Elam J. A comparison of the mouth-to-mouth and mouth-to-airway methods of artificial respiration with the chest-pressure arm-lift methods. New Engl J Med 1958;258:671–7.

[16] Safar P, Elam J. Manual versus mouth-to-mouth methods of artificial respiration. Anesthesiology 1958;19:111–2.

[17] Safar P. Ventilatory efficacy of mouth-to-mouth artificial respiration. Airway obstruction during manual and mouth-to-mouth artificial respiration. J Am Med Assoc 1958;167:335–41.

[18] Safar P. Introduction to respiratory and cardiac resuscitation. A documentary film of human volunteer research. Produced by the Walter Reed Army Institute of Research, Washington, DC. Army Film No. PMF 5349, 1957 and 1961.

[19] Ruben H, Elam JO, Ruben AM, Greene DG. Investigation of upper airway problems in resuscitation. Anesthesiology 1961;22:271–9.

[20] Gordon AS, Frye CW, Gittelson L. Mouth-to-mouth versus manual artificial ventilation for children and adults. J Am Med Assoc 1958;167:320–8.

[21] Zoll PM, Linenthal AJ, Norman LR. Treatment of unexpected cardiac arrest by external stimulation of the heart. New Engl J Med 1956;254:541–64.

[22] Zoll PM, Linenthal AJ, Gibson W. Termination of ventricular fibrillation by externally applied electric countershock. New Engl J Med 1956;254:727–32.

[23] Kouwenhoven WB, Jude JR, Knickerbocker GG. Closed chest cardiac massage. J Am Med Assoc 1960;173:1064–7.

[24] Jude JR, Kouwenhoven WB, Knickerbocker GG. Cardiac arrest: report of application of external cardiac massage on 118 patients. J Am Med Assoc 1961;178:1063–7.

[25] Safar P, Brown TC, Holtey WH. Ventilation and circulation with closed chest cardiac massage in man. J Am Med Assoc 1961;176:574–6.

[26] Benson DW, Jude JR, Kouwenhoven WB, Safar P, Hacket PR. Recent advances in emergency resuscitation, Maryland State Med J 1961;(August):398–411.

[27] Safar P. Community wide cardiopulmonary resuscitation. J Iowa Med Soc 1964;11:629–35.

[28] Harris LC, Kirimli B, Safar P. Ventilation–cardiac compression rates and ratios in cardiopulmonary resuscitation. Anesthesiology 1967;28:806–13.

[29] Lind B. Teaching mouth to mouth resuscitation in primary schools. Acta Anaesth Scand (Suppl) 1961;9:63.

[30] Lind B, Stovner J. Mouth to mouth resuscitation in Norway. J Am Med Assoc 1963;185:933–5.

[31] Gurvich NL, Yuniev SG. Restoration of a regular rhythm in the mammalian fibrillating heart. Am Rev Sov Med 1946;3:236.

[32] Lown B. Comparison of AC and DC electroshock across the closed chest. Am J Cardiol 1962;10:223–33.

[33] Pantridge JF, Geddes JS. Cardiac arrest after myocardial infarction. Lancet 1966;1:807–8.

[34] Pantridge JF, Geddes JS. A mobile intensive care unit in the management of muocardial infarction. Lancet 1967;2:271–3.

[35] Ibsen B. The anaesthetists viewpoint on treatment of respiratory complications in poliomyelitis during the outbreak in Copenhagen in 1952. Proc Roy Soc Med 1954;47:72–4.

[36] Safar P, De Kornfeld TJ, Pearson JW, Redding JS. The intensive care unit. A three year experience at Baltimore City Hospitals. Anaesthesia 1961;16:275–84.

# Henning Ruben
# The Ruben Valve and the AMBU Bag

Peter Baskett    John Zorab

Think of a man who has had a unique career as a member of the Danish fencing team, a professional dancer, magician and thought reader, dentist, doctor, anaesthesiologist, clinician, inventor, bon viveur and raconteur. There you have Henning Ruben (Fig. 1).

For the majority he will be remembered as an inventor—of the first constant-rate syringe pump, of the portable foot suction device, the Ruben non rebreathing valve, the self-inflating resuscitator and one of the first resuscitation manikins. But there is more, much more, to this remarkable man.

Henning Ruben was born in 1914 in Copenhagen into an orthodox Jewish family. At the age of 19 he began his studies to be a dentist at the Royal Dental College in Copenhagen, but he had many other talents.

As a professional dancer and dance teacher (the tango was reputedly his specialty) he toured the halls of Denmark with a well known singer [1] to amplify his allowance as a student (Figs. 2 and 3). He was an accomplished athlete, representing his country at fencing and was a member of the Danish team who gained a bronze medal at the World Championships in Monte Carlo in 1939 (Fig. 4).

Like his fellow Scandinavian anaesthesiologist Torsten Gordh, Henning was also a brilliant illusionist and thought reader, who was elected a member of the exclusive Danish 'Magisk Circel'. This talent was to stand him in good stead later in the crucial years after the second World War [1].

Ruben qualified in dentistry in 1938 and started a general dental practice in Copenhagen. He wanted to study medicine as well and enrolled in the University of Copenhagen Medical School. In 1943, however, when Denmark was occupied by the Nazi regime, his activities required him to leave the country very urgently one night in a fishing boat bound for neutral Sweden. As a refugee in Sweden for nearly two years, he continued to work as dentist, and a magician and thought reader in some of the bigger restaurants [1].

Returning home to Denmark at the end of the war, he completed his medical studies the next year, 1946, and decided to become an anaesthesiologist. Anaesthesia was then an under-developed specialty in Denmark. He wished to study in Sweden but travel and foreign money exchange were very difficult. His talents as a magician came to his rescue when he was able to visit Sweden as an invited guest of the Swedish Society of Illusionists at one of their special performances at a packed Stockholm Concert Hall [1]. During this visit he introduced himself to the anaesthetic leaders at Sabbatsberg Hospital and St. Ericks Hospital. As a result he was appointed to do neuroanaesthesia at the celebrated Serafimerlasarattet the next year, 1948, and during this time he started to publish [2,3] and was able also to visit leading centres of anaesthesia in the UK, including Oxford and Liverpool.

In 1949 he returned to Copenhagen to an appointment as an anaesthetist at the Gentofte Hospital and the Finsen Institute. He began a programme of research and invention that was to continue throughout his professional life and which was to have an enduring effect on the practice of anaesthesia and resuscitation. Hungry to broaden his experience even further, he negotiated a secondment for 6 months in 1951 to the Department of Anaesthesiology at the University of Iowa to work with the renowned Lucien Morris. They published together [4]. A fortuitous meeting with James Elam in Iowa during this time established their common interest in resuscitation and the start of an international collaboration that was to last until both men retired.

Around this time Ruben's inventive nature began to flourish. It started with a constant-rate, mechanical syringe pump, propelled by an electric motor and

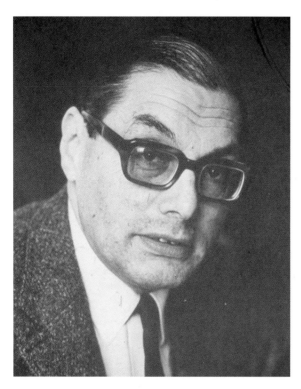

Fig. 1. Henning Ruben.

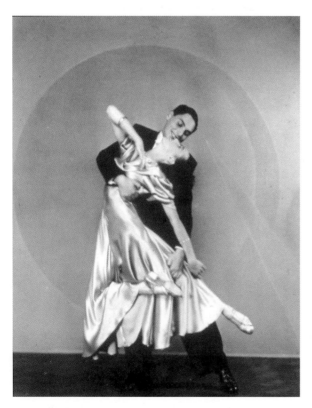

Fig. 2. Ruben—the professional dancer.

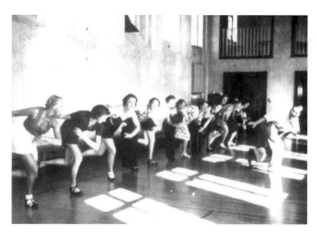

Fig. 3. Ruben—the professional dancer.

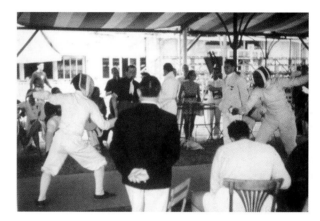

Fig. 4. Ruben—the international fencer.

controlled by an alarm clock mechanism. The succinct description of the simple and ingenious device amounted to one and a half pages and was published in Acta Pharmacology and Toxicology in 1953 [5]. A major venture was into the field of non re-breathing valves and this was to make him a household name in anaesthesia and resuscitation. Impressed with the Stephen–Slater valve, he tried to copy it from a drawing.

Henning says 'I misinterpreted the drawing so, by chance, I introduced changes in the design which resulted in my very first anaesthesia valve' [6]. The valve and its subsequent modifications were described in Scandinavian medical journals between 1950 and 1954 [7,8]. The early valves were delicate precision affairs made with rubies and springs from watch balances to support the moving shaft. As we recall they did not take kindly to being dropped on a hard operating room floor! Later these materials were substituted by more robust silicone membranes and a plastic casing. Over a million were made and Ruben's name became synonomous with the non re-breathing valve. One confused anaesthesiologist once even addressed him as Dr Valve!

In response to a contemporary need in Denmark and other countries for the practice of domiciliary anaesthesia for simple ear, nose and throat operations, Ruben designed a lightweight, simple, portable, foot suction apparatus in 1956 [9]. It was soon appreciated that this

258

"First description and publication of "Head tilt method", which was suggested by Henning Ruben in Buffalo, NY in January 1959.

*Reprinted from* THE LANCET, *August* 1, 1959, *p.* 69

RESCUE BREATHING

**A Modification**

A. RUBEN
Med. Lic. Stockholm
DIRECTOR, DEPARTMENT OF ANESTHESIOLOGY,
CENTRALLAZARETTET, KARLSKRONA, SWEDEN

J. O. ELAM
M. D. Johns Hopkins
DIRECTOR, DEPARTMENT OF ANESTHESIOLOGY,
ROSWELL PARK MEMORIAL INSTITUTE, BUFFALO 3,
N.Y., U.S.A.

H. RUBEN
Cand Med. Copenhagen
DIRECTOR, DEPARTMENT OF ANAESTHESIA,
THE FINSEN INSTITUTE, COPENHAGEN

Fig. 5. Landmark Paper on Rescue Breathing.

equipment had a very widespread application and it became virtually standard equipment on transfer trollies and ambulances world wide. Variations of this device are still in popular use today. The portable suction unit was the first collaboration between Ruben and the AMBU-TESTA company, which was founded in Copenhagen by Dr H. Hesse. This was a relationship that was to endure throughout Ruben's professional lifetime. There have been many copies of Ruben's suction unit manufactured by rival companies—imitation is really the sincerest form of flattery!

A chance occurrence led to the invention of a device that has probably saved more lives than anything else in anaesthesia, and emergency and pre-hospital medicine.

Henning says 'The Danish truck drivers bringing gasoline to the service stations went on strike. As a result, the lorries bringing oxygen to the hospital were forced to a standstill by lack of gasoline. When the strike was finally called off, almost no oxygen was left in several hospitals. This inspired me to the construction of the self-inflating bag resuscitator. I went to my bicycle mechanic, had him weld four bicycle spokes together, then manipulated the joined spokes into an anaesthesia bag. With the aid of an attached string, I obtained a global-shaped frame, which kept the bag expanded. When manual compression of the bag was interrupted, the re-expansion made the bag self-filling. It was followed by different metal frame constructions, filling the bag entirely with lumps of foam rubber—finally ending up by lining the bag with foam rubber, thereby leaving the centre of the bag free. With it my non re-breathing valve was used as an inflating valve, and an air inlet valve was put on its tail. And that was it [10]. Apparently my idea of the self-inflating bag was also considered a good one by others. I have been shown copies of it from almost everywhere in the world' [6].

It is a compliment to Ruben that the 'AMBU Bag' that he invented has become a generic term, regardless of the manufacturer, in much the same way as a 'Hoover' has become synonomous with a vacuum cleaner. In 1964 the Ruben AMBU resuscitator was declared to be 'one of the most significant advances in anaesthesiology of the last 25 years' by the American Society of Anaesthesiologists [11]. How right they were.

Ruben had maintained his association with James Elam, who now had moved from Iowa to Buffalo, New York where he was Professor and Chairman at the Roswell Park Memorial Institute. In 1958 Ruben joined Elam at the Institute as a research associate. Elam and Safar had shown recently that expired air ventilation was more effective than the old manual methods proposed by Silvester, Schafer and Holger Nielsen [12,13]. James Elam and Henning Ruben, together with Arne Ruben (no relation) from Karlskrona in Sweden, were able to demonstrate that head tilt was the essential element in establishing a clear airway. This was reported in landmark papers in the Lancet in 1959 [14], (a splendid one page article! Fig. 5) and in JAMA in 1960 with other American collaborators in a more extensive paper [15]. Ruben later went on to prove the point using X-ray studies [16]. He pointed out, perhaps ruefully, in a personal letter to one of the authors (JZ) in response to a request for personal details for a citation for election to the Fellowship of the Faculty of Anaesthetists of the Royal College of Surgeons.

'Take a look at my article in the Lancet in 1959, where I present my, then, new method of opening the air-passages by merely tilting the head backwards, a method now generally accepted, though it is forgotten (or not known), that I did in fact suggest this method.' Ruben believed that the mouth-to-nose route was superior to the mouth-to-mouth method with less risk of gastric inflation and the mouth-to-nose route was widely practiced in Denmark and central Europe for decades.

Henning Ruben had an early interest in training aids.

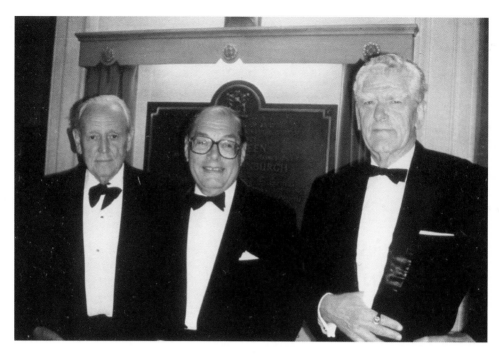

Fig. 6. Bjorn Ibsen, Henning Ruben and Ole Secher.

He wrote ' In 1957 I constructed the first manikin to make it possible to train people in the proper use of the resuscitator. Apart from imitating facial anatomy, I incorporated an airway mechanism which only allowed lung inflation when forward movement of the jaw and backward tilt of the head was accomplished. I tested it with the local Red Cross Chapter in my own community, Sollerød Røde Kors. One of its members, a painter, who was good in modeling, helped me to make its plaster head. In making the airway mechanism I was assisted by the bicycle mechanic who had helped me with my valves, as well as by the watch maker. Half a year later, hearing about experiments on expired air resuscitation, I also started using the manikin to teach mouth-to-mouth respiration. I began demonstrating and using it whenever I got a chance; for example in October 1958 at the meeting of the Swedish Anaesthesiology Association as well as at an international NATO meeting in Copenhagen. In November when I began an appointment in Buffalo in the United States, at the Roswell Park Memorial Institute I took the manikin with me. James O. Elam, the Director of the Anaesthesiology Department, was convinced of its essential teaching value, so we went together to a number of places in the United States to demonstrate it, including the Walter Reed Hospital in Washington' [6].

'After my return to Denmark we modified it to protect against cross infection' [6].

'In 1959 we suggested the nasal route of inflation as the first choice—experimental evidence had shown that the risk of gastric inflation was lower compared to mouth-to-mouth-breathing—and introduced the head tilt method [14].The manikin was additionally supplied with a gastric mechanism, so that it could be used for the training of the technique which lowered the risk of gastric inflation [17]. In 1960 the manikin had further mechanisms added for the training of closed chest cardiac massage. Another teaching aid which I introduced, the sagittal airway model, [17] had already been shown on Danish television in 1958 in a course on expired air resuscitation' [6].

This remarkable man continued to attempt to satisfy his almost insatiable appetite for research and invention in his 70s with new anaesthetic circuitry and valves [18–20].

Always a popular and entertaining speaker he was much in demand as a guest lecturer all over the world. He published prolifically. His papers were always succinct and simply explained and of the highest quality.

Henning Ruben was Chairman of the Danish Society of Anaesthesiologists from 1963 to 1965 and received their Honorary Award for his contributions to anaesthesiology. He delivered the prestigious Husfeldt lecture in 1977. He received many Honours including election to the Fellowships of the Faculty of Anaesthetists of the Royal College of Surgeons in Ireland and the Faculty of Anaesthetists of the Royal College of Surgeons of England. In addition he has been made an Honorary Member of the Danish Association of Anaesthesiology in 1990, European Resuscitation Council in 1994 [21], European Society of Intensive Care Medicine 1997, and was made a Knight of the Order of Danneborg in 1973.

Henning Ruben belongs to a select group of contemporary Danish anaesthesiologists who included

Bjorn Ibsen and Ole Secher, who have left a lasting mark on the specialty through their dedication and innovation (Fig. 6). It is quite fascinating to consider the enormous contribution made to resuscitation by Scandinavians in the 1950s, 1960s, and 1970s—names such as Bjorn Ibsen, Bjorn Lind, Ivar Lund, Asmund Laerdal, Ole Secker, Ole Lippman, Henning Poulsen, Stig Holmberg and Henning Ruben. They will all endure as Resuscitation Greats.

Henning Ruben will be remembered as one of the great inventors. For those of us who have the privilege of knowing him and his wonderful wife Vera personally, he was also a brilliant raconteur, a man of exquisite manners and modesty, a generous and charming host, and above all, always a joy to be with.

Perhaps the last word should go to the late Ole Secher 'Henning has always been interested in fast cars...but has never been a good driver. As he says himself... I am driving fast but not very well'.

He was pretty good at everything else.

## Acknowledgements

The authors would like to acknowledge the background material contained in the homage volume ' Henning Ruben on his 60th birthday—a biography, bibliography and a selection of publications 1948–1973' edited by Julie Knudsen and published by Mohr and Co, Copenhagen, 1974. They are grateful particularly to the late Sophus H. Johansen who describes himself as one of the 'Sorcerers Apprentices', for the information contained in the introduction to that volume.

## References

[1] Johansen SH. Introduction. In: Knudsen J, editors. Henning Ruben on his 60th Birthday—Biography, Bibliography and a selection of Publications 1948–1973. Copenhagen: M Mohr and Co; 1974.

[2] Ruben H. Traek fra den nyere anaesthesiologie. Ugeskr Laeger 1948;110:849–53 (in Danish).

[3] Ruben H. Anaesthetisten i neurokirurgica. Nord Med 1949;42:1503–8 (in Norwegian).

[4] Ruben H, Morris LE. Effect of cocaine on cardiac automaticity in the dog. J Pharmacol Exp Ther 1952;106:55–61.

[5] Ruben H. Simple and accurate infusion mechanism for syringes. Acta Pharmacol Toxicol 1953;9:199–200.

[6] Ruben H. Anaesthesia and Resuscitation Equipment I happened to be involved with. In: Ruprecht J, Van Lieburg MJ, Lee JA, Erdmann W, editors. Anaesthesia—Essays on its History. Berlin, Heidelberg: Springer; 1985.

[7] Ruben H. Multipurpose anaesthesia valve. Nord Med 1953;50:1242–3 (in Danish).

[8] Ruben H. New anaesthetic valve with possibilities for extensive application. Ugeskr Laeger 1954;116:297–300 (in Danish).

[9] Ruben H. Effective suction pump independent of installations. Ugeskr Laeger 1957;118:1252–4 (in Danish).

[10] Ruben H. A new apparatus for artificial ventilation. Ugeskr Laeger 1957;119:14–6 (in Danish).

[11] Editorial. American Society of Anesthesiology Newsletter, August, 1964.

[12] Safar P, Escarrage L, Elam J. A comparison of the mouth-to-mouth and mouth-to-airway methods of artificial respiration with the chest-pressure arm-lift methods. N Eng J Med 1958;258:671–7.

[13] Safar P, Elam J. Manual versus mouth-to-mouth methods of artificial respiration. Anesthesiology 1958;19:111–2.

[14] Ruben A, Elam JO, Ruben H. Rescue breathing. A modification. Lancet 1959;ii:69.

[15] Elam JO, Greene D, Schneider MA, Ruben H, Gordon AS, Hunstead RS, et al. Head tilt method of oral resuscitation. JAMA 1960;172:812–5.

[16] Ruben H, Bentzen N, Saev SK. X ray study of passage of air through the pharynx in anaesthetized patients. Lancet 1960;I:849–51.

[17] Ruben H, Ruben A, Elam JO, Benvister D. Artificial respiration. Improving laymens ability in the performance of artificial respiration without apparatus. Ugeskr Laeger 1960;122:215–9 (in Danish).

[18] Ruben H. New anaesthesia circle: intermittently closed system. Nord Med 1969;82:1316–8 (in Danish).

[19] Ruben H. Universal anaesthesia with automatic dumping. Ugeskr Laeger 1981;143:2719–21 (in Danish).

[20] Ruben H. Anaesthesia system with eliminated spill valve adjustment and without lung rupture risk. Acta Anaesthesiol Scand 1984;28:310–4.

[21] Baskett PJF, Henning Ruben. A Citation for Honorary Membership of the European Resuscitation Council. Resuscitation 1994;28:181–2.

# Kouwenhoven, Jude and Knickerbocker
# The introduction of defibrillation and external chest compressions into modern resuscitation

Pilar Acosta    Joseph Varon    George L. Sternbach    Peter Baskett

The development of cardiopulmonary resuscitation has been achieved by a combination of small contributions by multiple investigators. The re-introduction of closed-chest cardiac massage by William Kouwenhoven, Guy Knickerbocker and James Jude changed the outcome of patients with cardiac arrest profoundly (Fig. 1).

Sponsored by an electric company in 1926, William Kouwenhoven started by undertaking research on the effects of electrical currents on the heart. Experimenting first with rats and dogs, Kouwenhoven and co-workers developed internal defibrillation.

Internal defibrillation was used for the first time in humans by Claude Beck in 1947. The development of a closed-chest defibrillator combined with closed-chest cardiac massage came some years later. The description of closed-chest cardiac massage appeared in a landmark publication in the *Journal of the American Medical Association* in 1960. This technique has revolutionized the management of patients with cardiac arrest.

The development of cardiopulmonary resuscitation (CPR) cannot be attributed to a particular individual or team but has evolved rather as a result of contributions by many investigators. Over several centuries members of civilizations, old and new, have attempted to restart the heart, and recent researchers have added to the development of this aspiration. In the early years of the 20th century,

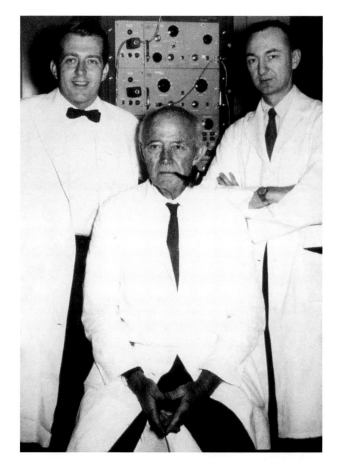

Fig. 1. Knickerbocker, Kouwenhoven and Jude.

electricity sparked the minds of the public around the world. Everyone wanted to have their offices and homes rewired to receive the convenience of this phenomenon. Electric companies enjoyed an expanding market, but recognized an increasing number of sudden deaths, as utility linemen suffered sudden death from ventricular fibrillation (VF), even with low voltage shocks. The increase of these tragedies encouraged the electric companies to fund research into electrical conduction of the heart [1–4].

The search started in 1925, motivated and sponsored by, Consolidated Edison of New York [2]. As a result, five investigations were initiated: at Columbia University by H.B. Williams, at Johns Hopkins School of Medicine by W.G. MacCallum, at the Harvard Engineering Committee by P. Drinker, at the Rockefeller Institute by W.J.V. Osterhout and at School of Hygiene and Public Health at Johns Hopkins University in Baltimore by W.H. Howell [3–5]. In 1926, the Edison Power Company selected the Johns Hopkins School of Hygiene and Public Health as its exclusive research site where Howell and co-workers researched the effects of electrical current on the heart and organized rhythms [3].

In 1933, the team of Hooker, Kouwenhoven and Langworthy from this laboratory in John's Hopkins University had published their work on the recovery of the heart after electric shock [6] the effect of alternating current on the heart in dogs [7] and the concept of resuscitation by counter shock [8].

Almost simultaneously the team at the Case Western Reserve University in Cleveland, Ohio, of Guthrie, Crile, Sollman, Stewart and led by C.J. Wiggers were undertaking similar work and published in 1936 and in 1940 [9].

From the mid 1930s, the investigations in Baltimore were led by William Kouwenhoven, an electrical engineer without any formal medical training and experience.

William Kouwenhoven was born on January 13, 1886 in Brooklyn, New York. He received his degree in electrical engineering in 1906 and obtained a masters degree in mechanical engineering in 1907 from the Polytechnic Institute of Brooklyn [5,10,11]. After he married, he moved to Germany and completed a doctoral degree in electrical engineering in 1913 [4,5]. In 1914, he joined the staff at Johns Hopkins University, serving as Dean from 1938 to 1954. In 1956, after working for several years in the laboratories at the Department of Surgery, Kouwenhoven became a lecturer in Surgery in the Johns Hopkins School of Medicine.

**Experiments that brought about modern resuscitation**

The official investigation into the effects of electricity at Johns Hopkins started in 1928. Co-working with Donald Hooker and Orthello Langworthy, an associate professor of neurology, Kouwenhoven embarked upon electrical conduction experiments. Using rats as experimental animals, these researchers observed the outcome of direct current (DC) and

alternating current (AC) shock applied to body surface electrodes. The current was passed from head to toe as well to electrodes on the limbs. The results of this preliminary study revealed that high voltage shocks applied to the head and one extremity stopped breathing and heart pump function. They also concluded that a lessor current was enough to cause fibrillation when applied in the head to toe direction [3,4]. Using the method recommended by Dr. Boehn of Germany, the chests of these animals were massaged, but this attempt only crushed their cervical spines, causing paralysis [2].

In 1930, this group of researchers started using dogs as experimental animals. Following Dr. Howell's recommendation, Kouwenhoven and Langworthy based their research on previous work on defibrillation published in 1899 by Prevost and Battelli [12]. In this paper, the authors showed that using a weak alternating current could induce ventricular fibrillation and the application of a higher intensity current would achieve defibrillation [7]. To their surprise, they found that providing a surge of electricity as low as 0.1 A applied directly to the surface of the heart caused ventricular fibrillation and, if applied a second time, a current of 0.8 A or more ("counter shock") was required to defibrillate the ventricles. They also concluded that if fibrillation remained for 2 min or more, the countershock would not be effective in producing a resumption of sinus rhythm. From this work came the primitive alternating-current internal cardiac defibrillator [2,3,5,13].

The intervention of World War II put a brake on CPR research for about 7 years. Soon after the war Kouwenhoven was transferred from the School of Hygiene and Public Heath to the School of Medicine, where he continued his studies under the sponsorship of Dr. Alfred Blalock who was Chairman of the Department of Surgery. Blalock gave him laboratory space to carry on his investigations [3,6].

In 1947, Claude Beck reported the first successful open-chest defibrillation in humans during chest surgery while working at Case Western Reserve University in Cleveland [14] There is no doubt he was influenced by the work of Kouwenhoven in Baltimore and clearly also by Wiggers working in his own University in Cleveland.

Susequently, the use of an internal defibrillator with open-chest cardiac massage became a standard method used in cardiac arrest [15]. Open-heart massage was not an innovation, being reviewed before by Charles White. Publications grew, as open-chest defibrillation was used more frequently in patients in cardiac arrest in emergency situations [3]. Several of these early thoracotomies were performed, not in actual cardiac arrests, but in apparent "arrests" caused by malfunction of electrocardiograph electrodes or simple syncopal episodes [3].

The Johns Hopkins Surgical Laboratory, headed by Vivien Thomas, started to build an open-chest defibrillator [3,4,16,17].

As open-chest CPR with internal defibrillation was not practical or suitable for the electrical industry, and because of the increase in frequency of electrocution in linemen, Con

Ed encouraged the development of a closed-chest defibrillator [6,15,16]. Kouwenhoven continued to investigate the effects of electricity on the heart and tried to develop a more functional defibrillator, which could be used without performing a thoracotomy.

In 1950, working with William Milnor, a cardiologist with a strong interest in biomedical engineering and cardiac problems, Kouwenhoven began to develop a closed-chest defibrillator [18,19]. The research focused on the development of a capacitor portable defibrillator. Kouwenhoven had succeeded in defibrillating dogs before with electrodes placed across the chest, but was aware that a higher current would be needed for humans [6]. At first, Kouwenhoven and associates discovered that an alternating current of 20 A that crossed the chest wall was required to arrest fibrillation in a dog [3,6,19]. However, when they placed one electrode on the suprasternal notch and another over the apex of the heart only 5 A were required to defibrillate the dog's heart [19].

Unknown to Kouvenhoven and Milnor, Gurwich and Yuniev (who published their original paper in a Russian language journal), had been ahead of them and had published a paper on defibrillation quite a long time before, in 1939 [20]. Kouwenhoven and Milnor were also beaten in the race to be first to report an external defibrillator for use in humans by Zoll and co-workers in 1956 who were working at Harvard University [21]. It is likely that Kouwenhoven and Milnor wanted to use their defibrillator appreciably earlier but their boss Dr. Blalock was nervous and told them to "run more tests" [1]. There is also a hint of poor Kouwenhoven's frustration when he described how, during the months while they were developing their own defibrillator, they visited Dr. Zoll at Harvard University several times [1]. It is interesting to speculate how much help Zoll may have had from Kouwenhoven during these visits.

It is also worth mentioning that Kouwenhoven, Knickerbocker and Becker described the first "diphasic" – now called biphasic – defibrillator in 1963 in an engineering journal that may have escaped the notice of the doctors [22].

## Team work

In 1954, Guy Knickerbocker, an electrical engineer joined the team. Knickerbocker, a Baltimore native who had just graduated from Johns Hopkins University, started working with Kouwenhoven and Langworthy [1]. In 1958, while experimental studies and tests were being performed trying to develop a portable defibrillator that would be useful for electric companies, Knickerbocker made the crucial observation that a momentary rise in the intra-arterial pressure trace occurred when the heavy electrodes were applied to the chest wall of the dog with ventricular fibrillation [23,24].

Knickerbocker's observation elicited an extensive series of experiments applying pressure to the sternum and to the sides of the chest. Several trials were done, which included the connection of strain gauges to the ventricle in order to find the most effective spot on the chest to apply the force. To verify the fact that the rhythmic chest compression provided circulatory support Kouwenhoven and his associates also used a blood flowmeter, which enabled them to find the optimal site for application of the force in the lower part of the sternum [6]. Blalock was especially interested in the observation of a rise in blood pressure during chest compression and he assigned Dr. James Jude, a clinician, to join the team. Jude was finishing his last year as a fellow in cardiac surgery, and had just returned from serving in Korea when he joined the team [6,10,13,15].

During the time they were together at the Johns Hopkins institution, Kouwenhoven, Jude and Knickerbocker performed additional studies, trying to improve the success of circulatory support with closed-chest cardiac massage. They substituted the electrode for a hand and applied rhythmical pressure to the sternum. They concluded that after 15–20 min of rhythmic chest massage over the distal part of the sternum with a force of 100 lb and a rate of 60 compressions per minute, they were able to defibrillate a dog from ventricular fibrillation, which recovered without any effect on the central nervous system [1,3,6,11,15]. It should be noted that there had been work done on closed-chest compression before, especially in Germany in the late 1880s and it had been practiced right up into the early 20th century, before being "forgotten"[25].

Many others assisted the team of researchers to establish what we now know as modern chest compression techniques. Henry Bahnson, another energetic investigator joined the group, due to his eagerness to try this technique in a human patient. The opportunity arrived soon when a 2-year-old child with VF was brought to the emergency department, and was successfully resuscitated with this new combined method of external cardiac compression and closed-chest defibrillation. The next day, Blalock obtained consent to use this 'new' technique in children when indicated [3,5,16]. That same year, Jude had the opportunity to apply closed-chest cardiac massage to a 40-year-old obese woman, who had presented to the emergency room with acute cholecystitis. This lady was taken directly to operating room for an emergency cholecystectomy and while undergoing anesthesia she developed VF. The resuscitation, using closed-chest compressions, was a success and this led Blalock to approve the use of this method for humans and the report was published in 1960.

Kouwenhoven, Jude and Knickerbocker began applying the technique in very precise situations. Some cases were better documented than others. Over a 10-month period, 20 cases of cardiac arrest were documented using closed-chest massage and three cases that required defibrillation [3,16]. The results provided the basis for the classic publication entitled "Closed-Chest Cardiac Massage" that appeared in the *Journal of the American Medical Association* in 1960 [23]. There followed a report, published in the next year, of the clinical use of closed-chest cardiac massage in 118 patients, that produced remarkable results in terms of

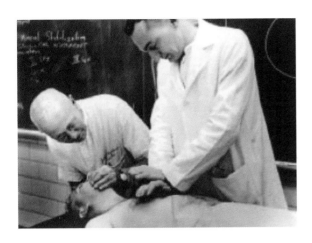

Fig. 2.

survival, when it is considered that ventilation was not part of the resuscitation process [26].

Peter Safar, who was also working in Baltimore at that time, sought to incorporate ventilation and oxygenation into the resuscitation process with external chest compressions [26]. The combination of external cardiac compression and mouth to mouth ventilation later became known as cardiopulmonary resuscitation with a sequence of 15 compressions to 2 ventilations for a single rescuer and 5 compressions to 1 ventilation for two rescuers [27].

In the early 1960s, Kouwenhoven, Jude and Knickerbocker travelled through the United States and Puerto Rico to make presentations and actual canine demonstrations of their technique [28] (Fig. 2). Their goal was to involve the public as much as possible. To achieve public awareness, they recruited the support of the Red Cross, which became deeply involved in the task of training the public by writing manuals, producing visual aids and training programmes. The innovative concept of closed-chest cardiac compression combined with artificial ventilation as the principle of basic life support in the management of cardiac arrest was widely acknowledged [3,29–34].

To acknowledge his contribution to medicine, William Kouwenhoven was awarded an honorary medical degree in 1969, this being the first such degree to be granted by Johns Hopkins University [1,4,5]. In addition, Kouwenhoven, Jude and Knickerbocker all received the Hektoen Gold Medal of the American Medical Association and in 1973 Kouwenhoven received the Albert Lasker Award for Clinical Medical Research. He died on November 10, 1975 [5,17].

Guy Knickerbocker served as a researcher in John Hopkins for 17 years following the publication of the technique. In 1972, he graduated with a doctorate in electrical engineering. The same year he moved to Philadelphia and worked in a non-profit Emergency Care Research Institute. He retired in 2000 [15].

In 1964, when Dr. Blalock retired from Johns Hopkins, James Jude moved to Miami, Florida and joined the Miami School of Medicine, where he is still on duty in private practice of thoracic and cardiovascular surgery [15].

Closed-chest CPR is practiced every day around the world. It was the work of engineers and a clinician that facilitated our modern understanding of this life-saving technique. The development emphasizes the importance of team work in the perfection of a medical technique.

## Acknowledgement

The authors would wish to thank Dr. Douglas Chamberlain for his contribution to the manuscript.

## References

[1] Kouwenhoven WB, Langworthy OR. Cardiopulmonary resuscitation: an account of 45 years of research. Johns Hopkins Med J 1973;132:186–93.
[2] Eisenberg MS. Cardiac Arrest. The science and practice of resuscitation medicine. In: Paradis NA, Halperin HR, Nowak RM, editors. The quest to reverse sudden death: a history of cardiopulmonary resuscitation. Baltimore: Williams and Wilkins; 1996.
[3] Sladen A. Closed chest massage, Kouwenhoven, Jude, Knickerbocker. JAMA 1984;251:3137–40.
[4] Bolling S. The introduction of closed chest cardiac massage. Ann Thorac Surg 1990;49:154–6.
[5] Milnor WR. William Bennett Kouwenhoven 1886. Johns Hopkins Med J 1976;138:109–10.
[6] Hooker DR. On the recovery of the heart in electric shock. Am J Physiol 1930;91:305–28.
[7] Hooker DR, Kouwenhoven WB, Langworthy O. The effect of alternating electric currents on the heart. Am J Physiol 1933;103:444–54.
[8] Kouwenhoven WB, Hooker DR. Resuscitation by countershock. Electr Engin 1933:475–7.
[9] Wiggers CJ. The physiological bases for cardiac resuscitation from ventricular fibrillation Method for serial defibrillation. Am Heart J 1940;20:413–22.
[10] Geddes LA. William Bennett Kouwenhoven, a pioneer biochemical engineer. Med Instrum 1976;10:141–3.
[11] Hosler R. History of cardiopulmonary resuscitation. Ohio State Med J 1979;75:701–3.
[12] Prevost JL, Battelli F. On some effects of electrical discharges on the hearts of mammals. Compt Rendu Acad Sci (Paris) 1899;129:1267.
[13] DeBard M. The History of Cardiopulmonary Resuscitation. Ann Emerg Med 1980;9:273–5.
[14] Beck CS, Pritchard WH, Feil HS. Ventricular fibrillation of long duration abolished by electric shock. JAMA 1947;135:985–6.
[15] Jude JR. Personal reminiscences of the origin of CPR. Am J Cardiol 2003;92:956–63.
[16] Criley M. Cardiopulmonary resuscitation research 1984 discoveries and advances. Ann Emerg Med 1984;13:756–8.
[17] Jude JR. Personal reminiscences of William Bennett Kouwenhoven. Med Instrum 1976;10:144–5.
[18] Kouwenhoven WB, Milnor WR, Knickerbocker GG, et al. Closed chest defibrillation of the heart. Surgery 1957;42:550–61.
[19] Jude J, Haroutunian LM, Folse R. Hypothermic myocardial oxigenation. Am J Physiol 1957;190:57–62.
[20] Gurvich N, Yuniev SG. Byulletin eksperimental biologii I midistiny. 1939;8:55–8. (Translated: restoration of a regular rhythm in the mammalian fibrillating heart.). Am Rev Sov Med 1946;3:236–9.

[21] Zoll PM, Linenthal AJ, Gibson W, Paul MH, Norman LR. Termination of ventricular fibrillation in man by an externally applied electric shock. N Engl J Med 1956;254:727–32.

[22] Kouwenhoven WB, Knickerbocker G, Becker L. IEEE Transpower Appar Syst 1963;69:1089.

[23] Kouwenhoven WB, Jude J, Knickerbocker G. Closed chest cardiac massage. JAMA 1960;173:1064–7.

[24] Safar PJ. Careers in anaesthesiology: an autobiographical memoir, vol. 5. Pub Wood Library—Museum Anesthesiology; 2000. p. 142.

[25] Koenig F. Lehrbuch der allegemeinen Chirurgie, Erste Abtheilung. Berlin: August Hirchwald; 1883.

[26] Jude JR, Kouwenhoven WB, Knickerbocker GG. Cardiac arrest; report of application of external cardiac massage on 118 patients. JAMA 1961;178:1063–71.

[27] Safar P, Brown TC, Holtey WJ, Wilder RJ. Ventilation and circulation with closed chest cardiac massage in man. JAMA 1961;176:574–6.

[28] Safar P, Brown TC, Holtey WJ, Wilder RJ. The history of cardiopulmonary resuscitation. Acute Care 1986;12:61–2.

[29] Harris LC, Kirimli B, Safar P. Ventilation-cardiac compression rates and ratios in cardiopulmonary resuscitation. Anesthesiology 1967;28:806–13.

[30] Sabanayagam T, Weil M, Rackow E. Cardiopulmonary resuscitation: a historical review. Acute Care 1986;12:63–94.

[31] Fye WB. Ventricular fibrillation and defibrillation: historical perspectives with emphasis on the contributions of John Mac Millan, Carl Wiggers, and William Kouwenhoven. Circulation 1985;71:858–65.

[32] Varon J, Sternbach GL. Cardiopulmonary resuscitation: lessons from the past. J Emerg Med 1991;9:503–7.

[33] Mitka M. Father of CPR, innovator, teacher humanist. JAMA 2003;281:2485–6.

[34] Benson DW, Jude JR, Kouwenhoven WB. External cardiac massage. Anesth Analg 1963;42:75–83.

# Sven-Ivar Seldinger: The revolution of radiology and acute intravascular access

Joseph Varon, Ulf Nyman

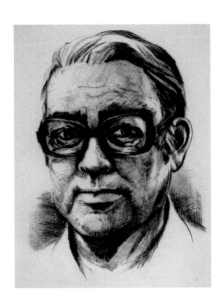

## Introduction

The history of modern medicine is the story of the continuing endeavours by physicians to apply the newest scientific medical methods to the care of their patients. This is particularly the case of the history of acute intravascular access. Over the past 1000 years access has been gained to the venous and arterial circulations using a variety of methods. In the late 1600s, Frederik Ruysch (1638–1731), described and perfected the method of injecting blood vessels.[1,2]

In emergency and critical care conditions, such as in the case of a cardiac arrest, practitioners commonly are required to place intravenous and intra-arterial lines. On many occasions the ''Seldinger technique'' is used for these procedures. In the field of radiology, acute medicine and cardiology the percutaneous intravascular access method developed by Sven-Ivar Seldinger (1921–1998) has had an enormous impact.[3]

## The development of an idea

Dr. Seldinger was born in Mora, Sweden in 1921. As a boy he spent many days with his grandfather who was a very talented mechanic and constructor of precision-tools.[4] He attended medical school at the Karolinska Institute in Stockholm from 1940 to 1948.[5] He began his radiology training in 1950 and remained at the Karolinska institute until 1966, time when he returned to his home in Mora. There he became the Chief of Radiology at the local hospital until his retirement in 1986.

In the early 1950s clinical angiography relied on (1) trans-needle injections of contrast media through direct puncture of, e.g. the carotid and femoral artery, and the lumbar aorta, or (2) vascular catheter access via surgical arteriotomy and catheter-through-needle techniques. The former technique precluded access to distant vessels and the latter were traumatic and could involve considerable blood loss.[5] Seldinger's idea was to use a smaller caliber needle, inserted through the catheter, to minimize vascular trauma and a larger caliber catheter to promote higher injection rates of contrast media, not least for aortic injections. Seldinger had several attempts at developing his now world-recognized technique. He first tried a catheter with a single side-hole located a short dis-

FROM THE ROENTGEN DIAGNOSTIC DEPARTMENT (DIRECTOR: PROFESSOR KNUT LINDBLOM), KAROLINSKA SJUKHUSET, STOCKHOLM, SWEDEN

## CATHETER REPLACEMENT OF THE NEEDLE IN PERCUTANEOUS ARTERIOGRAPHY

### A new technique

by

*Sven Ivar Seldinger*

The catheter method of angiography has become more popular in the past few years, as it provides the following advantages over the method of injecting the contrast medium by means of a simple needle:

1) The contrast medium may be injected into a vessel at any level desired.

2) Risk of extravascular injection of the contrast medium is minimised.

3) The patient may be placed in any position required.

4) The catheter may be left in situ without risk while the films are being developed, thus facilitating re-examination if necessary.

Until recently, however, the use of the catheter method was restricted because of the lack of a suitable flexible thin-walled catheter which could be used percutaneously. FARIÑAS, in 1941, described a method in which a urethral catheter was passed up into the aorta through a trocar inserted in the exposed femoral artery. In 1947, RADNER catheterized the exposed and ligated radial artery and performed vertebral angiography and later thoracic aortography. Since then, many authors have catheterized arteries for various purposes, by surgical exposure followed by ligature or resuturing of the artery. In 1949, JÖNSSON performed thoracic aortography after puncture of the common carotid artery by means of a blunt cannula provided with an inner sharp needle. The cannula, guided by a silver thread, was then directed downwards. Later

Briefly presented at the Congress of the Northern Association of Medical Radiology, Helsinki, June, 1952; submitted for publication, October 28, 1952.

tance from the tip. Through this hole, he placed a needle protruding from the tip of the catheter. The needle punctured the skin and vessel wall, and once the catheter was in place, he pushed it forward into the vessel and removed the needle.[6] However, the newly developed poly-ethylene tube he used was not rigid enough and was difficult to push through the skin and the vessel wall without kinking. He therefore introduced a piano wire to stiffen the catheter. Shortly thereafter he participated in the construction of a metal-spiral armed wire with a central core and, together with the company Stille-Werner, the modern guide wire was born. Still the technique was imperfect, with a possible risk of catheter rupture at the side-hole. After another failed attempt Seldinger one day stood depressed with the three items in his hand, the needle, the catheter and the guide wire. Then he was struck by what he himself described as a "severe attack of common sense". Within a split second he realized how to use the three items: needle in, guide-wire in through the nee-

the procedure was abandoned, partly because it was considered that the cannula might injure the aortic wall. This percutaneous method might have proved more useful if a technique for using a flexible catheter of adequate lumen had been available at the time.

The artery exposure technique of catheterization is time-consuming, troublesome and may present certain risks. The thin-walled polyethylene tube, however, makes percutaneous catheterization possible, as reported by PEIRCE in 1951, who passed in the tubing through a large bore needle. This method was suitable for aortography via the femoral artery. In the same year, DONALD, KESMODEL, ROLLINS and PADDISON, employing a similar technique, catheterized the common carotid artery in cerebral angiography. The method necessitates the use of a large bore needle which may make puncture difficult and limits its use to comparatively large arteries, hence PEIRCE's attempts to catheterize the brachial artery were disappointing. There is also extra damage to the artery and, as the hole in the artery is larger than the catheter, haemorrhage after removal of the needle may be troublesome. To prevent bleeding, the needle may be kept in situ during the investigation; this, however, increases the risk of injury to the patient during movement.

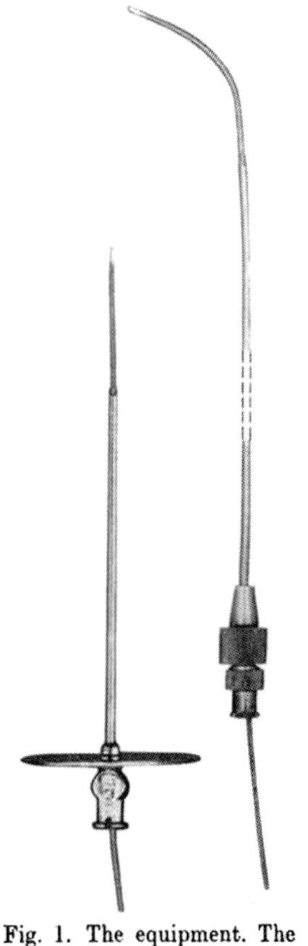

There is a simple method, however, of using a catheter the same size as the needle, and which has been used at Karolinska Sjukhuset since April 1952. The main principle consists in the catheter being introduced on a flexible leader through the puncture hole after withdrawal of the puncture needle. The details are as follows:

Fig. 1. The equipment. The stilette is removed and the leader inserted through the needle (left) and the catheter (right).

*Equipment.* (Supplied by A. B. Stille-Werner, Stockholm.)

1) A puncture needle with stilette.

2) A flexible rounded-end metal leader with increased flexibility of its distal 3 cm.

3) A polyethylene tube, of the same diameter as the needle, with an adapter for the attachment of a syringe.

26 - 530088. *Acta Radiologica. Vol. 39.*

dle, needle out, catheter in over the wire and finally removal of the guide wire. The next day the new technique was attempted. Following percutaneous puncture of the brachial artery the catheter was advanced to the subclavian artery for parathyroid angiography and a mediastinal parathyroid adenoma, missed at previous surgery, was disclosed.

The Nordic Association of Medical Radiology was to meet within a week in Helsinki, Finland, June 1952, and the deadline for submitting papers was far overdue. Seldinger, being only a 2-year resident in radiology, was to stay home and do the routine work. Instead his chief, Professor Knut Lindblom, with Seldinger's permission, presented the new technique (from Seldinger's personal history published in Swedish) (Figure 1).

Seldinger's work was extensive and comprehensive and showed that all arteries in the body could be reached from the femoral route if adequate shaped catheters were used. It enabled the development of, for example, selective coronary, cerebral, renal, and mesenteric angiography and of selective catheterisation of all four cardiac chambers by bloodless percutaneous catheter introduction. His own primary examples were demonstration of the renal and the parathyroid arteries. He also described transhepatic and - splenic catheterisation of the portal vein and pioneered percutaneous transhepatic cholangiography with this technique.

Seldinger's technique was originally published in *Acta Radiologica* (Stockholm) in spring 1953 and in his own writing it ''is simpler than appears on paper and after a little practice should present no difficulties'' (Figure 2).

The technique became widespread in Europe just a few years after its publication, especially in Scandinavia, except for the nearby Serafimer Hospital in Stockholm. It also took many year before the acceptance of this method in the United States.[7,8] Once in use by radiologists in the United States, the study of visceral structures and branches of the aorta was accelerated as this technique was simple, efficacious and did not involve an open surgical field.

Seldinger was very modest and in a personal communication to Professor Nordenström at the Karolisnka Hospital, he indicated that he had ''beginner's luck''.[9]

The success this technique had lead him to explore other areas of diagnostic and interventional radiology.[5] Seldinger never thought of the magnitude of clinical applications that his technique would have in the decades to follow his initial report.[5] Seldinger died in his home in Mora, Sweden on 21 February 1998.

## Implications for the acute care practitioner

The Seldinger technique is practiced every day in acute medicine. Its principal use in this field has been in central venous cannulation of adults and children. However, this guide-wire technique has also found to be useful in peripheral arterial cannulation, percutaneous transtracheal ventilations, chest tube insertion, and diagnostic peritoneal lavage.[10-12] Other applications of the Seldinger technique have included percutaneous placement of feeding gastrotomy tubes, cannulation of a diseased aorta, lumbar epidurography, percutaneous drainage of obstructed bile ducts and renal pelvis/ureters, abscesses and fluid collections and insertion of difficult to place ventricular catheters among others.[13-17] The Seldinger technique for central venous access has been proven useful in adult and pediatric populations in the context of cardiac arrest. Indeed, this is a commonly taught technique.[18] Dr. Seldinger's work has been truly a milestone and its significance is quite apparent in every day emergency and critical care practice.

## References

1. Seelig MG. Medicine: an historical outline. Baltimore: Williams & Wilkins; 1931. p. 110—1.
2. Varon J, Sternbach GL. Cardiopulmonary resuscitation: lessons from the past. J Emerg Med 1991;9:503—7.
3. Sternbach GL. Sven-Ivar Seldinger: catheter introduction on a flexible leader. J Emerg Med 1990;8:635—7.
4. Meyers MA. Science, creativity and serendipity. AJR 1995;165:755—64.
5. Doby T. A tribute to Sven-Ivar Seldinger. AJR 1984;142:1—11.
6. Seldinger SI. Catheter replacement of the needle in percutaneous angiography: a new technique. Acta Radiol (Stockholm) 1953;39:368—76.
7. Abrams HL. Selectivity in the study of the cardiovascular system. Calif Med 1962;96:149—55.
8. Conahan TJ, Schwatz AJ, Taggart Geer R. Percutaneous catheter introduction: the Seldinger technique. JAMA 1977;237:446—7.
9. Nordenström B. Testimonials to Seldinger: historical perspective. AJR 1984;142:9—10.
10. Daily RH. Use of wire-guided (Seldinger-type) catheters in the emergency department. Ann Emerg Med 1983;12:489—92.
11. Argall J, Desmond J, Mackway-Jones K. Seldinger technique chest drains and complication rate. Emerg Med J 2003;20:169—709.

12. Lazarus HM, Nelson JA. A technique of peritoneal lavage without risk or complication. Surg Gynecol Obstet 1979;149:889—92.
13. Halkier BK, Ho CS, Yee CAN. Percutaneous feeding gastrostomy with the Seldinger technique: review of 252 patients. Radiology 1989;171:359—62.
14. Khoynezhad A, Plestis KA. Cannulation in the diseased aorta; a safe approach using the Seldinger technique. Tex Heart Inst J 2006;33:353—5.
15. Hatten HP. Lumbar epidurography with metrizamide. Radiology 1980;137:129—36.
16. Stephenson TF, Guzzeta LR, Tagulinao OA. Ct-guided Seldinger catheter drainage of a hepatic abscess. AJR 1978;131:323—4.
17. Lam CH, Horrigan M, Lovick DS. The Seldinger technique for insertion of difficult to place ventricular catheters. Pediatr Neurosurg 2003;38:90—3.
18. Macnab AJ, Macnab M. Teaching pediatric procedures: the Vancouver model for instructing Seldinger's technique of central venous access via the femoral vein. Pediatrics 1999;103:1—4.

# Åsmund S. Lærdal

## Nina Tjomsland　　Peter Baskett

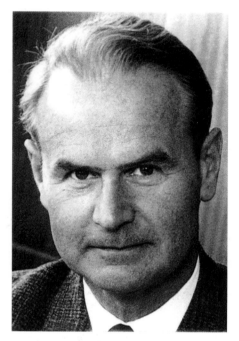

Fig. 1. Åsmund S. Lærdal

## 1. Introduction

In 1958, one of the most fortuitous meetings in the history of resuscitation occurred: Dr Peter Safar from the United States, and Dr Bjørn Lind from the Stavanger hospital, both attended a conference of Scandinavian anaesthesiologists, in Norway.

Together with Dr James Elam, Peter Safar, in a remarkable series of studies in Baltimore, had confirmed that life-saving resuscitation could be performed with expired air, mouth-to-mouth or mouth-to-mask [1,2]. But how to train people in this skill? The situation only arose as a dire life threatening emergency—not a time

for practical training by the uninitiated. There was a clear need for training manikins. Bjørn Lind had an idea: a Stavanger publisher and toymaker, Åsmund S. Lærdal, might be able to help (Fig. 1).

Actually, Åsmund Lærdal was favourably predisposed towards this challenge. He had saved his own 2-year-old son Tore from drowning, by grabbing him from the water just in time and clearing the boy's airways. He had designed and produced his first medical training aids, a series of very realistic imitation wounds. Discussing this concept with Dr Per Strömbäck, chief physician of the Swedish Red Cross, Åsmund had been told about the new mouth-to-mouth method that had been developed in the U.S.

Bjørn Lind felt that Åsmund Lærdal should go to the U.S. to discuss the making of a manikin with Peter Safar. Lærdal went in November, and the meeting resulted in an instant, life-long friendship. "We were like brothers, inspired by the same mission", said Safar later.

The task at hand was extremely complicated. A manikin must resemble an unconscious person, have airways that could be obstructed and cleared, a head that could be turned, a chest that could move with inflation, and be easy to transport. Another requirement was that many people should be able to practise in quick succession, without fear of contamination.

But not only did Åsmund Lærdal possess—and guard closely—a thorough knowledge of soft plastics: he had amply demonstrated his ability to develop an enterprise combining a very sound footing with a sense of purpose and meaning beyond profit and growth.

"Time is our most valuable asset, and we must use it well" he declared as a very young man, telling his fiancée about his dream of earning enough to be able to give half of it away. Right from the start of his own enterprise in 1940, he had identified important needs and then become the dominant supplier. Often several steps ahead, he habitually started developing new products long before the old ones were outdated. He discussed his visions with his employees, sought out professionals who could advise him, and made friends with quite a few of them.

Although he grew up in the the years of the depression, he invested in education, going to Copenhagen to study marketing and advertising. He always sought impressions and inspirations from other cultures: as a 20-year-old he went on his first bicycle trip abroad, all the way to Italy, and in 1936 he cycled alone to Moscow (Fig. 2).

His first business venture was commissioning and publishing books, most of all for children, and manufacturing wooden toys. There was plenty of wood in Norway.

In 1949, he flew to the States for the first time. Tourist class (Fig. 3). "It does not make sense to just sit away all that money", he said. He was looking for new opportunities, and found them in soft plastics. Although this new material was jealously guarded, he managed to bring it home and start experimenting.

Struggling to master the new medium, at first he baked samples in his wife's oven. Undaunted by endless complications, he had 'the doll sensation of the century' ready for production a year later. 'Anne' was a huge hit, all over toy-starved, post-war Europe (Fig. 4).

"Good toys are vitamins for children" he said. And followed up with the cheap, durable Tomte cars, also made of soft plastic (Fig. 5).

However, as competition grew, he looked around for new areas, applying the company knowledge of soft plastics to making the imitation wounds for the Civil Defence—and so we have reached the time of his trip to see Per Strömbäck in Gothenburg. The Swede inspired him to start experimenting with a resuscitation mask. He

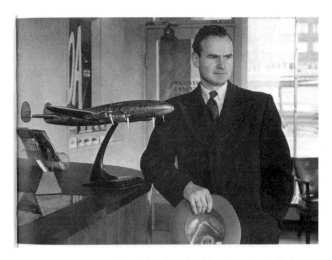

Fig. 3. With a model of the plane for his transatlantic flight.

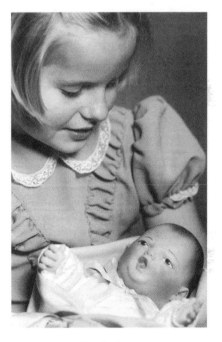

Fig. 4. Anne.

made a prototype, tried it on his wife and son, and decided he needed to learn more—just around the time when Safar and Lind met for the first time.

For long periods, Bjørn Lind and Åsmund Lærdal were in almost daily contact. Almost 2 years work went into the development of the manikin, which had to meet all requirements and at the same time be reasonably priced. It is much more meaningful to deliver 10,000 dolls at 1000 kroner each, than 1000 at 10,000 kroner each, Lærdal said later. The details of the design of the manikin were to be the reasons for its success in overcoming natural psychological retiscence. By the attitudes of the time the manikin had to be female. Men would be loathe to practice mouth to mouth ventilation on men. Åsmund chose the face modelled

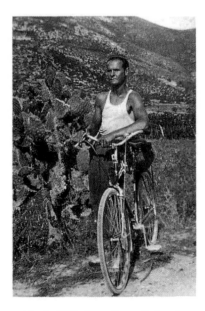

Fig. 2. With the well travelled cycle.

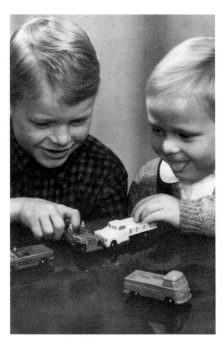

Fig. 5. Tomte cars.

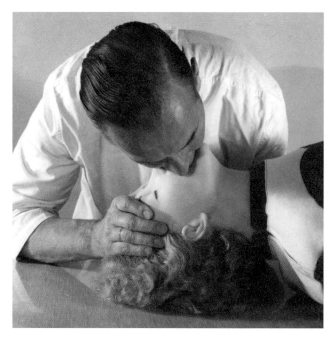

Fig. 7. Resusci Anne.

on the death mask of a renowned girl who had been found drowned in the River Seine in Paris. The death mask had become famous because of the girl's wistful, enigmatic and peaceful countenance. She was beautiful but not sexy. The clothes that the manikin was dressed in was also a master stroke—a track suit was attractive and embodied a concept of fitness. Putting the manikin in a dress would have been a disaster (Figs. 6–8).

By May 1960, Resusci Anne went to New York for the first time, and was presented to Peter Safar and the American Red Cross. At the same time, Åsmund Lærdal met another pioneer for the first time, Dr Archer Gordon.

The specialists were impressed by his product—but in this first year, Lærdal sold one doll in the U.S. At half price.

In Norway, however, things took off. Bjørn Lind and his colleague Ivar Lund joined forces to convince the profession of the importance of mass training in resuscitation. The breakthrough came when a group of banks donated 650 manikins to primary schools. Dr Lind followed the training and published his findings, that children learned just as well as their teachers [3].

This enterprise attracted international attention, and Norway emerged as a pioneering country in the history of life-supporting first aid.

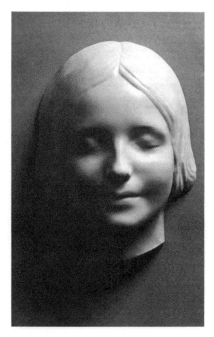

Fig. 6. The face of Resusci Anne.

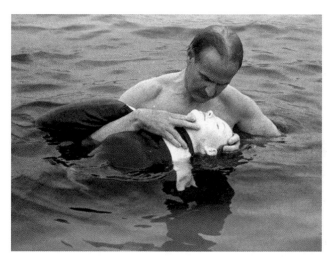

Fig. 8. Resusci Anne.

274

Within 10 years Resusci Anne had become a film star in America, when the Lærdal company cooperated with Archer Gordon to make several award-winning training films, among them 'Breath of Life'.

Meanwhile, Åsmund Lærdal was following closely new developments in the field. Import duties and competition from American manufacturers led him to establish a company in the U.S.—thus starting the transformation of the Stavanger company into the international Lærdal Medical (Fig. 9).

But there were still practical questions about Resusci Anne to be solved, most of all to do with the risk of cross-contamination. In August 1961 Lærdal, in close cooperation with Safar and German specialists, initiated and hosted the First International Symposium on Emergency Resuscitation. It was held in Stavanger, attended by specialists from all over the world. The results and recommendations were published in English as a special edition of the Acta Anaesthesiologica Scandinavia: mouth-to-mouth should be taught in all schools [4]. The ABC of life-saving should be as commonly known as the ABC of reading, as Åsmund Lærdal put it.

Three years after this symposium, the World Federation of Anaesthesiologists established a CPR committee; Peter Safar and Bjørn Lind were among its members.

Meanwhile, in the U.S. two engineers Guy Knickerbocker and William Kouwenhoven and Dr James Jude had made a landmark discovery. External chest compressions could provide a circulation of blood to the brain when the heart stopped beating, and increase greatly the possibility of revival [5,6]. Åsmund Lærdal saw the significance and potential: already in 1969,

several years before the authorities approved the general training in CPR, he applied himself and his company to the task of making a complete Resuci Anne for CPR, capable of being used to practise artificial ventilation and external chest compressions.

His natural interest in developing more equipment for first aid was coupled with a unique ability to understand specialists and teach them the technical and commercial possibilities and limitations.

In addition to the new Resuci Anne, a series of other products were developed. A Resusci Baby was produced (Fig. 10). A proposal from James Elam resulted in the Resusci Folding Bag with a new type of valve based on the 'duck bill' principle. The Arrhythmia Anne came as a response to a suggestion by Archer Gordon in 1969, the same year as the introduction of the Pocket Mask to protect the rescuer, and the Vacuum Mattress to protect the patient.

The disaster kit followed. Lærdal had always harboured an inherent and overwhelming desire to help his fellow man and he gave his whole hearted support to the emerging special interest in disaster medicine. He supported the Club of Mainz, subsequently to become the World Association for Emergency and Disaster Medicine, and later was created an Honorary Member of that organisation in recognition of his immense contribution.

In 1971, the Recording Resusci Anne was introduced, equipped with a printer giving instant feed-back to the

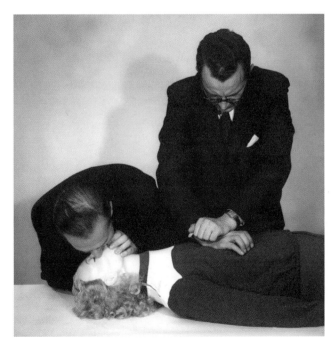

Fig. 9. Resusci Anne from Lærdal Medical in the United States.

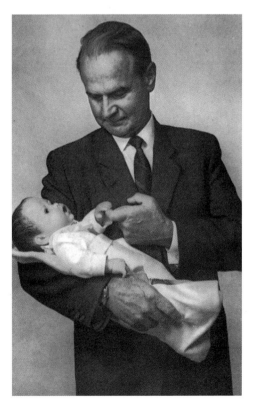

Fig. 10. Åsmund Lærdal with Resusci Baby.

trainee and at the same time providing important information about the efficiency of the training, and possible areas of improvement in the manikin.

Within 2 years, all objections in the U.S. had been overcome. The American Heart Association (AHA) recommended the teaching of CPR to all lay persons, and Lærdal helped to disseminate this recommendation, covering the cost of publishing a supplement to the Journal of the American Medical Association in 1974 [7]. In total, around 5 million copies were distributed. Lærdal provided support for the publication of all five subsequent revisions of the guidelines.

At home efforts went into developing a life-saving kit in the shape of a cushion for cars, complete with equipment and a self-training programme—yet another product that had been developed in close cooperation with physicians.

In 1978, Lærdal felt that his company had reached a crossroads. Toys had remained on the agenda. Over 100 million Tomte cars were spread around the world, and these cheap toys were still selling well. But Lærdal decided to concentrate all efforts on saving lives. Characteristically, this suited the spirit of the company—but it was also a wise policy for manufacturing in high-cost Norway.

The company's own presses continued to print information material for the medical sector in 15 languages, among them Chinese, Arabic and Russian.

Åsmund Lærdal always kept a very low profile in his home town. But having been highly respected in specialist circles, this modest, unassuming man came into the highlight himself. In 1978, he became the first non-physician to receive the International Award of the AHA. The same year he became an Honorary member of both the British Association for Immediate Care and the Norwegian Society of Anaesthesiologists. He was also honoured by the University of Pittsburgh.

By 1979, Lærdal was the established market leader, exporting 95% of the output from several production lines. Now he decided to channel some of his profits into a new foundation for acute medicine. The Lærdal family has continued to make grants to the Foundation so that the funds today represent more than 10 times the original capital of 10 million kroner. The Lærdal Foundation for Acute Medicine has funded a prodigious number of research projects and educational initiatives including several Utstein Guidelines meetings. Resuscitation Councils also have reason to grateful to this philanthropic Foundation for support in their creation and their ongoing activities.

But Åsmund Lærdal's time was running out. He died in Stavanger in November 1981. "We are links in chains, some strong, some weak. What counts is the overall plan". "Without Åsmund Lærdal, CPR would never have been implemented so rapidly and so widely", wrote Peter Safar at his death.

Time had come for the epitaph of this soft-spoken enigma of a man. Sensitive and generous, understanding, humble, and at the same time demanding and unshakably stubborn. Who made enormous demands on himself and his collaborators, and yet, recognizing his own limitations, harboured a deeply felt concern for the weaknesses of others. He was an unusual listener, and never spoke ill of anyone.

"The strangest man I have met in my life" wrote one of his closest collaborators. "The most modest and most immodest person I have known", declared another.

He had a deep sense of duty. Given his abilities, it was his duty to make the best possible use of them. One needs to dig to the bottom of the problem, and then dig underneath the bottom, he said. But he also had the lateral thinker's capacity for the daring leaps that are necessary for innovation.

With all of this, Åsmund S. Lærdal was a very private man. "Millions have been influenced by Lærdal's products, thousands by his thoughts. But only a privileged few by the twinkle in his piercing, loving blue eyes" wrote Peter Safar [8]—about his brother, who never stopped caring for 'hearts that are too good to die'.

## Acknowledgements

Figures 2–7 are taken from the book 'From Stavanger with Care' by Nina Tjomsland published by Lærdal. They are reproduced here with permission.

## References

[1] Safar P, Elam J. Manual versus mouth to mouth methods of artificial respiration. Anesthesiology 1958;19:111–2.

[2] Safar P, Escarraga L, Elam J. A comparison of the mouth to mouth and mouth to airway methods of artificial respiration with chest pressure arm lift methods. New Eng J Med 1958;258:671–7.

[3] Lind B. Teaching mouth to mouth resuscitation in primary schools. Acta Anaes Scand Suppl 1961;3:63–6.

[4] Poulson H, editor. International Symposium on Emergency Resuscitation. Stavanger, Norway, 1960, Acta Anaes Scand 1961;9:Suppl.

[5] Kouwenhoven WB, Jude JR, Knickerbocker CG. Closed chest cardiac massage. J Am Med Assoc 1960;173:1064–7.

[6] Jude JR, Kouwenhoven WB, Knickerbocker CG. Cardiac arrest: report of application of external cardiac massage in 118 patients. J Am Med Assoc 1961;178:1063–71.

[7] American Heart Association and the National Academy of Sciences—National Research Council. Standards for Cardiopulmonary Resuscitation (CPR) and Emergency Cardiac Care (ECC), J Am Med Assoc 1974;Suppl. 227:xii–xiv.

[8] Safar P. In Memoriam Åsmund Lærdal 1913–1981, J World Assoc Emerg Disaster Med 1985;1:Suppl. 1.

# Friedrich Wilhelm Ahnefeld

## Wolfgang F. Dick

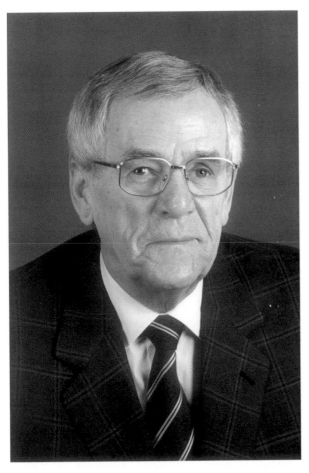

Whenever the '*Chain of Survival Concept*' or the '*Rescue Chain Concept*', the original name of the concept in Germany (1966-[1]) are mentioned, the name Friedrich Wilhelm Ahnefeld (FWA) invariably comes to mind [5]. Born on 12 January 1924 in Berlin, he spent his childhood and formative years there before going on to university in Poznan. No sooner had he begun his course of studies there than he was called into the German army and sent to the eastern front where he was severely injured. At the end of the war he was able to continue with his medical curriculum, first in Münster and later in Düsseldorf. With many young medical students returning from the battlefield and eager to continue their studies, medical schools were hopelessly over-crowded at that time. Ahnefeld soon found that the only chance to be accepted at university and to continue his medical studies, was by taking a somewhat different route. On learning that the catholic and protestant churches were looking for students to be trained for medical missionary work, he enrolled at the protestant faculty of theology of the University of Münster instead. But luck was on his side, and after only a short time he was able to get into medical school. Fortunately for medicine, this opportunity arose before he was able to think seriously about giving his life an entirely different direction as a clergyman.

For the final part of his undergraduate medical curriculum he enrolled at the Medical Academy of Düsseldorf, where he passed his medical examination and was later awarded a doctor's degree for his thesis on a topic which already reflected an early interest in emergency medicine. In order to do research on this topic, he joined a pharmacological working group at the company IG Farben-Werke, Wuppertal, headed by the famous pharmacologist Helmut Weese, the developer of Evipan (Hexobarbital), one of the first short-acting i.v. barbiturates used in anaesthesia.

After obtaining his doctoral degree, he applied to the Friedrich-Krupp Hospital in Essen and the Bergmann-sheil Hospital in Bochum, in order to study with one of the most famous surgeons of the time, Professor Bürkle de la Camp; training in surgery was then still customary for young trainee doctors, even for those wishing to specialise in anaesthesia. On graduating as a specialist in surgery he had already demonstrated a growing interest in intensive care medicine and, in particular, in the intensive care treatment of burn patients. This interest gave repeated impetus to a large number of clinical and experimental investigations at various institutions during his scientific career. These included animal experiments on the use of local therapeutics and their role in the development of organ failure in the treatment of burns, and the influence of colloidal volume replacement on the water and electrolyte balance in burn patients. Other investigations focussed on the improvement of the application of local therapeutics and local antibiotics to burned tissue, while studies on colloidal volume replacement solutions continued to be one major focus of Ahnefeld's scientific work.

At that time military hospitals still had the broadest experience in the treatment of burn patients, a reason why Friedrich Ahnefeld joined the Military Hospital in Koblenz in 1958, and soon thereafter the Department of Anaesthesiology in Mainz, where Rudolf Frey was appointed chairman in 1960. 'FWA' became one of the first trainees of Rudolf Frey.

In 1964 Friedrich Ahnefeld graduated as a specialist in anaesthesia and qualified as a university lecturer at the Faculty of Medicine of the University of Mainz on successful completion of his postdoctoral thesis titled 'Shock in burn patients, Clinical and experimental investigations'. The study of different aspects of shock remained one of Ahnefeld's major scientific interests throughout his clinical career.

A further scientific focus had already become apparent in his work during that period, i.e. the study of infusion therapy and parenteral nutrition. His fascination with this topic lead him to join the famous Institute of Physiological Chemistry of the University of Mainz to study under Professor Lang, an internationally recognised expert in the field. Infusion therapy and parenteral nutrition remained at the centre of his scientific interest in future years. In Mainz he began to concentrate in particular on the 'political' aspects of emergency medicine, and initiated studies aimed at improving and standardizing the frequently inadequate technical equipment of ambulances and mobile life support units, leading to the development of official standards (DIN) for ambulances, mobile life support units, doctors kits, etc.

An intense awareness of the need for the reorganisation of the emergency medical services in Germany has remained a matter of vital concern for him until today. Investigations into the improvement of lay training in first aid and resuscitation, on the adequacy or inadequacy of training programmes for emergency medical technicians (EMTs) and paramedics have given rise to much debate in the scientific community. However, the training concept for EMTs co-developed by Ahnefeld in this context was implemented by federal legislation as late as 1990.

The University of Ulm was founded in 1967, and it was only a year later when Ahnefeld left the Military Hospital in Koblenz and the department in Mainz for his new post as Chief of Anaesthesia at the Military Hospital in Ulm, a clinical teaching hospital at the new university. At the same time, he was also appointed Chairman of the Department of Anaesthesiology of the University Hospital. The focus of his scientific work in Ulm was initially on obstetric anaesthesia. He was primarily involved in the clinical work of the department of Obstetrics and Gynaecology there, where the chief, Professor Karl Knörr, and his staff encouraged and welcomed clinical cooperation with specialist colleagues in anaesthesiology. It was, however, not long until this example was followed by all surgical disciplines, after 'FWA' had convinced even those department heads who were less readily persuaded than others that anaesthesia was not only for the benefit of the patient, but also in the interest of the responsible clinicians.

When Ahnefeld also was appointed Chief of the Department of Anaesthesiology of the Municipal Hospital of Ulm, he carried the responsibility for three positions. At different times in the future he served as Dean of the clinical faculty of medicine, and was further appointed medical director of the entire university hospital (Around that time—in 1971—I had the pleasure of joining the department, working there until 1983).

The growing importance of anaesthesia for the various joint ventures and institutions led the university formally to establish a professorial chair of anaesthesiology, which was held by Ahnefeld following an academic election procedure in 1973. Among his many medical administrative posts, the position of medical superintendent of the German Red Cross for a period of 3 years during the time of the Vietnam war led him—as the person responsible for medical operations of the Red Cross Hospital Ship Cap Helgoland—to a variety of places in South Vietnam.

FWA gave a memorable demonstration of his organisational talents during the term as president of the German Society of Anaesthesia and Intensive Care Medicine, when he organised one of the most widely recognised and attended annual congresses in Wiesbaden in 1984, whose innovative programme attracted vast numbers of colleagues from all German speaking countries.

Despite a multitude of commitments and obligations, he continued and intensified his studies on the treatment of burn patients, and extended his efforts to the investigation of the controversially discussed administration of crystalloids vs. colloids in the prehospital treatment of emergency patients. Together with his research group he demonstrated conclusively that on-scene resuscitation (including intubation and stabilisation) of trauma patients improves outcome after trauma compared with the load-and-go concept. To give a full account of all of Ahnefeld's interests and concerns, would require the addition of a great number of additional accomplishments to this list—those mentioned here represent only a few of the scientific endeavours associated with the name of Friedrich Wilhelm Ahnefeld.

Since the early seventies, emergency medicine has constituted a compulsory part of the medical curriculum in Germany. It was first made an integral part of all training courses for medical students in basic and advanced measures of cardiac resuscitation, trauma care, etc. and was later also offered in the form of a practical course on the assessment and treatment of comprehensive medical emergencies. Throughout his career Ahnefeld has been committed to the idea of integrating emergency medicine into the curriculum and the clinical practice of anaesthesiology. His efforts have contributed to making it the one of the main responsibilities of anaesthesia to provide training in various aspects of emergency medicine to medical students in Ulm, Mainz, and at a number of other universities. While this concept has attracted many medical students to anaesthesia, induced young physicians to specialise in anaesthesiology and to become emergency physicians, it has not always been readily realised. Various university anaesthesia departments in Germany initially did not accept, and even opposed the innovative ideas of Ahnefeld and others.

Ahnefeld officially retired from his chair at the University of Ulm in 1992, but he has nevertheless continued to actively work in different functions, e.g. as the general secretary of the German Society of Anaesthesia and Intensive Care Medicine, or as the official advisor to eastern German universities on behalf of the government of the state of Baden-Württemberg after the unification of Germany etc. As the organiser of various workshops he took a firm stand on various important political issues. For instance, one workshop dedicated to an evaluation of the present and future needs of emergency medicine in Germany has led to the publication of a keystone paper on the documentation and development of emergency medicine in the 1990s [3]. Another initiative just 2 years ago was dedicated to the 'requirements of drugs and equipment of emergency medical services system (EMSS)' [2]. Even after he finished his work as the general secretary of the German Society of Anaesthesiology he still served on various committees, primarily related to the standardisation of equipment, the realisation of training programmes for EMTs and paramedics, and the development of EMSS in Germany [4].

Although Friedrich Wilhelm Ahnefeld celebrated his 78th birthday in January 2002, his keen interest in many medical, societal and political developments in health care, and particularly in the development of emergency medicine remains undiminished. Intensity has always been an integral part of his personality. It is, in fact, impossible to imagine him without continuous involvement, a multitude of different interests, and a lively creativity which brings forth new ideas and finds ways of realising them. The interest generated by his thought-provoking ideas and activities extends beyond the scientific community, and he has received the highest honours and recognition for his work. Among these are the Order of the Federal Republic of Germany by the Federal President of Germany, the Ernst von Bergmann Medal of Honour for his contributions to education and training of doctors in emergency medicine by the German Medical Council, the honorary doctoral degree of the Semmelweis-University Budapest in 1991, for assisting the Hungarian authorities in establishing an EMSS tailored to the needs of their country, and the Rudolf Frey Medal of the German Society of Anaesthesiology and Intensice Care medicine.

In addition to these honours, he was awarded honorary membership of the University of Ulm, the Germany Society of Anaesthesiology and Intensive Care Medicine, the European Resuscitation Council, and the German Interdisciplinary Association of Intensive Care and Emergency Medicine (DIVI).

The development of emergency medicine—not only in Germany—would hardly have been possible without the innumerable scientific, political and personal contributions made by FWA. It is wished and hoped by all concerned that his sustained emphasis on and involvement in emergency medicine may continue, even in the face of sometimes frustrating disappointments. Especially in view of the fact that it was FWA who spurned us on when frustration made us consider to halt our efforts, reminding us to look at what, in fact, had already been achieved, and to count our successes instead of the mishaps.

We cordially wish him many more years of good health spent with his wife, children and a growing number of grandchildren.

## References

[1] Ahnefeld FW, Schröder E. Preparations for disasters from a medical view(Rettungskette). Medicine et Hygiene 1966;24:1084.
[2] Dick WF Ahnefeld FW (Ed.) Ambulance equipment(German). Rescue Service Series of the Institute of Rescue Service of the German Red Cross 1999:22;1–227.
[3] Ahnefeld FW, Dick W, Schuster HP. Physicians responsibilities in German EMSS (German). Emergency Medicine (German) 1995;21:165–9.
[4] Ahnefeld FW, Knuth P. In: Dick WF, editor. Logbook of emergency medicine algorithms and checklists (German), 2nd ed.. Springer, 1999.
[5] Dick WF. Citation for Friedrich Wilhelm Ahnefeld, M.D., Dr.h.c. for Honorary Membership of the European Resuscitation Council. Resuscitation 28(1994) 179–180.

# Frank Pantridge and mobile coronary care

Thomas F. Baskett   Peter J.F. Baskett

In the mid 1960s, Frank Pantridge reflected on the appalling mortality following myocardial infarction, noting that most deaths occurred within 12 h of the onset of symptoms and the majority within 3 h. A study in Belfast had shown that the mean interval between the onset of symptoms and admission to hospital was 12 h [1]. From the 1950s, it had been recognized that sudden death associated with myocardial infarction was usually due to ventricular fibrillation. Furthermore, it had already been shown that ventricular fibrillation could be treated effectively by providing an electric shock to the heart through the intact chest [2].

Studies in Australia, UK and US had shown that the survival from cardiac arrest after myocardial infarction in general medical wards was poor; 5–10%, [3,4] whereas the mortality was reduced 5–7-fold, when these patients were admitted to intensive care units [5,6]. Putting these facts together, Pantridge concluded logically that the most effective way to reduce mortality was to provide intensive care facilities at the earliest opportunity for patients suffering myocardial infarction. Working with his senior house officer of the time, John Geddes, they established a mobile resuscitation team of nurses and junior medical staff within the Royal Victoria Hospital, Belfast in 1964. They found that when cardiac arrest occurred in an intensive care area of the hospital, the survival was 62%, but when arrest occurred in the general medical ward or casualty department, it was 31% [7]. As they said; 'the object of this report is to indicate that with adequate nursing instruction and a highly mobile resuscitation team, the chance of successful treatment, outside an intensive care unit, of cardiac arrest in patients with ischaemic heart disease, should be reasonably good' [7]. In the summary of this report they stated 'a highly mobile resuscitation team, operating over a wide area within the confines of a large general hospital, will save over a third of patients, who have a cardiac arrest after myocardial infarction'.

The results of this study led them to the conclusion; 'since the majority of deaths from cardiac arrest happen immediately after the onset of infarction, a mobile resuscitation team should be able to reach the patient in his own home'. It is briefly mentioned at the end of this article that; 'since January 1, a 'flying squad' based at this hospital, has been in action' [7].

The following year, they reported on the first 15 months experience with a mobile intensive-care unit in the management of myocardial infarction in the community (Fig. 2) [8]. They described the function of the mobile intensive care unit as follows:

'The mobile intensive-care unit consists of an ambulance, which carries routine monitoring and resuscitation equipment including a battery-operated D.C. defibrillator and bipolar pacing catheters. The personnel are found from the staff of the cardiac department. The signal from the general practitioner is given priority at the hospital telephone switchboard and immediately transmitted to the duty registrar or houseman and to ambulance control. The team proceeds with all possible speed to the patient. When the ambulance has arrived, the patient is immediately under intensive care. Monitoring and therapy in the patient's home may be required, before a stable rhythm is established. When it is considered safe, the patient is transferred to the ambulance and monitored continuously during transport to hospital. Haste or fuss during transit, are carefully avoided. The mobile unit is available to a population of approximately half-a-million in the Belfast area. About 100 000 live within a one-mile radius of the hospital [8].

Of 312 patients admitted to hospital with a suspected diagnosis of coronary thrombosis, none died in transit and ten were successfully resuscitated outside the hospital. This was in contrast to a study 2 years before in the same population, which showed that 102 of 414 patients brought to hospital were dead on arrival [8].

Pantridge and Geddes presented these results to the Association of Physicians of Great Britain and Ireland which met in Belfast on May 19, 1967. They received a cool reception, as Pantridge was

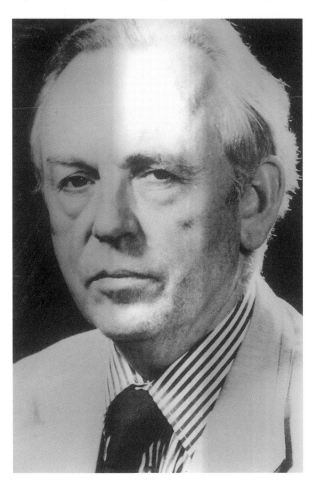

Fig. 1. Frank Pantridge [9].

The Lancet · Saturday 5 August 1967

### A MOBILE INTENSIVE-CARE UNIT IN THE MANAGEMENT OF MYOCARDIAL INFARCTION

J. F. PANTRIDGE
M.C., M.D. Belf., F.R.C.P.
PHYSICIAN-IN-CHARGE

J. S. GEDDES
M.D., B.Sc. Belf.
REGISTRAR

CARDIAC DEPARTMENT, ROYAL VICTORIA HOSPITAL, BELFAST 12

**Summary** The risk of death from myocardial infarction is greatest in the twelve-hour period after the onset of symptoms. Despite this, the hospital admission of a large proportion of patients is delayed for more than twelve hours, and many die in transit to hospital. A scheme has been described involving the use of a highly mobile unit which enables intensive care to reach the patient when he is at most risk. The unit has been used in the transfer of patients to hospital. No death has occurred in transit in a fifteen-month period. Ten examples of successful resuscitation outside hospital are reported. 5 of these patients are now alive and well. Thus it has been shown perhaps for the first time that the correction of cardiac arrest outside hospital is a practicable proposition.

Fig. 2. Title page of mobile intensive care unit paper.

later to describe 'we were disbelieved and indeed, to some extent, ridiculed. The unfavorable comments emphasized the lack of need for prehospital coronary care, the prohibitive costs and the danger to moving a patient who had a recent coronary attack' [9].

Though the attitude of physicians and administration in the UK to Pantridge was unenthusiastic, and pervaded by a 'cannot do' mentality (except for a few enlightened individuals such as Douglas Chamberlain in Brighton [10] and a team in Bristol [11]), the reception in the outside world was in sharp contrast. 'Immediate countershock' was the title of a leading article in Time Magazine in September 1967 [12] which observed that the sophisticated hospital coronary care unit was of little benefit, if one in four patients were dead on arrival. How much better it would be, if intensive care skills and equipment could be brought early to the patient in the community.

Leaders in US were quick to appreciate Pantridge's concept of prehospital coronary care and mobile units were set up by William Grace in New York [13] and Eugene Nagel in Miami [14] in 1968, by Leonard Cobb in Seattle in 1970 [15] and Richard Crampton in Charlottesville in 1972 [16]. Pantridge received accolades and honours galore in US, including a citation in the records of the House of Representatives — while at home in UK, the physicians did not offer official support until 1975 and the Department of Health dithered until the 1980s when Sir Donald Acheson, another Ulsterman by birth, became Chief Medical Officer in the UK.

Some idea of the creativity and common sense behind the whole operation comes from Pantridge's description in his autobiography *An Unquiet Life*; [9]

'The problem of dealing with the coronary victim outside hospital was that all available defibrillators were designed for use in hospitals. They operated from the mains electrical supply. What we needed was a portable defibrillator. In the winter of 1965, Alfred Mawhinney, a technician, John Geddes, a senior house officer and I converted a mains machine to operate from two 12-V car batteries through a static invertor, which converted the battery DC to 230 AC required by the defibrillator. The apparatus weighed some 70-kg and could hardly be described as portable. Nonetheless, patients could be defibrillated inside the ambulance and the machine could be manhandled into a patient's home. We obtained an old ambulance to carry the converted defibrillator, the drugs and other requirements normally available in a hospital coronary care unit. Trained personnel, a junior doctor and a nurse travelled in the ambulance. The unit went into action on January 1, 1966, … .A grant of £2300 from the British Heart Foundation financed the operation of the unit for the first year.'

Frank Pantridge was born in Hillsborough, County Down, Northern Ireland on October 3, 1916. After schooling in Hillsborough and the nearby market town of Lisburn, he started medicine at the Queen's University of Belfast in 1934. He qualified in medicine in the summer of 1939. In his final clinical medical examination, he made a diagnosis of pleural effusion but was told by the examiner that he was wrong; it was a case of pneumonia. Failure in this case would have cost Pantridge the entire examination. Convinced that he was right, he returned to the hospital that evening, performed a pleural tap, and took the resultant fluid from the effusion to the house of the Professor of Medicine to ensure that his correct diagnosis was acknowledged. He passed with honours. On August 1, 1939 he became a house physician in the Royal Victoria Hospital, Belfast. War was declared on September 3, 1939 and the following day Pantridge was among 11 of the 13 house officers at the Royal Victoria Hospital, who volunteered at the local recruiting office. He was posted to Malaya, as medical officer to the 2nd Battalion, The Gordon Highlanders (Fig. 3). He remained with the battalion during the Japanese invasion of Malaya and the ultimate fall of Singapore. During this campaign, Pantridge was awarded the military cross (MC) — a high honour rarely won by doctors in the field. The citation to support this award reads; 'during the operations in Johore and Singapore … as medical officer attached to the 2nd Gordons, this officer worked unceasingly under the most adverse conditions of continuous bombing and shelling and was an inspiring example to all with whom he came in

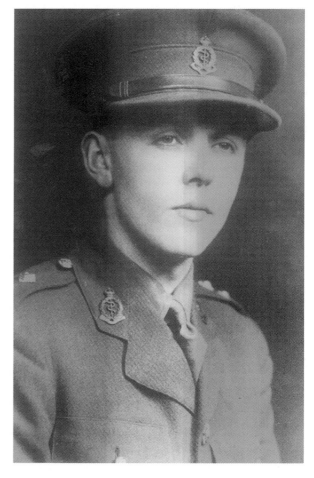

Fig. 3. Photograph of Frank Pantridge, 1939 [9].

282

contact. He was absolutely cool under the heaviest fire and completely regardless of his own personal safety at all times.

He was to survive the horror as a prisoner of war and medical officer in the slave labour camp of the Siam-Burma railway, and was one of the few to emerge from the infamous Tambayla Death Camp. Upon liberation, he was described by a fellow medical officer as follows; 'I found Pantridge in one of the many huts...The upper half of his body was emaciated, skin and bones. The lower half was bloated with the dropsy of berri berri. The most striking thing were the blue eyes that blazed with defiance. He was a physical wreck but his spirit was obviously unbroken. The eyes said it was indestructible...' He weighed just under 80 lbs.

After the war, Pantridge returned to Northern Ireland, 'God's own country' as he called it, and completed his houseman's year. He quickly acquired his MD and MRCP. He gained a scholarship to work at the University of Michigan with Frank Wilson, who was the world leader in electrocardiography at that time. He also acquired a good knowledge of electronics, which was invaluable in his development of the defibrillator in the 1960s. He returned to Belfast in 1949 and was appointed consultant physician in 1951. At that time, he only had six beds. Ultimately, he was to have 80 patients under his care in the Royal Victoria Hospital.

Pantridge's creation of a pre-hospital coronary care service in 1966 in Belfast, inspired others in the province to emulate him in Ballymena. Comparison with a similar town, Omagh, which at the time did not have a mobile coronary care unit, showed greatly improved mortality and morbidity in Ballymena [17]. Pantridge also showed that infarct size could be limited by early control of the autonomic disturbances in cardiac ischaemia [18] and that an initial shock 200 J from a monophasic defibrillator seemed to represent the best balance between successful conversion to a perfusing rhythm and the potential for myocardial damage [19].

One of his major contributions was to design and develop the first small portable defibrillator for use in prehospital care and within hospitals, making early defibrillation a much more practical proposition (Fig. 4).

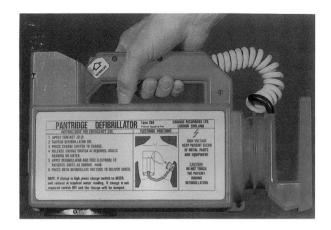

Fig. 4. Photograph of the Partridge defibrillator [9].

Frank Pantridge was affectionately known as Frankie P and both the authors served under him as students and house officers (PJFB in 1958 and TFB in 1964). We are proud to have done so and also to have been present, when he received honorary membership of the European Resuscitation Council in 1994 [20]. One of us (TFB) started as a houseman (intern) in the Royal Victoria Hospital in August 1964. These were the early days of Pantridge and Geddes' attempt to apply 'properly organized resuscitation methods in the treatment of cardiac arrest' [7]. This entailed the establishment of a mobile resuscitation team within the Royal Victoria Hospital. As a new houseman, I remember John Geddes gathering us together for about 1 h, showing us the equipment trolley and going through the steps of resuscitation and defibrillation. After that, we just got on with it for the rest of our houseman's year. As we lived in the hospital every day and all day, we became quite good in a mechanical sort of way. Towards the end of my year, I was houseman to the Professor of Medicine, Graham Bull. During the morning ward round a woman who had been admitted the night before with a myocardial infarction arrested in the bed next to us. The nurses and I went to work in what was now a well-established routine, quickly applied CPR, and soon had the woman intubated and defibrillated. After we had her stabilized, Professor Bull, who had watched the whole process with some bewilderment, took me aside and said 'well done Baskett, that was quite impressive. But, if I should ever have a heart attack and cardiac arrest in your presence, promise me that under no circumstances will you subject me to resuscitation'. He was deadly serious. The patient was discharged home 2 weeks later.

Frank Pantridge always acknowledged the considerable contribution of John Geddes, now a Professor of Cardiology at the University of Manitoba, in the organization and establishment of resuscitation services and the mobile ambulance at the Royal Victoria Hospital [21,22]. Writing in his autobiography of the development of acute coronary care in Belfast Pantridge said; 'these might not have come about if, Dr John Geddes, now in Canada alas, had not been in the Cardiac Department of the RVH from 1964 to 1987' [9]. Coming from Frank Pantridge, this is the verbal equivalent of a standing ovation.

Some 30 years on, it is impressive that the defibrillator has evolved from the 70 kg device in the Belfast ambulance to an implantable device weighing only a few grams [23,24].

Indeed, Pantridge and Mirowski had discussed the future of defibrillation on a train journey they made together between Gent and Amsterdam on March 6, 1976 [25]. The following extract describing the gist of their conversation is taken from a paper by Pantridge and Wilson on the history of prehospital coronary care published in the Ulster Medical Journal in 1996 [25].

"One of us (JFP), therefore, suggested that if small cheap defibrillators had a fail-safe mechanism like the safety catch on a pistol, the layman might defibrillate. It was reasonable to assume that anyone capable of doing CPR could use a fail-safe defibrillator. The possibility of the development of such an instrument certainly existed since Mirowski had described an automatic defibrillator. The implantable defibrillator depended on picking up the cardiac rhythm from the tip of a catheter in the right ventricle. When ventricular fibrillation appeared, the apparatus automatically delivered a defibrillating shock. One of us (JFP) discussed with Mirowski the possibility of using his circuit to pick up the rhythm from the chest surface so that a defibrillator might be produced which would deliver a shock only when VF was present. Mirowski was adamant that it was impossible. Artefact he thought, would be the problem. JFP was unconvinced about the impossibility of a fail-safe defibrillator and after a prolonged discussion with Cobb (Seattle) he suggested a Foundation for Immediate Resuscitation (FIR). Cobb agreed to contact the defibrillator manufacturers. Thus, the automatic external defibrillator was born."

Early defibrillation is now recognized world wide as the single most important treatment in sudden cardiac death [26]. The provision of defibrillation has now moved on from the exclusive prerogative of doctors, nurses and ambulance personnel to public access programmes in aircraft, airports, rail stations, shopping malls, sporting meetings and crowd events.

For once, the UK is back in the lead with a Government project placing over 700 automated external defibrillators in key strategic places in the community [27].

We think Frankie P will approve.

## References

[1] Mittra B. Potassium, glucose and insulin in treatment of myocardial infarction. Lancet 1965;2:607–9.

[2] Zoll PM, Linenthal AJ, Gibson W, Paul MH, Norman LR. Termination of ventricular fibrillation in man by externally applied elective countershock. New Engl J Med 1956;254:727–32.

[3] Nachlas MM, Miller DI. Closed-chest cardiac resuscitation in patients with acute myocardial infarction. Am Heart J 1965;69:448–59.

[4] McNicol MW. The intensive care of patients with myocardial infarction. Practitioner 1966;196:209–14.

[5] Julian DG, Valentine PA, Miller GG. Disturbance of rate, rhythm and conduction in acute myocardial infarction. Am J Med 1964;37:915–27.

[6] Day HW. Effectiveness of an intensive coronary care area. Am J Cardiol 1965;15:51–4.

[7] Pantridge JF, Geddes JS. Cardiac arrest after myocardial infarction. Lancet 1966;1:807–8.

[8] Pantridge JF, Geddes JS. A mobile intensive-care unit in the management of myocardial infarction. Lancet 1967;2:271–3.

[9] Pantridge JF. An Unquiet Life: Memories of a Physician and Cardiologist. Antrim: Greystone Books, 1989.

[10] Chamberlain DA, White NM, Binning RA, Parker WS, Kimber ER. Mobile coronary care provided by ambulance personnel (abstract). Br Heart J 1973;35:550.

[11] Baskett PJF, Diamond AW, Cochrane DF. Urban mobile resuscitation; training and service. Br J Anaesth 1976;48:377–85.

[12] Immediate countershock. Time Magazine. New York: September 1967.

[13] Grace WJ, Chadbourn JA. The mobile coronary care unit. Dis Chest 1969;55:452–5.

[14] Nagel EL, Hirschmann JC, Meyer PW, Dennis F. Telemetry of physiologic data: an aid to fire rescue in a metropolitan area. Southern Med J 1968;61:598–601.

[15] Cobb LA, Conn RD, Samson WE, Philbin JE. Early experiences in the management of sudden death with a mobile intensive/coronary care unit. Circulation 1970;42(Suppl 3):144.

[16] Crampton RS, Stillerman R, Gascho JA, et al. Prehospital care in Charlottesville and Adbemarle County. Va Med Mon 1972;99:1191–6.

[17] Wilson C. Effect of a medically-manned mobile coronary care unit on community mortality. In: Geddes JS, editor. The Management of the Acute Coronary Attack. The Frank J. Pantridge Festschrift. London: Academic Press, 1986:39–50.

[18] Pantridge JF, Adgey AAJ, Geddes JS, Webb SW. The Acute Coronary Attack. New York: Grune and Stratton, 1975:29.

[19] Pantridge JF, Adgey AAJ, Geddes JS, Webb SW. The Acute Coronary Attack. New York: Grune and Stratton, 1975:67–71.

[20] Baskett PJF. Citation for Frank Pantridge. Resuscitation 1994;28:183–4.

[21] Geddes JS, editor. The Management Of The Acute Coronary Attack: The J. Frank Pantridge Festschrift. London: Academic Press, 1986.

[22] Eisenberg MS. Belfast leads the way. In: Life in the Balance. New York: Oxford University Press, 1997:203–18.

[23] Mirowski M. Prevention of sudden arrhythmic death with implanted automatic defibrillators. Ann Intern Med 1982;97:606–8.

[24] Moss AJ, Hall WJ, Cannon DS, et al. Improved survival with an implanted defibrillator in patients with coronary disease at high risk for ventricular arrhythmia. New Engl J Med 1996;335:1933–40.

[25] A history of prehospital coronary care. Pantridge JF, Wilson C. Ulster Med Journal 1996;65:168–73.

[26] International Resuscitation Guidelines 2000. Resuscitation 2000;46:1–3.

[27] Davies S. The first Government scheme of its kind ... Defibrillation in Public Places. ABC Heartstart Magazine. Published by British Heart Foundation, London. 2000; (12). p. 2–3.

# Brian Sellick, Cricoid Pressure and the Sellick Manoeuvre

Peter J.F. Baskett     Thomas F. Baskett

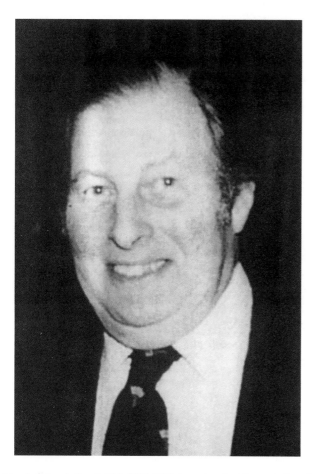

Fig. 1. Brian Arthur Sellick 1918–1996 (reproduced with permission of the Association of Anaesthetists of Great Britain and Ireland).

The induction of anaesthesia using either an intravenous barbiturate and muscle relaxant technique or an inhalational agent with a short-acting muscle relaxant are both fraught with the risk of regurgitation of stomach contents followed by pulmonary aspiration. Brian Sellick, an anaesthetist at the Middlesex Hospital, London, studied a potentially simple method of avoiding this regurgitation in the cadaver.

The manoeuvre consists in temporary occlusion of the upper end of the oesophagus by backward pressure of the cricoid cartilage against the bodies of the cervical vertebrae. In the cadaver it was found that when the stomach was filled with water and firm pressure was applied to the cricoid, as described below, a steep Trendelenburg tilt did not cause regurgitation of fluid into the pharynx. Moreover, the flow of water from the pharynx could be controlled by varying the pressure on the cricoid cartilage [1].

## Preliminary Communications

### CRICOID PRESSURE TO CONTROL REGURGITATION OF STOMACH CONTENTS DURING INDUCTION OF ANÆSTHESIA

WHEN the contents of stomach or œsophagus gain access to the air-passages during anæsthesia the consequences are disastrous. In spite of modern anæsthetic techniques—or sometimes, regrettably, because of them—regurgitation is still a considerable hazard during the induction of anæsthesia, particularly for operative obstetrics and emergency general surgery.[1-8]

By a simple manœuvre during induction of anæsthesia, regurgitation of gastric or œsophageal contents can be controlled until intubation with a cuffed endotracheal tube is completed. The same manœuvre may also be used to prevent inflation of the stomach (a potent cause of regurgitation) resulting from positive-pressure ventilation

1. De Lee, J. B., Greenhill, J. P. Principles and Practice of Obstetrics; p. 255. Philadelphia, 1951.
2. Mendelson, C. L. Amer. J. Obstet. Gynec. 1946, 52, 191.
3. Morton, H. J. V., Wylie, W. D. Anæsthesia, 1951, 6, 190.
4. Coleman, D. J., Day, B. L. Lancet, 1956, i, 708.
5. Edwards, G., Morton, H. J. V., et al. Anæsthesia, 1956, ii, 194.
6. Lancet, 1956, i, 734.
7. Rep. Publ. Hlth med. Subj., Lond. no. 97, 1957.
8. Reports on Confidential Enquiries into Maternal Deaths in England and Wales, 1952-54 and 1955-57. H.M. Stationery Office

Fig. 2. The Lancet 1961;2:404 (reproduced with permission).

The problem of regurgitation of acid stomach contents into the lungs was particularly dramatic in obstetric anaesthesia. The New York obstetrician, Curtis Mendelson, in a review of all cases at the New York Lying – in Hospital from 1932 to 1945 found an incidence of 1.5 per 1000 deliveries [2,3]. Acid aspiration, or Mendelson's syndrome as it came to be called, was a major cause of maternal death in the middle of the 20th century [4].

The anatomical rationale for Sellick's manoevure had previously been put forward previously by John Hunter in 1776 in his article *Proposals for the recovery of people apparently drowned* [5]. The essence of Hunter's treatment was 'blowing air into the lungs'. To ensure that air went into the lungs and not into the stomach he proposed the following: [5].

If during this operation the *larynx* be gently pressed against the *oesophagus* and spine, it will prevent the stomach and intestines being too much distended by the air, and leave room for the application of more effectual *stimuli* to those parts. This pressure, however, must be conducted with judgement and caution so that the *trachea* and the apparatus into the *larynx* may both be left perfectly free.

Sellick did not refer to Hunter's work so we do not know whether his own manoeuvre, aimed at preventing the opposite flow, from stomach to the airways, was inspired by Hunter's publication. As reported by Wilkinson [6], others, however, had noted Hunter's work. Charles Kite, of Gravesend in Kent, had noted that tracheal intubation was not a particularly easy technique but a nasal airway in conjunction with cricoid pressure was very effective [7]. James Curry, a general practitioner from Northampton, had formed his own society to "promote recovery from a state of apparent death" and had published a book on the subject which ran to two editions [8,9]. In these volumes his principle mission was to attempt to define the point of futility in attempting resuscitation but he also mentions the benefit of cricoid pressure in assisting with tracheal intubation so as to be able to administer the recently discovered "pure air or oxygen as the French chemists now call it [6]".

Sellick's description was simple and precise: [1].

During induction, the patient lies supine with a slight head-down tilt. The head and neck are fully extended (as in the position for tonsillectomy). This increases the anterior convexity of the cervical spine, stretches the oesophagus, and prevents its lateral displacement when pressure is applied to the cricoid......Cricoid pressure must be exerted by an assistant. The nurse or midwife accompanying the patient can be shown in a few seconds how to do it. Before induction the cricoid is palpated and lightly held between the thumb and the second finger; as anaesthesia begins, pressure is exerted on the cricoid cartilage mainly by the index finger. Even a conscious patient can tolerate moderate pressure without discomfort; but, as soon as consciousness is lost, firm pressure can be applied without obstruction of the patient's airway. Pressure is maintained until intubation and inflation of the cuff of the endotrachial tube is completed......During cricoid pressure the lungs may be ventilated by intermittent positive-pressure without risk of gastric distention.

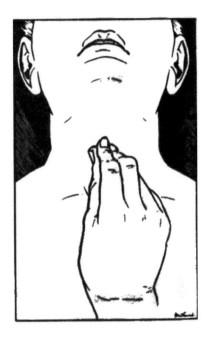

Fig. 3 The Sellick Manoeuvre for applying Cricoid Pressure (reproduced with kind permission of the Lancet 1961;2:404).

Sellick's manoeuvre has been adopted world wide in anaesthetic circles to reduce the risk of gastric regurgitation and pulmonary aspiration during rapid sequence induction of anaesthesia. The benefits are also clear during the resuscitation process and the technique has been advocated in airway management during resuscitation, including the most recent international guidelines, both to prevent gastric regurgitation and pulmonary aspiration, and to facilitate tracheal intubation [10].

Brian Arthur Sellick was born in Dorking, Surrey in 1918. A rugby football player of some note at school and medical school, he qualified in medicine from the Middlesex Hospital London in 1941. He went immediately into anaesthesia where there was a huge emergency workload arising from injuries inflicted by the Blitzkrieg on London. When asked how they coped with the phenomenal number of cases Brian replied "Well, the surgeons were much quicker in those days".

He was promoted to senior resident in anaesthesia at the Middlesex in 1942, passing the Diploma in Anaesthesia at the Royal College of Surgeons a year later. After service in the Royal Navy in the Oriental and Australian waters from 1944–1946, he returned to civilian life and was appointed as a member of the Honorary Consultant Anaesthetic Staff of the Middlesex Hospital and soon afterwards to Harefield Hospital and the Royal Masonic Hospital, also in London.

These posts did not carry any salary until the introduction of the National Health Service in 1948, so he also gave anaesthetics at the King Edward VIIth Hospital for Officers and at various sanatoria treating the epidemic of tuberculosis that followed the war [11,12].

Specialising initially in thoracic anaesthesia, he became drawn into cardiac anaesthesia in its very early days. He was impressed with the potential of hypothermia to allow a period of safe cardiac arrest to permit open heart surgery for relatively simple procedures such as repair of atrial secundum defects and correction of pulmonary and mitral stenosis. The technique of surface cooling to a core temperature of 30 °C, using ether and tubocurarine, that he developed after a visit to Swan and his colleagues at the University of Colorado proved to be highly effective. In his landmark paper, published in 1957, he reported the successful management of 32 cases without loss [13]. Ultimately the team at the Middlesex Hospital, using this technique, operated on over 400 patients with atrial secundum defects with only one death [11].

Brian Sellick took a very active role in the early days of academic anaesthesia at the Royal Society of Medicine and the Faculty (later to become the Royal College) of Anaesthetists, serving as Vice Dean there from 1972–1974. He received the Henry Hill Hickman Medal of the Royal Society of Medicine for his work on cricoid pressure. In the citation for that honour it was stated – .

"It is impossible to overestimate the benefit that this discovery has made to the safe conduct of anaesthesia, as it has undoubtedly saved many patients from serious post operative complications or death. Thirty years (now 43) years after its presentation, the technique is still in use world wide and has not been superseded by any other solution [11]".

Sellick's great contribution was also recognized by the award of the Gold Medal of the Royal College of Anaesthetists in 1989.

In his retirement in Devon in the southwest of England, he became chairman of the local conservation society, enjoyed the theatre and concerts and worked hard in his garden and at woodwork. He married Florence in 1943; they had three sons and ten grandchildren. He died suddenly in 1996 in his woodwork workshop.

"He was a happy and fulfilled man with a great sense of humour whose ready laughter was always full of glee" – so wrote Bill Pallister in his obituary of Brian Sellick [11].

On a personal note, one of us (PB), as an aspiring cardiac anaesthetist with an interest in resuscitation, remembers Brian as a humble and gentle, yet effective, person, always approachable and politely receptive to any modest (sometimes they were very modest indeed!) ideas one would have. He was a big man in every sense of the word, with a warm smile that has been captured in his photograph.

## References

[1] Sellick BA. Cricoid pressure to control regurgitation of stomach contents during induction of anaesthesia. Lancet 1961;2:404–6.

[2] Mendelson CL. The aspiration of stomach contents into the lungs during obstetric anaesthesia. Am J Obstet Gynecol 1946;52:1–205.

[3] Baskett TF. On the Shoulders of Giants: Eponyms and Names in Obstetrics and Gynaecology. London RCOG Press 1996; p. 147–8.

[4] Report on Confidential Inquiries into Maternal Deaths in England and Wales 1955–7. London: H.M. Stationary Office, 1959.

[5] Hunter J. Proposals for the recovery of people apparently drowned. Phil Trans R Soc Lond 1776;66:412–25.

[6] Wilkinson DJ. The development of resuscitation in the United Kindom. In: Atkinson RS, Boulton TB, editors. The History of Anesthesia. Pub Royal Society of Medicine Services and the Parthenon Publishing Company. London and New Jersey, 1989.

[7] Kite C. An essay on the recovery of the apparently dead. London 1788.

[8] Curry J. Popular observations on apparent death from drowning, hanging, suffocation etc with an account of the means to be employed for their recovery. Northampton, 1792.

[9] Curry J. Observations on apparent death from drowning, hanging, suffocation by noxious vapours, fainting fits, intoxication, lightning, exposure to cold, etc. and an account of the means to be employed for their recovery. London, 1815.

[10] The American Heart Association in collaboration with the International Committee on Resuscitation. Guidelines for Cardiopulmonary Resuscitation and Emergency Cardiac Care – A Consensus on Science. Resuscitation 2000;46(1–3):121.

[11] Pallister WK, Brian Arthur Sellick. (Obituary) Anaesthesia 1996;51:1194–5.

[12] Maltby JR. The Sellick Manoeuvre. In: Maltby JR, editor. Notable Names in Anaesthesia. London, RSM Press 2002; p. 196–8.

[13] Sellick BA. A method of hypothermia for open-heart surgery. Lancet 1957;1:443–6.

# Thomas Cecil Gray and Gordon Jackson Rees
# Major contributors to post-resuscitation care

John Ballance

The inclusion of these two great men in the roll of Resuscitation Greats comes about because of their contribution to post-resuscitation care. Before their work, ventilation was either spontaneous or 'assisted'. After the work with relaxants, ventilation could be completely controlled, and the patient allowed to recover in the best possible circumstances.

Professor Emeritus Thomas Cecil Gray was born on 11 March 1913, in a room above a public house in Scotland Road, Liverpool, where his father was the publican. He attended a preparatory school and then the famous Roman Catholic public school, Ampleforth College.

The latter was very influential in Cecil's life as he later became a novice monk there, for two months. Medicine, however, had a stronger influence and he enrolled as a student in the University of Liverpool. Thus began a long association with the University which saw the development of the techniques for which he is justly famous and his leading the Department of Anaesthetics and, later, the Medical School as Dean.

After his marriage and graduation in 1937, Cecil decided to become a General Practitioner and secured a partnership in a practice, later (1939) buying his own practice in Upper Parliament Street in Liverpool. The work entailed dispensing, surgeries and a domiciliary obstetric service in this poor and deprived area.

At the time, anaesthesia was administered by General Practitioners and other non-medically qualified staff and this single-handed practitioner decided to acquire some specialist knowledge. Accordingly, he attended the sessions of another famous General Practitioner and anaesthetist, RJ Minnitt. He was instructed on two afternoons a week by this prominent member of the Liverpool Society of Anaesthetists and shortly afterwards took the Diploma in Anaesthetics, which required the documentation of personal administration of 1000 anaesthetics.

On the outbreak of the Second World War, in September 1939, Cecil was turned down by the forces because of long-term asthma and so continued as a GP and part-time anaesthetist. As anaesthesia increased in importance as a speciality, he gave up the general practice aspect of the work and was appointed as a full time anaesthetist at the Northern General Hospital in Liverpool.

His persistence and desire to serve paid off, however, as he was accepted by the RAMC to work in a neurosurgical unit in North Africa as a Captain but was invalided home in 1944 after contracting bronchial pneumonia. Before this, Cecil describes the push up the desert to the sea by the 8th Army and the sight, as he crested the last dune, of most of the troops, senior officers and all, bathing stark naked in the Mediterranean.

Back in Liverpool, having recovered, Dr. Gray then proceeded to begin the pioneering work on curare, assisted by John (also known as Jack) Halton. John had two jobs—as anaesthetist to the thoracic surgical department at Clatterbridge Hospital and as a Medical Officer to the Royal Air Force. His latter employment put him in touch with the mess (social club) and doctors at the United States Air Force (USAF) base at Burtonwood near Warrington, Lancashire. Here, he learnt of the work of Harold Griffith in Montréal in using curare as a muscle relaxant, the first occasion being in January 1942, and the publication of a paper which popularised its use.[1]

Cecil and John persuaded the USAF to fly over some crude extract of *Chondrodendron tomentosum* which they put to use, initially experimentally on themselves, then on patients, realising that this South American arrow poison worked on the neuromuscular junction and could assist the surgeon by causing muscle relaxation.

Cecil's first experience of this was with a patient for abdominal surgery. Although the anaesthesia was described as 'lissive' (incomplete paralysis with assisted ventilation), the effect was "dramatic". When the initial supplies of the drug ran out, Curarine (d-tubocurarine chloride) was obtained from Doctor, later Professor, Rod Gregory, of the Physics Department in Liverpool University. This was a pure form of the alkaloid, with much more predictable effects.

Eventually, respiration was entirely controlled after an increase in the dose of the relaxant and reduction in the amount of the other anaesthetic agents (principally thiopentone and cyclopropane). The triad of light hypnosis, analgesia and relaxation was born. This Milestone in Anaesthesia was presented to the Royal Society of Medicine (RSM) on 1 March 1946 and was subsequently published in the Proceedings of the Society.[2]

It was, however, some years before the technique became universal and a paper published in 1949 outlined a more advanced technique using controlled respiration and reversal of paralysis, with prostigmine.[3] This spread into general use in the early 1950s.

After the award of an MD in 1947, Professor Gray went on, as Senior Lecturer, to head the newly formed academic Department of Anaesthesia in Liverpool, as Reader. He received considerable help from the Professor of Surgery, Charles Wells, and also from a newly appointed Demonstrator, Dr. Gordon Jackson Rees. 'Jack' or 'Jacko'

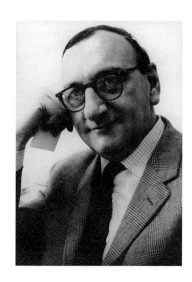

Fig. 1

adapted the Liverpool Technique for use in children, forming a department at Alder Hey Children's Hospital and teaching a basic method to thousands of national and international anaesthetists. The friendship between Jack and Cecil lasted for many years, until the former's death in 2001.

The name of Dr. Gordon Jackson Rees (Fig. 1) is inextricably linked with that of Cecil Gray because of their lifelong friendship and also by virtue of the involvement of Jacko at an early stage in the refinement of the 'Liverpool Technique' or triad.

Jack was born in 1918 and educated at Shrewsbury School. He entered the Liverpool University Medical School in 1937 and qualified in 1942. As this was wartime, he was soon called up as a Station Medical Officer in the Royal Air Force and then detached to the Radliffe Infirmary in Oxford, under Professor Sir Robert Macintosh and William Mushin.

Having acquired the Diploma in Anaesthetics in 1946, he was appointed as a consultant anaesthetist to the Royal Liverpool Hospitals and part-time Demonstrator in Cecil Gray's new department. With paediatric surgeon Isabella Forshall, he developed the use of the Liverpool Technique in paediatric anaesthesia. This pioneering work between surgeon and anaesthetist continued until she retired, in 1965. This combination produced much research in this field, taking a more humane approach to surgery in children and that surgery could not develop in the absence of first-rate anaesthesia.

Jack's innovations included the use of heavy premedication, the application, with muscle relaxation, of the 'triad of anaesthesia' to children and infants and the use of intravenous induction instead of the unpleasant open ether. A 1950 paper on neonatal anaesthesia heralded greatly improved results of surgery and the development of more complicated operations. This was so widely read that Jack was asked to travel extensively to demonstrate it.

The arrival of Peter Rickham in Liverpool heralded developments in neonatal anaesthesia and surgery, including thoracic and open-heart work, with cardiopulmonary bypass. Also included was some early work into the sensitivity of neonates to d-tubocurarine hydrochloride and the publication of the first textbook of paediatric anaesthesia.

Anaesthetists from across the world would beat a path to Alder Hey Children's Hospital in Liverpool to be taught a standard, safe technique for children. The author has first hand experience of this and can still squeeze the tail of a Jackson Rees modification to the Ayre's T-piece, while opening a glass ampoule with the other hand!

Jack Rees began his association with the Department of Anaesthetics in Liverpool in 1947, when he was appointed Part-time Demonstrator. He followed this by becoming Honorary Demonstrator, Honorary Lecturer, Honorary Lecturer in Paediatric Anaesthesia, Honorary Clinical Lecturer and, last, Honorary Director of Studies in Paediatric Anaesthesia.

During a long career, Jack was also appointed as Consultant Adviser to the Royal Navy and served a term as President of the Tri-service Anaesthetic Society, as well as being appointed to many Fellowships and Presidencies of august bodies.[4]

The Author has been influenced by Jack Rees and it was with joy that my last meeting with him was at an Association Dinner. Dr. Gordon Bush, Jack and I wandered back to their hotel where Gordon confessed his weariness and asked that I should not ''tire the old boy out!'' Nothing of the sort occurred, of course, and several whiskies later, the author retired in a weary state! This was reminiscent of another occasion when I had invited the great man to the annual meeting of the Association of Operating Department Practitioners, where he was mobbed by an adoring crowd.

Professor Gray was invited to be a founder member of the newly established Faculty of Anaesthetists of the Royal College of Surgeons in 1948 and was President of the Section of Anaesthetics of the Royal Society of Medicine in 1955. From 1957 to 1959, he was President of the Association of Anaesthetists of Great Britain and Ireland (AAGBI).

In 1959, Cecil was given a personal chair in Liverpool University and, after a time as Postgraduate Dean, became Dean of the Faculty of Medicine, holding this post until retirement.

A brilliant teacher and always approachable, Cecil has been a mentor and friend to the author and countless others. His front door in Formby, Lancashire is always open to the many who wish simply to meet or to interview him and a glass of gin will sometimes be proffered!

Cecil retired from anaesthesia and academia in 1976 but continues his attendance at functions of the AAGBI, as well as the Royal Society of Medicine and the Tri-Service Anaesthetic Society. In 2003, in Birmingham, the author was delighted to be asked to give the Cecil Gray Eponymous Lecture to this latter Society. I chose the title DTC, TCG and me, recalling the enormous amount of help afforded to me by this kind man and also because I knew his collaborator, John Halton, when he anaesthetised in the dental chair for my father, a dentist in Lancashire. Cecil sat in the front row and told me that I had acquitted myself well!

When Dean of the Faculty, Cecil was instrumental in setting up a meeting, in 1964, between members of the Council of the AAGBI and the Association of Operating Theatre Technicians. This began a long association between the AAGBI and Operating Theatre Technicians (OTT), later Operating Department Assistants (ODA) and Operating Department Practitioners (ODP). The AAGBI has, from that date, supported the registration of these colleagues and Cecil's drive has considerably assisted in this.

In January 1965, Cecil brought to the attention of Council the fund raising activity of the World Federation of Societies of Anaesthesiologists (WFSA) and encouraged funding of this organisation.

Over a long career, Cecil has published many papers and, in retirement, he has written a biography of the founder of the Liverpool School of Medicine.

Sadly, while at the Winter Scientific Meeting of the Association of Anaesthetists in January 2001, I was informed by an ODP colleague that Jack Rees had died, on the 19th at the age of 82. The afternoon began with a two minutes silence to recognise a great loss to the world of anaesthesia, to a life well lived but, sadly, cut short.

Happily, Professor Cecil Gray is still very much with us and continues to live in Formby, Merseyside, where he welcomes visitors from across the world. On 11 March 2003, many friends gathered in Formby for Cecil's 90th birthday party. Many tributes were given, as well as gifts. Perhaps the most interesting was a fake car number plate commemorating his research, made and presented by a grateful colleague. The plaque visible in the photograph (Fig. 2) reads:

*1846. Morton, WTG used the inhalation of ether vapour to prevent the agony of surgery.*

*1946. Gray, TC and Halton, JA established the use of d-tubocurarine chloride in general anaesthetic practice.*

*Two giant leaps for mankind.*

In 2003, on 19 March, the Sir Ivan Magill Medal of the AAGBI was awarded to Professor Gray, at the Anniversary Dinner of the Royal College of Anaesthetists, by Dr. Peter Wallace, President (Fig. 3).

The names of Thomas Cecil Gray and Gordon Jackson Rees are remembered by anaesthetists across the world. Their work on relaxants and the setting up of a system of anaesthesia, far better than what preceded, has benefited huge numbers of patients. We salute them here for their contribution to post-resuscitation care.

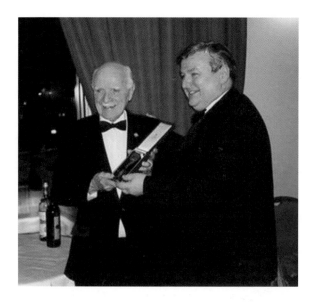

**Fig. 3**

## References

1. Griffith HR, Johnson GE. The use of curare in general anaesthesia. Anesthesiology 1942;3:418—20.
2. Gray TC, Halton J. A milestone in anaesthesia (d-tubocurarine chloride). Proc Roy Soc Med 1945-1946;39:400—10.
3. Gray TC. Modern anaesthesia. Transact Med Soc London 1949;65:80—7.
4. Bush GH. Obituary. Anaesthesia 2001;56(4):370—1.

## Further reading

Boulton TB, The Association of Anaesthetists of Great Britain and Ireland, 1932—1992.
Anaesthesia News 2003; No. 188: March.
Anaesthesia News 2003; No. 190: May.
Interviews with Dr. Max Blythe, Oxford, MSVA 138, 139, 144, 145, 164.
The Times Short Obituary, Dr. Jackson Rees, February 8, 2001.

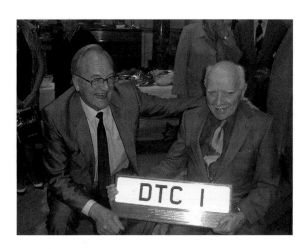

**Fig. 2** Cecil Gray presented with DTC 1 to mark his work with d-tubocurarine chloride.

# Bjørn Ibsen

## John Zorab

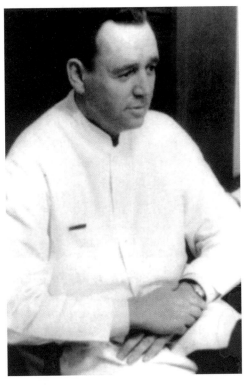

Fig. 1. Professor Bjørn Ibsen (by kind permission of Bjørn Ibsen).

## 1. Introduction

Bjørn Ibsen (Fig. 1) has been described as the father of intensive therapy as we know it today. This description is fitting, since his interests and contributions stretch far beyond the introduction of positive pressure ventilation in the management of poliomyelitis for which he is probably best known. Ibsen was born on 30th August, 1915 and graduated from the University of Copenhagen in January 1940. Two Danish surgeons, one of whom was Erik Husfeldt (Fig. 2) had taken up thoracic surgery and needed well-trained anaesthetists but none were available. Ole Lippmann (Fig. 3) was

director of a Danish firm selling medical instruments and he had visited the US and bought a McKesson anaesthetic machine (Fig. 4). It was Lippmann who, in 1939, gave the anaesthetic for Husfelt's first pneumonectomy [1]. That was also the year that Ibsen, as a medical student, gave his first anaesthetics. He had obtained a post in a provincial Danish hospital where he gave the majority of the anaesthetics. His equipment comprised a Wanscher bag filled with 100 ml of ether, a Young's tongue forceps and Heister's mouth-opener (Fig. 5). There was no oxygen, no tubes, no absorbers and no suction and even if there had been, Ibsen would not have known what to do with them. At that time in Denmark, anaesthetics were administered by anyone and everyone under the supervision and responsibility of the surgeon. It could be a nurse or even the surgeon's secretary. After graduation, Ibsen obtained a post in a provincial hospital in Jutland. Here, one of the practi-

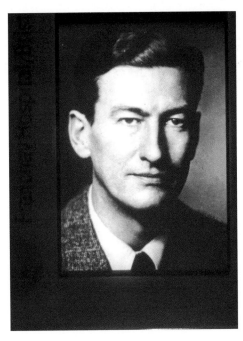

Fig. 2. Erik Husfeldt, thoracic surgeon and Director of the WHO course (by kind permission of Henning Ruben).

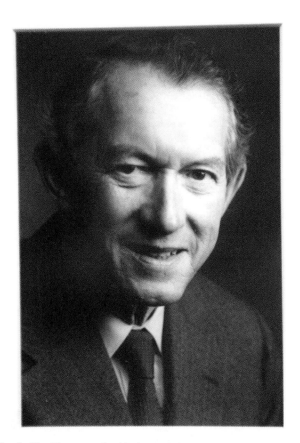

Fig. 3. Ole Lippmann (by kind permission of 'The Special Forces Club', London).

tioners in the city came and gave all the anaesthetics using an Ombrédanne inhaler. Later, Ibsen served in the departments of radiology, surgery, pathology and gynaecology. Eventually, he came to work in the department of chest surgery in the Rigshospitalet in Copenhagen (Fig. 6). It was here that he came to realise the essential role that the anaesthetist played in the surgeon's work. Thus it was, he decided to explore the possibilities of a future in anaesthesiology. To do this, however, it was necessary to look outside Denmark.

## 2. Massachusetts general hospital

On 1st February 1949, Ibsen started as assistant resident anaesthetist in the department of anaesthesia at the Massachusetts General Hospital (Fig. 7) under H.K. Beecher (Fig. 8). This presented him with a different world. Hospital organisation in Danish hospitals before World War II, as in most continental hospitals, resembled the old-fashioned Prussian system with the Professor at the top of a pyramid of all the other staff. It was quite an experience for Ibsen to come from the recently occupied Denmark to the Massachusetts General hospital. There seemed to be no shortage of money and the medical staff had almost complete

clinical freedom to do as they wished in whatever branch of medicine they wished. The background for all anaesthetic teaching was open-drop ether and all medical students were required to administer at least two inductions with open-drop ether. Because of some bad experiences with pentothal during the war, it was only permitted to administer the drug in 25 mg increments. The young American doctors expressed themselves freely and were much more self-assured than the Danish doctors in their hierarchical system. For foreign doctors, language was sometimes a problem. Ibsen recalls that a French anaesthetist who had come for training, worked for 3 months in a surgical department before the surgeons discovered that he had come for anaesthetic training! [1]. Postoperative complications were freely discussed but usually put down to 'bad luck' and, generally speaking, no anaesthetic records were kept. Nevertheless, for Ibsen, and for many before and after, the Massachusetts General provided an excellent training.

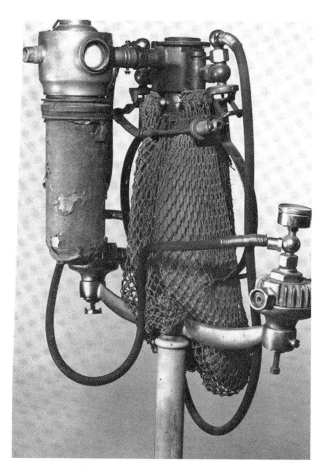

Fig. 4. McKesson anaesthetic machine (from K. Bryn Thomas, The Development of Anaesthetic Apparatus) (by kind permission of The Association of Anaesthetists of Great Britain and Ireland).

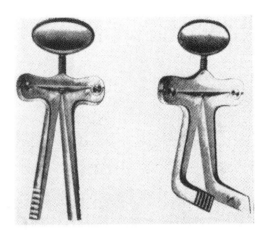

Fig. 5. Heister's mouth opener (from Sykes W.S. vol I, by kind permission of Churchill Livingstone). (Described by Sykes as a brutal instrument only suitable for removing refractory wheels from old railway trucks. A fearsome instrument of tremendous leverage).

## 3. The World Health Organisation (WHO) anaesthesiology training centre in Copenhagen

After his return from the Massachusetts General in 1950, Ibsen worked for the next 3 years at the Rigshospitalet in Copenhagen as a free-lance anaesthetist. There was an uneasy relationship with the surgeons and it was not always easy to persuade them of the anaesthetist's point of view. Ibsen relates a nice exchange when his surgeon once expressed the view that he could not see any difference between the Massachusetts General and Copenhagen. Ibsen's reply was 'I was away a year and I have been back 3 weeks. We talk about the Mass. General every day but, while I was away, we never mentioned the Rigshospitalet'! [1]. However, the WHO training course in anaesthesiology had started in 1950, initiated by the thoracic surgeon, Erik Husfeldt who became the Course Director, a position he held throughout the duration of these courses (1950–1973). Even so, at that time, the choice of anaesthetic was still not that of the anaesthetist but that of the surgeon and ether was still the preferred agent. Amongst the distinguished anaesthetists from overseas who came to teach on the first WHO course in 1950 were Stuart Cullen from Iowa City and Ralph Waters from Wisconsin. On one occasion, the surgeon was using cautery to open the chest during a cyclopropane anaesthetic, Cullen left the operating room. When the surgeon asked him later why he had left, Ibsen was instructed to say he had left because his insurance company would not cover that type of risk! But the WHO course was greatly appreciated by Ibsen and his colleagues and all those who attended as students or teachers. In Fig. 9, Cullen can be seen administering what was probably a cyclopropane anaesthetic using a British Oxygen Company (BOC) 'Centanaest' anaesthetic machine which they had donated to WHO.

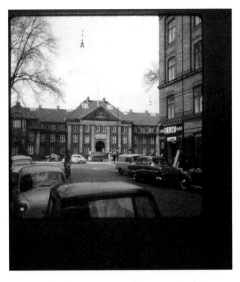

Fig. 6. Rigshospitalet entrance, Copenhagen (1965) (by kind permission of John Zorab).

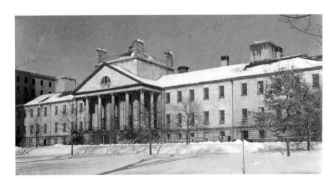

Fig. 7. Massachusetts General Hospital, Boston (by kind permission of the Wood Library Museum).

Both Ibsen and Secher have recorded their gratitude to Erik Husfeldt and to all who participated in these training courses, which took place at a time when anaesthesiology was virtually non-existent as a specialty. The names of those who came to Copenhagen to teach on the courses read like a 'Who's Who' in anaesthesia in the 1950s. Fuller accounts have appeared elsewhere [2,3]. Fig. 10 shows John Severinghaus and Henning Ruben attending one course and Fig. 11 shows the students on the 1953 course when Sir Robert Macintosh was among the instructors. Although not a formal instructor, the writer was both fortunate and proud to spend 3 months in Copenhagen at that time and, like others, made friendships that lasted throughout his professional life—including with Bjørn Ibsen.

## 4. The Copenhagen polio epidemic, 1952

However, in 1952 the terrible poliomyelitis epidemic struck Copenhagen. While at the Massachusetts General, Ibsen had observed patients being treated in a tank

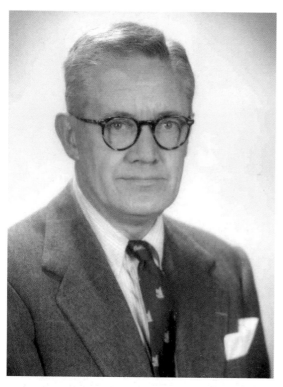

Fig. 8. H.K. Beecher, Director of Department of Anesthesia, Massachusetts General Hospital (by kind permission of the Wood Library Museum).

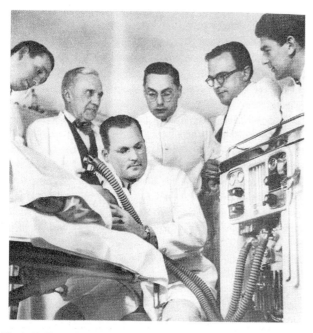

Fig. 9. B. Ibsen, R. Waters, S. Cullen, H. Ruben, W. Andersen and O. Secher at WHO course in Copenhagen (1950) (from Looking Back to Find the Future by Mona Frederiksen, by kind permission of the publishers).

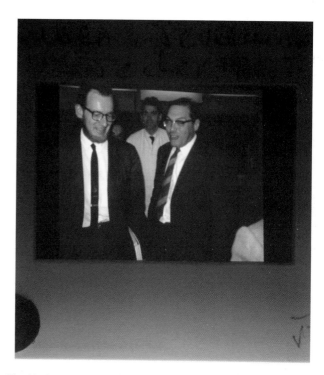

Fig. 10. J. Severinghaus, H. Ruben and O. Secher at WHO course (by kind permission of John Zorab).

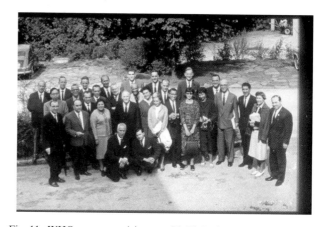

Fig. 11. WHO course participants with Sir Robert Macintosh (fourth from right) (by kind permission of John Zorab).

respirator (Fig. 12). After his return to Copenhagen, Ibsen was giving an inhalation anaesthetic 1 day to a patient who already had a tracheostomy and he realised how easy it was to ventilate a patient who already had a free airway. While Ibsen was at the Massachusetts General, Beecher did not allow the use of curarising agents so Ibsen had no experience of managing patients with respiratory paralysis. However, in 1950, Bower et al. [4] had published the results of their treatment of respiratory insufficiency in bulbar poliomyelitis. Within 3 years, the mortality was brought down from 88 to 20% by the early use of tank respirators. At the same time, in Europe, in Lubeck, a 10-year-old boy with poliomyelitis had been kept alive for 2 weeks with artificial ventilation by the Holger-Nielsen method, given by the doctors involved. At the start of the polio epidemic in Copenhagen in August 1952, Ibsen wrote to Bower and obtained a reprint of his article. When Ibsen was first called to the

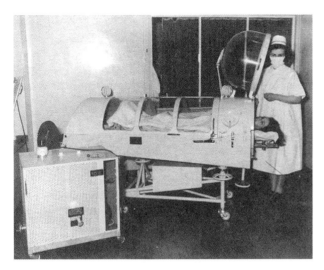

Fig. 12. Tank respirator (from the Proceedings of the First World Congress of Anaesthesiology) (by kind permission the International Anesthetic Research Society).

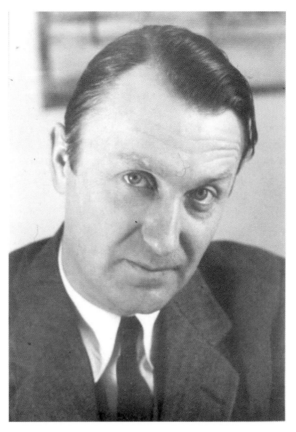

Fig. 13. H.C. Lassen, epidemiologist, Copenhagen, 1952 (by kind permission of Medinsk–historisk Museum, Copenhagen).

Blegdam Hospital in Copenhagen to see a polio patient with incipient respiratory paralysis, he quoted Bower's article and pointed out that some improvement in the patient's condition was possible by the use of a tank respirator. It was argued, however, that the reason why Bower's results were so good was that the patients were put into respirators very early and the improved ventilation helped to protect against pulmonary complications. Keeping the patient out of the tank respirator too long allowed pulmonary complications to develop with sometimes fatal results. At the outbreak of the epidemic, Copenhagen had one tank respirator and six cuirass respirators. But between 50 and 60 new patients were being admitted *every day*! Ibsen's first suggestion was to perform a tracheostomy. This was rejected on the grounds that it had been tried earlier in 17 consecutive patients, all of whom had died. Later, Lassen (Fig. 13) published a preliminary account of the epidemic [5] and reported that 2722 patients with poliomyelitis had been admitted to the Blegdam hospital, 866 with paralysis. In the first month of the epidemic, 31 patients were admitted with respiratory paralysis of whom 27 died and it was at this time that Ibsen was consulted. Copenhagen was in a state of siege. The following is an abbreviated quotation from a lecture given by Ibsen to the Section of Anaesthetics of the Royal Society of Medicine in London in May, 1953 [6].

*"In August 25 1952, I was called as anaesthetist for consultation by the epidemiologist, Professor Lassen. Within the preceding 3 weeks 31 patients with bulbar poliomyelitis and been treated in respirators-iron lungs as well as the cuirass. 27 had died. With enthusiastic encouragement from Lassen, I demonstrated, on a patient, how sufficient ventilation could be achieved without a respirator. The patient was a*

*12 year old girl with quadriplegia and atelectasis of the left lung. She was gasping for air, cyanotic and drowning in her own secretions. Using local anaesthetic, a tracheostomy was done immediately and a cuffed endotracheal tube put in place. During the procedure, she became unconscious. A to and fro absorption system was connected directly to the tube with good endotracheal suction. Even then it was impossible to inflate the lungs, partly due to the secretions and partly due to bronchospasm. In this desperate situation, I gave her 100 mg of pentothal in the hope that I could stop her struggling. She collapsed, her own respiration stopped and I found that I could now inflate her lungs"*

Ibsen continued his lecture by describing the patient's turbulent course with the development of hypovolaemic shock and a grossly raised $CO_2$. These problems were managed by manual ventilation and fluid infusion. An X-ray revealed that the atelectatic left lung had been completely inflated. The patient improved and was put back in the tank respirator. All the signs of underventilation returned and she became cyanotic. She was given oxygen and her colour improved but her $CO_2$ continued to rise. Manual ventilation improved her again. In this patient, manual ventilation had to be continued since the tank respirator did not provide adequate ventilation. This patient enabled Ibsen and Lassen to formulate the principles of treatment of bulbar poliomyelitis. This involved the mobilisation of all anaesthetists and many medical students and, after 8 days, a big organisation was working. All patients with respiratory problems were collected in a special department where the treatment team could observe them. The team comprised an epidemiologist, ENT surgeon and an anaesthetist with help from laboratory staff and, later, radiologists and physiotherapists. Some 50–60 patients were being admitted every day and then transferred to the special department when they showed signs of respiratory impairment. During the epidemic, the principle was adopted that help should go to the patient and not wait for the patient to come to the hospital. Thus, teams went out by ambulance or air to prepare the patient for transfer to the hospital. This was pre-hospital care on the grand scale and long before the term had been coined. The UK was not oblivious to the lessons to be learned from the Copenhagen epidemic and an editorial in the British Journal of Anaesthesia suggested that, in case a similar polio epidemic should strike the UK, a decision needed to be taken as to whether negative or positive pressure ventilation should be adopted as the main line of treatment and that, if it were to be the latter, positive pressure machines should be produced in sufficient quantity to deal with a crisis [7]. The foregoing can only be a brief account of the major role Ibsen played in the Copenhagen polio epidemic, but the technique he introduced of long-term manual positive pressure ventilation of patients in respiratory failure laid the foundations of intensive therapy as it is known today. This episode also provided an impetus for the development of mechanical respirators, one of the first being described by Claus Bang at another hospital in Denmark [8].

## 5. The Kommunehospital

After the polio epidemic had subsided, one of the surgeons at the Kommunehospital appointed Ibsen there as one of his assistants to organise the anaesthetic service for his department. Ibsen started there on 1st April, 1953 and opened a ten-bedded recovery room 3 months later and here he began his work in what became known as intensive therapy. A year after his appointment, a separate department of anaesthesiology was established with Ibsen as its chief. The decision that chief anaesthesiologists should receive the same salary as chief surgeons gave Ibsen a degree of financial independence that was a great help in pursuing his interest in intensive therapy. In that year, Ibsen was called to see a 10-year-old boy with tetanus. The boy was clearly dying. With some trepidation, Ibsen decided to 'convert' the

disease, for treatment purposes, from tetanus to polio. Earlier, a neonate with tetanus had been treated with D-tubocurarine for 10 days and ventilated on a rocking bed. The 10-year-old boy was anaesthetised, curarised and ventilated manually for 17 days with nitrous oxide and oxygen with a to-and-fro system. As with the polio epidemic, a team was formed to continue manual ventilation round the clock in 4 h shifts. The boy made a complete recovery. Other tetanus cases occurred and this led to the formation of tetanus units. The UK had already begun to establish polio units after the Copenhagen epidemic and soon began to follow suit with what were known, at first, as tetanus units and, later, as respiratory units. Ibsen's influence was beginning to spread far beyond Denmark. In Copenhagen, however, Ibsen soon realised that it was inefficient and uneconomic to create units requiring specialised knowledge and equipment for one or two specific diseases. And so, on 1st August, 1953, the first general intensive therapy unit was opened in the Kommunehospital [9]. This innovation opened the way for similar units to be opened in major hospitals all over the world.

In 1956, a decision was taken to found the journal Acta Anaesthesiologica Scandinavica and the first editorial board was appointed which included Ibsen. The first issue of the new journal appeared in 1967 and Ibsen remained a member of the editorial board until 1971. Ibsen's interest in intensive therapy soon led him to develop an increasing interest in monitoring. In 1975 he wrote '.....and the future will require more and more

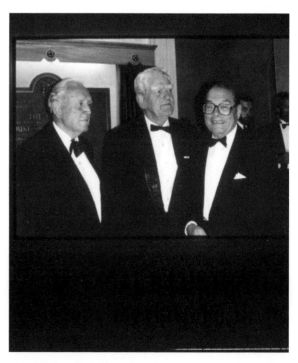

Fig. 14. B. Ibsen, O. Secher, H. Ruben (at the meeting of the Society of Anaesthetists of the South Western Region (of UK) in 1990) (by kind permission of John Zorab).

monitoring devices-also during anaesthesia'. An amazingly prescient observation. But this man, with a restless and enquiring mind, did not stop there. The problems of managing shock, fluid balance, humidification all occupied his attention. In about 1975, the function of the Kommunehospital was due to undergo a fundamental change. Acute medicine was largely moved out and the hospital was designated to receive patients, not for treatment, but for nursing care. Not wishing to transfer to a new department of anaesthesiology, Ibsen began to explore the field of chronic pain and pain clinics. A field in which he became pre-eminent in his own city. Indeed, pain clinic work became his major interest in the final years of his clinical work. At the time of writing, Ibsen is 87 and, throughout his life, has been one of the major figures in Danish anaesthesiology. As already mentioned, the writer spent 3 months in Copenhagen during his training years, including visits to Sweden, providing him with the golden opportunity to get to know many of the leading Scandinavian anaesthesiologists. Therefore, it gave him particular pleasure when a joint meeting was arranged in 1990 between the Danish Society of Anaesthesiologists and his own Regional Society (The Society of Anaesthetists of the Southwestern Region). But an even greater pleasure was in store when he was invited to deliver the 'Husfeldt Lecture' (the first occasion that this lecture had been given outside Denmark). The high spot was that, in the audience, were his

three old Danish friends, Bjørn Ibsen, Ole Secher and Henning Ruben who were guests at the society's dinner that evening (Fig. 14).

It is not surprising that the writer believes that, 'Bjørn Ibsen, Father of Intensive Therapy' is not an inappropriate description of this remarkable man.

## References

[1] Ibsen B. Ibsen. From Anaesthesia to Anaesthesiology, Acta Anaesthesiologica Scandinavica 1965;Suppl. 61.
[2] Secher O. Anaesthesia, In: Rupreht et al., editors. Essays on its History, Anaesthesia Centre, Copenhagen (Springer Verlag).
[3] Proceedings of the World Congress of Anaesthesiologists, Scheveningen, The Netherlands, 1955. (International Anesthesia Research Society).
[4] Bower AG, Bennett VR, Dillon JB, Axelrod B. Investigation on the care and treatment of poliomyelitis patients. Annals of Western Medicine and Surgery 1950;4:563.
[5] Lassen HCA. Preliminary report on the 1952 epidemic of poliomyelitis in Copenhagen with special reference to the treatment of acute respiratory insufficiency, The Lancet (Jan 3, 1953).
[6] Ibsen B. The anaesthetist's viewpoint on the treatment of respiratory complications in poliomyelitis during the epidemic in Copenhagen. Proceedings of the Royal Society of Medicine 1952;47:72–4.
[7] British Journal of Anaesthesia Editorial, 26. 81 (March, 1954).
[8] A new respirator, The Lancet (April 11, 1953) 723–26.
[9] Ibsen B. Intensive therapy: background and development. Int Anesth Clin 1966;4:277–94.

# Peter J. Safar. Part Two. The University of Pittsburgh to the Safar Centre for Resuscitation Research 1961–2002

Peter J.F. Baskett

In 1960 Peter Safar felt it was time to move on from Baltimore where he had inspired the birth of CPR [1]. He aspired to lead an academic department to provide physician based anaesthesiology, teach and inspire medical students and young graduates, and develop research programmes in anaesthesiology, critical care, emergency medical services (EMS), resuscitation medicine and disaster reanimatology.

He was appointed Chairman and Professor of Anaesthesiology and Critical Care at the University of Pittsburgh in 1961—being interviewed for the post personally by the Chancellor of the University. The offer and acceptance of the post was entirely verbal. Nothing was put on paper. The salary was not discussed. "I trusted it would be fair ... I considered it poor taste to talk about money ... it often spoiled collegiality and friendships" [2]. He was 36 years old and has stayed in Pittsburgh ever since (Fig. 1).

His mission at Pittsburgh as the founding University Chairman and Professor in Anaesthesiology and Critical Care was complex and many thought impossible. Five hospitals in the city had university affiliation—but there were only three physician anaesthesiologists between them—all the rest were nurse anaesthetists—just over 70 people in all. To integrate these to form a cohesive academic department was a tall order. He set about an ambitious programme to convert the anaesthetic service to physician control and participation, to establish training programmes in physician anaesthesia, critical care medicine, resuscitation, pain control, respiratory therapy, EMS, specialist neuro and cardiothoracic anaesthesia and, of course, clinical and laboratory research. Recruitment to Pittsburgh at that time was not easy. It was a steel city renowned for grime and air pollution. Only some years later, with the demise of the steel industry there, did it become transformed into one of the more attractive American cities with hilltops overlooking the meeting point of three rivers.

Over the years he achieved his mission, not only in the field of anaesthesia, but also ensuring that physician anaesthesiologists expanded their talents outside the operating room to encompass resuscitation, critical care medicine, emergency and disaster medicine and basic and clinical scientific research. Safar had a talent for selecting gifted colleagues and research fellows from the length and breadth of the United States and from all over the world. Many have become household names in their own right. They include Bjorn Lind, Ake Grenvik, Miroslav Klain, Peter Winter, Paul Berkebile, Bulent Kirimili, Robert Hingson, Maurice Albin, Nancy Caroline, Sven Erik Gisvold, Ron Stewart, Nicholas Bircher, Ernesto Pretto, Pat Kochanek, Acheil Bleyaert, Erga Cerchiari, Fritz Sterz, Per Vaagenes, Norman Abramson and countless others too numerous to list.

Throughout this feverish period of activity Peter remained true to his inherent sensitivity, experiencing happiness and tragedy to the full. Tragedy struck in 1966 when his beloved daughter, Elisabeth, always a frail child, died in status asthmaticus, aged 12.

Her death inspired Peter to increase his efforts to develop intensive care and research into cerebral resuscitation and encourage organ donation—then in its infancy. He joined in the debate of the time on brain death and, with Grenvik, formed a group in Pittsburgh to address the problem. They wisely came up with the concept of brain death equating to actual death without relating the diagnosis to potential organ donation, unlike the Harvard group who published their recommendations a year later. He and Grenvik also addressed the problem of the persistent vegetative state and allowing patients to die in futile situations, placing the responsibility and decision making clearly on the physician, and introduced the concept of titrating critical care in appropriate cases. They were invited to give guidance to the US Presidential Commission and to Harvard University guideline group on the subject.

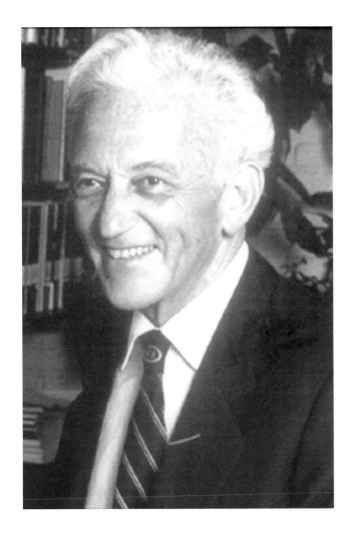

In the field of resuscitation, with the help and inspiration of Asmund Laerdal and Bjorn Lind [3], Safar, Winchell and Berkebile in 1964 [4] studied the acquisition of basic life support skills on a manikin developed by Laerdal—Resusci Anne. This potentially opened the door for citizen CPR which had been advocated by Claude Beck in Ohio. Sadly the American Heart Association refused to endorse citizen CPR training at that time. It was not until the early 1970s that that organisation responded positively and then with a rather detailed and rigid training programme that could only be reached by relatively few people. Only recently has it been realised that the simplicity in training such as advocated by Safar using a basic manikin and flip chart yields the best results [5–7].

On the international stage however, things were moving on. The World Federation of Societies of Anaesthesiology through its CPR committee commissioned Safar to write a CPR instructor manual in 1968 which blossomed into a booklet in 1982, both published by Laerdal in Stavanger. It became a landmark comprehensive text book on Cardiopulmonary Cerebral Resuscitation coauthored by Nicholas Bircher in 1988

[8]. I had the honour to be Chairman of the committee at that time (Figs. 2 and 3).

Despite the enormous clinical and teaching activity time was found for basic scientific research. By his own admission Safar had a naïve attitude towards funding of 'get it started and later look for the money to finish it' [9] that somehow worked. Blood flow studies during CPR were difficult in the early days [10,11] as Safar sought to enhance the meagre output produced by standard chest compressions. Gradually his research moved increasingly towards investigating the potential reversibility of the dying process whether this was caused by asphyxia, primary cardiac arrest, exsanguination or pulmonary failure. At this stage he became involved with Negovsky of Moscow and reproduced and confirmed some of his experimental work on exsanguination cardiac arrest [12,13]. He was almost unique in cooperating with scientists behind the 'Iron Curtain' at this time.

Safar's early foray into cerebral resuscitation on 'brains too good to die' involved Bjorn Lind, on sabbatical from Stavanger in 1970–1971. Together with Jim Snyder, they were among the first to study cerebral blood flow and metabolism after prolonged cardiac arrest [14]. They demonstrated the transient cerebral hyperaemia followed by protracted hypoperfusion. The efforts of Safar, and many others have been

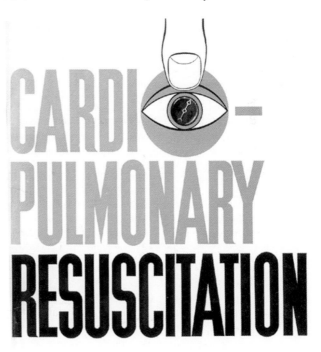

A MANUAL FOR PHYSICIANS AND
PARAMEDICAL INSTRUCTORS
PREPARED FOR THE WORLD FEDERATION
OF SOCIETIES OF ANAESTHESIOLOGISTS

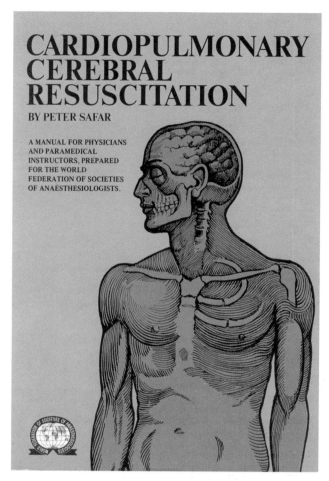

Fig. 3. The third edition of the WFSA CPCR manual.

concentrated on overcoming this viscious and destructive sequence.

In 1978, after much reflection Peter decided to relinquish the Chairmanship of the Academic department at the University of Pittsburgh to concentrate on research. His position at the university was filled by Peter Winter in 1979. To mark his enormous achievement for the University of Pittsburgh he was appointed Distinguished Professor of Resuscitation Medicine—a rare honour.

In 1979 Safar, decided to found the International Resuscitation Research Centre (IRRC) at 3434 Fifth Avenue, Pittsburgh. To take this remarkable step into the dark required an enormous amount of courage and dedication. The Centre was housed on the site of an old coffin (casket) factory. Peter quipped that it was a move 'from resurrection to resuscitation'. He obtained priming funding from the Pennsylvania Department of Health and the Rippell Foundation and ongoing running costs from the University at Pittsburgh, the National Institute of Health (NIH) and the Laerdal Foundation. His research there has mainly centered around brain resuscitation. Starting with a monkey (caught in the wild) model, Safar and Gisvold changed

to custom-bred dogs. "I felt that even the food chain cannot justify shortening the lives of animals so close to us ... shortening the lives of custom bred dogs seemed easier to justify ... the reasoning was that, without research, these dogs would not exist" [15]. Large rooms, not cages, were used for holding the animals and I got the impression when I visited the centre that concern for the animals welfare was high on Safar's list of priorities.

The output of scientific papers from the IRRC has been phenomenal, too many to cite here. They included studies of brain metabolism and the influence of hypertensive fluid infusion, cardiopulmonary bypass, barbiturates and calcium channel blockers on brain recovery after cardiac arrest. All of these investigations showed great promise but, sadly, the goal of proven significantly improved outcome has, so far, eluded the researchers. But the background scientific knowledge that has been acquired forms a rock solid foundation for future research that will probably prove successful.

Safar has been interested in the protective and therapeutic effects of induced hypothermia since the 1960s [16] and carried out further enlightening studies in the 1980s [17–19]. The process of inducing moderate hypothermia after cardiac arrest to improve cerebral outcome has always shown promise but the practicalities of producing rapid cooling in the clinical situation had proved difficult. Only now (2000–2002) has the technique returned to the realm of clinical possibility [20,21] and it is likely that the induction of moderate hypothermia will find its way into the official guidelines for post resuscitation care in the near future. With Sam Tisherman and Pat Kochanek, Safar continues to lead investigations into brain protection during cardiac arrest after trauma using profound hypothermia induced rapidly by cold saline infused via an intraaortic balloon catheter. The project has attracted substantial grant funding from the US military.

Safar has always had a strong leaning towards disaster medicine. Perhaps influenced by his experiences between 1939 and 1945, but more likely driven by his love and feeling for his fellow man, his horror of the carnage arising from 'natural' and 'man made' disasters has been channeled into studies of disaster reanimatology. A founder member of the Club of Mainz with Rudolf Frey in 1976, he had studied injuries after earthquakes in Peru [22], Italy [23], and Armenia [24–26]. He and his colleagues, particularily Miroslav Klein and Ernesto Pretto, were able to show that simple first aid by uninjured co-victims had a strong life saving potential—probably more than advanced trauma life support. The Club of Mainz ran, as its successor the World Association for Disaster and Emergency Medicine (WADEM) still runs, biannual congresses. Safar hosted the 1981 congress in Pittsburgh, and during my time as Honorary Secretary of the Association and his Presidency created the journal Disaster Medicine in

302

1983. This was later to become the Journal of WADEM in 1985 and subsequently Prehospital and Disaster Medicine under the continuing editorship of Marvin Birnbaum in Madison, Wisconsin.

Despite cordial (and research) relationships with the military throughout his career Safar is a pacifist at heart and was a leading member of the International Physicians for the Prevention of Nuclear War (IPPNW). This group encouraged a reduction in nuclear arms (that has now been achieved to some extent) and Safar urged the military to divert some of their efforts, at least, towards assistance with non military mass disasters.

In 1994 Safar (then aged 70) retired from the leadership role at the IRRC and handed over the reins to Pat Kochanek, his collaborator for many years. To mark the occasion Pat Kochanek renamed the institution the 'Safar Centre for Resuscitation Research' to highlight the contribution that both Peter, and his beloved wife of over 50 years, Eva, had made. Safar continues to work productively in the centre. Peter Winter gave up the Chairmanship of the University Department in 1996 and was succeeded by Leonard Firestone as the "Peter and Eva Safar Chairman of Anesthesiology and Critical Care Medicine". In 2002 this position was assumed by John Williams. Safar is less than impressed with modern management involvement in medicine in the United States. He calls it "mismanaged care for managed profit by non professional middlemen" [27].

Peter Safar is a world renowned figure not just because of his personal research and discoveries, but also because of his inspiration and practical help to colleagues and friends throughout the length and breadth of the world. There are few places that he has not visited, there are few places where he has not been honoured. He fostered professional and friendly relations with colleagues in many countries behind the 'Iron Curtain' during the Cold War when it was difficult and unfashionable to do so. He visited Vietnam before the catastrophic war there and, sadly to no avail, advocated peace and cooperation with Ho Chi Minh [28]. He has been influential and hugely supportive in Latin America, the Orient and Africa. He has been a regular and sought after speaker in Australasia and in virtually every country in Western Europe (Fig. 4).

He has published over 1000 scientific papers and is still active at his beloved Safar Center for Resuscitation Research.

Few people have packed more into their life than Peter Safar—the family man, the lover of music and the arts, the inspired creator of ideas, the courageous exposer of the false and the bogus, the great lover of his fellow human beings. I have wonderful personal memories of his boundless energy and enthusiasm, of his simple but capacious plastic shoulder bag packed with an impossible amount of paper, his Viennese accent that never changed in over 50 years of life spent in the United

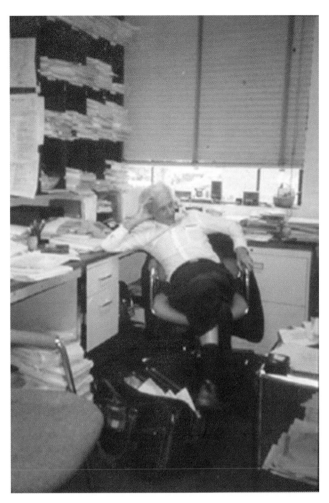

Fig. 4. Peter Safar in his office at the Safar Centre for Resuscitation

States, his exuberant dancing with Eva to a Strauss waltz in Vienna, and above all, his eyes twinkling with friendship that is beyond words.

## Acknowledgements

Many of the facts recounted in this article has been gleaned from Peter Safar's Autobiographical Memoir in the series Careers in Anesthesiology, Volume V, published by the Wood Library Museum of Anesthesiology in 2000 and from citations written in relation to his Honorary Degree in Magdeburg, his award of the Austrian Cross of Honour in Vienna, and his election to Honorary membership of the European Resuscitation Council. Aside from those books and documents, Peter has given me a copy of his 120 page Curriculum Vitae and I have had the pleasure of spending many hours with him over the past quarter of a century. I would also like to acknowledge the help given to me by Ake Grenvik, John Zorab and Tore Laerdal with details for the final manuscript.

# References

[1] Baskett PJF. Resuscitation Great. Peter J Safar, The Early Years 1924–1961, The Birth of CPR. Resuscitation 2001;50:17–22.

[2] Safar PJ. An Autobiographical Memoir. In: Careers in Anesthesiology, vol. V. Published by the Wood Library Museum of Anesthesiology, 2000, p. 167.

[3] Tjomsland N, Baskett PJF. Resuscitation Great. Asmund S Laerdal. Resuscitation 2002;53:115–9.

[4] Winchell SW, Safar P. Teaching and testing lay and paramedical personnel in cardiopulmonary resuscitation. Anesthesia Analgesia Curr Res 1966;45:441–9.

[5] Berkebile P, Benson D, Ersoz C, Safar P. Public education in heart–lung resuscitation. Evaluation of three self-training methods in teenagers. Critical Care Med 1973;1:115–6.

[6] Safar P, Berkebile P, Scott MA, Esposito G, Medsger A, Ricci E, Malloy C. Education Research on life supporting first aid (LFSA)and CPR self training systems (STS). Critical Care Med 1981;9:403–4.

[7] Braslow A, Brennan RT, Newman MM, Bircher NG, Batchellor AM, Kaye W. CPR training without an instructor: development and evaluation of a video self-instructional system for effective performance of cardiopulmonary resuscitation. Resuscitation 1997;34:207–20.

[8] Safar P, Bircher NG. Cardiopulmonary-cerebral resuscitation. An introduction to Resuscitation Medicine. World Federation of Societies of Anaesthesiologists. 3rd ed. Published WB Saunders, London, 1988.

[9] Safar PJ. An Autobiographical Memoir. In: Careers in Anesthesiology vol. V. Published by the Wood Library Museum of Anesthesiology, 2000, p. 213.

[10] Harris LC, Kirimli B, Safar P. Ventilation-cardiac compression rates and ratios in cardiopulmonary resuscitation. Anesthesiology 1967;28:806–13.

[11] Harris LC, Kirimli B, Safar P. Augmentation of artificial circulation during cardiopulmonary resuscitation. Anesthesiology 1967;28:730–4.

[12] Kirimli B, Kamptschulte S, Safar P. Cardiac arrest from exsanguination in dogs, evaluation of resuscitation methods. Acta Anaesthesiol Scand (Suppl) 1968;29:183–9.

[13] Kirimli B, Kamptschulte S, Safar P. Resuscitation from cardiac arrest due to exsanguination. Surg Gynae Obstet 1969;129:89–97.

[14] Lind B, Snyder J, Safar P. Total brain ischaemia in dogs: cerebral, physiological and metabolic changes after 15 minutes of circulatory arrest. Resuscitation 1975;2:97–113.

[15] Safar PJ. An Autobiographical Memoir. In: Careers in Anesthesiology, vol. V. Published by the Wood Library Museum of Anesthesiology, 2000, p. 257.

[16] Rosomoff HL, Safar P. Management of the comatose patient. In: Safar P, editor. Respiratory Therapy. Philadephia: FA Davis Co, 1965:244–58.

[17] Leonov Y, Sterz F, Safar P, Radovsky A, Oku K, Tisherman S, Stezoski SW. Mild cerebral hypothermia during and after cardiac arrest improves neurologic outcome in dogs. J Cerebral Blood Flow Metabolism 1990;10:57–70.

[18] Kuboyama K, Safar P, Radovsky A, Tisherman SA, Stezoski SW, Alexander H. Delay in cooling negates the beneficial effect of mild resuscitative cerebral hypothermia after cardiac arrest in dogs. A prospective, randomised, controlled study. Critical Care Med 1993;21:1348–58.

[19] Safar P, Xiao F, Radovsky A, Tanigawa K, Ebmeyer U, Bircher N, Alexander H, Stezoski SW. Improved cerebral resuscitation from cardiac arrest in dogs with mild hypothermia plus blood flow promotion. Stroke 1996;27:105–13.

[20] The Hypothermia after Cardiac Arrest Study Group. Mild therapeutic hypothermia to improve the neurologic after cardiac arrest. NEJM 2002;346:549–556.

[21] Bernard SA, Gray TW, Buist MD, Jones BM, Silvester W, Gutteridge G, Smith K. Treatment of comatose survivors of out-of-hospital cardiac arrest with induced hypothermia. NEJM 2002;346:557–63.

[22] Safar P, Ramos V, Mosquera J, Ames A. Anecdotes on resuscitation potentials following the earthquake of 1970 in Peru. Prehospital Disaster Med 1987;3:124(abstract).

[23] Safar P, Kirimli N, Agnes A, Magalini S. Anecdotes on resuscitation potentials following the earthquake of 1980 in Italy. Procedings Fourth World Congress on Emergency and Disaster Medicine June 1985, Brighton, UK.

[24] Other members of the Disaster Reanimatology Study Group, Klain M, Ricci E, Safar P, Semenov V, Pretto E, Tisherman S, Abrams J, Comfort L. Disaster reanimatology potentials. A structured interview study in Armenia I. Methodology and Preliminary Results. Prehospital Disaster Med 1991;4:135–54.

[25] Other members of the Disaster Reanimatology Study Group, Ricci EM, Pretto EA, Safar P, Klain M, Angus D, Tisherman SA, Abrams J, Crippen D, Comfort L, Semenov V. Disaster reanimatology potentials. A structured interview in Armenia II. Methods. Prehospital Disaster Med 1991;6:159–66.

[26] Other members of the Disaster Reanimatology Study Group, Pretto EA, Ricci E, Klain M, Safar P, Semenov V, Abrams J, Tisherman S, Crippen D, Comfort L. Disaster reanimatology potentials. A structured interview in Armenia III. Results, conclusions and recommendations. Prehospital Disaster Med 1992;7:327–37.

[27] Safar P. An Autobiographical Memoir. In: Careers in Anesthesiology, vol. V. Published by Wood Smith Library of Anesthesiology, 2000, p. 289.

[28] Safar P. An Autobiographical Memoir. In: Careers in Anesthesiology, vol. V. Published by the Wood Library of Anesthesiology, 2000, p. 302.

# Eugene Nagel and the Miami paramedic program

## Mickey S. Eisenberg

Though known primarily for its sandy beaches and sunny weather Miami, Florida is also home to the first paramedic program in the US. In addition to pioneering paramedical personnel, the Miami program is noteworthy for its use of telemetry that allowed physicians to supervise care from a remote base station hospital. Today we take for granted the delivery of paramedic staffed emergency medical services throughout all urban and suburban areas of the US and in many other countries. But this was not always the case. Innovations require visionaries able to recognize a problem and seek a solution. In the US the problem was sudden cardiac arrest due to ventricular fibrillation and one of the visionaries was Eugene Nagel.

The chain of events leading up to the innovative program in Miami began 40 years ago. Like many chain of events it was comprised of equal parts serendipity and preparation. In Nagel's case, it involved CPR, an invitation to speak at a rescue association, a stubborn fire chief, a colleague named James Hirschman, and a dogged determination to do what needed to be done.

In 1962, Eugene Nagel was 38 years old and finishing a residency in anesthesia at Columbia-Presbyterian Hospital in New York City. He had graduated from Washington University School of Medicine in St. Louis 3 years earlier. During his residency one of the senior doctors suggested he look into something new in the medical field called 'CPR.' Nagel followed the advice and learned what there was to learn about the new procedure. From residency Nagel took an academic position at the University of Miami working as an instructor in anesthesiology at Jackson Memorial Hospital. Nagel's knowledge of CPR earned him membership on the CPR committee at the hospital and this led to an invitation to speak at the International First Aid and Rescue Association meeting in January 1964 at Miami Beach. CPR was a hot topic, and it seemed that Nagel was the local 'expert.'

Shortly after the association meeting, Nagel came to Fire Station No. 1 and offered to teach CPR to the firemen. 'They were like eager sponges, willing to learn anything that made some sense to them. They knew almost as much as I did about the art of CPR. But there were facets of the resuscitation management, the airway particularly, that they were a little bit 'foggy' on, and we worked together very well,' said Nagel. The connection with the fire department was one he thoroughly enjoyed (see Fig. 1).

While this was taking place, other events were happening in Nagel's life. For one thing, he had originally intended to come to Miami for just 2 years, in order to pass his boards. He did so in 1965. By then, the young doctor who was not sure he would like doing academic research was in the midst of two different such efforts. His work with the Miami Fire Department was connected to his first research program, in resuscitation. His other was in communication and physiology of dolphins, and it was becoming a major avenue of research [1,2]. The dolphin work would lose out to his resuscitation interest and become the fork in the road not taken.

An event in Nagel's personal life that may have affected his professional work was the birth of his first child. He and his wife Joan had married in early 1963, and his daughter had been born late that year. She was a very premature infant, weighing only about 1000 g at birth. In 1963 1000-g birth-weight infants had less than a 3% chance of surviving. Linda Nagel beat the odds, but it was touch and go for the first 3 months. 'Her weight dropped to 700 g,' Nagel said, 'and she had many apneic spells—that is, she stopped breathing numerous times during those first 3 months. She had to be rock-resuscitated (the infant was rocked forward and backward to assist breathing)—I do not know if they did mouth-to-mouth.' Nagel today does not believe his daughter's return from death through resuscitation affected his professional choices—at least not consciously. His interest in resuscitation had started at Columbia-Presbyterian. But he admits that the connec-

305

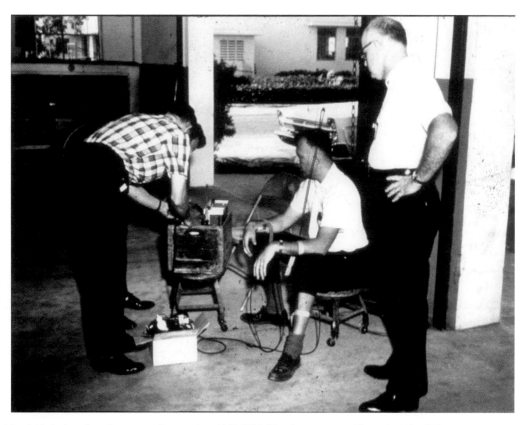

Fig. 1. Eugene Nagel (sitting) testing telemetry equipment circa 1968. With Nagel are personnel from the Miami Fire Dept. Communications Dept.

tion with his daughter's health strengthened that interest.

Because of Nagel's persistence and support, the fire department began to initiate CPR in the field routinely and then bring the patient to the emergency department. But this only created larger problems since the rescue personnel invariably faced a disinterested physician. Few, if any, patients with cardiac arrest were saved. Nagel observed, 'We had them bring in, in ventricular fibrillation, and very often the doctor in the ER would not even put the patient on the monitor. The docs in the ER, I would say 75%, when you rushed one in doing CPR, would tell you to quit and say he is dead. Disgustedly he would say this and ask 'Why are you bothering me?' This was very discouraging to the rescue guys.' Just as stultifying was the very poor CPR given to those cases in which the emergency department would take over. Nagel described these cases, 'The firemen would come in trying to do 60 chest compressions a minute, interposed with a breath every five compressions—(they would) immediately get elbowed aside and somebody would be pushing with about as much compression as would dent a grape on the sternum and the ventilation would be abysmal.'

Nagel was convinced that the only way to save cardiac arrest victims was to have firefighters defibrillate at the scene and he set out to sell the Miami fire chief on the idea. Though Nagel had good camaraderie with the firefighters, rescue personnel, and their immediate superiors, his relationship with the chief was not terribly simpatico. Nagel describes his encounter, 'I told the fire chief that I wanted to train the guys in defibrillation. A big, tall, 6 ft 3 in. Irishman by the name of Lawrence Kenny, he had been quite tolerant of me up to now. He took his finger and he punched me in the chest and drove me back about 3 ft with his one finger. He said, 'This is a fire department, not a hospital; these are firemen and not doctors. I do not want you to forget that.' Every time he would say something, he would punch me again in the chest with his finger, which hurt a lot. I think that I probably got the idea.'

In 1967, Nagel became aware of the work of Pantridge and Geddes in Belfast [3]. He believed that the Belfast model of a doctor-staffed prehospital mobile cardiac care unit (MCCU) was not going to work for the US in general or for Miami in particular. The Belfast model was primarily based on treating myocardial infarction and whether the MCCU arrived at the scene in 5 or 12 min made little difference, in general. But Nagel was focused on cardiac arrest and minutes were crucial. Given the role of the fire department in providing prehospital emergency care Nagel became convinced that firefighters could be trained to do much of what physicians could do for cardiac arrest.

Despite the chief's opposition, Nagel moved incrementally toward his goal of paramedic defibrillation. He did not think he could initially sell the idea of paramedics working alone, even if they had authorization to perform medical procedures signed by physicians. 'I saw no hope of a standing operating procedure,' he recalled. 'That would have been a major jump, and I did not think I could sell it to anybody. But the fact that I, or a doctor like me, could be on the radio and give specific verbal orders to a fireman to perform a specific maneuver he had been trained to do—well, that seemed semi-OK to the medical school and the fire chief.'

So Nagel's first step was radio and telemetry [4,5]. Refined in the space program, telemetry allowed mission control in Houston to monitor each astronaut's heart rate. With minor modifications, it was just the technology Nagel needed to make his case. Jim Hirschman, a cardiologist who was an experienced amateur radio expert and who was interested in Nagel's telemetry effort, joined Nagel. But before he could sell the need for defibrillation and medications, Nagel had to prove that ventricular fibrillation was the cause of sudden collapse in the community—and he had to prove that the ECG signal could be sent from the field to the hospital. Telemetry was something the fire chief could accept because it seemed unlikely to hurt the patient or embarrass the department. The firefighters on the rescue squad could not do anything else, though—no drug administration, no defibrillation. It was one step at a time for Nagel, and it worked. 'What we did in Miami was to gradually systematize a lot of situations. Eventually, we gave the paramedics permission to do a number of things without radio contact,' explained Nagel. 'That included IVs, obviously, and then certain drugs in certain sequences.' But for the first couple of years, it was one small step at a time.

Nagel's decision to use telemetry was the Trojan Horse that would get around the legal impediments stopping firefighters from defibrillating and administering medications. If the fire department could transmit the ECG signal to the hospital, the firefighters (with special training) could then be authorized by the physician to administer needed drugs and procedures prior to arriving in the emergency department. He believed a paramedic at the scene was a legal extension of a physician. He recalled later, 'We saw telemetry as the key to extending our treatment to outside the hospital where hitherto trying to legislate it was the dark side of the moon in those days.'

During the initial experiments with telemetry, the signal from the rescue unit went through the fire department voice channel and by phone line to Nagel's office in Jackson Memorial Hospital. When the practicality of the system was proven, the receiving terminal was transferred to the post-anesthesia recovery unit where residents were on call 24 h a day. Nagel and Hirschman as supervisors alternated being on call every other night. The telemetry was an ECG-modulated voice channel, and Nagel became accomplished at the art of using his ear to interpret the sound signal coming over the phone without even looking at the ECG pattern. According to Nagel there was no mistaking the absolutely unique sound pattern of ventricular fibrillation— once likened by him to a mezzo-soprano being goosed with an icicle during an aria. The telemetry documented the rhythm causing the cardiac arrest, but for the first year there was no means to defibrillate the patient.

By the beginning of 1968, the fire rescue squads had a year of experience using telemetry and radio contact. Nagel in turn had a solid year's worth of telemetry data to use for his ongoing sales pitches to the fire chief and his superiors. 'Whereas in 1966 I got punched in the chest; in 1968 I got a lot of lecture and a lot of moaning and groaning, but he finally said OK.'

With that as background, Nagel began training firefighters in the use of defibrillators. At about the same time, he snagged a grant from the Florida Heart Association and used it to purchase additional defibrillators. By 1969 Nagel and the fire rescue squads were going 'full-bore' (as he phrased it). The Miami Rescue Unit quickly expanded to three trucks, and the annual number of rescue calls jumped from 8000 to 15 000. Nagel took the next step: he asked the chief to authorize the paramedics to initiate intravenous lines. This sales job involved a dramatic presentation, Nagel recalled. 'I let a paramedic start an IV in me, lying on a table in front of the city commissioners at a public meeting,' he said. 'There were a lot of people in the audience including the chief. I told the commissioners that these men had been well trained, and that I had as much confidence in them as I did in most of the people at the hospital. And that did it. They accepted it.' Once the struggle for intravenous lines had been won, Nagel surprisingly had no difficulty convincing the chief to allow medications.

Nagel had a more difficult job selling the chief on intubation (the placement of a tube down the throat and into the trachea). To Nagel as an anesthesiologist, the need for intubation was obvious. Though intubation is not without risk Nagel was confident in his skills and knew he could teach the procedure. To overcome Chief Kenney's reluctance, Nagel trained nine paramedics using manikins and visited the morgue to practice on unclaimed bodies. He then set up a demonstration to prove his paramedics could perform the skill. Nagel recalled the event, 'I enlisted one of our residents, Harry Heinitsch. We sprayed each other with topical anesthetic. I then intubated Harry, awake, demonstrating the technique. All nine paramedics then intubated Harry successfully. Harry then intubated me and the paramedics followed his lead.' Nagel describes himself as a prodigious gagger, claiming 'even looking at a tongue blade makes me gag.' But liberal amounts of anesthetic got him through the evening, and neither Nagel nor the resident reported even so much as a sore throat. It is doubtful that a mere sore throat or even laryngitis could have stopped Nagel's determination. The following morning he made a 'bee-line to the chief's office' and presented the results of the evening's training. The chief remonstrated weakly but finally conceded that the paramedics had demonstrated proficiency, and allowed them to intubate.

It should not be surprising that the medical directors of the various paramedic programs would remember the first resuscitation in their city. Nagel vividly recalled the first save of the Miami paramedic program. The collapse occurred near Station 1, on the fringe of downtown Miami, where the smart part of town meets the underside. He reminisced, 'There was a well known alcoholic named Dan Jones who was then about 60 years old. He lived in a rooming house near our rescue unit. Dan Jones was familiar to the guys since they had hauled him to Jackson Memorial Hospital on several occasions. In June of 1969 they got a call—man down. It was Dan Jones. They put the paddles on him, he was in VF, started CPR, zapped him, he came back to a regular rhythm, brought him to the ED, and 3 days later he was out and walking around. In gratitude, about a week later, he came down to Station 1, which he had never done before, and he said he would like to talk to the man who saved his life. They told me they had never seen Dan Jones in a clean shirt and sober, both of which he was that day. He would periodically come to the firehouse and just say hello and he seemed to be sober. In my talks in those days I said this was the new cure for alcoholism.'

Nagel's efforts to establish prehospital coronary care in Miami earned him a place as one of the founding fathers in EMS. Why did he take the initiative to visit Station 1 and offer his services to the fire department in 1964? Reflecting on that decision, Nagel answered, 'I come from a small Midwestern town of about 5000 (Clinton, Missouri). Neighbors in that town meant something, friends meant something. The town was sort of a social group—you did not like everyone in the town, but it was so small that there was a feeling of community, and I liked that. If you are from a big city, you tend to be much more reserved, I think, much more careful about whom you form relationships with. I think that possibly had something to do with it.'

Nagel, who was not really certain that academic work was for him, continued to have an extremely distinguished academic career. From Miami he became chair of the department of anesthesiology at Harbor General Hospital in Torrance, California and then at Johns Hopkins Hospital in Baltimore, Maryland. In 1980 he returned to Florida and worked as professor of anesthesiology at University of Florida and University of South Florida until 1996. He authored 41 peer-reviewed articles and 14 book chapters on resuscitation related topics. Nagel was also adept at bridging academia and the real world. For 6 years, from 1974–1980, during formative years in paramedic services, Nagel wrote a column in *Emergency Medical Services*, an influential trade journal. From 1972–1980 he was chair of the medical advisory committee to the International Association of Fire Chiefs. Since 1975 he has served as chair of the medical committee for American Red Magen David, the American support organization for emergency medical services in Israel [6]. Though officially retired, Nagel is as active today at age 78 as when he first walked into Fire Station No. 1 over 40 years ago. Miami and the world are better off for it.

## References

*Parts of the bibliographic profile of Eugene Nagel are derived from a profile of his work in Eisenberg, MS, Life in the Balance: Emergency Medicine and the Quest to Reverse Sudden Death.* 1997, Oxford, New York, pgs. 225–232. Quotes from Eugene Nagel are from interviews conducted on July 2, 1989 and July 6, 1989.

[1] Nagel EL, Morgane PJ, McFarland WL. Anesthesia for the bottlenose dolphin (tursiops truncatus). Science 1964;146:1591–3.
[2] Nagel EL, Morgane PJ, McFarland WL. Anesthesia for the bottlenose dolphin. Vet Med 1996;61:229–33.
[3] Pantridge JF, Geddes JS. A mobile intensive-care unit in the management of myocardial infarction. Lancet 1967;ii:271–3.
[4] Nagel EL, Hirschman JC, et al. Telemetry of physiologic data: an aid to fire-rescue personnel in a metropolitan area. South Med J 1968;61:598–602.
[5] Nagel EL, Hirschman JC, et al. Telemetry medical command in coronary and other mobile emergency care systems. JAMA 1970;214:332–8.
[6] Hadas E, Eisenberg MS, Nagel EL. Emergency medical services in Israel. Am J Emerg Med 1984;2:366–7.

# Stig Holmberg—A visionary giant in cardiopulmonary resuscitation

## Johan Herlitz

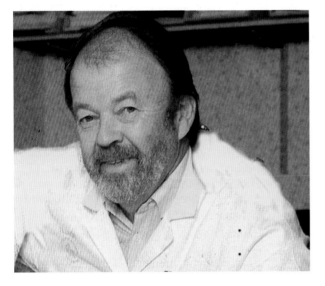

"How does it feel to be so small?" This question was addressed to Stig on the day of his retirement, when a couple of hundred people had assembled to acknowledge his skilful work over the years. "I don't understand what you mean", was the reply. "It's you guys who are unnecessarily tall."

Stig was born in 1927 and started his medical career as a surgeon in the north of Sweden. He came to Sahlgrenska University Hospital in Göteborg in 1962 at the age of 35. Here, he started working in internal medicine but switched to cardiology in 1963 and continued as a cardiologist at this hospital until he retired in 1992.

I first heard about Stig Holmberg a few months after having started to study medicine in 1969. My older brother, who was 3 years ahead of me, had come to study internal medicine. There he heard of a physician who always had a knife in his belt. He used it, as my brother said, "to open the chest of people who were dying". My brother was quite right. For many years, Stig Holmberg had a personal pager and each time there was a presumed cardiac arrest and pulseless electrical activity in the hospital, he was called upon to "open the chest" and do "internal chest compressions". These happenings were mostly major events and a great many people were involved. Later on, as a junior cardiologist, I was allowed to "feel the heart beat with my own hands" during such events.

As a junior cardiologist at the coronary care unit, it was routine to call Stig even at night when there were problems, even if he was not on call. That was the way he wanted it to be.

As the person who built up the Coronary Care Unit at Sahlgrenska University Hospital, he was keen to teach the nurses to defibrillate ventricular fibrillation as early as possible. He, therefore, introduced the concept of "one Holmberger", which was the maximum allowed time from the onset of ventricular fibrillation until defibrillation. It corresponded to the length of an ECG strip (50 mm/s) from top to toe.

Stig was an elite gymnast. One morning, when he was walking into the coronary care unit, he was stopped by the cleaning woman who said that the floor had just been polished. Stig, however, was not put off and walked on his hands through the department.

Stig was very competitive. When we had just started a pre-hospital study with fibrinolysis in 1986 and I arrived at the Coronary Care Unit with the first recruited patient, I met Stig and he asked me immediately how soon after the onset of symptoms we had started infusion. "After 37 minutes," I said. He replied, "37 minutes—you have broken the world record!"

Stig introduced the Mobile Coronary Care Unit to Sweden with an enormous amount of energy and stubbornness. When this goal had been achieved, he and Bertil Wennerblom performed a unique study in the late 1970s. They instructed the dispatchers to use envelope randomisation to allocate patients with a presumed acute myocardial infarction to be transported by a mobile coronary care unit or by a standard ambulance. At that time, the treatment available in the mobile care unit was morphine, furosemide, atropine, lidocaine and defibrillation. They were able to demonstrate improved survival among patients transported by the Mobile Coronary Care Unit during 5 years of follow-up—a unique documentation for the future.

His great mission, for which he will always have a specific place in Swedish medical history, is his life-long work on resuscitation. In 1987, he suggested to the Swedish Cardiac Society that a working group for resuscitation should be set up. He was the Chairman of this group until 2005. With great support from his colleague Lars Ekström and a number of nurses, led by Marianne Jarlöv, he initiated education in cardiopulmonary resuscitation in Sweden, according to the cascade principle. Stig has been the brain behind the large number of Swedish pioneering educational programmes in cardiopulmonary resuscitation. These programmes were often created in collaboration with Laerdal (an example of how fruitful collaboration between the medical profession and industry can be at its best).

Stig's vision was that knowing how to perform CPR should be as natural as knowing how to swim. Today, 20 years later, he can harvest the fruits of his efforts.

Among patients suffering from bystander-witnessed, out-of-hospital cardiac arrests in Sweden, cardiopulmonary resuscitation is started by a bystander prior to the arrival of the ambulance in about 50% of cases.

In 1990, Stig persuaded the majority of ambulance chief physicians in Sweden to create a National Registry of out-of-hospital cardiac arrests in the country. Today, 15 years later, this registry includes about 45,000 patients suffering from out-of-hospital cardiac arrest.

In the same year (1990), again with Lars Ekström and Marianne Jarlöv, he started a development project designed to improve the treatment of patients suffering from in-hospital cardiac arrest at his own hospital. He demanded resources from the hospital management committee in order to create special training for employees for this purpose. He threatened to sue the hospital management for every single case of cardiac arrest within the hospital where an unnecessary delay until the start of treatment could be demonstrated.

This work has resulted in an effective organisation with very high survival after in-hospital cardiac arrest.

During the last few years, he has (he is now 77 years old) conducted national surveys of how various hospital organisations in Sweden function with regard to the handling of patients with in-hospital cardiac arrest.

With regard to this work, he has recently sent a report, supported by his data, to the Swedish National Board of Health and Welfare to inform them that, in all probability, at least 600 patients die each year in various hospitals in Sweden from in-hospital cardiac arrest due to unnecessary delay until the start of treatment, a delay which could be prevented if hospitals introduced automated external defibrillators in non-monitored wards. He is still waiting for a reply.

Over the years, Stig has been involved with a large number of patients suffering from cardiac arrest. Here is a brief description of the most spectacular case.

In 1987, Stig was working temporarily as a general practitioner in the north of Norway. One busy morning, a 50-year-old woman presented at the surgery with thoracic pain, which she had developed during Christmas shopping. She was immediately taken to the ECG room, where she developed a cardiac arrest with ventricular fibrillation. In 1987, not all surgeries were equipped with defibrillators and, in this case, the closest defibrillator was situated eight Swedish miles (80 km) away in a mine. Stig, who had obviously anticipated that the situation could occur at some-time in his career, remembered the times when all the defibrillators used alternating current, and quickly instructed two colleagues to perform CPR and sent a nurse to the nearby department store to buy aluminium foil. He himself took to dismantling a lamp cord to which he attached two electrodes made of aluminium foil. He quickly put the plug in and out of the electrical socket. Initially, there was no effect on the life-threatening rhythm, but after a while sinus rhythm was restored and the woman regained consciousness. She was then transferred to a secondary centre and was treated for her myocardial infarction. She was alive and well at least 15 years after this event.

Stig was one of the founders of the European Resuscitation Council. He was the first chairman of the Basic Life Support Working Group, which published the first educational programme on CPR. As a sign of his attention to detail several days were spent describing the best way of placing the victims arms in the ''recovery position'' This was a ''classical event'' in the history of the ERC.

He is still a member of the ERC executive com-mittee and continues to have a major input into resuscitation in Sweden and Europe.

Stig is still very active, but he has problems leav-ing his main area of interest. He is truly a visionary giant in the field of cardiopulmonary resuscitation.

## Suggested further reading

1. Wennerblom B, Holmberg S, Wedel H. The effect of a mobile coronary care unit on mortality in patients with acute myocardial infarction or cardiac arrest outside hospital. Eur Heart J 1982;3(6):504—15.
2. Holmberg M, Holmberg S, Herlitz J, Gårdelöv B. Survival after cardiac arrest outside hospital in Sweden. Resuscitation 1998;36:29—36.
3. Holmberg M, Holmberg S, Herlitz J. Effect of bystander CPR in out-of-hospital cardiac arrest in Sweden. Resuscitation 2000;47:59—70.
4. Holmberg M, Holmberg S, Herlitz J. Incidence, duration and survival of ventricular fibrillation in out-of-hospital cardiac arrest patients in Sweden. Resuscitation 2000;44:7—17.
5. Holmberg M, Holmberg S, Herlitz J. Factors modifying the effect of bystan-der-CPR on survival in out-of-hospital car-diac arrest patients in Sweden. Eur Heart J 2001;22:511—9.
6. Holmberg M, Holmberg S, Herlitz J. Low chance of sur-vival among patients requiring adrenalin or intubation after out-of-hospital cardiac arrest in Sweden. Resuscitation 2002;54:37—45.

# Harold Hillman

## A. Lowenthal, D. Karcher

Harold Hillman is a remarkable scientist. While his research concentrated primarily on the field of the neurosciences his endeavours have embraced a broader field of ethical principles, humanitarian aid and academic freedom and standards. Much of his work in the neurosciences had an application to resuscitation and to promulgate this aspect he founded this journal in 1972 and remained the Editor-in-chief until 1985 when he relinquished that post to John McCabe.

Harold Hillman was born in 1930 and, after national service with the Royal Air Force where he was an operating theatre assistant, he studied medicine at the Middlesex Hospital Medical School in London. After qualification he embarked upon a research career but always retained a clinical interest and contact with patients as a part-time general practitioner and emergency physician.

As a medical doctor, he attended various laboratories in London and Gothenburg and in so doing developed and refined his experimental knowledge and technique. He always emulated the high standard provided in his early days by the neurochemist Professor Henry McIllwain at the Institute of Psychiatry in London to whom he owed a great deal of his scientific development. Hillman developed primarily experimental studies. He started first to apply resuscitation methods to animals and subsequently examined animals with hypothermic cardiac arrest neurologically. He became reader in physiology in 1968 at the University of Surrey. His research and his teachings were centred on the application of neurochemistry to the interpretation of diagnosis and therapy.

Harold Hillman is among those who engaged in this type of research when it was still at a rudimentary stage. Many times we discussed with great pleasure and interest particular aspects of Hillman's endeavours. His scientific work started from a very moving event. His mother, a general practitioner had several episodes of myocardial infarction, some with prolonged unconsciousness. This led Hillman to study methods of resuscitation in particular from coronary disease and the application of hypothermia in prolonging organ survival. He tells us that in 1954, his mother's heart stopped for 23 min in the hospital. This was a key event for him.

He had two guidelines primary experimental design and the development of techniques based theoretical principles. He never accepted — and this principle persisted all through his career — research which was neither precise nor reproducible. At all times, he required total dedication in his personal studies, and those submitted to him for publication.

Early in his research, he noticed that some of his colleagues indulged in some doubtful practices. These included fabricating data, not reporting findings which did not agree with the hypothesis which the research project was testing, not doing control experiments, using inappropriate calibrations, etc. He was very shocked by these practices, especially when his analysis of a well-known biochemical technique threw into doubt the results of many standard publications. This led him to worry about how he would react, if some other research worker demonstrated, beyond reasonable doubt, that his life work has been based on wrong assumptions, and was of little use.

Therefore, he made two decision. Firstly, that he would always work on two entirely different research projects, so that if anyone 'pulled the rug out' from beneath him, in respect of one project, he could abandon it and continue to work on the other one, without losing his intellectual integrity and life work. Consequently, in 1964, he began working both in experimental resuscitation and in cell biology. His second decision was to determine that no work carried out by him or emanating from his laboratory, would ever contain any corner-cutting or casuistry.

He subsequently devised the concept of 'parafraud'. This terrn covers a series of common practices, which are misleading, but not fraudulent — for example, not doing the necessary control experiments, not reporting findings which fail to support one's hypothesis, refereeing of papers for publication or applications for grants in a hostile manner because they threaten the value of one's own, not reading manuscripts or applications with sufficient care, not answering proper questions about one's research, etc., etc. Subsequently, he published several papers on integrity in research.

He also proposed that in order to improve the quality of research, all students should be taught not only statistics, but also logic, the philosophy of science, and semantics, because all of these must be brought to bear in considering the value of research findings. His questioning attitude to much research led him into discussions with such well-known research workers as, Professors Ernest Chain, Christian de Duve, Hans Krebs and Sir Aldous Huxley. He often stuck to scientific beliefs which were not popular. He was always particularly worried about the effects of his criticism on the self respect and careers of young research workers, so he decided never to criticise them or ask them awkward questions in public; he would discuss their projects privately at tea or coffee time.

In physiology and in pharmacology among the many techniques, he studied anaesthesia very thoroughly in experimental animals and in man. He studied recovery from hypothermic, cardiac arrest in animals, and devised the technique of 'abdominal pumping', a finding of Dr Paul Rogers in Hillman's laboratory in the late 60s. Rats would recover frequently from hypothermic cardiac arrest, if their abdomens were compressed; they called this 'abdominal pumping'. They used the anaesthetised frozen rat firstly to design methods of increasing the incidence of recovery from cardiac arrest and, secondly to analyse the biochemistry of the brain and the blood, and thirdly, to analyse the neurology of recovery of function as one needed large numbers for statistically valid experiments; the use of larger animals would have been too expensive. Dr Charles Babbs and his colleagues at Purdue University, USA later found that 'interposed abdominal compression' in animals increased the chance of recovery, and they collaborated with clinical trials with patients.

Dr Hillman's interests in dying, death and resuscitation, led him to being asked to give evidence and submit affidavits to American courts in respect of prisoners being executed by the electric chair. The current view among the penal authorities was that electrocution results in instant unconsciousness, so that the subjects suffers no pain. Hillman brought evidence from animal slaughter research, accidental electrocution in patients and autopsies of people who had been executed by the electric chair, that the prisoner suffers extreme pain before becoming unconscious. This involvement in the physiology of the electric chair led him to an interest in the effects of stunning during slaughter of animals. Due to his straight forwardness and abiding principles, Hillman became a remarkable person in his field. His scientific rigour was known to all and gave him his charisma.

Since 1970, he has directed the Unity Laboratory of Applied Neurobiology at Surrey University, but has also been a sought after lecturer in other centres in the UK, Europe and Africa. He published prolifically with over a dozen books and chapters to his name and more than 20 significant papers on the subject of hypothermia and resuscitation alone. He also translated the Russian work of Academician A.V. Palladin, little known in Western Europe. His main topics were the study of cardiac arrest, and of the cellular structure of the nervous system from animal and human post mortem material. He focused his attention on the cardiovascular system and the central nervous system. His anatomical and histological studies led to a better understanding of the functions of the membranes, and intracellular movements.

On the ethical and humanitarian side he has served the Schizophrenia Society of Great Britain, War on Want, The Council for Academic Freedom & Standards, Physicians for Human rights

UK, Freedom to Care, British Amnesty and Burrow Hill School for Educationally Subnormal Children.

All of us who have an interest in resuscitation owe a debt to Harold Hillman who founded this journal in 1972 to fill a vacuum in the Scientific literature. It says much for his foresight that the journal goes from strength to strength and remains the only peer reviewed scientific journal in the world entirely devoted to resuscitation. We thank him for that.

## Key References in Hypothermia and Resuscitation

[1] Feldman H, Hillman H. A clinical description of death in rats and the effect of various conditions on the time until cessation of ventricular contraction following section between the brain and spinal cord, Br J Exp Path 1969;50:158–64.

[2] Rogers P, Hillman H. The increased recovery of spontaneous respiration in cats following profound hypothermia, J Appl Physiol 1970;29:58–63.

[3] Shorrock JET, Hillman H. The viscosity of rat blood between 2 and 35°C, Cryobiology 1969;5:324–327.

[4] Rogers P, Hillman H. Increased recovery of anaesthetised hypothermic rats by intracarotid infusions, Nature 1970;228:1314–5.

[5] Hillman H. The biology of dying and death, Archiv. Fndtn Thanatol 1971;2:194–8.

[6] Rogers P, Hillman H. Biochemical changes in the blood during hypothermia cardiac arrest and recovery of rats, Resuscitation 1972;1:25–30.

[7] Hillman H, Loupakine J, Fullbrook P. The clinical history of cardiac arrest and recovery of anaesthetised hypothermic rats, and their reproduction, Resuscitation 1972;1:51–60.

[8] Hillman H, Aldridge T. Towards a legal definition of death, Solicitors J 1972;116:323–6.

[9] Hillman H, Stollery S, Fullbrook P, Saunders C. Metabolic studies on rats recovering from 30 min cardiac arrest due to profound hypothermia, Resuscitation 1972;1:143–8.

[10] Hillman H, The treatment of hypothermia in general practice, General Practitioner 1972;3(11):14.

[11] Hillman H. The hazards of cold. Mountain Life 1972;1:22–24.

[12] Leonard C, Hillman H. The degree of recovery and biochemical changes in the brains of rats during cooling and recovery from cardiac arrest. Resuscitation 1972;1:335–47.

[13] Hillman H, Dying and Death, Teach-in, 1974;3:31–6.

[14] Wigley G, Stokes JJ, Hillman H. Time for death to become irreversible, Resuscitation 1973;2:140.

[15] Hillman H. Medical, ethical and social consequences of widespread resuscitation, Long Range Planning 1977;10:47–53.

[16] Hillman H. Boxing, Resuscitation 1980;8:211–5.

[17] Hillman H. Execution, New Scientist 1983;100:276–8.

[18] Hillman H. Abdominal pumping — a promising new technique, In: Manni C, Magalini SI, editors. Emergency and Disaster Medicine. Berlin: Springer, 1984, p. 404–410.

[19] Hillman H, Jarman D, Britton J. Perspectives in resuscitation, Farmers Weekly 1986;105:39.

[20] Hillman H. Hypothermia, Nursing Times 1987;Jan 28:19–20.

[21] Hillman H. The possible pain experienced during execution by different methods, Perception 1993;22:745–753.

[22] Hillman H. Abdominal pumping, Ann Emergency Med 1994;1:478–81.

[23] Hillman H. Certainty and Uncertainty in Biochemical Techniques. Surrey University Press, 1972. p. 1–126.

[24] Hillman H. Death, In: Stephenson HS, editor. Cardiopulmonary Resuscitation. St Louis: Mosby, 1974. p. 28–34.

# Leon Chameides: A gentle giant and the father of pediatric resuscitation

## Linda Quan

Many would say Leon Chameides, MD, is the father of pediatric resuscitation, and they would say it in many languages. This pediatric cardiologist speaks many languages himself. After learning these, Chameides laid the framework of what would become the language of pediatric resuscitation. He was, and continues to be, instrumental in developing and revising every major pediatric resuscitation program. His programs have trained tens of thousands, have been translated into even more languages encompassing five continents, and have ultimately affected the lives and quality of life of children around the world. How was it that as a pediatric cardiologist, he focused on education, first aid, basic life support, and prevention of arrest, and especially that he directed it to non-physicians? How was he able to develop so many programs, establish them as the standard of care, and get so many organizations to support and adopt them? His life work is a lesson in leadership, vision, and tenacity (Figure 1).

Leon Chameides was born in 1935 in Katowice, Poland. The son of a Rabbi, he would live in this town and with his family only a few years as the winds of hate and war blew across Eastern Europe. He learned to speak Polish from his nanny and this became especially useful when his native German was prohibited in Poland. Just days before the beginning of World War II, his family fled eastward to the Russian half of then divided Poland. At age 7, he learned to live without his family who placed him in a Ukrainian monastery for his safety. A school aged boy, the now Levko Chaminski had to learn to speak Ukrainian and to pray in Church Slavonic in the Ukrainian Greek Catholic church until Poland's liberation by the Soviet army in 1944.

At age 9, he became an assistant to the man who took care of the many wounded soldiers brought to the monastery; Chameides' job was to wash bandages and replenish the supply by going into the woods to remove bandages from dead soldiers. He quickly learned the odors and colors of wounds that predicted death. Perhaps this experience contributed to his future focus on prevention of cardiac arrest, rather than just reanimation.

Chameides immigrated to the United States in 1949, following several years in Britain where he learned English. Living in New York City, he finished high school at age 16 followed by attendance at

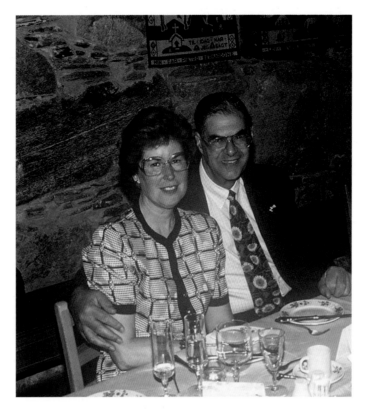

**Figure 1** Leon Chameides with his wife, Jean, in Stavanger, 1995.

Yeshiva University to reclaim his culture and learn Hebrew and Yiddish. In 1955, he graduated Yeshiva College with a B.A. and then the Teacher's Institute with a Hebrew Teacher's Diploma. This educational focus would forever direct his medical interests.

He entered the first class (1959) at the Albert Einstein College of Medicine in New York, NY. He subsequently completed two years of pediatric residency at Strong Memorial Hospital, University of Rochester in Rochester, NY, USA, and then a year of pathology at Boston Children's Hospital, Boston, MA, USA. Military duty also contributed to his later focus, as he served in the US Public Health Service Heart Disease Control Program. He completed his medical training with a pediatric cardiology fellowship at Strong Memorial Hospital in 1967.

As is often true, a single clinical experience during medical training proved a memorable, seminal event in his career. On July 1, 1959, the first day of his internship, at 8 a.m., a mother rushed into the emergency room of the clinic with her apneic 10-day old. Unsupervised, Chameides had no idea what to do. He quickly realized that no one else knew either and that, furthermore, the clinic's emergency room was unprepared for such an event. He stated that they "muddled through" a not-yet-defined resuscitation process, and miraculously the baby survived.

Once fully trained, Chameides directed what would be lifelong efforts to improve his environment. Seeing an opportunity for growth, he joined Hartford Hospital in Hartford, CT in 1967 as their first pediatric cardiologist. He soon began to build a program, which now consists of six pediatric cardiologists, and he remained Chief of Pediatric Cardiology for 30 years.

Chameides' abilities to build and lead a program soon became apparent. Starting in 1971, and for the next 10 years as Chief of Pediatrics at Hartford Hospital, he built the hospital's neonatology, intensive care, and ambulatory service, oversaw enlargement of the pediatric residency program, and recruited other pediatric subspecialists. He was part of a community-wide effort to consolidate the care of children that in 1996 resulted in the opening of a children's hospital, the Connecticut Children's Medical Center. In the early 1970s, he noted that there was no organized approach to resuscitation of newborns, despite the fact that many were born with apnea due to heavy maternal sedation. Neonatal resuscitation consisted of slapping the neonate or blowing high-pressure oxygen in its face. Chameides recounts that one of his pediatric residents was bodily removed from the delivery room when he attempted to intervene. Chameides reasoned that if this problem existed in an institution with approximately 5000 deliveries a year, it must be a national problem, and that the solution had to be national and not local. Addressing the absence of resuscitation training programs and designated providers with resuscitation skills would become his lifelong passion.

Chameides became involved with the newly formed University of Connecticut School of Medicine (1968) and was part of a committee that developed its first cardiovascular curriculum; he became a founding member of its faculty and rose to the rank of Professor in 1985. He has published over 60 papers and chapters in pediatric cardiology; he is most proud of his *New England Journal of Medicine* article that identified maternal lupus as a cause of neonatal heart block.[1] Chameides enjoys the fact that this observation was made clinically in an office setting. This same clinical acumen and experience would be critical in developing the resuscitation guidelines.

Chameides' active involvement in pediatric resuscitation guideline development sprung from early participation in the American Heart Association (AHA). In the early 1970s, Chameides was appointed as a member of the Executive Committees of the Council on Rheumatic Fever and Congenital Heart Disease (now known as the Council on Cardiovascular Disease in the Young) and to the Committee on Professional Medical Education. In

1975, he was asked to answer a question posed by a pediatric cardiologist in Boston about the council's recommendation on the appropriate defibrillation energy dose in infants and children. To address this question, Chameides put together a task group consisting of Grace E. Brown, RN, John R. Raye, MD, David I. Todres, MD, and Peter H. Viles, MD, to review the issue and write a position paper. This resulted in the first AHA pediatric position paper, "Guidelines for Defibrillation in Infants and Children."[2] The only other existing pediatric resuscitation guideline consisted of a table of drugs.

While working on the defibrillation dose issue, Chameides became aware that an ACLS course was being developed; however, there was no similar focus on pediatrics! His goal was to have pediatric input. So he reconvened the previous task group and added Richard Melker, MD, a pediatric intensivist and emergency physician trained in pediatric anesthesiology and cardiology, to write pediatric guidelines for the 1979 National conference. Thus, although he was the sole pediatric representative at that conference, the first Pediatric Basic Life Support standards and guidelines for Neonatal life support came out of the 1979 Conference.[3–6] The American Academy of Pediatrics (AAP) initially questioned why the AHA had developed guidelines for children, especially for the newborn, but a "turf war" was avoided by a series of meetings

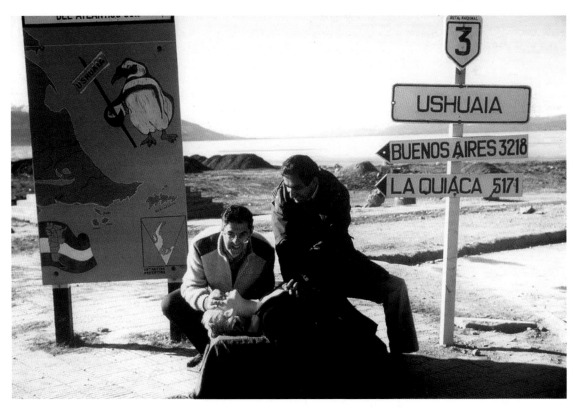

**Figure 2**   Teaching in 1984 in Ushaia, Argentina, the southernmost town in the world.

between Chameides and representatives of the AAP, who ended up endorsing all the guidelines and the courses.

By 1981, pediatrics had a seat at the AHA ECC table. Chameides' band of pediatricians officially had become a subcommittee of the Emergency Cardiac Committee (ECC), and he became the sixth member of the ECC. Chameides' goal was to develop a training course to teach, disseminate, and put into practice the pediatric guidelines. In 1983, under the auspices of the AHA, he chaired a National Conference on Pediatric Resuscitation in Dallas to develop as broad a base of support as possible for the guidelines and eventually the courses. Representatives from all the major organizations dealing with children's health participated in the conference. The Conference was a major success, concluding with consensus that guidelines were needed in Pediatric Basic Life Support, Pediatric Advanced Life Support, and Neonatal Life Support, and that courses should be developed in each of these (Figures 2—4).[7–9]

Chameides considered a neonatal course to be of primary importance because of its potential to do the most good. The need for neonatal resuscitation was much more common than pediatric resuscitation yet delivery rooms were far less prepared for them than emergency departments. One

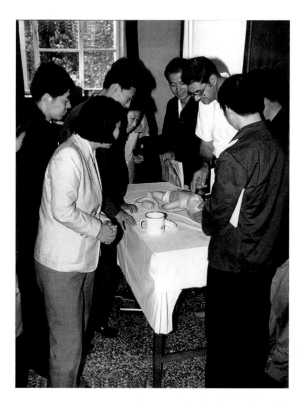

**Figure 3**  Teaching in China, 1983.

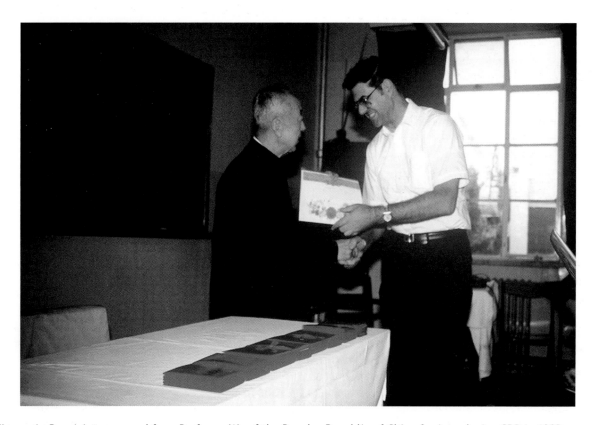

**Figure 4**  Receiving an award from Professor Wu of the Peoples Republic of China for introducing CPR in 1983.

of his challenges was to show the ECC how neonatal resuscitation fitted into their mission. This was one of the few times when a predicament was enough for Chameides to be ''kept up nights.'' By drawing a parallel between the emergency department and the delivery room, and by stressing the need for preparedness to handle life-threatening conditions, Chameides was able to get ECC support for a neonatal resuscitation curriculum. Aware that Ron Bloom, MD, and Catherine Cropley, RN, MSN, had NIH funding to develop a competency-based national neonatal resuscitation program, Chameides worked with them to incorporate AHA program guidelines and to develop what ultimately became the Neonatal Advanced Life Support (NALS) program. Importantly, he was able to forge a partnership with the AAP so that the course was and continues to be co-sponsored by the AHA and AAP. Neonatologists John Raye, MD, and Bill Keenan, MD, provided key leadership at the AHA and AAP. NALS debuted in 1985 and was very well received. Now called the Neonatal Resuscitation Program (NRP), it has been translated into many languages and has been taught all over the world to an estimated two million health care providers under AAP leadership.

Chameides also chaired the group that included Jim Siedel, PhD, MD, Arno Zaritsky, MD, Robert Luten, MD, James McCrory, MD, and Richard Melker, MD, which developed the PALS course. Their shared goal was to make sure it provided an educational experience based on adult learning principles that attempted to reduce the traditional lecture format used in courses such as ACLS; to achieve this, they made the PALS course scenario based. By 1985–1986, they had developed a trial course; by 1988, PALS courses were offered in three places throughout the country in order to train the first group of instructors. Chameides edited the first *PALS Textbook*.[10] Pediatric resuscitation training was a reality and a success, as an enjoyable teaching experience for participants. Using PALS as a model, the ACLS course would change its format to a scenario base educational format over a decade later. Concurrently, with the help of Gary Lapidus, MPH, Chameides developed the first Pediatric Basic Life Support Course (PBLS), which emphasized injury prevention and infant/child CPR.

At the 1986 AHA National Conference, Chameides was one of four pediatric representatives and neonatal, PBLS, and PALS guidelines were developed. Much of the initial planning for the written guidelines was done sitting on his hotel bed with a small group that he coerced into this task through his personal persuasion and with a member's infant on whom some skills were refined. He remained the Chair of the Pediatric Task Force/Committee for 12 years and was asked to resume its leadership after a hiatus of two years. He agreed to do so only on condition that Mary Fran Hazinski, RN, be brought on as Co-Chair and succeed him. This was unprecedented, since no ECC committee had previously been chaired by a non-physician; in fact, there were still discussions as to whether nurses could serve as course directors. Together Chameides and Hazinski edited the second *PALS Textbook*.[11]

With AHA PBLS, PALS, and NRP programs in full swing, Chameides wanted to ensure pediatric representation in the developing International Liaison Group that involved the resuscitation groups of Europe, South Africa, and Australia. Reminiscent of his prior formulae for developing a pediatric presence, Chameides chaired the first International Pediatric resuscitation conference, held in 1994, in Washington DC under the auspices of the AHA. A pediatric subcommittee of the International Liaison group was formed and cemented in the conference process.[12]

In 1999, ECC leadership approached Chameides with a proposal that he lead a group to develop Guidelines in First Aid, followed by the first evidence-based course in First Aid aimed at industry. Leon brought together experts with diverse backgrounds, assisted them in examining and discussing the science, in reaching consensus to distill the science down to what is important for patient care. The first evidence-based guidelines were published in 2000.[13] Bill Hamill, MD, pediatric cardiologist and chair of the First Aid committee states, ''the resulting First Aid course has been wildly successful, one of the most successful courses launched by AHA and adopted by numbers organizations beyond expectations.'' Its accompanying video has won several prestigious prizes (Figure 5).[14–16]

Chameides' success can be measured in many ways, including those whom he has mentored and brought into the ''resuscitation family.'' These include Mary Fran Hazinski, RN, Arno Zaritsky, MD, and Vinay Nadkarni, MD. An outstanding mentor, he has done so deftly, kindly, and respectfully supporting many of us who were unaware we were even being mentored. Mary Fran Hazinski, RN, points out, ''Leon launched us but was the first in line to give credit and the last in line to take credit.'' In addition to the love and respect of his mentorees, he has received many awards and honors, including the Hans Dahll Award for Distinguished Contributions in the Field of Science and Education in Resuscitation from the Citizen CPR Foundation (1996), and the Establishment of and presentation of the first Leon Chameides, MD, Lifetime Achievement Award by Pediatric House Staff, University of Connecticut

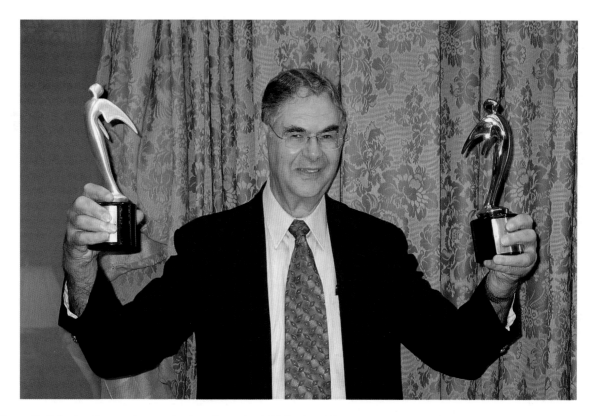

**Figure 5** Winning first and second prizes from the AHA for his videos accompanying the First Aid Course in 2003.

Health Center and Connecticut Children's Medical Center (1997). He was named an Honoree "Giants of Resuscitation" by the American Heart Association Emergency Cardiovascular Care, (2000) and elected as Honorary Member of the European Resuscitation Council (2000); he also received a Yeshiva College Alumni Association Bernard Revel Memorial Award for Professional Achievement (2002).

Chameides is thrilled that there is now a growing literature in the science of pediatric resuscitation, and continuing, expanding interest. He cannot choose his favorite program or most exciting achievement, noting that he is passionate about each project, and then moves on. He sees the real challenge as building a scientific basis for the guidelines. He is pleased, however, to note that many of the pediatric guidelines have endured and still make sense, although lacking science and formulated through discussions in an airport hotel room over two decades ago. However, as Mary Fran Hazinski, RN, elucidates, "Chameides is never satisfied with the status quo and will continue to strive for simplification and distillation of the guidelines to make them even more useful."

Despite continuing efforts to address the needs of pediatric resuscitation training, Chameides has few frustrations; he is pleased with what he has accomplished and the enormous support the AHA has provided. However, he points out that we still do not know how best to do CPR. The "ballet" of CPR is difficult, and people are too intimidated to dance. He believes much of the reluctance on the part of the public to perform CPR is related to individual psychology rather than teaching technique. The challenge is to understand how to get people to increase their self-confidence so that they will act and perform CPR when the need arises.

Focused on ventilation, chest compressions, and first aid, Chameides is unique as a pediatric cardiologist interested in resuscitation. However, it was his first resuscitation experience at the start of internship, his recognition of the unmet needs of the newborn, and his teaching background that drove his resuscitation interest, not pediatric cardiology with all its seductive technologies. He never had an illusion or a belief in reanimation; for him, resuscitation was not about saving children who were in cardiac standstill, but about raising the level of reaction and intervention before cardiac arrest. He sees the frontline health care providers, emergency medical technicians, and emergency department-based providers, as the key players in the mission to prevent cardiac arrest. His vision has been to develop national standards that will establish a culture that would filter down to local providers. Using his remarkable leadership skills, he has worked from a top down approach with organizations that facilitated his vision.

How did Chameides' achieve such long-standing, continued success at building programs? He enjoys the process of bringing different views together, finding common threads, and developing solutions that everyone can live with, solutions that make everyone "the most happy." He attributes his success to his ability to listen carefully; he interjects his opinions but does not insist on them. (He grins when declaring that he was early on a proponent of ventilation-only CPR.) Vinay Nadkarni, MD, describes Chameides as a "gentle giant", "a man who embodies trust, peace, and justice. He has a sense of history and intense intellectual honesty, and has mentored the field of pediatric and neonatal resuscitation science and practice with a kind and gentle, but firm, approach." Zaritsky notes, "he easily could have written the 1992 book, *"Getting to Yes"* since he clearly understood its basic principle of first seeking to understand the point that someone is making before attempting to make your point. Anyone who has worked with Leon recognizes his humility and his interest in focusing on what is in the best interest of helping children rather than promoting his own career. This approach has served Chameides well and is certainly one of the important lessons he imparted to those who were fortunate enough to work with him." His focus on the objective rather than being right has worked at the individual, committee, and organizational level. He has been a master at getting organizations' support to establish, engage, and nurture program development and production. He is almost always the man behind the scenes: setting the goal, identifying the key players, allowing the creative pot to boil with only an occasional stir while keeping his ego out of it. As proof, he is unable to identify issues for which he "had to go to the mat." In true fashion, eloquently and elegantly, Dr. Chameides sums up his astounding career that has aided so many children and their health care providers in all corners of the earth, as "I just arranged the deck chairs."

Chameides retired from active clinical practice at age 62 in order to translate his father's newly discovered essays from German and Polish into English and to study the history of his native Jewish community.[17] However, Chameides pursues his commitment to resuscitation even into his retirement. Most recently, he was editor and writer of the 2005 AHA Pediatric and First Aid Guidelines, once again using his skills to bring clarity, conciseness, and consensus to the written guidelines.[18]

While Chameides always looks forward, not backwards, he continues a longstanding interest in the history of medicine. He is most interested in 18th century resuscitation history because it was an era when Holland and England established Royal Societies to address fires and drowning at a societal level. These have been the visions of his interest in resuscitation: centralized standards of care, ubiquitous, provided at home, on the street, in hospital. A Renaissance man of arts and letters, with values based in the18th century of societal concerns, and a 20th century leader, Chameides is fully a man of the 21st century because what he has led and overseen has become the basis for care provided not just for a region, or a nation, but the world.

## References

1. Chameides L, Truex RC, Vetter V, Rashkind WJ, Galioto Jr FM, Noonan JA. Association of maternal systemic lupus erythematosus with congenital complete heart block. N Engl J Med 1977;297(22):1204—7.
2. Chameides L, Brown GE, Raye JR, Todres DI, Viles PH. Guidelines for defibrillation in infants and children. Circulation 1977;56:502A.
3. Chameides L, Melker R, Raye JR, Todres DI, Viles PH. Basic life support in infants and children. Standards and guidelines for cardiopulmonary resuscitation and emergency cardiac care. JAMA 1980;244:472.
4. Chameides L, Melker R, Raye JR, Todres DI, Viles PH. Advanced life support in neonates. Standards and guidelines for cardiopulmonary resuscitation and emergency cardiac care. JAMA 1980;244:494.
5. Chameides L, Melker R, Raye JR, Todres DI, Viles PH. Resuscitation of infants and children. In: Textbook of Advanced Life Support. Dallas, TX: American Heart Association; 1981.
6. Chameides L, Melker R, Raye JR, Todres DI, Viles PH. Resuscitation of the newborn. In: Textbook of Advanced Life Support. Dallas, TX: American Heart Association; 1981.
7. Standards and Guidelines for Cardiopulmonary Resuscitation (CPR) Emergency Cardiac Care (ECC). Pediatric basic life support. JAMA 1986;255:2954.
8. Standards and Guidelines for Cardiopulmonary Resuscitation (CPR) and Emergency Cardiac Care (ECC). Pediatric advanced life support. JAMA 1986;255:2961.
9. Standards and Guidelines for Cardiopulmonary Resuscitation (CPR) and Emergency Cardiac Care (ECC). Neonatal advanced life support. JAMA 1986;255:2969.
10. Chameides L, editor. Textbook of Pediatric Advanced Life Support. Dallas, TX: American Heart Association; 1988.
11. Chameides L, Hazinsky MF, editors. Textbook of Pediatric Advanced Life Support. 2nd ed. Dallas, TX: American Heart Association; 1994.
12. Zaritsky A, Nadkarni V, Hazinsky MF, Foltin G, Quan L, Wright J, et al. Recommended guidelines for uniform reporting of pediatric advanced life support: the pediatric Utstein style. A statement for health care professionals from a task force of the American Academy of Pediatrics, the American Heart Association, and the European Resuscitation Council. Resuscitation 1995;30:95—115.

13. Chameides L, Berlin P, Cummins R. New guidelines for first aid. Circulation 2000;102:177—85.
14. Chameides L, editor. Heartsaver First Aid. Dallas, TX: American Heart Association; 2002.
15. Chameides L, editor. Heartsaver First Aid with CPR and AED. Dallas, TX: American Heart Association; 2002.
16. Chameides L, editor. Heartsaver First Aid Instructor Manual. Dallas, TX: American Heart Association; 2002.
17. Chameides L. Rabbi Kalman Chameides: one of the last spiritual leaders of Katowice. A tribute. In: Wodzinski M, Spyra J, editors. Jews in Silesia. Cracow: Ksiegarnia Akademicka. University of Wroclaw Research Center for Culture and Languages of Polish Jews; 2001.
[18]. American Heart Association Guidelines for Cardiopulmonary Resuscitation and Emergency Cardiovascular Care. Circulation 2005;112(Suppl. IV):112.

# Leonard Cobb and Medic One

## Mickey S. Eisenberg

I was an intern in 1971 and Leonard Cobb was my attending physician in the coronary care unit at Harborview Medical Center. Daily we visited patients on the ward resuscitated from out-of-hospital ventricular fibrillation by the Seattle Fire Department paramedics. It seemed so ordinary at the time—I assumed all CCUs contained survivors of sudden cardiac arrest. Little at the time did I appreciate how astounding this was and the unique role Leonard Cobb played in making such events possible. In 1971 the Seattle paramedic program (Medic One as it was known locally) was 1 year old and it was one of the first of its kind in the world.

In the US prehospital care for out-of-hospital cardiac emergencies was an idea imported from Europe. The seminal work of Frank Pantridge and John Geddes in Belfast, Northern Ireland was published in *The Lancet* in 1967 [1]. Their idea was to turn an ambulance into a mobile intensive care unit and provide care directly at the scene of a suspected heart attack. The Pantridge/Geddes model required staffing by physicians and nurses. Although similar programs were initiated a few years later, by William Grace in New York City [2] and Richard Crampton in Charlottesville, Virginia [3], the idea of sending doctors and nurses was essentially a nonstarter in the US. Instead a handful of innovative physicians in five American cities developed an alternative program based on the Pantridge/Geddes model and created the paramedic. Almost simultaneously paramedic programs were started by Eugene Nagel and Jim Hirschman in Miami [4], James Warren and Richard Lewis in Columbus, Ohio [5], Michael Criley in Los Angeles [6], Leonard Rose in Portland, Oregon [7], and Leonard Cobb in Seattle [8,9]. The initial programs trained fire fighters as paramedics though later programs used non-fire fighters. The paramedic/fire fighter made sense in the US as, historically, much of pre-

hospital emergency medical care was provided by fire departments. An emphasis of these early programs was on the treatment of cardiac arrest. The Belfast program was designed primarily for the early and rapid management of acute coronary syndromes and, of course, sometimes cardiac arrest occurred and was treated. The paramedic programs had a primary goal to treat cardiac arrest and thus were designed to get to the scene within minutes, yet another reason to base the programs in fire departments.

Cobb, and the other innovators mentioned above, all deserve a place in the Pantheon of Resuscitation Greats. However, Cobb's place is assured for two other crucial innovations. He devised the tiered response system and he began community-wide citizen CPR training thus making citizens a crucial link in the chain of survival.

Leonard Arthur Cobb was born on June 23, 1926 in St. Paul, Minnesota. At age 17 he enlisted in the Navy. Much of his naval service took place in the US, but he did spend some time in the Philippines working with the construction battalions on Samar. Cobb rose to the rank of Electronics Technician's Mate Third Class, and was honorably discharged in 1946.

Like many young returning veterans, Cobb plunged straight into college after the war. He entered the University of Minnesota in 1946 and then went on to medical school, graduating in 1952. He then completed an internship at the University of Iowa and a residency in internal medicine at the University of California, San Francisco. In 1953, Cobb travelled to Switzerland, where he studied metabolism at the University of Zurich. He returned to the US the following year and completed a fellowship in cardiology in Boston, and Stanford. In 1957, he accepted a teaching position at the University of Washington in Seattle. By 1963, Cobb was appointed to Director of Cardiology at Harborview Hospital in Seattle and became Professor of Medicine in 1971.

Cobb's early research focused on valvular heart disease [10]. One particularly striking piece of research

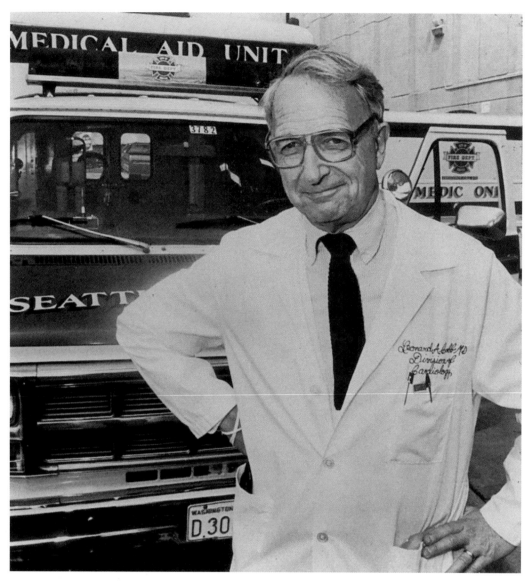

Fig. 1. Leonard Cobb

involved a double-blind evaluation of internal mammary artery ligation for coronary artery disease [11]. At the time, 'everyone' believed the artery ligation to be effective and, I suspect, several prominent surgeons questioned the need for such a study. The study, however, revealed the technique to be worthless. This classic study, his fourth scientific work to be published, already reveals a key trait of his character, namely scepticism of conventional wisdom. This trait would serve him well throughout his professional career and would lead him to begin new programs when 'everyone' said it couldn't be done. It would also lead to research that questioned established dogma.

As a cardiologist, Cobb was well aware of the problem of sudden cardiac arrest. In 1967 he came across the article written by Pantridge and Geddes in *The Lancet*. Pantridge's article energized Cobb to embark on a completely different type of research he had been conducting. 'I remember reading their report,' Cobb recalls, 'I think it was the first time anyone had come forth with an organized effort to provide pre-hospital care for patients with cardiac disease.' Cobb knew the Seattle Fire Department was already involved in first aid. He looked up Fire Chief Gordon Vickery and discovered the fire department had a system in place for documenting first aid runs carefully. Cobb realized that this system could provide scientific documentation for the efficacy (or lack thereof) of Pantridge's suggestions. Herein lies a second key trait to his character, namely, the desire to innovate. With the full and active support of Chief Vickery, Cobb and several medical colleagues first sought a grant in 1967 to fund a program in Seattle using a paramedic staffed mobile intensive care unit. It was turned down. They tried again the next year, and succeeded. The grant came from the Washington/Alaska Regional Medical Program, one of

Lyndon Johnson's Great Society programs. They were awarded $450 000 for a 3-year period. The funding primarily paid the salaries for 15 firefighters to be trained as paramedics. Salaries then were approximately $10 000 a year. Their first goal was to save lives. Their second goal, and here is the innovation, was to see if non-physicians really could carry out resuscitation and management of cardiac arrest. This would be a major change in the role of a fire department. Their third goal was to try and learn more about sudden cardiac death and see if the program really achieved its goals. The third goal reveals Cobb's third trait as a resuscitation great, namely, rigorous scientific investigation. Cobb had little desire to merely create a new program. In some ways, that was the easy part. He wished, in addition, to study the program, to see if it worked and to understand the factors associated with successful resuscitation.

Cobb ran into considerable opposition from his own colleagues. Some members of the King County Medical Society and the Red Cross thought Cobb's idea was a waste of time. Cobb and Vickery pressed ahead, however. With money from the grant, the fire department purchased a mobile coronary care unit and one of the deputy fire chiefs personally drove it from the Midwest back to Seattle. The 'mobile unit' they got was actually a large motor home with rounded sides, an Oldsmobile Toronado engine, and front-wheel drive. It had a kitchen sink, hot and cold running water, a refrigerator and freezer, and a toilet. The mobile unit soon acquired several nicknames—the most endearing being Moby Pig.

The toilet soon came out and other equipment went in. The conversion from motor home to mobile cardiac care unit was all done by intuition and inspiration. Neither Cobb nor Vickery—nor any of their associates—had ever designed a mobile coronary care unit. The mobile unit ended up with a huge coronary-care console installed. It carried then-state-of-the-art portable DC defibrillators and all the necessary respiratory equipment and medications. The first group of trained medics helped construct the mobile unit. They also took part in devising the protocols for treatment, copying much from then-current practices in hospital CCUs.

In mid-1969, Vickery began asking for firefighter volunteers for the new mobile unit, and in October, he helped select Seattle's first 15 paramedics. Cobb personally supervised their training. At the time it wasn't exactly clear what to teach the firefighters since there was no precedent to follow. Today detailed curricula are available, but not back then. Cobb put together a commonsense curriculum that included ECG rhythm interpretation, defibrillation, emergency administration of medications, and IV use. The training lasted several months.

In March 1970, the first class of paramedics took to the streets of Seattle. The mobile unit—and there was only one at first—was stationed outside the Harborview Hospital emergency room. As Cobb himself points out, the mobile unit was not the real innovation. Rather, it was the concept of a 'tiered response' to medical emergencies. The idea was 'that we would get someone out there quickly'—via the fire department's already-existing mobile first aid units—'and then a secondary response would come from the mobile intensive coronary care unit.' The beauty of the tiered response system was the efficient use of fire department personnel. The system allowed aid personnel to reach the scene quickly, in an average of 3 min, to start CPR. Then a few minutes later the paramedics arrived to provide more definitive care such as defibrillation. In this way the brain could be kept alive until the electric shock converted the heart to a normal rhythm. After the patient was stabilized the paramedics would transport the person to the hospital. Subsequent research has demonstrated that tiered response systems achieve a higher cardiac arrest survival compared to single tiered systems—undoubtedly due to the more rapid provision of CPR [12].

One of the first persons to be resuscitated in the Seattle program was a 17-year-old boy, with cardiomyopathy. Cobb remembered the event vividly. 'The boy was downtown in his father's office. After he went to the bathroom, somebody went in and found him slumped over unconscious. They called the unit and he had VF.' After a successful resuscitation, 'He was very slow to wake up; it took 10 days. He went back to finish high school and went skiing the following winter.'

For the first 9 months, the paramedics had a doctor on board their emergency runs. Cobb used the physicians as a kind of safety net and a reassurance to the medical community. It was always his intent to run the program with paramedics. Before the year was out, the paramedics were on their own. The physician was miles away at the base station hospital, though voice connection by radio or phone was always an option. The paramedics learned by watching and doing, and took over. One critical skill learned from working with the doctors was how to put in tracheal tubes. This was not part of the initial training, but it soon became apparent that tracheal intubation was a vital resuscitation skill. Despite some initial concerns, it was obvious that it worked just fine without doctors on the runs. Cobb devised standing orders signed by him which authorized the paramedics to provide defibrillation, perform tracheal intubation, start an intravenous line and administer medications for the management of cardiac arrest. For routine cases, not involving resuscitation, the paramedics contacted the base station physician by radio or phone prior to administering any medication. But for cardiac arrest, speed was everything—start the resuscitation, perform the critical procedures, and then contact the base station physician.

During the first year the Medic One program resuscitated and admitted 61 patients to the hospital; 31 were discharged. One of those made national news, on CBS's 60 Minutes. The 60 Minutes crew came to Seattle to film a segment on the burgeoning citizen CPR program and rode with the Seattle mobile unit, filming several resuscitations. The one that made the program was a resuscitation of a woman with multiple sclerosis. The 60 Minutes show was sufficiently impressed with what they witnessed to call Seattle 'the best place in the nation to have a heart attack'.

Word of the program was starting to spread nationally. But within Seattle the program was in jeopardy. Problems with funding occurred even before the program celebrated its third anniversary. The initial funding grant had to absorb a 25% cut, leaving the total grant of $450 000 over $100 000 short. The city would not make up the difference and, in fact, reminded Cobb that the grant had promised funding for a full 3 years. Vickery and Cobb decided on a fund-raising program. Rather than go the usual route of seeking corporate or institutional contributions, Vickery and Cobb decided on a nickel and dime grass roots approach. They reasoned that the program was for the community and in 2 years had garnered good publicity and strong local support. Nevertheless, Cobb was initially sceptical of the strategy. He later recalled, 'Initially I said, oh my God, we've got to go out with a hat on the corner and beg people to allow us to stay in business. In retrospect it was okay, but at the time it sure didn't seem like that was a very good idea.' The newspapers supported the effort with front-page thermometers showing the progress of the campaign. It was a real grass roots campaign—barbers donated a day's earnings, car dealers donated money, teenagers put on walk-a-thons in the city, donation jars were set up in malls. Over $200 000 was raised, double the amount needed to keep the program in business.

The Seattle paramedic program did more than pioneer paramedics and develop a tiered-response system. It was the first program in the world to make citizens an active part of the emergency system. Cobb knew from data the program had collected that the sooner CPR was started, the better the chances of survival. He reasoned that the best way to ensure early initiation of CPR was to train the bystanders. Thus Cobb, along with the support of Vickery, began a citizen CPR training program in 1972, the first of its kind in the world. Its goal was to train over 100 000 people in Seattle when and how to do CPR. Cobb recalled how the idea was first proposed. "One day he (Vickery) said, 'Look, if it's so important to get CPR started quickly and if firemen come around to do it, it can't be that complicated that other folks couldn't also learn—fire-

men are not created by God to do CPR. You could train the public.' I said, 'That sounds like a very good idea.' Shortly afterwards things started." Cobb decided to use an abbreviated course of training. He later described how the course was set up. 'We weren't going to do it by traditional ways where they had to come for 20 h or thereabouts. So they had to do it at one sitting—how long will people participate?—well, maybe 3 h. And that's pretty much the way it was. It was basically a notion that we had to do the training at one sitting.' At the time, Cobb had no idea know how long it would take to train 100 000 people, since such an undertaking had never before been attempted. In fact it took only a few years. By the 20th anniversary of the program, over 500 000 people in Seattle and the surrounding suburbs had received CPR training. This community wide citizen CPR training program is the sole reason Seattle and surrounding King County, Washington have the highest rates of bystander CPR in the world.

There were sceptics of the mass citizen training in CPR. Many felt the potential for harm was too great to allow such a procedure to be placed in the hands of laypeople. The sceptics had the support of some national medical organizations. When CPR was first promoted in the early 1960s, it was clearly defined as a 'medical procedure.' In a 1962 editorial in *Circulation* signed by the American Heart Association and the American Red Cross, CPR was to be applied only by carefully trained physicians. By 1965 this view had already changed. In another editorial in *Circulation*, CPR was reclassified as an 'emergency procedure.' It was recommended that training be widely disseminated to physicians, dentists, nurses, and ambulance personnel. Training of the general public was not recommended. Finally, in 1973, the American Heart Association at its national conference (with the results published in 1974) recommended training of the general public.

If Cobb had waited for official blessing, the entire citizen training effort would have been delayed 3 years. The sceptics were silenced thanks to some fortunate saves. Cobb recalled one resuscitation, involving a 54-year-old man, soon after the CPR training program began: 'In March'73 there were these kids playing golf at Jackson Park. They came across a victim a quarter of a mile from the clubhouse—so these kids had taken the CPR course over at the local high school. Two or three of them began doing CPR and the other kid ran off and phoned the fire department. Shortly they came with the aid car and Medic One screaming over the fairways.' The man was in ventricular fibrillation and required three shocks to be converted to a regular heart rhythm. Cobb concluded the story, 'They got him started up again. He survived; he's alive today (1990). That was a very convincing story. I didn't mind it being written up in the Reader's Digest.'

Cobb was never one to suffer official pronouncements or official dogma. The sceptics never seemed to bother him. 'I think,' he said, 'there were sceptics all along who didn't have much belief in CPR, resuscitation, or even CCUs. Basically we took stuff that was on the shelves already and did some packaging of it and made some modifications. We didn't have to develop CPR—CPR was done in 1960; we didn't have to develop a portable defibrillator—it was already there. We just put a good package together. It wasn't easy. There are all kinds of reasons why not to do it. It does take a lot of persistence. I think you have to realize that probably it's going to work. The two questions that we originally posed were, can you save lives? And, can you develop lay people to carry out this function of medical care? Both of those questions were answered affirmatively.'

Cobb modestly thinks the Medic One program and the citizen CPR programs were low-cost social experiments. 'Probably our major contribution in Seattle was in marshalling the necessary resources and people to see if something will work. It didn't cost a whole lot if it didn't work. If Medic One didn't save any lives, all we would be out would be the $450 000. That wasn't so bad.' It was a good investment. By Cobb's own calculations it cost $3000 to save a life in 1970. The mathematics were simple: $150 000 to run the program and 50 lives saved.

The Medic One program was, and is, an outstanding success. It continues to receive widespread community support. In the mid 1970s the program was emulated in the surrounding suburbs of Seattle. The Seattle Medic One and King County EMS system now serves 1 700 000 people. Since its inception the program was supported by tax dollars. All care and transportation are free to the citizen. In 1976 a series of county-wide levies was passed by voters to fund the program. The annual cost to the citizen is approximately 25 cents for every $1000 of assessed property valuation. In 2001 a levy vote to support the program for an additional 6 years was passed with 81% in favor.

In 1993 Cobb stepped down as Medical Director of the Medic One program and turned the directorship over to Dr Michael Copass. But Cobb has never been more active. He continues to serve as President of the Medic One Foundation (whose mission is to fund innovative programs in prehospital emergency medicine) and he remains as productive as ever as a researcher with 22 peer-reviewed publications in the past 5 years. His questioning of conventional wisdom continues to shine. In 1999 he published a study comparing persons in ventricular fibrillation receiving immediate defibrillation to those receiving 90 s of CPR prior to defibrillation [13]. The results suggested that those with CPR prior to defibrillation did better, thus calling into question whether defibrillation should always be the first therapy for VF. Cobb is the first to admit the study is not conclusive since it is an observational study without randomization of the intervention. Nevertheless, it suggests there may be a better way, a way different from perceived wisdom.

That is the essence of Cobb—scepticism, innovation, and meticulous research. These traits have served him well—to start one of the world's first paramedic program, to document its effectiveness, to create a tiered response system and citizen CPR training, to continually question how to do things better, and how to save more lives.

Parts of the bibliographic profile of Leonard Cobb are derived from a profile of his work in Eisenberg, M.S., *Life in the Balance: Emergency Medicine and the Quest to Reverse Sudden Death*. 1997, Oxford, New York, pp. 232–238.

Quotes from Leonard Cobb are from an interview conducted on February 2, 1993.

## References

[1] Pantridge J.F., Geddes J.S.. A mobile intensive-care unit in the management of myocardial infarction. Lancet 1967;ii:271–3.

[2] Grace W.J., Chadbourn J.A.. The mobile coronary care unit. Diseases of the Chest 1969;55:452–5.

[3] Crampton R.S., Aldrich R.D., Gascho J.A., et al. Reduction of pre-hospital, ambulance, and community coronary death rates by the community-wide emergency cardiac care system. Am J Med 1975;58:151–65.

[4] Nagel E.L., Nirschman J.C., Nussenfeld S.R., Rankin D., Lundblad E.. Telemetry-medical command in coronary and other mobile emergency care systems. JAMA 1970;214:332–8.

[5] Stand J.M., Keller M.D., Lewis R.P.. Mobile pre-hospital coronary care, Columbus, Ohio. In: Adgey A.A., editor. Acute Phase of Ischemic Heart Disease and Myocardial Infarction. The Hague: Martinus Hijhoff, 1982:99–118.

[6] Criley J.M., Lewis A.J., Ailshie G.E.. Mobile emergency care unite, implementation and justification. Advances in Cardiology 1975;15:9–24.

[7] Rose L.B., Press E.. Cardiac defibrillation by ambulance attendants. JAMA 1972;219:63–8.

[8] Baum R.S., Alvarez H., III, Cobb L.A.. Survival after resuscitation from out-of-hospital ventricular fibrillation. Circulation 1974;50:1231–5.

[9] Cobb L.A., Baum R.S., Alvarez H., III, Schaffer W.A.. Resuscitation from out-of-hospital ventricular fibrillation: four year follow-up. Circulation 1975;51 & 52(III):223–8.

[10] Dexter L., Harken D.E., Cobb La, Novack P., Schlant R.C., Phinney A.O., et al. Aortic stenosis. Arch Intern Med 1958;101:254–6.

[11] Cobb La, Thomas G.E., Dillard D.H., Merendino K.A., Bruce R.A.. An evaluation of internal mammary artery ligation by double-blind technique. N Engl J Med 1959;260:1115–8.

[12] Eisenberg M.S., Horwood B.T., Cummins R.O., Reynolds-Haertle R., Hearne T.R.. Cardiac arrest and resuscitation: a tale of 29 cities. Ann Emerg Med 1990;19:179–86.

[13] Cobb L.A., Fahrenbruch C.E., Walsh T.R., Copass M.K., Olsufka M., Breskin M., et al. Influence of cardiopulmonary resuscitation prior to defibrillation in patients with out-of-hospital ventricular fibrillation. JAMA 1999;282:1182–8.

# Bjørn Lind—the ground-breaking nurturer

Nina Tjomsland     Tore Laerdal     Peter Baskett

"My first appointment as a trained anaesthesiologist was in Stavanger in 1956. Because of this, I came by chance to contribute to the beginnings of cardiopulmonary resuscitation, and to an important part of its development. This was a unique opportunity, which has given me great satisfaction in my further career", says Bjørn Lind.

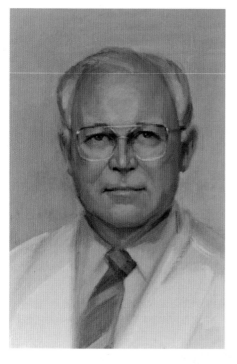

Fig. 1.  Bjørn Lind.

The Stavanger story, of the conception of the Resusci Anne training manikin, is well-known history. But, seen in retrospect, the concept was a highly unlikely one. Anaesthesiology was a very young profession in Norway. Lind was the 13th physician to enter the speciality, and the first and only in the field while working in Stavanger—a provincial town with about 50,000 inhabitants and two hospitals (Fig. 1).

Chiefly because of its long coast, Norway had a long-standing tradition of teaching resuscitation in schools. In 1939, the Holger–Nielsen method – back pressure arm lift – was included in the primary school curriculum and subsequent reports indicated that people would use it without hesitation. But when Peter Safar told the Congress of the Scandinavian Society of Anaesthesiologists at Gausdal in 1958 about his own work on mouth-to-mouth resuscitation, based on his own and James Elam's findings, Bjørn Lind and his colleagues were fascinated, and discussed the possibility of replacing the arm lift back-pressure practice with this new method [1]. The question was how the method could be taught, and whether people would be willing to use it. The Norwegian Association of Anaesthesiologists wanted to introduce mouth-to-mouth ventilation, and established a resuscitation committee to study the problems. From 1959, all manuals and pamphlets distributed by the Norwegian Red Cross and the Norwegian Civil Defence included the new method [1]. Individual members also worked hard to promote mouth-to-mouth ventilation. Bjørn Lind taught the method to colleagues at hospital meetings in Stavanger, using as subjects anaesthetised patients undergoing minor operations, but without much acceptance. He even used his wife – anaesthetised for the occasion – as a patient for one of these meetings.

Then, one day, the toy manufacturer Åsmund S. Lærdal called at his office. Lærdal was making wound imitations for the Red Cross in Sweden and Norway. Having heard about the new method from the medical adviser to the Swedish Red Cross, Dr. Per Stroemback, he saw the need for a training aid. Åsmund Lærdal had had international success with the life-like Anne doll, and thought that a life-size, life-like training manikin would be preferable, especially for psychological reasons. Could Dr. Lind help him address this challenge?

"This meeting decided the track of my career", says Bjørn Lind.

## 1. Designing the Resusci Anne

For a whole year, the two were in almost daily contact, working to make every detail simulate the key parts of the anatomy and physiology as realistically as possible. In the process, they became close friends. When the prototype Resusci Anne was finished in May 1960, two major points had to be proved: that the manikin was an effective training aid, and that people would accept the method and be willing to use it.

In September 1960, Bjørn Lind demonstrated the manikin to Professor Ronnie Woolmer in London, who was his friend and very interested in the topic. Woolmer immediately appreciated the great training potential of the manikin.

Back in Norway, Lind showed the manikin to the Director General of the Health Services, and obtained the go-ahead for a pilot project in the county of Rogaland. Together with the County Counsellor for physical training, he started teaching some 200 6th and 7th graders (13–14-year-olds),

using the manikin, with a control group being shown only an instruction film.

The time had come to show the manikin to Peter Safar. Safar immediately grasped its potential, and suggested a metal ring inside the chest, to include training in external compression as well.

The following year, in August 1961, Bjørn Lind and Ivar Lund hosted the First International Symposium on Resuscitation in Stavanger, on behalf of the Norwegian Society of Anaesthesiology. Dr. Woolmer chaired the meeting, and among the attending resuscitation pioneers from Europe and the United States were Peter Safar, James Elam, Archer Gordon, Henning Ruben and Rudolf Frey (Figs. 2 and 3).

Bjørn Lind presented the results of the school trial, and training with the new manikin. Seventy-three percent of the children who had worked with the manikin, achieved satisfactory ventilation, compared to 37% of the pupils who had only seen the film. The symposium concluded that the entire population should learn mouth-to-mouth ventilation, while external chest compressions should be reserved for helpers who had had special training. These recommendations were published as a supplement to the Acta Anaesthesiologica Scandinavia [2]. The supplement raised a great deal of interest in many parts of the world. Bjørn Lind was invited to several European meetings, and even to Cuba to demonstrate the new method and the Resusci Anne manikin.

By October 1960, Norwegian savings banks had donated 650 manikins to primary schools, of which 42 were placed in Rogaland. Bjørn Lind trained 31 first aid instructors, who then

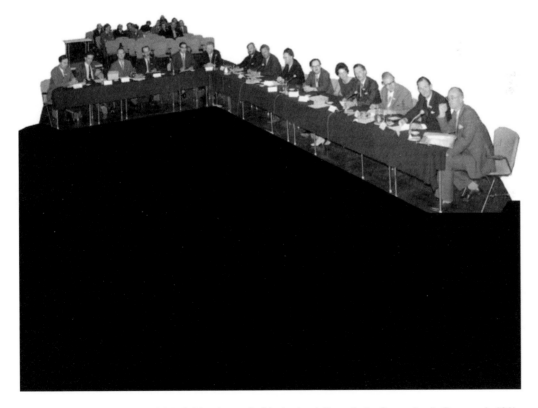

Fig. 2. Bjørn Lind (no. 3 from right) chairing the panel of the landmark Resuscitation Symposium in Stavanger in 1961.

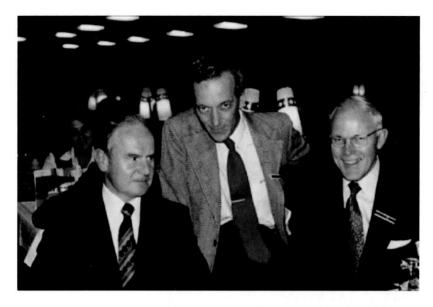

Fig. 3. Three "Resuscitation Greats" and great friends; from right: Bjørn Lind, Peter Safar and Åsmund S. Lærdal.

taught 765 school teachers how to instruct the children. This made possible the training of 6900 pupils, who represented 80% of their age group, by the spring of 1961. At the same time, a similar programme was started nationwide. This made Norway the pioneer in teaching mouth-to-mouth ventilation to an entire population.

## 2. Published in JAMA

Two years later, Lind and his colleague Jacob Stovner presented evidence that the Norwegian population had indeed accepted the method. At that time, the newspapers took a keen interest in resuscitation. Press clippings over two years showed that 40 of 85 reported resuscitation attempts – most of them drowning – had been successful. Interviewing the rescuers, Lind and Stovner found that only six had hesitated to start resuscitation for hygienic reasons. This analysis was published in *JAMA* in 1963 [3]. Nevertheless, in that same year, when Lind and Lund presented heart–lung resuscitation to the national medical society, the reception was lukewarm, not least among the cardiologists. One declared that if he were ever to suffer a cardiac arrest, he most certainly wanted no attempts at external chest compressions.

In 1967, Lind and Lund organised the second international symposium on resuscitation for the Norwegian Association of Anaesthesiology. To promote CPR around the world, the World Federation of Societies of Anaesthesiologists published a manual written by Peter Safar on cardiopulmonary resuscitation, in accordance with the guidelines from this symposium. This manual was printed in more than 300,000 copies, in 16 different languages [4]. The manual went on to further editions in 1981 and 1987 [5,6] (Fig. 4).

Bjørn Lind would never accept any fee from Åsmund S. Lærdal for his contribution. So one day, when they were on a professional visit in London, the industrialist took him into

a musical instrument dealer's and presented him with a rare cello. Now in his mid-80s, Lind still enjoys playing this very cello, and has decided that his treasure will eventually go to the Oslo Philharmonic Orchestra (Fig. 5).

## 3. Inspired by a who-done-it

World War II interrupted higher education in Norway. Bjørn Lind was 28 years old when he graduated from medical school in 1948. Actually, it was a film that pulled him into the field of anaesthesiology. Serving as an intern at the Trondheim hospital, he wanted initially to specialise in ophthalmology—until he saw the thriller "Green for Danger", where bottles of oxygen and carbon dioxide were switched during an operation. One of the main protagonists was an anaesthesiologist. This was young Lind's first glimpse of an anaesthetist at work, and he was fascinated. "This seemed the closest you could come to a physiology lab. I was very interested in physiology and pharmacology, and decided to make this my specialty."[1]

After spending one year as an intern in the anaesthesiology department at the Ullevål hospital in Oslo, Lind went to Copenhagen to study at the WHO Centre of Anaesthesiology. Here he made important contacts. In 1952, with just two years experience of anaesthesiology, he spent six months during the Korean war at the Norwegian field hospital, "Normash". On the plane going there, he felt inadequate, wondering "what on earth am I, with my slight background, going to do in the middle of the war zone?" he recalled, over 40 years later.[2] But the experience was to stimulate his interest in acute medicine, and in teaching. A study period in Bristol, England, was followed by six months in the anaesthesiology department of

---

[1] Kjell Erik Strømskag: Et fag på søyler, p. 189. Tano Aschehoug 1999.
[2] Strømskag, p. 189.

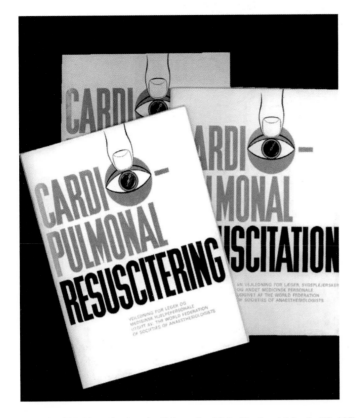

Fig. 4. The CPR Manual written by Safar and published by Lærdal for the World Federation of Societies of Anaesthesiology.

the Norwegian state hospital, Rikshospitalet, before he took on a second assignment in Korea. Returning home, he first served as senior registrar at the Haukeland hospital in Bergen, before moving to Stavanger in 1956.

## 4. Into acute medicine

As the lone anaesthesiologist in town, he came to work with Åsmund S. Lærdal on top of a very heavy hospital schedule. And yet, while this apparently unassuming man involved himself in a lengthy struggle with the hospital management, to improve work conditions, he also found the time to play a part in the development of the ambulance service.

During his internship in Trondheim in 1949, he had shown a pioneering interest in patient transportation, which strengthened his leaning towards acute medicine. In emergency cases, people living along the coastline and on small islands were offered transport by the Air Force with slow-moving fixed wing aeroplanes as an alternative to sea transportation in small boats. Lind compared transportation time, cost, comfort, and not least flying conditions in relation to the severity

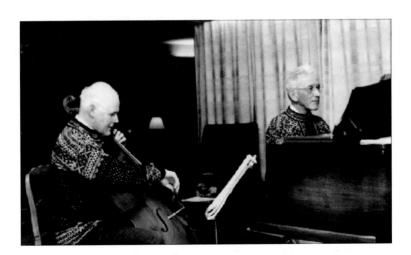

Fig. 5. Sharing a passion for patient care as well as chamber music; Bjørn Lind and Peter Safar.

331

of the patients' condition [7]. His survey addressed the main questions around the establishment of the Norwegian air ambulance, several decades later.

In 1959, Bjørn Lind took an interest in the ambulance service in Stavanger. He reviewed the records of 1596 patients brought to hospital by ambulance over a 12-month period, to see how many were in need of competent help before or during transportation, and arrived at the number of 107 patients. He also corresponded with colleagues in Sweden, Denmark and Germany, only to find that conditions were similar in these countries. This work promoted demands for trained ambulance personnel, plus sufficient space and appropriate equipment in the ambulances [8]. His work led the health authorities to take an interest in the ambulance services, and Bjørn Lind was appointed chairman for a departmental committee on the issue. This committee submitted its recommendations in 1963. However, these recommendations were not implemented until the early 1970s.

In 1972, the Norwegian parliament decided that qualified ambulance services must be capable of reaching 90% of Norway's population within 50 min.[3]

By then, Bjørn Lind had continued his development in acute medicine working with Peter Safar in Pittsburgh, in 1970–1971. When it became clear in the late 1960s that Norway was about to lag behind the other Scandinavian countries in the field of anaesthesiology, Bjørn Lind was a member of a committee set up to survey the situation. Norway had no academic positions in anaesthesiology or emergency medicine, and consequently lacked focus on research and the teaching of students. Denmark had three times as many anaesthesiologists per head of population as Norway, and in Sweden, the figure was two and a half. In 1972, Ivar Lund was appointed lecturer in anaesthesiology, and the following year Jacob Stovner was appointed to Norway's first chair in anaesthesiology. Bjørn Lind was appointed a senior lecturer in anaesthesiology in 1977, in connection with medical students' training at the Aker hospital and Sentralsykehuset i Akershus, and took on a professorship in 1979. By then he had served on a committee of three to set up a general plan for anaesthesiology in Norway. The result was the first systematic study of the specialty's status and perspectives, as seen in the context of needs and developments in other fields of medicine.

## 5. Promoting pain treatment

In addition to numerous articles on resuscitation and ambulance services, Bjørn Lind has contributed several studies on pharmacological themes.[4] From 1956, he ran a small evening clinic giving treatments by various nerve blocks. This led to further studies and developments, and in 1959, he lectured at a post-graduate course on alcohol blocks for trigeminal neuralgia, a therapeutic option that Lind was the sole physician to practise in Norway at that time. He also played an important part in the introduction of epidural pain relief in Norway, and published a small book, *Hvordan behandler vi de fødende* – How do we treat women giving birth? – in 1970.

These endeavours resulted in a breakthrough; in 1966, the Norwegian association of Anaesthesiologists devoted an entire autumn meeting to pain and pain management. Inspired by Lind, and two years of training with Peter Safar in Pittsburgh, his colleague Harald Breivik was to become the pioneer of pain treatment in Norway, one of the founding members of the International Association on the Study of Pain (IASP), in 1973, and a central figure in the establishment of the Scandinavian association, SASP, three years later.

Clearly, nurturing – in numerous ways – has been a key trait in the life of Bjørn Lind. In his retirement, he still lives at Fjellhamar, close to the university hospital in Akerhus where he invested 25 of his working years. And possibly, since his nurturing no longer involves daily contacts with patients, the plants in his winter garden benefit from even more generous doses than before—as is witnessed by productive vines and ebullient geraniums.

Sailing and chamber music are other passions that fill the time of this active man since his retirement.

However, Dr. Lind's passion for resuscitation keeps burning. At the age of 84, and with the exception of his three years abroad, he has missed only two Autumn Scientific Update meetings of the Norwegian Society of Anaesthesiology over the last 50 years. Stimulated by Bjørn Lind's pioneering work around 1960, Stavanger today has one of the most active EMS systems in Europe, with a particularly well-functioning chain of survival. No wonder, Bjørn Lind – who was then 83 years old – was the obvious choice as an invited lecturer for the opening session of the Scandinavian Congress of Resuscitation held in Stavanger in 2003.

## Acknowledgement

The authors would like to thank John Zorab for additional information in the preparation of this manuscript.

## References

[1] Lind B. Recent history of resuscitation in Norway. In: Joseph Ruprecht, Marius Jan von Lieburg, John Alfred Lee, Wilhelm Erdmann, editors. Anaesthesia—essays on its history. Berlin: Springer-Verlag; 1985.

[2] Lind B. Teaching mouth to mouth resuscitation in primary schools. Acta Anaesthesiol Scand 1961;9(Suppl):63.

[3] Lind B, Stovner J. Mouth to mouth resuscitation in Norway. J Am Med Assoc 1963;185:933.

---

3 Strømskag, p. 190.
4 Strømskag, p. 318.

[4] Safar P. Cardiopulmonary resuscitation. 1st ed. In: Prepared for the World Federation of Societies of Anaesthesiologists. Stavanger: Asmund S. Laerdal; 1968.

[5] Safar P. Cardiopulmonary cerebral resuscitation. 2nd ed. In: Prepared for the World Federation of Societies of Anaesthesiologists. Stavanger: Asmund S. Laerdal; 1981.

[6] Safar P, Bircher NG. Cardiopulmonary cerebral resuscitation. 3rd ed. In: Prepared for the World Federation of Societies of Anaesthesiologists. Stavanger: WB Saunders, Asmund S. Laerdal; 1987.

[7] Lind B. Ambulanseflyvning i Sør-Trøndelag. Tidskr Nor Laegeforening 1950;70:483–5.

[8] Lind B. Våre ambulanser. Tidskr Nor Laegeforening 1962;82:427–31.

# Nancy Caroline—from Mobile Intensive Care to Hospice

Peter Baskett     Peter Safar

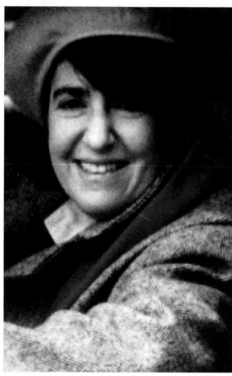

Nancy Caroline

Nancy Caroline made a fundamental contribution to the development of the modern day E.M.S. system with emergency medical technicians (EMT) and paramedics in the United Stated in the early 1970s. A brilliant writer, educator, communicator and motivator, she led from the front and was one of the few doctors in the US to experience prehospital care in the streets at first hand.

Never one to be content with success, she left the US in the late 1970s, took her considerable talents to Israel to bring A.L.S. to the Magen David Adom, and then to Africa to bring help to those who most needed it. At the turn of the century, in the final episode of her all too short life, she established a virtual hospice back in Metulla in her beloved Israel. Fittingly, this was at the site of the Good Fence, supposedly the bridge of good will and peace at the much fought over Golan Heights on the Lebanese border—Nancy's great hope and longing was that there would be peace in the Middle East. She was known there affectionately as 'Israel's Mother Theresa' [1].

Nancy Caroline was born in Boston, Massachussets, in June 1944. A highly intelligent girl, she received her College education at Harvard and went on to study medicine at Case Western Reserve University in Cleveland, Ohio. In 1973 she was appointed as a fellow in critical care medicine in Peter Safar's department in Pittsburgh. Peter Safar had started the Freedom House Ambulance project some six years earlier in 1967. The concept behind the project was to create an opportunity for African Americans from the underprivileged districts of Pittsburgh to train and work as EMTs and paramedics. At that time, prehospital care throughout Pittsburgh was very primitive—a 'scoop and run' policy by the police with precipitous transport in the back of a 'paddywagon' to the closest hospital. Avoidable deaths were occurring in great numbers. The position was not much better anywhere else in the United States.

*"Dr Peter Safar was looking for a proving ground to test new methods of resuscitation outside the hospital and for an opportunity to upgrade emergency care in Pittsburgh.*

*In the community, a biracial group of concerned citizens was looking for a means of encouraging Black enterprise. In the ghettos the Blacks were looking for work.*

*And it was out of this mix that the audacious, improbable idea of Freedom House ambulance service took shape. Take forty people—off the street corners—out of the pool halls—and train them to provide the most sophisticated emergency medical care possible, to provide this care not in the hospital, but at the emergency. And not just any forty people. Each applicant must fulfill two prerequisites; he or she must be Black; and he or she must be considered otherwise unemployable.*

*It was madness. Back in 1967, it was hard enough to persuade anyone that a layman could be trained to give sophisticated resuscitative care. Why load the dice against the experiment and choose laymen least likely to succeed? That is what Freedom House proposed to accomplish— and did."* [2]

Despite the apparent futility of the project, Safar ensured that the training programme got under way as a pilot project for the ambulance guidelines that he had initiated for the US National Research Council. In 1967 forty-four blacks, ranging from 18 to 60 years of age were enrolled. Many had not completed high school and were without employment prospects. The course was exacting and consisted of around 400 hours of theoretical and supervised clinical work, driver training and concurrent general adult education. Nine months later the successful trainees started to provide an ambulance service in two districts of Pittsburgh. The standard of care was far beyond anything that the city had known before.

However, the early success was also tainted by problems of finance and local administrative and police opposition. Successive medical directors had to leave for other posts and in 1974 the project was dying and Safar had all but given up. As a last effort in 1975, Safar offered Nancy Caroline the post of Medical Director. That was a master stroke. Nancy set about the task with her characteristic enthusiasm and dedication. Her mentors were Peter Safar [3–5] and Eugene Nagel.

When Safar was asked to create a manual for paramedics for the US department of Transportation he turned over the task to Nancy Caroline. Her manual, designed specially for EMTs and paramedics, was called 'Emergency Care in the Streets' (Fig. 1) [6]. It remained the only text book for paramedics for a decade and ran to five editions. Almost immediately this textbook was complemented by a work-book for self learning and self assessment to enhance the learning process. This concept was well ahead of the time and is only now becoming commonplace. Subsequently Nancy produced another landmark textbook with James McClintock entitled 'Ambulance Calls' based on their own unique experience in working in urban prehospital care (Fig. 2) [7]. Both books became 'bibles' for paramedic instructors and trainees—not just in North America but in other countries of the world where prehospital care was developing [8]. Later she wrote 'Emergency Medical Treatment' to complement the earlier books (Fig. 3) [9].

To the initial surprise of many of us, she abandoned a now sparking career and potential riches in the US in 1977 to work full time in her beloved Israel. She became an Israeli citizen and accepted the post of Medical Director of the Magen David Adom, the Israeli Ambulance Service, at a very modest salary indeed. On reflection, however, this move was entirely in character with Nancy's deeply held beliefs. She had

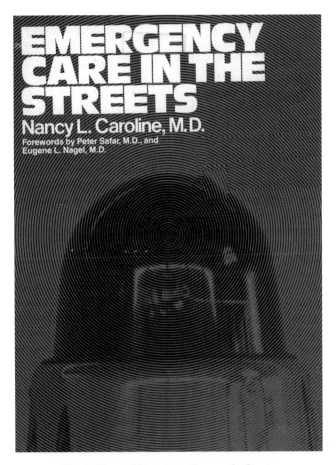

Fig. 1. Photo of Emergency Care on the Streets

been a civil rights supporter during her time as a medical student and unwaveringly dedicated her life to the care of the needy and underprivileged. I (PB), remember vividly talking long into the night when she stayed at my home in Bristol. Her passion for selfless and complete donation of all she had to give shone through that night, and I was left feeling rather inadequate and mundane in comparison to this super human being.

In Israel, Nancy set about upgrading the Magen David Adom. The organisation had at that time only very basic ambulances and equipment and virtually no advanced training. Her persistence that training and equipment would have to be improved to advanced life support standards ruffled feathers badly. Nevertheless her tenacity prevailed in the end and paramedic courses were introduced with improved vehicles and equipment.

Nathan Kindinsky, now head of paramedic training at the MDA, was a graduate of that first course "She carried out a revolution in MDA. She introduced Israel to paramedics. As a result of her work, treatment of trauma patients and other emergency patients presumably changed" [1]. Nancy herself perceived the need for change from the grass roots. "I was very much involved with day-to-day EMS—including, unfortunately, more mass casualty incidents than I would have seen in a

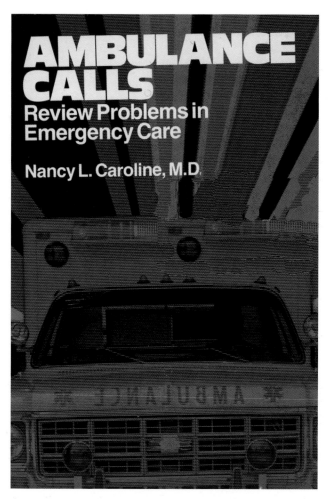

Fig. 2. Photo of Ambulance Calls

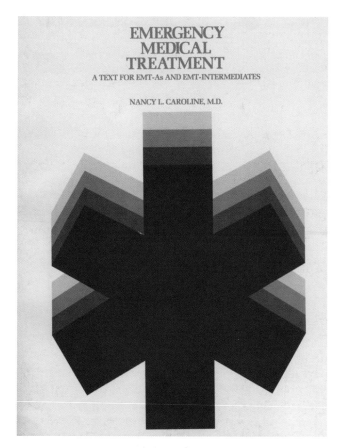

Fig. 3. Photo of Emergency Medical Treatment

lifetime in the United States" [2]. While in Israel Nancy maintained her links with the University of Pittsburgh as a member of the visiting faculty, and "I made it my business to ride rescue in Pittsburgh and Boston ... so I kept in touch with what was happening in the streets of the USA" [2]. She had many imaginative ideas including fluid therapy with chicken soup [10].

Life supporting first aid—the self acquisition of skills—was a concept put forward by Asmund Laerdal and Peter Safar in the 1960s. Nancy had proved herself as an eloquent and articulate writer. Her mastery of good English was superlative and it was therefore no surprise she was selected by the League of Red Cross and Red Crescent Societies and the CPR Committee of the World Federation of the Societies of Anaesthetists to write 'Life Supporting Resuscitation and First Aid' on their behalf [11]. Published in 1981, this excellent manual was really the blueprint of today's Basic Cardiac and Basic Trauma Life Support manuals. Little has changed to make the book much out of date today. As Chairman of the WFSA Committee at the time, the task of one of us (PB) was to edit the manuscript. It was a

simple task for the English was perfect and the style and clarity were quite enviable and an example to all.

In the 1980s Nancy surprised us once more. Her mission in Israel completed, as it had been in Pittsburgh a decade before, she took stock of her role. Once again she asked herself—what can I give rather than what can I receive? To her the answer was clear—thousands were dying in the famine inflicting the Horn of Africa, in Ethiopia in particular—not for want of sophisticated emergency care but for want of basic nutrition, hygiene and simple medicine. This was where she would go. As she had done before with deprived blacks in Pittsburgh, she helped people to help themselves, not only through training them in basic medicine. She learned simple techniques of agriculture and in turn passed them on to members of the native population. Conversations with her at that time revealed her passionate belief that the only way forward out of the disaster, for disaster it was, was to help people help themselves. Her quite extraordinary motivational skills stood her in good stead and once again she achieved her mission of leaving the place in a better state than she found it.

Moving on to Kenya, she raised funds through the University of Pennsylvania for the 'Clothesline to Africa' programme. In Kenya she trained and established 'bush doctors'—non physicians based in small communities, much in the same way as anaesthesiologist Mads Gilbert and his colleagues from Norway have done more recently in other parts of the world. Once again, she achieved her mission in large part but her efforts were clouded by her perceived corruption and misuse of funds by the local authorities in Kenya. This did not go down well at all and she was forced to flee the country—possibly in fear of her life. This was an opportunity missed by a country in dire straights—sadly a not uncommon story in the sad and beautiful continent of Africa. As ever, those whom she taught and worked with adored and worshipped her. Her forced departure from Kenya led her back to Israel. There she settled in Metulla in the 1990s to begin what was to be the final chapter of her life of variety and achievement. She helped to run the emergency medicine course at Kiryat Shumona during the Katyusha engagement. Realising that the country had little in the way of palliative care, she set about studying oncology and care of the terminally ill. Her anaesthetic background helped with the knowledge of pharmacology and therapeutic interventions required. As always she led from the front and trained local nurses to give palliative care in the community. Her strength of character and fierce enthusiasm ensured once again that the project was a success and greatly appreciated by the people of Metulla—a small town in the extreme north of Israel on the border with Lebanon. A section of that border has been called the 'Good Fence'—a term created in the hope that fighting and animosity will be replaced by tolerance and understanding—visiting the simply marked site is an emotional experience. It is fitting, perhaps, that Nancy's last place of work should be associated with hope for a better world, for that is what she strove to achieve in every episode of her life.

Nancy died in Metulla in December 2002 at the early age of 58 from rapidly growing multiple myeloma. She was cared for in the end by members of her hospice team who loved her dearly. She is survived by her mother, Zelda Caroline, in Boston, her brother Peter who lives in Arizona, and her husband Lazarus Astracham, formerly of Cleveland. Nine months before her death, the University of Pittsburgh set up a Research Fellowship in Emergency and Critical Care Medicine—a fitting tribute to a very special person who made a lot of good things happen for a lot of people who needed it.

Nancy Caroline, 'Israel's Mother Theresa', deserves the acknowledgement of a life truly dedicated to others. Her contribution to resuscitation is one of innovation surely, but also one of making it happen. That will be her epitaph. Her like may never come again.

## References

[1] Israel's Mother Theresa to be buried in Boston. Jerusalem Post. December 15, 2002.
[2] Caroline NL. Emergency. Pittsburgh April 1977. p. 43.
[3] Baskett PJF. Peter Safar. Part 1 The Early Years 1924–1961. The Birth of CPR. Resuscitation 2001;50(1):17–22.
[4] Baskett PJF. Peter Safar Part 2. The University of Pittsburgh to the Safar Centre for Resuscitation Research 1961–2002. Resuscitation 1961;55(1):3–7.
[5] Safar PJ. From Vienna to Pittsburgh for Anaesthesiology and Acute Medicine. An autobiography. Careers in Anesthesiology, vol. V. In: Fink BR, McGoldrick KE, editors. Wood Library—Museum of Anesthesiology. Illinois: Park Ridge, 2000.
[6] Caroline NL. Emergency Care in the Streets, first edition. Boston: Little, Brown and Co., 1979.
[7] Caroline NL. Ambulance Calls. Review Problems in Emergency Care, 1st Edition. Boston: Little, Brown and Co., 1981.
[8] Bledoe BE, Sanders MJ, A tribute to Nancy Caroline and Emergency care in the Streets. Journal of Emergency Medical Services 2002. June p. 127.
[9] Caroline NL. Workbook on Emergency Medical Treatment. Boston: Little, Brown and Co., 1982.
[10] Caroline NL, Schwartz H. Chicken soup rebound and relapse of pneumonia: report of a case. Chest 1975;67(2):215–6.
[11] Caroline NL. Life Supporting Resuscitation and First Aid. A Manual for Instructors of the Lay Public. Published by the League of Red Cross Societies and the World Federation of Societies of Anaesthesiologists Geneva 1982.

# Douglas Chamberlain
## —A man for all decades of his time

Peter Baskett

Without doubt Douglas Chamberlain has been a leading international light in the world of cardiac emergencies and resuscitation for the past 40 years (Figure 1). In each decade since the 1960s he has introduced something unique and valuable to the field of resuscitation and indeed, though now in his mid 70s, continues to do so with apparent remarkable ease. His contributions range from studying the early beta blocking drugs to pre-hospital care, from dual chamber cardiac pacing to the clinical introduction of automated external defibrillators, from the principles of education and training to the ethics of research and the history of resuscitation.

Douglas Chamberlain was born in Cardiff in 1931, the son of a successful coal merchant. His early school career was not promising—he frequently was given a score of 0/100 in writing and spelling and got so used to failure that at the end of class he would hold out his hand voluntarily to receive a slap with a ruler from his intemperate and frustrated school mistress in Cardiff. In some desperation his parents sent him away to be a boarder at Ratcliffe College in Leicester, where a caring and sage schoolmaster realised that that there was something specifically wrong that might be rectifiable, in this otherwise very bright child. He realised that the underlying problem lay in Douglas's inability to comprehend the written word easily and diagnosed a reading problem, well before dyslexia was a recognised condition by the psychologists and educationalists. This intelligent and far-sighted schoolmaster did his utmost to help and encourage Douglas who responded by a remarkable improvement, sufficient to pass the entrance examination to Queens' College, Cambridge. He had wanted to study medicine since the age of three when his mother had taken him to see the doctor in Cardiff. In the corner of the doctor's office was a human skull on a bookcase, wearing a hat and with a cigarette in its mouth. The subject fascinated Douglas and he never deviated from his chosen career thereafter.

One day when attempting to cycle a prodigious distance back from College he encountered a severe headwind. A bit exhausted, he paused to rest for a few hours. Never one to do nothing while awake, Douglas read a book on the physiology of the heart. This was to influence his choice of specialty.

At Cambridge he had mixed talents. He rowed with prowess in the Queens' College VIII. The rowing club had an intensive daily training programme, which coincided with anatomy dissection in the afternoons. This absence from study, combined with his great difficulty in differentiating between his left and his right side, made his prowess in anatomy, to be at best, poor. For many years, he had to check the top pocket of his jacket to know left from right.

At his final viva voce examination in surgical anatomy he felt that he was doomed to fail. He

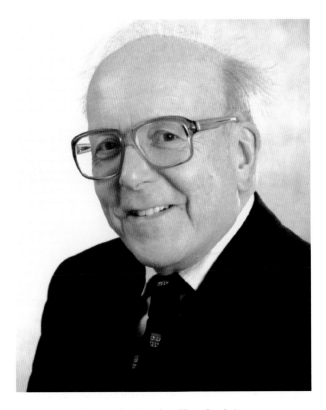

**Figure 1**  Douglas Chamberlain.

had a viva from two of the local examiners and did not get many questions right. They left the room, anxious to have coffee. However, the rather genial external examiner had jumped to the conclusion that Douglas Chamberlain was the son of a famous surgeon, who was his contemporary and friend, stayed and asked a simple question at the end. *"This is a tibia. It is the bone that joins the thigh bone to the ankle bone"*. *Douglas said he knew that. "But can you tell me if it is the left tibia or the right one?" Douglas struggled for the answer....* Now the conversation became entirely devoted to friendly enquiries, stories of old times together and messages of good will to be conveyed to his father. Douglas tried to say that he was not the son of the famous surgeon but was too polite to interrupt the charming gentleman in full flow to tell him the disappointing news that he was not at all related to the surgeon's old friend. Eventually, the bell rang to indicate that the time for the viva had elapsed and they parted company in a most cordial fashion. Douglas passed the examination in surgical anatomy and went on to qualify as a doctor. There is no doubt that the genial old surgeon got it absolutely right, for had he not acted as he did, medicine might have been deprived of one of its richest talents.

The author, who was a freshman at Queens' College in Douglas's final year tried to know Douglas but Douglas, by his own admission, was much too important to be dealing closely with such junior undergraduates! It was to be two decades before we got together with our common interest in resuscitation.

Douglas continued his studies at St. Bartholomew's Hospital in London and qualified as a doctor in 1956. He was appointed a House Physician at St. Bartholomew's for 6 months, which went well, and then a House Surgeon there, which did not go so well. Indeed his consultant surgical boss asked his junior surgical colleague to take Douglas out to lunch to inform him that he was the worst house surgeon he had ever encountered! This led Douglas to pursue a career in medicine and cardiology at St. Bartholomew's and later in the army during his national military service and in various teaching hospitals in London. In one of these posts in chest medicine Douglas found his consultant boss's lectures so boring that he went to sleep and fell off his chair, causing a commotion and great displeasure to the tedious speaker. Douglas realised that he was not making progress in this post and accordingly a week or two later offered 1 month's notice, indicating that he he wished to leave the post. On hearing this news, the irate and incensed consultant phoned Douglas immediately to say he was to leave his post with disgrace forthwith. Fortunately, that evening Douglas received a phone call offering him a research post in cardiology at St. Bartholomew's to start work immediately.

His research centred on drugs and cardiac pacing. Were it not for hapless delays by a drug company processing Douglas's work, he would have been among the first to describe the clinical applications of the drugs that were later to be called beta blockers.[1–6] He determined the dose of atropine (3 mg) to induce full vagal blockade[7]—a principle adhered to in the guidelines of today.

He studied various techniques of dual chamber cardiac pacing,[8–11] techniques that also have stood the test of time.

Appointed a consultant cardiologist in Brighton in 1970, he continued his pacing and pharmacological research. He was one of the first to investigate the use of amiodarone in clinical practice.[12]

A chance encounter in 1970, was to change the practice of the ambulance service at home and abroad.

*"I was doing a consultation visit in the patient's home. As I examined the chest he apparently died. I started vigorous chest compressions and patient looked up at me and struck me a severe blow on the chin. Nevertheless I continued the chest compressions and commanded his wife to dial 999 (the*

*emergency number in the UK) for the ambulance which arrived after a protracted time with a defibrillator that took two men to lift. When it was turned on it exploded and caught fire. I thought we ought to be able to do better...''*

In the aftermath of that event Douglas teamed up with William Parker (the Medical Officer of Health responsible for the ambulance service at that time) to start training selected ambulance personnel and to equip a number of ambulances for pre-hospital care. Within a year Brighton was to become the Seattle of the UK.[13–19] It was to be a long haul to gain acceptance of paramedics by the ministry of health. Frank Pantridge had experienced similar difficulties and obstructions in the earlier years from his own specialty with his doctor manned ambulance with a defibrillator in Belfast.[20]

Defibrillator technology was developing fast and the devices were being automated to make their use simple and safe. Unlike others in the United States and elsewhere, Douglas seized on the possible applications and was the first to use an automated defibrillator in the clinical situation and was the first to introduce Public Access Defibrillation, before the term was brought into use.[21] He trained station staff at Victoria Station in London (where the train from Brighton arrived) and staff of the British Caledonian Airline (based at Gatwick Airport close to Brighton) and at Brighton and Hove football ground.[22,23] It is interesting to note that when British Caledonian Airlines was taken over by British Airways (BA), a much larger organisation, they withdrew defibrillators from the Caledonian aircraft as they were not convinced that it was worth it to equip the much larger BA fleet. That is until Douglas became advisor to BA, then eventually all BA aircraft were fitted out with automated external defibrillators (AEDs).

Training was of the essence. Douglas had set up a the first organised community training scheme in Brighton.[24] He had been impressed with the performance of an ambulance man in Brighton, Dusty Miller, on his first fateful encounter with pre-hospital coronary care and attempted defibrillation in the home. Douglas trained Dusty to become the very first Resuscitation Training Officer (RTO) in Brighton. The concept spread like wild fire around the UK, so that now every district hospital has at least one post and many large institutions have several. The RTO takes charge of hospital and some community resuscitation training and the hospital resuscitation equipment and service. The concept is envied by many in continental Europe.

In the 1970s resuscitation training for laypersons was piecemeal and both the curriculum and standards varied between the volunteer services, such as St. John, St. Andrew and the British Red Cross, the charitable organisations, such as the British Heart Foundation, and a multitude of entrepreneurs who saw training for industry staff as a good way of generating an income. Douglas was, as ever, a catalyst and in 1981 a self appointed group from the relevant specialty interests of cardiology (himself), anaesthesia (the author), emergency medicine (John McNae and Roger Sleet), paediatric anaesthesia (David Zideman), general practice (Judith Fisher and Rodney Herbert) and life saving from water (Mark Harries) sat down to address the problem. As always matters were discussed over a drink, and within 1 h the group had founded the Community Resuscitation Advisory Group (CRAG) soon to become the Community Resuscitation Council (CRAC), which sounded more impressive. Each member of the group was able to gain the support of their specialist societies and academic bodies for the project. The first flip chart and booklet ''Resuscitation for the Citizen'' was produced a few months later with the help of Laerdal Medical and was an enormous success as it brought together a consensus drawn from all the relevant medical specialities and authorities for the first time. The CRAC set about organising scientific meetings. In 1983, as advanced life support was included, the CRAC became the Resuscitation Council UK (RC [UK]) with Judith Fisher as its first Chairman and Douglas, who never wished for power or glory, as its principal mentor. The RC [UK] started to produce guidelines[25] and has never looked back. It is now the authority acknowledged by all in medicine and government in the UK. It also enjoys considerable admiration and respect internationally.

With increasing co-operation within Europe politically and medically, there was a clear case for creating a European Resuscitation Council with the aim of unifying training and practice in the European countries. With the late Lars Mogensen of Denmark, Douglas approached the European Society of Cardiology (ESC) to act as the parent body for a European Resuscitation Council. To their great disappointment the ESC turned down the proposal (with hind sight this was a bit like turning down an offer to manage the Beatles!). Undaunted, Douglas and Lars gathered some proponents together, including Leo Bossaert of Belgium, Paul Hugenholtz of Switzerland and John Camm from the UK. Once again over a drink, they agreed that the concept should be pursued, but this time on an independent, multidisciplinary basis, because the European Regional Section of Anaesthesia, for example, had a thriving CPR committee of its own. In the manner of the creation of the RC (UK), self appointed enthusiastic representatives from several countries and specialities gathered together in Antwerp in 1988 and formed the European Resuscitation Council (ERC).[26] Once again Laerdal had supported the concept and enabled colleagues from various countries to meet together.

Douglas was an enormous driving force within the ERC, setting up working groups to address specific aspects of resuscitation.[27,28] He negotiated with Elsevier, the publishers, to make the ailing journal *Resuscitation* the Official Journal of the ERC, and was appointed Editor-in-Chief in 1990. Thanks to his worldwide contacts, who held him in the highest regard, and, working tirelessly, he took publication from an erratic half yearly to quarterly and finally bimonthly over a period of 7 years.

With his international contacts and friends, particularly Richard Cummins and others in the American Heart Association (AHA), he was able to bring together the ERC, the AHA, the Australian Resuscitation Council (ARC), the New Zealand Resuscitation Council (NZRC), the Resuscitation Council of Southern Africa and the Resuscitation Council of Latin America (CLAR) to form the International Liaison Committee on Resuscitation

(ILCOR).[29] The term ILCOR was suggested by Dr. Walter Kloeck from Johannesburg and was immediately accepted as a suitable catchy abbreviation for the activities of the organisation and, as a bonus, also conveniently conveyed the concept of a "sick heart". Through masterly persuasion and diplomacy, Douglas ensured that the ILCOR collaboration flourished. The first task was to create a uniform system for reporting the results of scientific studies. This was named the Utstein Style after the abbey near Stavanger where the first meeting had taken place (Figure 2).[30]

Subsequently, ILCOR produced a periodic international consensus on science that produced guidelines for resuscitation 1997[31–33], and later in 2000 and 2005. To supplement the guidelines he initiated and chaired ILCOR Working Groups to address specific topics that included research methods and education, training and assessment[34]. Dyslexic or not, Douglas is masterful with words.

Back in the UK he continued to be the principle driving force and acknowledged doyen of resuscitation[35], being a leading advisor to the British Heart Foundation and the Department of Health. In this role he introduced and

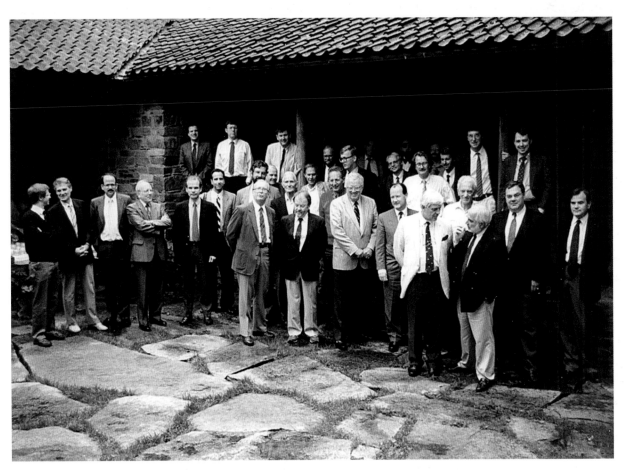

**Figure 2**  The first Utstein meeting in 1990 (photo courtesy of Tore Laerdal).

masterminded the most comprehensive national PAD programme of its time,[36,37] which served as an example to many others.

He established, with Tom Evans and Alan Macintosh, the Joint Royal Colleges Ambulance Liaison Committee, which brought a multidisciplinary approach to training, education, standards and practice in the UK ambulance service.

He was appointed Professor of Resuscitation Medicine at the University of Wales in Cardiff in 1997. This is an honorary post in that he is not paid a salary, but Douglas is always one to give his time and efforts quite selflessly. He led an active team in Cardiff that produced landmark publications on basic life support and automated defibrillation and the influence of education and assessment on performance.[38,39] He is also Visiting Professor of Cardiology at the University of Brighton and remains an Honorary Consultant Cardiologist at the Royal Sussex County Hospital.

Author of literally hundreds of scientific papers, a sought after lecturer in all corners of the globe, and a highly respected researcher, Douglas has been widely honoured—by the Pope in 1987 and by the Queen in 1988, and by numerous professional, academic and august bodies. These include conferment of Honorary Doctorates from the University of Sussex and the University of Hertford, Fellowships in the American College of Cardiology, the European Society of Cardiology, and the Royal College of Anaesthetists. He is an Honorary Member of the Association of Anaesthetists of Great Britain and Ireland, the Resuscitation Council (UK) and the ERC. He has received awards from the AHA, the Citizen CPR Foundation, the British Cardiac Society, the British Association for Immediate Care and the UK Ambulance Service.

Douglas continues his research and teaching endeavours undaunted and remains highly respected as an opinion and wise counsel. Very few have contributed more to resuscitation worldwide during the last 40 years.

## Acknowledgements

The author is grateful to Sarah Mitchell, Judith Fisher, and David Zideman for help with the precise early history of the RC (UK) and to Tore Laerdal for permission to publish Figure 2.

## References

1. Chamberlain DA, Howard J. The haemodynamic effects of beta-sympathetic blockade. Br Heart J 1964;26:213—7.
2. Apthorp GH, Chamberlain DA, Hayward. The effects of sympathectomy on the electrocardiogram and effort tolerance in angina pectoris. Br Heart J 1964;26:218—26.
3. Chamberlain DA. Effects of beta adrenergic blockade on heart size. Am J Cardiol 1966;18:321—8.
4. Chamberlain DA. The haemodynamic effects of beta-adrenergic blockade in man. In: Proceedings of the Symposium on Propranolol, Cardiologia Suppl II, vol. 49. 1966. p. 27—42.
5. Chamberlain DA, Davis WG, Mason DF. Effects of beta-blockade on coronary flow. Lancet 1967;2:1257.
6. Julian D, Chamberlain DA. Mechanisms for early mortality reduction produced by beta-blockers started early in acute myocardial infarction: ISIS-1. Lancet 1988;1:545—9.
7. Chamberlain DA, Turner P, Sneddon JM. Effects of atropine on heart rate in healthy man. Lancet 1967;2:12—5.
8. Leinbach RC, Chamberlain DA, Kastor JA, Harthorne JW, Sanders CA. A comparison of the haemodynamic effects of ventricular and sequential A—V pacing in patients with heart block. Am Heart J 1969;74:502—8.
9. Chamberlain DA, Leinbach RC, Vassaux CE, Kastor J, DeSanctis RW, Sanders CA. Sequential atrioventricular pacing in heart block complicating acute myocardial infarction. New Engl J Med 1970;282:577—82.
10. Chamberlain DA, Leinbach RC, Sanders CA. The effect of paired atrial pacing on left atrial and ventricular performance in the dog. Cardiovasc Res 1970;4:116—26.
11. Chamberlain DA, Leinbach RC. Electrical pacing in heart block complicating acute myocardial infarction. Br Heart J 1970;31:2—5.
12. Wheeler PJ, Puritz R, Ingram DV, Chamberlain DA. Amiodarone in the treatment of refractory supraventricular and ventricular arrhythmias. Br Heart J 1979;55:1—9.
13. Chamberlain DA, White NM, Binning RA, Parker WS, Kimber ERC. Mobile coronary care provided by ambulance personnel. Br Heart J 1973;35:550.
14. White NM, Parker WS, Binning RA, Kimber ER, Ead HW, Chamberlain DA. Mobile coronary care provided by ambulance personnel. Br Med J 1973;881:618—22.
15. Chamberlain DA, Williams JH. The Brighton Experiment. An appraisal of a coronary ambulance. Health 1975:11—5.
16. Chamberlain DA, Williams JH. Immediate care of cardiac emergencies. Anaesthesia 1976;31:758—63.
17. Briggs RS, Brown PM, Crabbe ME, et al. The Brighton resuscitation ambulances: a continuing experiment in pre-hospital care by ambulance staff. Br Med J 1976;2(6045):1161—5.
18. Macintosh AF, Crabbe ME, Grainger R, Williams JH, Chamberlain DA. The Brighton resuscitation ambulances: review of 40 consecutive survivors of out-of-hospital cardiac arrest. Br Med J 1978;40:124—30.
19. Macintosh AF, Crabbe ME, Brennan H, Williams JH, Chamberlain DA. Hospital resuscitation from ventricular fibrillation in Brighton. Br Med J 1979;1(6162):511—3.
20. Baskett TF, Baskett PJF. Frank Pantridge and mobile coronary care. Resuscitation 2001;48:99—105.
21. Jaggarao NS, Heber M, Grainger R, Vincent R, Chamberlain DA, Aronson AL. Use of an automated defibrillator—pacemaker by ambulance staff. Lancet 1982;2:73—5.
22. Jaggarao NS, Sless H, Grainger R, Vincent R, Chamberlain DA. Defibrillation at a football stadium: an experiment with Brighton and Hove Albion. Br Med J Clin Res Ed 1982;284:1451—3.

23. Cummins RO, Chapman PJ, Chamberlain DA, Schubach JA, Litwin PE. In flight deaths during commercial air travel. How big is the problem? J Am Med Assoc 1988;259:1983—8.

24. Vincent R, Martin B, Williams G, Quinn E, Robertson G, Chamberlain DA. A community training scheme in cardiopulmonary resuscitation. Br Med J Clin Res Ed 1984;288:617—20.

25. Chamberlain DA. Guidelines for resuscitation. Revised recommendations of the Resuscitation Council (UK). Br Med J 1989;299:446—8.

26. Chamberlain DA. The European Resuscitation Council. Resuscitation 1992;24:99—101.

27. Guidelines for basic life support. A statement by the Basic Life Support Working Party of the European Resuscitation Council 1992. Resuscitation 1992;24:103—10.

28. Guidelines for advanced life support. A statement by the Advanced Life Support Working Party of the European Resuscitation Council 1992. Resuscitation 1992;24:111—21.

29. Chamberlain DA (Co-ordinator). Compiled by the Founding Members of the International Liaison Committeeon Resuscitation. The International Liaison Committee on Resuscitation (ILCOR)—past and present. Resuscitation 2005;67:157—61.

30. Cummins RO, Chamberlain DA, Abrahamson NS, et al. Recommended guidelines for uniform reporting of data from out-of-hospital cardiac arrest: the Utstein style. Circulation 1991;84:960—75.

31. Chamberlain DA, Cummins RO. Advisory statements of the International Liaison Committee on Resuscitation (ILCOR). Resuscitation 1997;34:99—100.

32. Kloeck W, Cummins RO, Chamberlain DA, et al. The universal ALS algorithm: an advisory statement by the Advanced Life Support Working Group of the International Liaison Committee on Resuscitation (ILCOR). Resuscitation 1997;34:109—12.

33. Cummins RO, Chamberlain DA, Hazinski MF, et al. Recommended guidelines for reviewing reporting and conducting research on in-hospital resuscitation: the in-hospital Utstein style. Resuscitation 1997;34:151—84.

34. Chamberlain DA, Hazinski MF, on behalf of the European Resuscitation Council, the American Heart Association, the Heart and Stroke Foundation of Canada, the Australasia and New Zealand Resuscitation Council, the Resuscitation Council of Southern Africa, the Consejo Latino-Americano de Resuscitacion. ILCOR advisory statements. Education in resuscitation. Resuscitation 2003;59:11—43.

35. Chamberlain DA, Handley AJ, Colquhoun M. Time for change? Editorial. Resuscitation 2003;58:237—47.

36. Davies CS, Colquohoun M, Graham S, Evans T, Chamberlain DA. Defibrillators in public places: the introduction of a national scheme for public access defibrillation in England. Resuscitation 2001;50:27—37.

37. Whitfield R, Colquohoun M, Chamberlain DA, Newcombe R, Davies CS, Boyle R. The Department of Heath National Defibrillator Programme: analysis of downloads from 250 deployments of public access defibrillators. Resuscitation 2005;64:269—77.

38. Assar D, Chamberlain DA, Colquohoun M, et al. Randomised controlled trials of staged teaching of basic life support. Resuscitation 2000;45:7—15.

39. Woollard M, Smith A, Whitfield R, et al. To blow or not to blow: a randomised controlled trial of compression-only and standard CPR instructions in simulated cardiac arrest. Resuscitation 2003;59:123—31.

# A history of mechanical devices for providing external chest compressions

Russell Harrison-Paul

## Introduction

The development of the Lund University Cardiopulmonary Assist System (LUCAS), has interested the resuscitation community as it is hoped that this device may lead to an increase in survival from cardiac arrest.[1] It has been subjected to a number of clinical trials and is currently being used by some ambulance services. However, the use of mechanical means to compress the chest is not a new phenomenon. A recent review reported on 15 automatic or manual mechanical devices that are, or have been, available for use during resuscitation attempts.[2] A recent literature search has revealed some further inventions, and it is interesting to trace the history of these devices and consider why they failed to become an accepted adjunct during resuscitation attempts.

Long before Jude, Kouwenhoven and Knickerbocker produced their seminal paper on closed chest compressions, Pike et al. had recorded in 1908 a method of 'Extra-thoracic massage' that they had studied on dogs.[3] They noted that compressing the chest of a dog was 'exceedingly laborious and often cannot be kept up for a sufficiently long time'. With the help of Professor J.L. Kessler they developed a machine to massage the heart both externally and internally. However, they reported that applied externally it was no better than manual methods and applied internally it was less effective.

For the next 50 years opening the chest and giving internal cardiac massage was the only technique used during cardiac arrest and the idea of using any type of mechanical device appears to have been forgotten. However, as soon as closed chest massage was reported in the early 1960s, so ideas about using mechanical devices to assist with this procedure also developed. A brief chronological list of some of these devices will now be related.

## 1961

Harkins and Bramson[4] reported on an electro-pneumatic machine which Bramson had designed to overcome the disadvantages that they perceived in giving external chest compressions manually. Designed to fit over a standard hospital stretcher it required compressed gas to drive a spring-loaded piston with a force of between 60 and 75 pounds (27—34 kg), onto the patient's sternum (Figure 1). In addition to this machine being used in a cardiac arrest, they also suggested that it could be used to assist a failing heart as it was possible to synchronise it with an ECG monitor.

Dotter et al. [5] devised an artificial circulator which consisted of a thrusting mechanism mounted on a supporting frame (Figure 2). This was powered by an electric motor which was set to operate at 60 strokes/min. They describe testing the device on an adult cadaver and using it on a 75-year-old male who had suffered a cardiac arrest. Unfortunately, the patient died and they note that the post mortem showed multiple rib fractures which indicated 'inexperience with, or limitations of, the methods employed'. They also indicated that they were working on a second model which would use a smaller motor. A literature search did not reveal any references relating to this subsequent model.

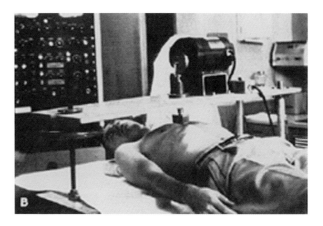

**Figure 2** Sources:[5].

## 1962

Nachlas and Siedband[6] described the development of a portable pneumatic pump for external chest compression (Figure 3). They reported that they were developing a different version which would be lighter in weight and available from the Westinghouse Electric Corporation. They recorded the successful use of this device during experiments with dogs and also that they had used it during resuscitation attempts with three patients. They did not indicate whether these attempts resulted in a successful outcome, however in the summary of this article they refer to recording arterial pressures in 'three recently deceased persons'.

In the United Kingdom, Michael et al.[7] described a machine designed by Warltier[8] which was intended to overcome the difficulties of providing chest compressions manually. They described this as an exhausting procedure calling for several changes of operator and wasteful of the energies of specialised personnel. They claimed that

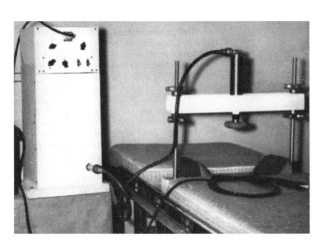

**Figure 1** Sources:[4].

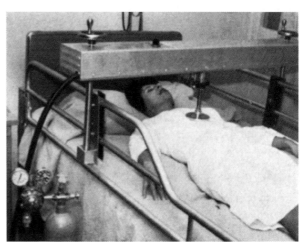

**Figure 3** Sources:[6].

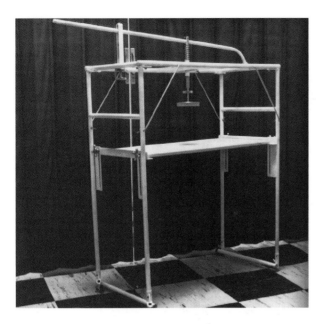

**Figure 4** Sources:[8].

this device was simple to use, cheap to produce and could also be made available to works medical teams. Designed to fit over a bed or couch it required an individual to pull a lever which operated a plunger placed on the patient's chest (Figure 4). They reported that an adequate femoral pulse was obtained in 17 out of 18 cases where it had been used. They had patented this device and it was being manufactured by a company in Sussex.

Tocker et al.[9] described their device, the 'Rodriguez Tocker Automatic External Cardiac Massage machine' (Figure 5), which had a number of distinctive features. Whilst these were not related in detail, they included sounding an alarm when the heart rate became inadequate and automatically activating when ventricular tachycardia or bradycardia were detected. This was achieved by synchronising the device with an ECG monitor.

Birch et al.[10] studied the effects of applying various forces to the sternum during chest compression. In doing so, they used a mechanical device, which had been developed at their hospital specifically for use during transport to hospital from the scene of a cardiac arrest. This was the 'Butterworth-LSI External Cardiac Compressor' (Figure 6). The main focus of their article is the work on the force, rate and duration of compression and little is related of the device itself.

## 1963

Safar et al.[11] evaluated the 'Beck—Rand External Cardiac Compression machine' a battery powered,

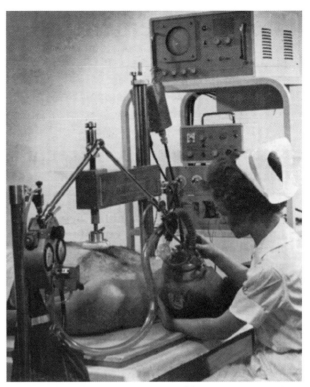

**Figure 5** Sources:[9].

portable device weighing 32 kg. They concluded that the time spent in obtaining, applying and adjusting the machine precluded its use at the start of the resuscitation. They also believed that it would only be valuable in cases where there was a need for prolonged resuscitation and that possibly it could be used by ambulance personnel.

Another device which was available at this time was the pneumatic external cardiac massage machine which was mentioned by Stewart in 1965.[12] He records that Dilcox had submitted a

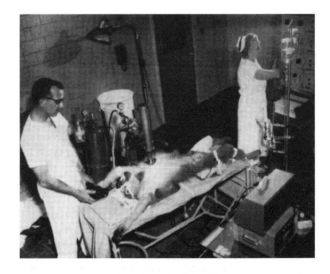

**Figure 6** Sources:[10].

patent for this in 1963 but there is no further detail as to how it worked. However, the application for a patent was never followed up (personal communication Brit. Lib.), and there appears to be no further references to it in any literature.

## 1964

Bailey et al.[13] described a machine they had designed which was powered by an oxygen cylinder and they claimed that it was fully portable and simple to operate, even by semi-skilled people (Figure 7). They reported the successful use of this device in a series of experiments on dogs and also on the 'recently dead' on whom they found it produced a good pulse without damaging the chest. This device was also patented and was being manufactured by a company in Warwickshire.

Knight[14] reported on an apparatus which he recommended be used in place of manual compressions, which he concluded had many disadvantages. His device needed no power source as it was operated by hand. Someone was required to push down on a bar, which had another bar attached to it covered by a sponge that had to be placed in the correct position over the sternum. This effort by the individual resulted in the sponge covered bar compressing the chest. He reported that there had been one successful use of this device.

## 1965

Nachlas and Siedband[15] wrote about mechanised cardiac massage and compared five commercially

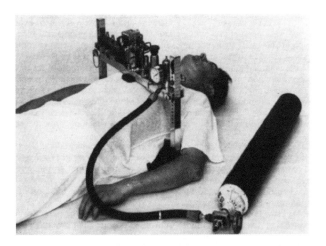

**Figure 7** Sources:[13] . *Note*: The requirement is for the wording 'reproduced with permission from the BMJ Publishing Group' to be placed adjacent to the picture.

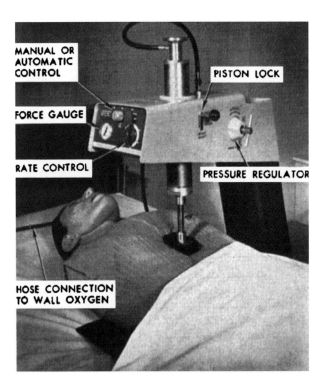

**Figure 8** Sources:[15].

available mechanical units with one they had devised (Figure 8). Their device was powered by oxygen and there was a different version which was for use in ambulances. They believed that one advantage of a mechanical device was the consistency of depth and force which was applied. They felt this was superior to the inadequacies of the 'timid physician' who would apply too little force and the 'robust enthusiastic house officer' who will do the opposite. They remark on the deficiency of the other devices, those designed by Bramson, Dotter et al., Birch et al., Tocker et al. and Beck et al., and stated that these did not compare favourably with their own. In critiquing these other designs they possibly give some clues as to why these devices failed to become widely used. They believed that those which required an electrical or battery power source were not portable enough, whilst some were too cumbersome or had unnecessary and complicated controls which meant that vital time would be lost when setting them up.

## 1966

In this year Pearson et al.[16] carried out a study of four mechanical devices for closed chest massage, the Cardio-Massager and Cardio-Pulser, both manually operated, and the Iron Heart and Baxter H-L-R, both powered by oxygen. They concluded that all of these took too long to set up and overall were generally inadequate. They supported the simplicity and effectiveness of massage performed by the human hand. Supporting their report, Jude, one of the pioneers of closed-chest massage, stated that 'we must guard against innovations that are without true purpose and with marginal positive benefit, if any at all'. Also, in this year an 'Ad Hoc' committee on resuscitation in the United States published what could be regarded as the first 'formal' guidelines.[17] These acknowledged that external cardiac compression machines could be used in cases of prolonged resuscitation or transportation, but recommended that the manual method should always be used first.

## 1973

The *Journal of Health Devices*[18] evaluated four mechanical cardiac compressors that were available at the time. These were the Bowen Pulsator and the Rentsch Press, both of which were operated by someone using a lever, and the Life Aid model 1004 and Travenol HLR50-90 both of which were powered by oxygen. Whilst not finding any great failings with these machines they did suggest that the purchase of them should be given a lower priority than other resuscitation equipment. They also stated that without effective training in the use of the compressor itself and frequent clinical use or practise, the external cardiac compressor could not fulfil its intended purpose. They reported that at least seven devices had been available in 1965 but commented that several of these were poorly conceived and ineffective. They warned against the use of some of these devices which, although no longer manufactured, may still have been in service.

## 1974

The Standards for Cardiopulmonary Resuscitation and Emergency Cardiac Care were published in this year and commented on both manual and automatic chest compressors. Regarding the latter, they recommended that they be used only by well-trained and experienced personnel and that their performance was comparable to the manual method.[19]

## 1980s

Following this initial enthusiasm to devise mechanical chest compressors there appears to be a waning in their popularity during the late 1970s and early 1980s. The potential use of such devices however was still referred to in most resuscitation guidelines produced at the time.[20] One model to endure throughout this time was the 'Thumper', introduced in 1965 by Michigan Instruments and continually redesigned since then.[21] The '1005 Model' was one which the author recalls using at that time during his work in an emergency department.

In the mid-1980s there was a new development in the design of mechanical aids, which was vest-CPR.[22] This system consisted of an inflatable vest which could be placed around the thorax and inflated and deflated rapidly. At the time it was suggested that this device showed great promise for improving survival in humans. The more recent version of this type of device is the Auto-Pulse CPR load-distributing band.[23]

## 1990s

In 1990, a chance intervention led to a renewed interest in the use of devices to assist with cardiac massage. A lay-person used a toilet plunger in an attempt to resuscitate his father, which proved to be successful.[24] This prompted speculation as to how this procedure may have assisted with improving both circulation and ventilation and led to the development of the Active Compression–Decompression device (ACD–CPR).[25] This device received varying reports on its effectiveness and it was suggested in 1995 that it not be adopted until it had clearly produced an improvement over manual CPR.[26]

## Discussion

The mechanical devices currently available have recently been reviewed[27] and it would appear that the evidence relating to their ability to improve survival from cardiac arrest is inconclusive and conflicting. Whilst many would regard these devices as something new they have in fact evolved from others that have been devised over the past 45 years. One can speculate as to why these earlier models failed to gain acceptance amongst those involved in resuscitation. The devices invented in the early 1960s were developed at a time when resuscitation medicine was in its infancy. There were some at that time who questioned the value of closed-chest massage[28–30] and resuscitation did not have the status of a speciality that it does today. Given these circumstances it may be that the reports of these devices met with little interest or support from the wider medical community. Certainly at that time, the dissemination of these reports through a variety of journals and media was not available and therefore they would have become known to a very limited number of people who potentially could have supported their use.

Until the 1970s, there were no recognised guidelines which would have had an influence on the likelihood of these devices being used in a cardiac arrest. Even when guidelines were produced they never fully endorsed the regular use of mechanical aids over manual methods.[19,20] Also at this time there were no organisations such as the Resuscitation Council (UK) and the European Resuscitation Council which could have reviewed and perhaps recommended the use of these devices.

Other factors not present when many of these devices were being suggested were evidence-based medicine and randomised controlled trials. The articles reporting these devices, which were being tested on the 'recently dead' and 'cadavers' for example, give no indication of any recognised research methodology or ethical approval. Whilst the culture of medicine at that time may not have required this, it is possible that many were unwilling to adopt a device that had no great evidence base to support it.

The mechanical devices being promoted and used at the present time do not face these obstacles and it could be that one of them proves to be a valuable aid in the struggle to improve survival from cardiac arrest. That such a device is not currently an accepted component of resuscitation practice is due to a number of factors. It is also interesting to note that some of these historical papers also suggested the setting up of resuscitation teams, and produced brief guidelines for staff to follow when dealing with a cardiac arrest.[7] Here is another example of ideas which failed to become widespread practice at the time but which are universally taught and recommended practice today. Chamberlain wrote recently of those components of resuscitation that were suggested long before they eventually became accepted practice.[31] It would seem that mechanical devices for providing chest compressions are another example of such innovations that were, in his words, 'never quite there'.

## Acknowledgements

To Dr. Stephen Timmons, for advice and support; Mrs. B. Warltier, for personal correspondence relating to her late husband; Dr. A.W. Warltier, who devised one of the earliest mechanical devices; the British Library Intellectual Property Enquiries Department, for information regarding patents.

## References

1. Steen S, Liao Q, Pierre L, Paskevicius A, Sjoberg T. Evaluation of LUCAS, a new device for automatic mechanical compression and active decompression resuscitation. Resuscitation 2002;55:285.
2. Wik L. Automatic and manual mechanical external chest compression devices for cardiopulmonary resuscitation. Resuscitation 2000;47:7.
3. Pike FH, Guthrie CC, Stewart GN. Studies in resuscitation: the general conditions affecting resuscitation, and the resuscitation of the blood and of the heart. J Exp Med 1908;10:371—418.
4. Harkins G, Bramson M. Mechanized external cardiac massage for cardiac arrest and for support of the failing heart. J Surg Res 1961;1:197—200.
5. Dotter C, Straube K, Strain D. Circulatory arrest: manual and mechanical means for emergency management. Radiology 1961;77:426—33.
6. Nachlas MM, Siedband MP. A simple portable pneumatic pump for external cardiac massage. Am J Cardiol 1962:107—9.
7. Michael TD, Taylor D, Warltier A. The management of cardiac arrest in a general hospital. Postgrad Med J 1962;38: 560—70.
8. Warltier A. A machine for giving external cardiac massage. Triangle 1963;20:63—6.
9. Rodriguez Tocker L, Tocker A, Hammond R, Givner D. Cardiac arrest: automatic ECG synchronised external cardiac massage machine. J Kans Med Soc 1962;63:420—1.
10. Birch L, Kenney L, Doornbos F, Kosht D, Barkalow C. A study of external cardiac compression. J Mich State Med Soc 1962;61:1346—52.
11. Safar P, Harris L. The Beck—Rand external cardiac compression machine. Anesthesiology 1963;24:586—8.
12. Stewart J. Advances in the management of cardiac arrest. J R Coll Physicians Edinb 1965;10:85—101.
13. Bailey RA, Browse NL, Keating V. Automatic external cardiac massage: a portable pneumatic external cardiac compression machine. Br Heart J 1964;26:481—9.
14. Knight I. New apparatus for intermittent cardiac compression. BMJ 1964;1:894.
15. Nachlas MM, Siedband MP. Clinical experiences with mechanised cardiac massage. Am J Cardiol 1965;15:310—9.
16. Pearson J, Navarro R, Redding J. Evaluation of mechanical devices for closed-chest massage. Anesth Analg 1966;45:590—8.
17. Ad Hoc Committee on Cardiopulmonary Resuscitation. Cardiopulmonary resuscitation. JAMA 1966;198:372—9.
18. Anon. External cardiac compressors. Health Devices 1973;6:136—48.
19. American Heart Association Committee on Cardiopulmonary Resuscitation and Emergency Cardiac Care. Standards for Cardiopulmonary Resuscitation (CPR) and Emergency Cardiac Care (ECC). JAMA 1974;227:833—66.

20. American Heart Association Committee on Cardiopulmonary Resuscitation and Emergency Cardiac Care. Standards for Cardiopulmonary Resuscitation (CPR) and Emergency Cardiac Care (ECC). JAMA 1980;244:453–509.
21. Kern KB, Carter AB, Showen RL, et al. Comparison of mechanical techniques of cardiopulmonary resuscitation: survival and neurologic outcome in dogs. Am J Emerg Med 1987;5:190–5.
22. Halperin HR, Guerci AD, Chandra N, et al. Vest inflation without simultaneous ventilation during cardiac arrest in dogs: improved survival from prolonged cardiopulmonary resuscitation. Circulation 1986;74:1407–15.
23. Timerman S, Cardoso LF, Ramires JAF, Halperin H. Improved hemodynamic performance with a novel chest compression device during treatment of in-hospital cardiac arrest. Resuscitation 2004;61:273.
24. Lurie K, Lindo C, Chin J. CPR: the P stands for plumber's helper. JAMA 1990;264:1661.
25. Cohen TJ, et al. Active compression–decompression. A new method of cardiopulmonary resuscitation. JAMA 1992;267:2916–23.
26. Halperin HR, Weisfeldt ML. New approaches to CPR. Four hands, a plunger, or a vest. JAMA 1992;267:2940–1.
27. Deakin C. Mechanical devices for external chest compression. Resuscitation Counc Newslett 2006:13–5.
28. Harley HR. Reflections on cardiopulmonary resuscitation. Lancet 1966;2:1–4.
29. MacKernzie GJ, Taylor SH, McDonald AH, Donald KW. Haemodynamic effects of external cardiac compressions. Lancet 1964;18:1342–5.
30. Nayak S. External cardiac massage. Lancet 1964;1:223.
31. Chamberlain D. Never quite there: a tale of resuscitation medicine. Resuscitation 2004;60:3–11.

# Never quite there: a tale of resuscitation medicine

## Douglas Chamberlain

Resuscitation Medicine is of its nature multi-disciplinary and perhaps for that reason something of an orphan. That may account for the long delay in its development as an effective branch of medicine for it started a little over 40 years ago, within my own professional lifetime and very much within my memory. Even now, it can be only a secondary interest for a few individuals with other mainline principal specialties.

These days, it is frequently the older members of our profession who become interested in history. To a degree this is understandable: it is easier to cope with the reassuringly static past than with the frenetic pace of modern progress. But one should not make excuses for such an interest. William Osler was a very wise man, and he saw fit to endorse a view [1] that contains much wisdom:

'History maketh a young man to be old, without either wrinkles or grey hairs, privileging him with the experience of age, without either the infirmities or inconvenience thereof.'

One can commend the notion of seeking the advantages of age before being vulnerable to its drawbacks. Heed well, therefore, the lessons of history.

Amongst the precepts that drive progress in science and in medicine are four that are manifestly true yet call for vigilance and wisdom if a correct balance is to be maintained between them: first, the willingness to accept new ideas that are supported by good evidence, but more importantly the determination to discard quickly those that have none; secondly, the defence of practices that are demonstrably successful, and their rejection only for others that are truly better; thirdly, the acceptance that heterodox views are not necessarily wrong, and an appreciation that valid ones

are often particularly important; fourthly, an awareness that fashion may be a more potent force than science. My review of some aspects of the history of resuscitation reveals past failures in all these respects, tendencies at least as likely today as in the past.

We will consider how the various components of resuscitation began, and how in the end they were integrated into procedures that eventually proved their value for preserving or restoring life. But many current practices that we regard as relatively new were first introduced long ago. Often they came close to acceptance - some indeed had a brief vogue - only to be abandoned or forgotten by our forebears. They were not quite there. In retrospect it seems surprising that progress faltered so frequently. Even now, however, good scientific evidence is either being ignored or is accepted into clinical practice far too slowly. We might well ask ourselves why so little progress has been made in resuscitation medicine over the last 40 years – but that is a question for another day. We too do not learn - and we are still not quite there.

For convenience and clarity I will consider the history of resuscitation not in a strictly sequential way but separately for the individual components of artificial ventilation, cardiac massage and chest compression, electrical pacing, defibrillation, and—briefly—of aftercare (or advanced life support).

## 1. Artificial Ventilation

Biblical references apart, the history of artificial ventilation is usually regarded as beginning with the 16th century anatomist Andreas Vesalius [2]. Vesalius was born in Brussels but undertook his most important work in Padua where our own William Harvey studied about 60 years later. Although he was not strictly the first in the 16th century to describe artificial ventilation, Vesalius must be considered the true father both of modern anatomy and of resuscitation. He published De humani corporis fabrica [3] in 1543 at the age of 28 and described in it how the lungs of animals

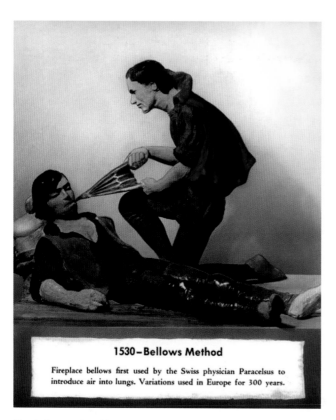

**1530—Bellows Method**

Fireplace bellows first used by the Swiss physician Paracelsus to introduce air into lungs. Variations used in Europe for 300 years.

Fig. 1. Is reproduced by permission of the Chicago Museum of Science and Industry.

collapsed after the chest was opened and that the heart was then affected. But he also wrote

'... that life may... be restored to the animal, an opening must be attempted in the ... trachea, into which a tube of reed or cane should be put; you will then blow into this, so that the lungs may rise again and the animal take in air... I have seen none... that has afforded me greater joy!'

Sadly, his heterodox views were widely condemned. To avoid execution, allegedly for conducting an autopsy on a nobleman whose heart was seen to be beating, he set out on a pilgrimage to the Holy Land but died before he was able to return.

As is so often the case, a new idea emerges almost simultaneously from more than one source. The illustration on the use of bellows for artificial ventilation (Fig. 1) is from the front-piece of the 1974 American Heart Association publication on standards for cardiopulmonary resuscitation [4]; it has a notation that the method dates from 1530. It was in that year, 13 years before the publication of Vesalius's great work, that Paracelsus [5] was said to have used the technique in an apnoeic patient. But he, too, was a controversial figure, driven out of Basel to wander through Europe, eventually to meet a violent death. He had much less influence on subsequent events than did Vesalius. Indeed, no firm evidence exists to confirm the belief that Paracelsus was responsible for the use of bellows for ventilation or indeed wrote on the topic at all [6].

Bellows could hardly have been very effective, but success does seem to have been achieved in a simpler way in 1732 when Tossach [7] used mouth-to-mouth ventilation effectively to resuscitate a miner in Scotland who had been declared dead as a result of a fire. He found 'not the least pulse in either heart or arteries, and not the least breathing could be observed'. He also wrote:

'... he was to all appearance dead. I applied my mouth close to his, and blew my breath as strong as I could, but having neglected to stop his nostrils, all the air came out of them; wherefore, taking hold of them... blew again my breath as strong as I could, raising his chest fully with it, and immediately I felt six or seven very quick beats of the heart... the pulse was felt soon after...'

Tossach adds that after about an hour the rescued man began to yawn and to move. He walked home four hours afterwards, one imagines somewhat unsteadily! Tossach seems to have had a modest view of what he had achieved though it was apparently witnessed by three or four hundred people.

John Fothergill, a London practitioner, certainly did appreciate its importance. When he learned about the incident in 1745 [8], he declared in relation to this discovery that for facts of such great importance it is the duty of everyone 'to render them as extensively public as it is possible'. And so indeed he did, with a list of indications for its use that included suffocation in water. Drowning was by then a matter of great and growing concern. Fothergill was influential in the formation in 1767 of a Society for the Recovery of Drowned Persons in Amsterdam, later called the Humane Society. Mouth-to-mouth artificial ventilation was recommended with other treatments of more doubtful efficacy including insufflation of tobacco smoke into the rectum which indeed became a standard treatment for about 50 years.

Efforts to prevent death from drowning were clearly effective. Herholdt and Rafn [9] reported in an landmark publication of 1796 that 990 lives had been saved by 1793, with a survival rate over the previous nine years of 50%. Saving life meant, however, rescue from drowning rather than resuscitation from apparent death, so we need not be concerned that we cannot now claim comparable success! But we should not belittle the efforts that were made; they showed commitment and ingenuity. The amphibious craft illustrated in Herholdt and Rafn's book (Fig. 2) was used to move quickly over rough ice to reach drowning victims; if the ice gave way the rescuer himself would not be at risk because he had a save haven all around him. The value of postural drainage to empty the lungs was, however, more controversial, especially as it was recognized that the lungs in even fatal cases might remain relatively dry. An appreciation of Herholdt and Rafn as 'two unsung heroes from Denmark' by Baskett [10] also pays tribute to Henning Poulson of the Scandinavian Society of Anaesthetists for instigating in 1960 the translation into English of the remarkable 18th century monograph.

Other Humane Societies followed, including the Royal Humane Society of London in 1774, but here

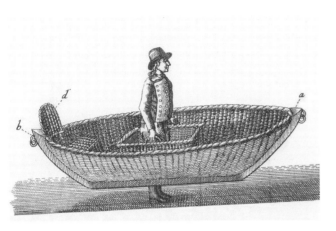

Fig. 2.

mouth-to-mouth ventilation was viewed less enthusiastically. This was partly on aesthetic grounds, a consideration even today; but also because Priestley had discovered by 1774 that the composition of expired air was different from that which was inhaled — and therefore 'unfit to enter any lungs again'. It did remain an option for a while, however, as is shown by the third verse of a poem written by one of the founders of the London Society [11]:

'And if you'd see, what you so much desire,

The object of you care again respire

Let one mouth and either nostril close,

While th'inflating bellows up the other blows.

The air with well-adjusted force convey,

To put the flaccid lungs again in play.

Should bellows not be found, or found too late,

Let some kind soul with willing mouth inflate.

Then lightly squeeze — awhile compress the chest,

That the excluded air may be exprest.' [sic]

Other verses addressed the benefits of heat, friction, the rectal tobacco smoke, and even electricity.

Occasional recommendations for mouth-to-mouth ventilation continued through the 19th and early 20th centuries [12] but it was well out of fashion and virtually forgotten. William Hunter considered it to be 'a method practised by the vulgar' [13], and even Herholdt and Rafn considered in their 1794 monograph [9] that it was 'a very toilsome and loathsome act' and of only little use.

So it was that the Royal Humane Society in 1782, less than 20 years after it had been formed, recommended bellows once again in preference to mouth-to-mouth ventilation [14]. By this time, the technique had been developed and refined. In 1776, John Hunter (the brother of William Hunter who guided his early career) had presented to the Society the results of experiments using double bellows designed to

be introduced into one nostril whilst at the same time the other nostril and the mouth were occluded. Its mechanism generated both positive and negative pressure [15,16]. But using bellows to blow into the nose was clearly not satisfactory, nor universally accepted. The Vesalius technique of tracheal intubation was becoming fashionable again, even while bellows and the mouth-to-mouth methods were still in vogue. There were very full details of the technique in a letter from Dr William Cullen to the President of the Board of Police in Glasgow [17] dated 1776 and posted in every parish:

'Dr Monro informs me, it is very practicable to introduce directly into the glottis and trachea a crooked tube such as a catheter used for a male adult'

Dr Monro, a professor of anatomy, was clearly an expert in such matters, for in the same letter we read:

'Whether blowing in is done by a person's mouth or by bellows, Dr Munro opines, that the air is ready to pass by the gullet into the stomach, but that this may be prevented, but pressing the lower part of the larynx backwards upon the gullet. To persons of little knowledge of anatomy it is to be observed, that the pressure should be only on the cricoid cartilage, by which the gullet may be flattened, while the passage through the lungs is not obstructed.'

Cricoid pressure became accepted in anaesthesia and in resuscitation 185 years later after its description by Sellick [18] but he and others subsequently became aware of Dr Munro's earlier recommendation [19].

In 1788 there was published a very accurate account of the care of the airway by Kite [20] — it would pass muster today except perhaps for the choice of tube:

'If any difficulty should arise in distending the lungs. . . we shall generally remedy the inconvenience by bringing the tongue forwards, which being connected to the epiglottis by inelastic ligaments, must of course be elevated. Should any further impediment however occur, the crooked tube, bent like a male catheter should be introduced through the mouth or one nostril into the glottis. . . When every attempt to inflate the lungs has been made in vain, tracheostomy is the very last expedient, and ought to be performed as soon as it becomes necessary'

But although all this was so accurate and potentially so valuable, other counsels prevailed. By 1855 the recommendations of the Royal Humane Society made no mention at all of artificial ventilation [21].

Surprisingly, electricity had also played a role in artificial ventilation by this time. The possibility of using phrenic stimulation had been mentioned in 1756, experiments were recorded from 1818 and by 1872 there were said to be impressive series of successes [22]. The principal protagonist was a Frenchman called Duchenne [23] who wrote a comprehensive treatise on the many uses for electrical stimulation. He believed that 'electric excitation' of the phrenic nerves was the best solution for asphyxia.

But mouth-to-mouth ventilation, intubation, and phrenic electrotherapy were all considered loathsome or dangerous or too complex. Attention therefore turned to much less effective methods of artificial ventilation performed by external manipulation of the chest wall, such as the Sylvester and Schäfer methods, in an attempt to increase and decrease lung volume. Things had seemed to be going in the right direction, but we were not quite there. And it all went wrong for a long time.

## 2. Cardiac Massage and Chest Compression

We now turn to cardiac massage and chest compression. By a narrow margin, the closed technique of chest compression was attempted in man before open cardiac massage. It may have been used first by John Hill, a British dentist, in 1868 [24]. Boehm in 1878 described successful experiments in cats [25]. I am not sure that I understand fully where I would place my hands if I were to attempt to follow what he described, but it did involve rhythmical compression of the thorax over the heart which could result in restoration of both heart beat and ventilation. The technique was quickly translated into the clinical arena. Koenig who worked as a surgeon in Göttingen from 1875 developed external cardiac massage using compressions over the heart. He described his method in a textbook of surgery in 1883 [26], and mentioned that the technique had saved six patients in whom pulses had been absent. He achieved his successes despite combining chest compressions with relatively ineffective methods of artificial ventilation. His assistant, Maass, published a report in 1892 [27] of two successful resuscitations of cases of chloroform syncope using compressions at 120 per minute. The account of the first of them illustrates the excitement of the occasion:

'...I now had to regard the patient as dead. In spite of this, I returned immediately to the direct compression of the region of the heart and, indeed, in my excitement applied it very forcefully and rapidly. The pupils again became rather quickly constricted... A few gasping respiratory movements, too, returned. When approximately 50 minutes after the beginning of the syncope had elapsed, peculiar movements returned in the region of the heart. Recovery took place very slowly. The patient was discharged completely well after 10 days of stupor.'

External chest compressions survived, at least in Germany, for several more decades [28] and continued to be used in association with the inefficient methods of artificial ventilation by then in vogue. Why, then, did we forget? Perhaps if mouth to mouth ventilation had also persisted, then success would have been compelling and resuscitation would have been commonplace nearly 100 years

earlier than was eventually achieved. We were not quite there...

Open cardiac massage might have seemed a more obvious strategy for re-starting the heart, but only in 1874 was its experimental use described by Moritz Schiff [29].

'When... the heart becomes flaccid, neither artificial ventilation nor Galvanic current can cause the heart to beat again. If, however, one opens the thorax while one slowly blows into the lungs, making methodical compressions with the hand around the heart in order to expel the blood... then the heart can thump and show new movements after 1–2 min.'

Leaving aside the experience of Vesalius who opened the chest of a man whose heart was seen to be beating – leading directly to his exile (I am not clear if that was vivisection or resuscitation!), the first recorded attempt at direct chest massage in man was by Niehans in Berne – recorded by a colleague in 1903 [30]. The first definite success occurred in Tromso a little over a hundred years ago but it was described only after Igelsrud told a colleague of it when he visited the United States [31].

'... Total abdominal hysterectomy was performed. When the operation was almost finished the patient passed into collapse; artificial respiration, lowering of the upper portion of the bed, faradization, and the other usual means were used for about three or four minutes. The heart was then laid bare by a resection of parts of the 4th and 5th ribs. The pericardium was opened and the heart seized between the thumb and fore and middle fingers on the anterior and posterior surfaces. Quite strong and rhythmical pressure was made for about one minute, when the heart began to pulsate of itself. Then observing that the pulsations were becoming weaker, massage of the heart was practiced (sic) for about one minute more. From that time the pulse was perceptible and the contractions of the heart became regular. The patient was discharged from hospital after 5 weeks.'

Interest continued for a while. Green in 1906 reviewed heart massage as a means of restoring the heart beat [32]. He described 40 cases that were by then in the literature, of which 9 had been 'entirely successful' and 8 others with transient recovery of pulse and respiration. But we did not learn. We were not quite there. For many years, attempts at cardiac massage were made only infrequently. Few were interested in resuscitation.

## 3. Electrical Pacing

Electrical pacing of the heart also has a longer history than most appreciate. Its origin is doubtful because there are a number of accounts of resuscitation by electricity in which mechanisms of recovery are at best speculative. Here is one from Hernholdt and Rafn in 1796 [9]:

354

'An electric shock applied across the chest from the right side to the left side, directly over the large blood vessels of the heart and lungs - such a shock of suitable strength, applied when the lungs are filled with pure atmosphere of vital air, is the best cardiacum in a drowned person.'

I confess that I do not know the meaning of cardiacum but I take it to be a good thing! It seems unlikely, however, that a single electric shock across the chest could do much other than elicit a protest if the victim were conscious...

Aldini [33], Galvani's nephew, recommended the use of 'galvanic power externally to the diaphragm and to the region of the heart' for drowned persons, but only after the lungs had been inflated – sound enough advice. The strength of the shocks should be increased gradually and passed through the chest in different directions to achieve the best effect. Although he claimed that shocks administered in this way 'cannot fail', we have no idea how often these and other 19$^{th}$ century suggestions for electrical stimulation were indeed successful.

There is no such doubt about Steiner's work [34]. The stimulus for development in resuscitation of earlier centuries had been drowning, but by now it had passed to the deaths under chloroform and ether anaesthesia that were all too common and equally tragic. Later the stimulus would come from death by electrocution, then coronary disease. But for now the need experimentally was to investigate the mode of death under anaesthesia and its effective treatment. The variety of animals used by Steiner in 1871 is, however, surprising! He successfully paced the chloroform-arrested hearts of 1 donkey, 10 dogs, 14 cats, and 6 rabbits using direct current pulses applied to a needle thrust into the heart via the chest. But he was unsuccessful in 1 patient!

But very soon afterwards it did work in man... Green [35] treated 7 patients with chloroform asystole by the intermittent application of a galvanic current from hand-held electrodes placed over the lower ribs and the neck on the left side. The stimulating current is calculated to have been about three times more than currently used for closed chest pacing. The neck would have provided a good electrical pathway through the great vessels, and coincident phrenic nerve stimulation may well have achieved diaphragmatic movement. The cases are described graphically—especially the five who recovered of which one was an elderly man:

'A small quantity of chloroform had been given when the pulse suddenly stopped and the man appeared dead. The Galvanic apparatus was near and was instantly used. A deep and rapid inspiration, succeeded by a strong noisy expiration like a loud groan, was the immediate result, and at the same time he started up into the sitting position. The circulation was at once restored and he entirely recovered.'

One wonders in such a case who was more surprised by this dramatic result, the patient or the physician...

The great McWilliam—who did much to uncover the secrets of fibrillation–also carefully studied closed chest pacing and made recommendations [36] for its use that could well be followed today:

'In order that such excitation should be as effective as possible... one electrode should be applied in front over the area of the cardiac impulse, and the other over the region of the fourth dorsal vertebra behind, so that the induction shocks may traverse the organ.'

He recommended large electrodes with saline to enhance conduction, and emphasised the need for simultaneous artificial respiration. He urged that this should become a routine emergency procedure, yet mysteriously it was forgotten.

Its later rediscovery is usually ascribed to an American, Albert Hyman [37] whose classic paper was published in 1932. His interest had started when he believed that he had restarted a heart by a direct needle prick. What then was more obvious than to enhance the efficacy of the stimulus by applying electricity through a needle that had been passed through the chest and into an arrested heart. He did seem to know about atrio-ventricular block so I am not sure why he aimed for the right atrium lest it was for the sake of prudence. Hyman does seem to have been the first to use the term 'artificial pacemaker' and he did build three dedicated machines which are fully described and illustrated in an article published in 2001 [38]. He also pioneered a bipolar electrode. But there were problems reproducing his successes, and he was declared to be a 'clumsy fraud' by the Siemens company that had been interested in his devices. His position would have been stronger if he had kept clinical records, especially of the two patients for whom he claimed good results, and possibly if he had been more determined to stimulate the right ventricle...

Although clearly deserving of recognition, we have other evidence that Hyman was careless in his record keeping. He had generously credited an Australian called Gould for having reported at the Australasian Medical Congress of the British Medical Association in 1929 the successful resuscitation of a child using a technique similar to his own. Gould could never be traced, but a recent determined attempt to solve the mystery [39] led to the realization that one Mark Lidwell of Melbourne was the real name of the pioneer who had presented his ideas and experience at the Congress – which did involve *ventricular* stimulation. Perhaps he might now share the accolade for bringing clinical pacing into the 20th century. But we had to wait until 1952 for external pacing to be accepted [40]—though the first commercial units were produced in 1950 to the design of Bigelow, Callaghan, and Hopps [41,42]—and until early 1959 for intracardiac pacing [43]. We were almost there 80 years earlier, so why did we forget?

## 4. Defibrillation

There are surprises too in defibrillation. Not everyone would agree, but I really thing we have to go back to 1775 for the start of this story... It is about a remarkable Danish veterinarian who was a man of many talents, and about his chickens. Abildgaard does seem to well known in his native Denmark, and has more than one statue in his honour. But he deserves wider acclaim. An excellent account of his role in defibrillation and a translation from Latin of his relevant writings were published to commemorate the bicentennial of his experiments [44]. Having read the translation with interest, I believe that Abildgaard probably did fibrillate and defibrillate hearts. He used cocks and hens only because his assembly of 10 Leiden jars did not provide a sufficient capacity discharge to kill a horse. So it was:

'I took a hen, which I knocked down with the first shock directed to the head...it lay without feeling as if completely dead and was unable to be aroused by any stimulus...

I tried an electric shock directed through the chest to the spine ...it rose up and, set loose on the ground, walked about quietly on its feet.

...after the experiment was repeated rather often, the hen was completely stunned, walked with some difficulty, and did not eat for a day and night; then later it was very well and even laid an egg.'

Why did he do such an experiment, and indeed was the hen really dead? Here are extracts from what followed in his account that address these questions:

'...all reports of men, slain by a bolt of lightning, state that nothing in such bodies, when dissected, was found which was sufficient to be called the cause of death...'

'I took a different hen, along with the same cock, upon which I had conducted the second experiment. I left both on the ground...made lifeless by one shock... But on the next morning I found them completely dead and very cold, and I was unable to revive them with the electrical machine with any amount of trying.'

It is noteworthy that whilst the capacitor discharge to the head was capable of killing a chicken, revival needed a discharge across the thorax.

His work did not go un-noticed at the time, with at least two subsequent references in the literature including an anonymous comment in 1779 [45] that was particularly prescient: that Dr Abidgaard's experiments may lead to conjectures 'as to the cause of death from lightning, but also, perhaps, to important discoveries with respect to the means of recovery in such a case'.

But credit for the discovery of defibrillation is usually given to much later work. Prevost and Batelli worked in Geneva on high strength electric currents on dog hearts — with their main objective to show that these could stop any effective heart beat. It has been said that defibrillation was mentioned only in a footnote [46], but this is not wholly correct. Their scientific interest in the restoration of the heart beat is clear from at least one of their several papers [47].

'...we asked ourselves what would be the effect of applying a high voltage current on a dog whose heart had just been put into a state of ventricular tremulation. We worked on 6 dogs, in three of which we noticed that the heart that had been paralysed with ventricular tremulation started to beat again and the pressure rose and stayed up after the application for 1–2 s of a 4800 volt current applied from the head to the feet.'

The language is also persuasive in that the word 'saved' is used:

'In the dog... one can—if a high voltage current is applied in time—stop the tremulation caused by the low voltage current. A dog which had been lost due to paralysis of the heart can be saved in this way.'

But it does seem that they did not understand the implications of their findings in relation to sudden death in humans. This is curious and unfortunate, because 10 years earlier McWilliam had made important observations on the pathology of ventricular fibrillation in man that he believed to be the usual mechanism of sudden death [48]. Once more we were so very nearly there, but not quite... Man had to wait 48 more years. Why did we forget?

I will not comment on the seminal work of Kouwenhoven and his group [49], nor that of Gurvich and Yuniev [50], nor of Zoll [51] in relation to the development of clinical defibrillation because my purpose is to stress opportunities missed rather than notable achievements.

But one aspect of Kouwenhoven's work does deserve comment because it was indeed forgotten and even now is little known. I refer to the introduction of biphasic defibrillation – the use of a discharge that is in effect one cycle of alternating current. This was introduced in modern medicine for implantable defibrillators only after1989 when it had been appreciated that lower energies were required and that therefore smaller capacitors could be used [52]. Clinical evidence that the same held true for out-of-hospital external defibrillation followed [53]. But Kouwenhoven had worked with alternating current and progressively reduced the number of cycles to one – originally he called it a diphasic discharge – and regarded this as optimal. Indeed it was used in a portable defibrillator described in 1963 [54] that could be operated using 6- or 12-volt dry batteries. It was many years ahead of its time and therefore ignored. Perhaps independently, our colleagues in Eastern Europe had the lower energy and probably more effective biphasic units at least 33 years before we did in the West [55]. So why did we take no notice or forget? We were still not quite there.

## 5. After Care: Advanced Life Support

I turn finally to after-care or advanced life support. I will take as examples two therapies, one now accepted as an important advance, and the other a promising development that still requires further testing. Neither are new, but both were long forgotten, even by most with an interest in resuscitation.

The first is therapeutic hypothermia that came sharply to the fore in 2002 when two studies were published in the same issue of the New England Journal of Medicine [56,57]. The data are convincing for victims of cardiac arrest who have delayed resuscitation. The improvement in survival and in cerebral function is impressive; the importance of hypothermia is underscored because we have few other treatment options of any value for post-resuscitation syndromes. But therapeutic hypothermia has been well known for almost 50 years [58]. Although it found most applications in cardiac surgery and neurosurgery, attempts were made to develop its use for resuscitation as early as the 1950s [59,60], and one group in particular continued to recommend this treatment strategy [61]. Yet major clinical trials have only recently been completed. One can believe that many opportunities were lost for preserving adequate neurological function in some survivors of cardiac arrest.

The second example, thrombolysis was used experimentally to show improved survival after cardiac arrest [62] as early as 1956 by Crowell and Smith, three years before the first clinical paper on its use for pulmonary embolus and myocardial infarction [63] (which also went largely unheeded at the time). The rationale is prescient:

> '...blood coagulates in the small vessels for some unknown reason when blood flow through the body of a dog is stopped by fibrillating the heart... Since heparin has no effect once a clot is formed, a fibrinolytic agent was used in the present studies...'

The experiment was a striking success, with one survivor of 15 control dogs, but 12 of 14 treated with streptokinase and plasma before cardiac arrest was induced. Later observations confirmed benefits in terms of cerebral flow and cerebral function [64]. Only in recent times have a series of observational studies suggested that survival from resuscitation may be better for patients who have had a cardiac arrest after infarction if a fibrinolytic is used in subsequent management [65–67]. Moreover, a pilot study of thrombolysis as primary treatment for refractory cardiac arrest showed very promising results [68]. Yet even now thrombolysis is regarded as contraindicated after prolonged cardiopulmonary resuscitation. The opposite may well be demonstrated in the future: large randomized multicentre study is likely to start in 2004. It could have been so much earlier. We were nearly there.

## 6. Questions from the past, implications for the future

The modern era of resuscitation is regarded—appropriately — as having started in the years 1947 to 1960. But might the first human internal defibrillation have been shortly after 1899 [47], not 1947 [69]? Might the first human external pacing been in 1872 [35], not 1952 [40]? Would it have been possible for mouth-to-mouth ventilation to have become established from the 18th century [7,8] so that it did not have to be re-introduced in 1958 [70]? And might closed chest cardiac massage have been accepted in the 1890s [27] instead of in 1960 [71]? We could have had cricoid pressure from the 18th century, and more realistically biphasic defibrillation from 1967. We could have – maybe should have – investigated properly in the 1960s both therapeutic hypothermia and thrombolysis for resuscitation.

We must not be complacent even now. Over the past 25 years the success rate of out-of-hospital resuscitation has improved little. This is because we are 'never quite there' in another sense: not there with a defibrillator for immediate use when an individual collapses in ventricular fibrillation. The importance of time in relation to success has recently been highlighted in a re-presentation of data from a Seattle cardiac rehabilitation programme [72]: whereas the survival rate was almost 100% if patients with ventricular fibrillation are treated at once, the success rate falls to 15 to 40% by 4 to 5 min, and to 5 to 10% by 8 to 15 min. Most cases of cardiac arrest can never be reached within five minutes even by the best emergency system. This might seem an insuperable barrier to any major improvement in the outlook from sudden premature death. But I believe that defibrillation could probably be more successful than current data would suggest. I predict with some confidence that the time-window for successful resuscitation will have widened 10 years from now and that clues suggesting how this might have been achieved earlier will be recognized as having been in the public domain for many years.

There are lessons to be learned from the history of resuscitation. Progress in all disciplines can be hastened if new ideas are welcomed but always evaluated critically, if old practices are not discarded until they can be replaced by others that are demonstrably better, if we have more enthusiasm for why we should change our practices than for why we should not, and if we recognize that dogma must never be above scrutiny. So often our predecessors 'did not learn' when it seems in retrospect they should have done, and so often they were 'never quite there' for developments that then had to wait many years. These and other sound precepts were not followed, but we share the same frailties and are not doubt guilty of the same sorts of errors. History will be our judge too.

## Acknowledgements

My appointment at the Medical College of the University of Wales in Cardiff is supported by a grant (expenses only) from the Laerdal Foundation. I am grateful for suggestions and help with some of the references to Dr Colin Robertson, Dr Mickey Eisenberg, Dr Leo Chameides, and Dr Luke Davidson. I would have missed other important references had my attention not been drawn by Dr Arthur Holman to The History of Cardiology by Louis J Acierno (Parthenon Publishing, 1994). Valuable assistance was given by the librarians and archivists at the Postgraduate Medical Centre, Brighton, The Royal Humane Society, the Royal Society of Medicine, and the Wellcome Foundation – which made my task much easier than it might have been.

## Suggested sources for general reading

Eisenberg MS. Life in the balance. Emergency Medicine and the quest to reverse sudden death. p 182. Oxford University Press. New York, 1997.

Safar P. History of cardiopulmonary-cerebral resuscitation. In Cardiopulmonary resuscitation. Kaye W, Bircher NG Editors. Churchill Livingstone New York, 1989.

Safer P. On the history of modern resuscitation, Crit Care Med 1996; 24 (Suppl): S3–S11.

Böhrer H, Goerig M Early proponents of cardiac massage. Anaesthesia 1995;50:869–71.

Geddes LA. Two unsung heroes of closed-chest cardiac pacing: Green and McWilliam. Pace 1994;17:1320–2.

Ksouwenhoven WB, The development of the defibrillator. Ann Int Med 1969;71:449–57.

Fye WB Ventricular fibrillation and defibrillation: historical perspectives with emphasis on the contributions of John MacWilliam, Carl Wiggers, and William Kouwenhoven. Circulation 1985;71:858–65.

Vallejo-Manzur F, Perkins Y, Varon J, Baskett P. The Resuscitation Greats. Andreas Vesalius, the concept of an artificial airway. Resuscitation 2003;56:3–7.

Davies JE, Sternback GL, Varon J, Froman RE The Resuscitation Greats: Paracelsus and mechanical ventilation. Resuscitation 2000;47:3–5.

Driscol TE, Ratnoff OD, Nygaard OF. The remarkable Dr. Abildgaard and countershock. The bicentennial of his electrical experiments on animals. Ann Int Med 1975;83:872–82.

## References

[1] Osler W (after Fuller). A note on the teaching of the history of medicine. Brit Med J 1902;ii:93.

[2] Vallejo-Manzur F, Perkins Y, Varon J, Baskett P. The Resuscitation Greats. Andreas Vesalius, the concept of an artificial airway. Resuscitation 2003;56:3–7.

[3] Vesalius A. De humani corporis fabrica. Libri Septum 1543, Cap XIX, p658, Basel. (See Ref 2 and Safar P. History of cardiopulmonary-cerebral resuscitation. In Cardiopulmonary resuscitation. Kaye W, Bircher NG Editors. Churchill Livingstone New York, 1989.)

[4] Standards for Cardiopulmonary Resuscitation (CPR) and Emergency Cardiac Care (ECC). JAMA 1974;227 (Supplement): 833–868.

[5] Davies JE, Sternback GL, Varon J, Froman RE. The Resuscitation Greats: Paracelsus and mechanical ventilation. Resuscitation 2000;47:3–5.

[6] Baker AB. Artificial respiration, the history of an idea. Med Hist 1971;15:336–51.

[7] Tossach WA. A man dead in appearance recovered by distending the lungs with air. Med Essays and Observations 1744;5:605–8.

[8] Fothergill J. Observations on a case published in the last volume of the medical essays, etc., of recovering a man dead in appearance, by distending the lungs with air. Phil Trans Roy Soc London 1745;43:275–81.

[9] Herholdt JD, Rafn CG. An attempt at an historical survey on life-saving measures for drowning persons and information on the best means by which they can again be brought back to life. Printed H Tikiob's, Bookseller, with M Seest. 1796.

[10] Baskett PJF. The Resuscitation Greats. JD Herholdt and CG Rafn: two unsung heroes from Denmark. Resuscitation 2003;58:283–8.

[11] Hawes W. The Royal Humane Society, Annual Report, p 9, 1796.

[12] Woods RH. On artificial respiration. Trans Roy Acad Med Ir 1906;24:137–41.

[13] Hunter W. Quoted by Keith A (ref 15).

[14] Bishop RJ. A Short History of the Royal Humane Society to Mark its 200th anniversary. London: the Royal Humane Society, 1974.

[15] Hunter J. Proposals for the Recovery of People Apparently Drowned. Phil Trans R Humane Soc, London, 1776.

[16] Keith A. Three Huntarian lectures on the mechanism underlying the various methods of artificial respiration (Lecture I). Lancet 1909;i:745–9.

[17] Cullen WA. A letter to Lord Cathcart, President of the Board of Police in Scotland concerning the recovery of persons drowned and seemingly dead. Medical Tracts, London 1776.

[18] Sellick BA. Cricoid pressure to control regurgitation of stomach contents during induction or anaesthesia. Lancet 1961;2:2404–6.

[19] Saliem MR, Sellick BA, Elam JO. The historical background of cricoid pressure in anaesthesia and resuscitation. Anaesthesia and Analgesia 1974;53:230–2.

[20] Kite C. An essay on the Recovery of the apparently dead, p146, London. C Dilly in the Poultry, 1788.

[21] Keith A. Three Hunterian lectures on the mechanism underlying the various methods of artificial respiration. (Lecture II). Lancet 1909;I:825–8.

[22] Schechter DC. Application of electrotherapy to noncardiac thoracic disorders. Bull NY Acad Med 1970;46:932–51.

[23] Duchenne G. De l'Électrisation Localisée et de son Application a la Pathologie et à le Thérapeutique, 3rd ed. Paris, Baillière, 1872.

[24] Hill J. Br J Dent 1868;11:335.

[25] Boehm R. Arbeiten aus dem pharmakologischen Institut der Universität Dorpat. 13. Ueber Wiederbelebung nach Vergiftungen und Asphyxie. Archiv für experimentelle Pathologie und Pharmakologie 1878;8:68–101.

[26] Koenig F. Lehrbuch der allgemeinen Chirurgie, Erste Abthuilung. Berlin. August Hirchwald, 1883;64.

[27] Maass. Die Methode der Wiederbelebung dei Herztod nach chloroformeinathmung. Berliner Klinische Wochenschrift 1892;29:265–8.

[28] Böhrer H, Goerig M. Early proponents of cardiac massage. Anaesthesia 1995;50:869–71.

[29] Schiff M. Recueil des mémoires physiologiques 1874 iii. Quoted by Green TA (ref 31).

[30] Zesas DG. Über Massage des freigelegten Herzens beim Chloroformkollaps. Zentralblatt für Chirurgie 1903;30:452–64.

[31] Keen WG. A case of total laryngectomy (unsuccessful) and a case of abdominal hysterectormy) successful) in both of which massage of the heart for chlroroform collapse was employed, with notes of 25 other cases of cardiac massage. Therepeutic Gazette 1904 20 (third series): 217–30.

[32] Green TA. Heart massage as a means of restoration in cases of apparent sudden death, with a synopsis of 40 cases. Lancet 1906;ii:1708–14.

[33] Aldini J. Essai Théorique et Experimantal pour le Galvinsime. Paris 1804, Fournier fils. Cited in Acierno LJ. The History of Cardiology. Parthenon London, New York 1994.

[34] Steiner F. Ueber die Electropunctur des Herzens als Wieder-belebungsmittel in der Chloroformsyncope. Archiv fur klin Chir 1871;12:748–90.

[35] Green T. On death from chloroform: its prevention by galvanism. Br Med J 1872;i:551–3.

[36] McWilliam JA. Electrical stimulation of the heart in man. Br Med J. 1889;I:348–50.

[37] Hyman S. Resuscitation of the stopped heart by intracardiac therapy. Arch Intern Med 1932;50:283.

[38] Furman S, Jeffrey K, Szarka G. The mysterious fate of Hyman's pacemaker. Pace 2001;24:1126–37.

[39] Mond HG, Sloman JG, Edwards RH. The first pacemaker. Pace 1982;5:279–82.

[40] Zoll PM. Resuscitation of the heart in ventricular standstill by external electrical stimulation. New Engl J Med 1952;247:768–71.

[41] Bigelow WG, Callaghan JC, Hopps JA. General hypothermia for for experimental intracardiac surgery. The use of electrophrenic respirations, an artificial pacemaker for cardiac standstill, and radiofrequency re-warming in general hypothermia. Ann Surgery 1950;132:531.

[42] Hopps JA. The development of the pacemaker. Pace 1981;4:106–8.

[43] Furman S, Schwedel JB. An intracardiac pacemaker for Stokes-Adams seizures. New Engl J Med 1959;261:943–8.

[44] Abildgaard PC. Tentamina electrica in animalibus instituta. Societatis Medicae Havniensis Collectanea 1775;2:157–61. Translation in Driscol TE, Ratnoff OD, Nygaard OF Editors. The remarkable Dr. Abildgaard and countershock. The bicentennial of his electrical experiments on animals. Ann Int Med 1975;83:872–82.

[45] Anonymous. Medical and Philosophical Commentaries by a Society in Edinburgh, p 255. London. J. Murray, 1779;6:252–5.

[46] Eisenberg MS. Life in the balance. Emergency Medicine and the quest to reverse sudden death. p 182. Oxford University Press. New York, 1997.

[47] Prevost J-L, Battelli F. La mort par les courants électriques – courants alternatifs a haute tension. J Physiol et Pathol Gen 1899;ii:427–42.

[48] McWilliam JA. Cardiac failure and sudden cardiac death. Br Med J. 1889;I:6–8.

[49] Kouwenhoven WB. The development of the defibrillator. Ann Intern Med 1969;71:449–58.

[50] Gurvich N, Yuniev SG. Byulletin eksperimentalnoi biologii i miditsiny 1939;8:55–8. Translated: Restoration of a regular rhythm in the mammalian fibrillating heart. Amer Review of Sov Med 1946;3:236–9.

[51] Zoll PM, Linenthal AJ, Gibson W, Paul MH, Norman LR. Termination of ventricular fibrillation in man by an externally applied electric shock. N Engl J Med 1956;254:727–32.

[52] Winkle RA, Mean RH, Ruder MA, et al. Improved low energy defibrillation efficacy in man with the use of a biphasic truncated exponential waveform. Am Heart J 1989;117:117–22.

[53] Schneider T, Martens PR, Paschen H, Kuisma M, Wolcke B, Gliner BE, et al. Multicenter, randomized, controlled trial of 150-J biphasic shocks compared with 200- to 360-J monophasic shocks in the resuscitation of out-of-hospital cardiac arrest victims. Circulation 2000;102:1780–7.

[54] Kouwenhoven WB, Knickerbocker GC, Becker EM. Portable defibrillator. IEEE Trans Power Appar & Systems, no. 69, December 1963, pp. 1089–93. Quoted in Ref 37.

[55] Gurvich NI, Makarchev VE. Defibrillation of the heart with biphasic electrical impulses. Kardiologya 1967;7:109–12.

[56] Bernard SA, Gray TW, Buist MD, Jones BM, Silvester W, Gutteridge G, et al. Treatment of comatose survivors of out-of-hospital cardiac arrest with induced hypothermia. N Engl J Med 2002;346:557–63.

[57] The Hypothermia After Cardiac Arrest (HACA) study group. Mile therapeutic hypothermia to improve the neurologic outcome after cardiac arrest. N Engl J Med 2002;346:549–56.

[58] Smith MS, Stetson JB. Medical Progress: therapeutic hypothermia (concluded). N Engl J Med 1961;265:1147–51.

[59] Williams GR, Spencer FC. Clinical use of hypothermia after cardiac arrest. Ann Surg 1958;148:462–8.

[60] Benson DW, Williams GR, Spencer FC. The use of hypothermia after cardiac arrest. Anesth Analg 1959;38:423–8.

[61] Safar P. Cerebral resuscitation after cardiac arrest: research initiatives and future directions. Ann Emerg Med 1993;22:324–49.

[62] Crowell JW, Smith EE. Effect of fibrinolytic activation on survival and cerebral damage following periods of circulatory arrest. Am J Physiol 1956;186:283–5.

[63] Fletcher AP, Sherry S, Alkjaersig N, Smyrniotis FE, Jick S. The maintenance of a sustained thromblytic state in man. II. Clinical observations on patients wit myocardial infarction and other thrombo-embolic disorders. J Clin Invest 1959;38:1111–9.

[64] Lin S, O'Connor MJ, Fischer HW, King A. The effects of combined dextran and streptokinase on cerebral function and blood flow after cardiac arrest an experimental study on the dog. Invest Radiol 1978;13:490–8.

[65] Ruiz-Bailen M, Aguayo de Hoyos R, Diaz Casteleanos MA. Role of thrombolysis in cardiac arrest. Intensive Care Med 2001;27:438–41.

[66] Lederer W, Lichtenberger C, Pechlaner C, Kroesen G, Baubin M. Recombinant tissue plamsinogen activator during cardiopulmonary resuscitation in 108 patients with out-of-hospital cardiac arrest. Resuscitation 2001;50:71–6.

[67] Schreiber W, Gabries D, Sterz F, Muellner M, Duerkciyan I, Holzer M, et al. Thrombolytic therapy after cardiac arrest and its effect on neurological outcome. Resuscitation 2002;52:63–9.

[68] Böttiger BW, Bode C, Kern S, Gries A, Gust R, Glätzer R, et al. Efficacy and safety of thrombolytics thererapy after initially unsuccessful cardiopulmonary resuscitation: a prospective clinical trial. Lancet 2001;357:1583–5.

[69] Beck CS, Pritchard WH, Feil HS. Ventricular fibrillation of long duration abolished by electric shock. JAMA 1947;135:985.

[70] Safar P, Escarrage LA, Elam JO. A comparison of the mouth-to-mouth and mouth-to-airway methods of artificial respiration with the chest-pressure arm-lift methods. N Engl J Med 1958;258:671–7.

[71] Kouwenhoven WB, Jude JR, Knickerbocker CG. Closed-chest cardiac massage. J Amer Med Assoc 1960;173:1064–7.

[72] Weaver WD, Peberdy MA. Perspective: Defibrillators in Public Places—One Step Closer to Home. NEJM 2002;347:1223–4.

# Index